FOURTH EDITION

BD Chaurasia's

HUMAN ANATOMY

Regional and Applied
Dissection and Clinical

VOLUME 3
Head, Neck and
Brain

10/09 : *40 :

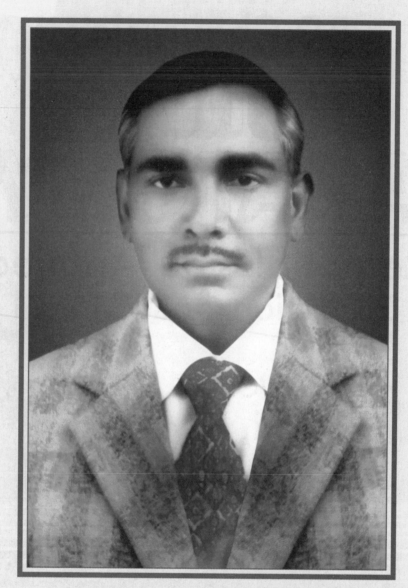

Late Dr BD Chaurasia

1937–1985

FOURTH EDITION

BD Chaurasia's
HUMAN ANATOMY

Regional and Applied
Dissection and Clinical

VOLUME 3
Head, Neck and Brain

CBS

CBS PUBLISHERS & DISTRIBUTORS
NEW DELHI • BANGALORE

Medical knowledge is constantly changing. As new information becomes available, changes in treatment, procedures, equipment and the use of drugs become necessary. The author and the publisher have, as far as it is possible, taken care to ensure that the information given in this text is accurate and up to date. However, readers are strongly advised to confirm that the information, especially with regard to drug usage, complies with the latest legislation and standards of practice.

BD Chaurasia's
HUMAN ANATOMY
Regional and Applied
Dissection and Clinical
Volume 3   4/e

Copyright © Publishers and Author

ISBN : 81-239-1157-2

Fourth Edition: 2004
Reprinted: 2005, 2006

First Edition: 1979
Reprinted: 1980, 1981, 1982, 1983, 1984, 1985, 1986, 1987, 1988

Second Edition: 1989
Reprinted: 1990, 1991, 1992, 1993, 1994

Third Edition: 1995
Reprinted: 1996, 1997, 1998, 1999, 2000, 2001, 2002, 2003, 2004, 2005

Editor:
The fourth edition has been revised by Dr Krishna Garg, Ex-Professor and Head, Department of Anatomy, Lady Hardinge Medical College, New Delhi.

Production Director : Vinod K. Jain

Published by :
Satish Kumar Jain for CBS Publishers & Distributors,
4596/1-A, 11 Darya Ganj, New Delhi - 110 002 (India)
E-mail : cbspubs@vsnl.com
Website : www.cbspd.com

Branch Office :
Seema House, 2975, 17th Cross, K.R. Road,
Bansankari 2nd Stage, Bangalore - 560070
Fax : 080-26771680 • E-mail : cbsbng@vsnl.net

Typeset at :
CBS P&D Typesetting Unit.

Printed at :
Diamond Agencies Pvt Ltd, Noida (UP), India

dedicated to
my teacher

Shri Uma Shankar Nagayach

FOURTH EDITION

BD Chaurasia's
HUMAN
ANATOMY

Regional and Applied
Dissection and Clinical

VOLUME 1
Upper Limb and Thorax

VOLUME 2
Lower Limb, Abdomen
and Pelvis

VOLUME 3
Head, Neck and Brain

ABOUT THE EDITOR

Dr. Krishna Garg joined Department of Anatomy, Lady Hardinge Medical College, New Delhi, in 1964 and learnt and taught anatomy till 1996 except for a brief stint at Maulana Azad Medical College. She has been decorated as Fellow of Indian Medical Association-Academy of Medical Specialists, Member of Academy of Medical Sciences and Fellow of International Medical Science Academy. She recieved Appreciation Award in 1999 from Delhi Medical Association and Excellence Award in Anatomy on Doctors Day in 2004. Krishna Garg is the co-author of Textbook of Histology and Neuroanatomy. Having revised BD Chaurasia's Hand Book of General Anatomy in 1996, she has now revised and brought out the 4th edition of the three volumes of BD Chaurasia's Human Anatomy.

This human anatomy is not systemic but regional
Oh yes, it is theoretical as well as practical
Besides the gross features, it is chiefly clinical
Included in anatomy, it is also histological

Anatomy is not only of adult but also embryological
It is concise, comprehensive and clinical

Surface marking is provided in the beginning
To light the instinct of surgeon-in-the-making

Lots of tables for the muscles are provided
Even methods for testing are incorporated
Numerous coloured illustrations are added
So that right half of brain gets stimulated

Hope these volumes turn highly useful
The editor's patience and perseverance prove fruitful

Preface to the Fourth Edition

In July 1996, I had gone to the office of CBS Publishers and Distributors to hand over the manuscript of the third edition of our *Textbook of Histology*, when Mr SK Jain, Managing Director of CBS, requested me to shoulder the responsibility of editing the three volumes of their extremely popular book *BD Chaurasia's Human Anatomy*, the third edition of which was earlier edited by respected Prof. Inderbir Singh. This was a 'God given gift' which I accepted with great gratitude. This had also been the wishful thinking of my son, now a nephrologist in the US.

The three volumes of the fourth edition of this book are extremely student-friendly. All out efforts have been made to bring them closer to their hearts through serious and subtle efforts. Various ways were thought of, which I discussed with my colleagues and students, and have been incorporated in these volumes.

One significant method suggested was to add 'practical skills' so that these volumes encompass theoretical, practical and clinical aspects of various parts of human body in a functional manner. The paragraphs describing human dissection, printed with blue background, provide necessary instructions for dissection. These entail identifying structures deeper to skin which need to be cut and separated to visualise the anatomic details of various structures.

Dissection means patiently clearing off the fat and fasciae around nerves, blood vessels, muscles, viscera, etc. so that their course, branches and relations are appreciated. This provides the photogenic memory for the 'doctor-in-making'. First year of MBBS course is the only time in life when one can dissect at ease, although it is too early a period to appreciate its value. Good surgeons always refresh their anatomical knowledge before they go to the operation theatre.

Essential part of the text and some diagrams from the first edition have been incorporated glorifying the real author and artist in BD Chaurasia. A number of diagrams on ossification, surface marking, muscle testing, in addition to radiographs, have been added.

The beauty of most of the four-colour figures lies in easy reproducibility in numerous tests and examinations which the reader can master after a few practice sessions only. This makes them user-friendly volumes. Figures are appreciated by the underutilised right half of the cerebral cortex, leaving the dominant left half for other jobs in about 98% of right-handed individuals. At the beginning of each chapter, a few introductory sentences have been added to highlight the importance of the topic covered. A brief account of the related histology and development is put forth so that the given topic is covered in all respects. The entire clinical anatomy has been put with the respective topic, highlighting its importance. The volumes thus are concise, comprehensive and clinically-oriented .

Various components of upper and lower limbs have been described in a tabular form to revise and appreciate their "diversity in similarity". At the end of each section, an appendix has been added wherein the segregated course of the nerves has been aggregated, providing an overview of their entire course. These appendices also contain some clinicoanatomical problems and multiple choice questions to test the knowledge and skills acquired. Prayers, patience and perseverance for almost 8 years have brought out this new edition aimed at providing a holistic view of the amazing structures which constitute the human anatomy.

There are bound to be some errors in these volumes. Suggestions and comments for correction and improvement shall be most welcome: These may please be sent to me through e-mail at cbspubs@del3.vsnl.net.in.

KRISHNA GARG

Preface to the First Edition

The necessity of having a simple, systematized and complete book on anatomy has long been felt. The urgency for such a book has become all the more acute due to the shorter time now available for teaching anatomy, and also to the falling standards of English language in the majority of our students in India. The national symposium on "Anatomy in Medical Education" held at Delhi in 1978 was a call to change the existing system of teaching the unnecessary minute details to the undergraduate students.

This attempt has been made with an object to meet the requirements of a common medical student. The text has been arranged in small classified parts to make it easier for the students to remember and recall it at will. It is adequately illustrated with simple line diagrams which can be reproduced without any difficulty, and which also help in understanding and memorizing the anatomical facts that appear to defy memory of a common student. The monotony of describing the individual muscles separately, one after the other, has been minimised by writing them out in tabular form, which makes the subject interesting for a lasting memory. The relevant radiological and surface anatomy have been treated in separate chapters. A sincere attempt has been made to deal, wherever required, the clinical applications of the subject. The entire approach is such as to attract and inspire the students for a deeper dive in the subject of anatomy.

The book has been intentionally split in three parts for convenience of handling. This also makes a provision for those who cannot afford to have the whole book at a time.

It is quite possible that there are errors of omission and commission in this mostly single handed attempt. I would be grateful to the readers for their suggestions to improve the book from all angles.

I am very grateful to my teachers and the authors of numerous publications, whose knowledge has been freely utilised in the preparation of this book. I am equally grateful to my professor and colleagues for their encouragement and valuable help. My special thanks are due to my students who made me feel their difficulties, which was a great incentive for writing this book. I have derived maximum inspiration from Prof. Inderbir Singh (Rohtak), and learned the decency of work from Shri SC Gupta (Jiwaji University, Gwalior).

I am deeply indebted to Shri KM Singhal (National Book House, Gwalior) and Mr SK Jain (CBS Publishers and Distributors, Delhi), who have taken unusual pains to get the book printed in its present form. For giving it the desired get-up, Mr VK Jain and Raj Kamal Electric Press are gratefully acknowledged. The cover page was designed by Mr Vasant Paranjpe, the artist and photographer of our college; my sincere thanks are due to him. I acknowledge with affection the domestic assistance of Munne Miyan and the untiring company of my Rani, particularly during the odd hours of this work.

Gwalior
February, 1981

BD CHAURASIA

Acknowledgements

I am grateful to Almighty for giving me the opportunity to edit these three volumes, and further for sustaining the interest which many a times did oscillate.

When I met Mr YN Arjuna, Publishing Director in CBS, in May 2003, light was seen at the end of the tunnel and it was felt that the work on the volumes could begin with definite schedule. He took great interest in going through the manuscript, correcting, modifying and improving wherever necessary. He inducted me to write an introductory paragraph, brief outlines of embryology and histology to make it a concise and complete textbook.

Having retired from Lady Hardinge Medical College within a fortnight of getting this assignment and having joined Santosh Medical College, Ghaziabad, my colleagues there really helped me. I am obliged to Prof. Varsha Katira, Prof.Vishram Singh, Dr Poonam Kharb, Dr Tripta Bhagat (MS Surgery), Dr Nisha Kaul and Ms Jaya. They even did dissection with the steps written for the new edition and modified the text wherever necessary.

From 2000–03, while working at Subharti Medical College, Meerut, the editing of the text continued. Dr Satyam Khare, Associate Professor, suggested me to write the full course of nerves, ganglia, multiple choice questions, etc. with a view to revise the important topics quickly. So, appendices have come up at the end of each section. I am grateful to Prof. AK Asthana, Dr AK Garg and Dr Archana Sharma for helping me when required.

The good wishes of Prof. Mohini Kaul and Prof. Indira Bahl who retired from Maulana Azad Medical College; Director-Prof. Rewa Choudhry, Prof. Smita Kakar, Prof. Anita Tuli, Prof. Shashi Raheja of Lady Hardinge Medical College; Director-Prof. Vijay Kapoor, Director-Prof. JM Kaul, Director-Prof. Shipra Paul, Prof. RK Suri and Prof. Neelam Vasudeva of Maulana Azad Medical College; Prof. Gayatri Rath of Vardhman Mahavir Medical College; Prof. Ram Prakash, Prof. Veena Bharihoke, Prof. Kamlesh Khatri, Prof. Jogesh Khanna, Prof. Mahindra Nagar, Prof. Santosh Sanghari of University College of Medical Sciences; Prof. Kiran Kucheria, Prof. Rani Kumar, Prof. Shashi Wadhwa, Prof. Usha Sabherwal, and Prof. Raj Mehra of All India Institute of Medical Sciences and all my colleagues who have helped me sail through the dilemma.

I am obliged to Prof. DR Singh, Ex-Head, Department of Anatomy, KGMC, Lucknow, for his constructive guidance and Dr MS Bhatia, Head, Department of Psychiatry, UCMS, Delhi, who suggested the addition of related histology.

It is my pleasure to acknowledge Prof. Mahdi Hasan, Ex-Prof. & Head, Department of Anatomy, and Principal, JN Medical College, Aligarh; Prof. Veena Sood and Dr Poonam Singh of DMC, Ludhiana; Prof. S Lakshmanan, Rajah Muthiah Medical College, Tamil Nadu; Prof. Usha Dhall and Dr Sudha Chhabra, Pt. BD Sharma PGIMS, Rohtak; Prof. Ashok Sahai, KG Medical College, Lucknow; Prof. Balbir Singh, Govt. Medical College, Chandigarh; Prof. Asha Singh, Ex-Prof. & Head, MAMC, New Delhi; Prof. Vasundhara Kulshrestha, SN Medical College, Agra; and Dr Brijendra Singh, Head, Department of Anatomy, ITS Centre for Dental Science and Research, Muradnagar, UP, for inspiring me to edit these volumes.

I am obliged to my mother-in-law and my mother whose blessings have gone a long way in the completion of this arduous task. My sincere thanks are due to my husband Dr DP Garg, our children Manoj and Rekha, Meenakshi and Sanjay, Manish and Shilpa, and the grandchildren, who challenged me at times but supported me all the while. The cooperation extended by Rekha is much appreciated.

I am deeply indebted to Mr SK Jain Managing Director of CBS, Mr VK Jain, Production Director, Mr BM Singh and their team for their keen interest and all out efforts in getting the volumes published.

I am thankful to Mr Ashok Kumar who has skillfully painted black and white volumes into coloured volumes to enhance clarity. Ms Deepti Jain, Ms Anupam Jain and Ms Parul Jain have carried out the corrections very diligently. Lastly, the job of pagination came on the shoulders of Mr Karzan Lal Prashar who has left no stone unturned in doing his job perfectly.

Last, but not the least, the spelling mistakes have been corrected by my students, especially Ms Ruchika Girdhar and Ms Hina Garg of 1st year Bachelor of Physiotherapy course at Banarsidas Chandiwala Institute of Physiotherapy, New Delhi, and Mr Ashutosh Gupta of 1st Year BDS at ITS Centre for Dental Science and Research, Muradnagar.

May Almighty inspire all those who study these volumes to learn and appreciate CLINICAL ANATOMY and DISSECTION and be happy and successful in their lives.

Delhi
April 2004

KRISHNA GARG

Contents

Section 1
HEAD AND NECK

Nahum

Section 2
BRAIN

Section 1

HEAD AND NECK

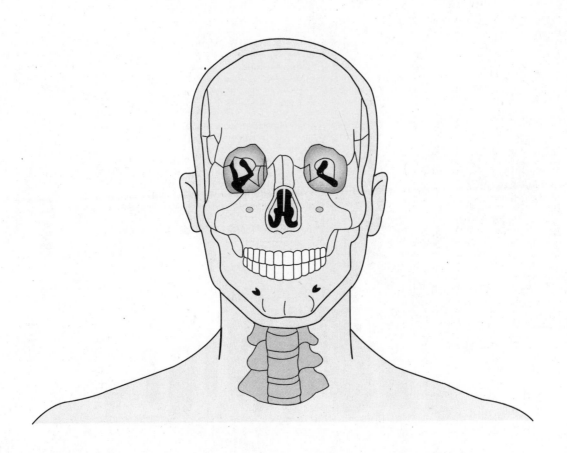

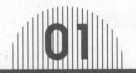

Osteology of the Head and Neck

Bones of head and neck include somatic bones, the skull, i.e. skull with mandible, seven cervical vertebrae and the hyoid, developed from the second and third branchial arches. The skull cap formed by frontal, parietal, squamous temporal and a part of occipital bones, develop by intramembranous ossification, being a quicker one-stage process. The base of the skull in contrast ossifies by intra-cartilaginous ossification which is a two-stage process (membrane-cartilage-bone). The joints in the skull are mostly sutures, a few primary cartilaginous and only a pair of synovial joint the temporomandibular joint. This mobile joint permits us to speak, eat, drink and laugh.

Skull lodges not only the brain, but also special senses like cochlear and vestibular apparatus, retina, olfactory mucous membrane, and taste buds. The weight of the brain is not felt as it is floating in the cerebrospinal fluid. Our personality, power of speech, attention, concentration, judgement, and intellect are because of the brain that we possess and its proper use, for our own good and for the good of the society as well.

THE SKULL : INTRODUCTION

Terms

The skeleton of the head is called the *skull*. It consists of several bones that are joined together to form the *cranium*. The term skull also includes the mandible or lower jaw which is a separate bone. However, the two terms skull and cranium, are often used synonymously.

The skull can be divided into two main parts: (a) The *calvaria* or *brain box* is the upper part of the cranium which encloses the brain, (b) the facial skeleton constitutes the rest of the skull and includes the mandible.

Bones of the Skull

The skull consists of the 22 bones which are named as follows.

(A) The calvaria or brain case is composed of 8 bones.

Paired	Unpaired
1. Parietal	1. Frontal
2. Temporal	2. Occipital
	3. Sphenoid
	4. Ethmoid

(B) The *facial skeleton* is composed of 14 bones.

Paired	Unpaired
1. Maxilla	1. Mandible
2. Zygomatic	2. Vomer
3. Nasal	
4. Lacrimal	
5. Palatine	
6. Inferior nasal concha.	

Skull Joints

With the exception of the temporomandibular joint which permits free movements, most of the joints of the skull are immovable and fibrous in type; these are known as sutures. A few are primary cartilaginous joints. During childhood the sutures can open up if intracranial tension increases. In adults, the bones are interlocked and the sutures cannot open up. In old age, the sutures are gradually obliterated by fusion of the adjoining bones; fusion begins on the inner surface of the skull between the ages of 30 and 40 years; and on the outer surface between 40 and 50 years.

Anatomical Position of Skull

The skull can be placed in proper orientation by considering any one of the two planes.

1. Reid's base line is a horizontal line obtained by joining the infraorbital margin to the centre of the external acoustic meatus, i.e. auricular point.

2. The Frankfurt horizontal plane of orientation is obtained by joining the infraorbital margin to the upper margin of the external acoustic meatus.

Methods of Study of the Skull

The skull can be studied as a whole. This is of greater practical importance and utility than knowing the details of individual bones.

A. The whole skull can be studied from the outside or externally in different views:

1. Superior view or norma verticalis.
2. Posterior view or norma occipitalis.
3. Anterior view or norma frontalis.
4. Lateral view or norma lateralis.
5. Inferior view or norma basalis.

B. The whole skull can be studied from the inside or internally after removing the roof of the calvaria or skull cap:

1. Internal surface of the cranial vault.
2. Internal surface of the cranial base which shows a natural subdivision into anterior, middle and posterior cranial fossae.

C. The skull can also be studied as individual bones.

EXTERIOR OF THE SKULL

NORMA VERTICALIS

Shape

When viewed from above the skull is usually oval in shape. It is wider posteriorly than anteriorly. The shape may be more nearly circular.

Bones Seen in Norma Verticalis

1. Upper part of the frontal bone anteriorly.
2. Uppermost part of the occipital bone posteriorly.
3. A parietal bone on each side.

Sutures

1. *Coronal suture.* This is placed between the frontal bone and the two parietal bones. The suture crosses the cranial vault from side to side and runs downwards and forwards (Fig. 1.1).

2. *Sagittal suture.* It is placed in the median plane between the two parietal bones.

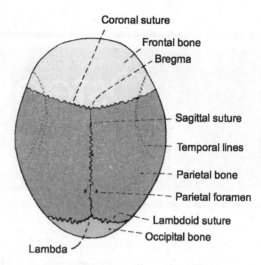

Fig. 1.1: *Norma verticalis.*

3. *Lambdoid suture.* It lies posteriorly between the occipital and the two parietal bones, and it runs downwards and forwards across the cranial vault.

4. *Metopic suture.* This is occasionally present in about 3 to 8% individuals. It lies in the median plane and separates the two halves of the frontal bone.

Some other Named Features

1. The *vertex* is the highest point on the sagittal suture.

2. The *vault* of the skull is the arched roof for the dome of the skull.

3. The *bregma* is the meeting point between the coronal and sagittal sutures. In the foetal skull, this is the site of a membranous gap, called the anterior fontanelle, which closes at eighteen months of age (Fig. 1.2).

4. The *lambda* is the meeting point between the sagittal and lambdoid sutures. In the foetal skull, this is the site of the posterior fontanelle which closes at two to three months of age.

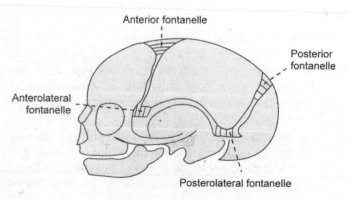

Fig. 1.2: *Fontanelles of skull.*

5. The *parietal tuber (eminence)* is the area of maximum convexity of the parietal bone. This is a common site of fracture of the skull.

6. The *parietal foramen,* one on each side, pierces the parietal bone near its upper border, 2.5 to 4 cm in front of the lambda. The *parietal* foramen transmits an emissary vein from the veins of scalp into the superior sagittal sinus.

7. The *obelion* is the point on the sagittal suture between the two parietal foramina.

8. The *temporal lines* begin at the zygomatic process of the frontal bone, arch backwards and upwards, and cross the frontal bone, the coronal suture and the parietal bone. Over the parietal bone there are two lines, superior and inferior. Traced anteriorly, they fuse to form a single line. Traced posteriorly, the superior line fades out over the posterior part of the parietal bone, but the inferior temporal line continues downwards and forwards.

NORMA OCCIPITALIS

Norma occipitalis is convex upwards and on each side, and is flattened below.

Bones Seen

1. Posterior parts of the parietal bones, above.

2. Upper part of the squamous part of the occipital bone below (Fig. 1.3).

3. Mastoid part of the temporal bone, on each side.

Sutures

1. The *lambdoid suture* lies between the occipital bone and the two parietal bones. Sutural bones are common along this suture.

2. The *occipitomastoid suture* lies between the occipital bone and the mastoid part of the temporal bone.

3. The *parietomastoid suture* lies between the parietal bone and the mastoid part of the temporal bone.

4. The posterior part of the *sagittal suture* is also seen.

Other Features

1. *Lambda, parietal foramina* and *obelion* have been examined in the norma verticalis.

2. The *external occipital protuberance* is a median prominence in the lower part of this norma. It marks the junction of the head and the neck. The most prominent point on this protuberance is called the *inion.*

3. The *superior nuchal lines* are curved bony ridges passing laterally from the protuberance. These also mark the junction of the head and the neck. The area below the superior nuchal lines will be studied with the norma basalis.

4. The *highest nuchal lines* are not always present. They are curved bony ridges situated about 1 cm above the superior nuchal lines. They begin from the upper part of the external occipital protuberance and are more arched than the superior nuchal lines.

5. The *occipital point* is a median point a little above the inion. It is the point farthest from the glabella.

6. The *mastoid foramen* is located on the mastoid part of the temporal bone at or near the occipitomastoid suture. Internally, it opens at the sigmoid sulcus. The mastoid foramen transmits an emissary vein, and the meningeal branch of the occipital artery.

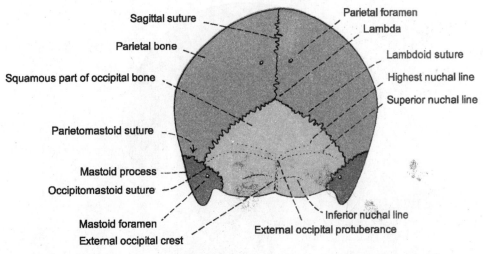

Fig. 1.3: *Norma occipitalis.*

7. The *interparietal bone* is occasionally present. It is a large triangular bone located at the apex of the squamous occipital. This is not a sutural or accessory bone but represents the membranous part of the occipital bone which has failed to fuse with the rest of the bone.

Attachments

1. The upper part of the external occipital protuberance gives origin to the *trapezius*, and the lower part gives attachment to the upper end of the *ligamentum nuchae* (see Fig. 1.15).

2. The medial one-third of the superior nuchal line gives origin to the trapezius, and the lateral part provides insertion to the *sternocleidomastoid* above and to the *splenius capitis* below.

3. The highest nuchal lines provide attachment to the *epicranial aponeurosis* medially, and give origin to the *occipitalis* or occipital belly of occipitofrontalis muscle laterally (Fig. 1.4).

NORMA FRONTALIS

The norma frontalis is roughly oval in outline, being wider above than below.

Bones

1. The *frontal* bone forms the forehead. Its upper part is smooth and convex, but the lower part is irregular and is interrupted by the orbits and by the anterior bony aperture of the nose (Fig. 1.5).

2. The right and left *maxillae* form the upper jaw.

3. The right and left *nasal* bones form the bridge of the nose.

4. The *zygomatic* bones form the bony prominence of the superolateral part of the cheeks.

5. The *mandible* forms the lower jaw.

The Norma Frontalis will be studied under the following heads: (a) Frontal region; (b) orbital opening; (c) anterior piriform-shaped bony aperture of the nose; and (d) lower part of the face.

Frontal Region

The frontal region presents the following features:

1. The *superciliary arch* is a rounded, curved elevation situated just above the medial part of each orbit. It overlies the frontal sinus and is better marked in males than in females.

2. The *glabella* is a median elevation connecting the two superciliary arches. Below the glabella the skull recedes to the frontonasal suture at the root of the nose.

3. The *nasion* is a median point at the root of the nose where the internasal suture meets with the frontonasal suture.

4. The *frontal tuber* or *eminence* is a low rounded elevation above the superciliary arch, one on each side.

Orbital Openings

Each orbital opening is quadrangular in shape and is bounded by the following four margins.

1. The *supraorbital margin* is formed by the frontal bone. At the junction of its lateral two-thirds and its medial one-third, it presents the supraorbital notch or foramen.

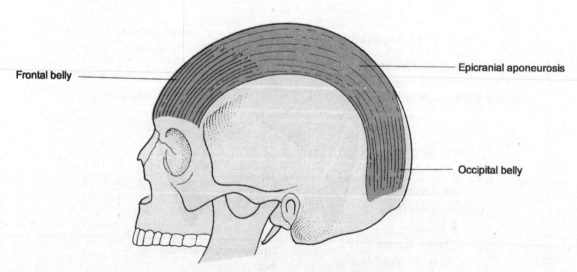

Fig. 1.4: *Attachments of the occipitofrontalis muscle.*

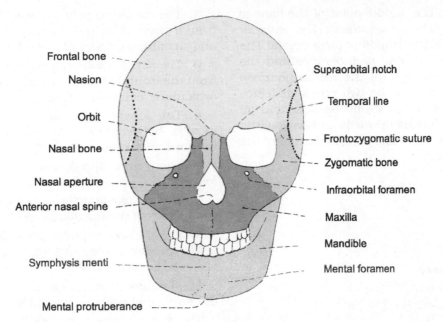

Frontal bone
Nasion
Orbit
Nasal bone
Nasal aperture
Anterior nasal spine
Symphysis menti
Mental protruberance

Supraorbital notch
Temporal line
Frontozygomatic suture
Zygomatic bone
Infraorbital foramen
Maxilla
Mandible
Mental foramen

Fig. 1.5: *Norma frontalis.*

2. The *infraorbital margin* is formed by the zygomatic bone laterally, and the maxilla medially.

3. The *medial orbital margin* is ill-defined. It is formed by the frontal bone above, and by the lacrimal crest of the frontal process of the maxilla below.

4. The *lateral orbital margin* is formed mostly by the frontal process of zygomatic bone but is completed above by the zygomatic process of frontal bone. *Frontozygomatic suture* lies at their union.

Anterior Bony Aperture of the Nose

The anterior bony aperture is pear-shaped, being wide below and narrow above.

Boundaries

Above: by the lower border of the nasal bones.
Below: by the nasal notch of the body of the maxilla on each side.

Features

Note the following.

1. *Articulations of the nasal bone:* (a) *Anteriorly,* with the opposite bone at the internasal suture, (b) *posteriorly,* with the frontal process of the maxilla, (c) *superiorly,* with the frontal bone at the frontonasal suture, and (d) *inferiorly,* the upper nasal cartilage is attached to it.

The *nasal bone is one of the most commonly fractured bones of the face.*

2. The *anterior nasal spine* is a sharp projection in the median plane in the lower boundary of the piriform aperture (Fig. 1.4).

Lower Part of the Face

Maxilla

Maxilla contributes a large share in the formation of the facial skeleton. The anterior surface of the body of the maxilla presents (a) the *nasal notch* medially; (b) the *anterior nasal spine;* (c) the *infraorbital foramen,* 1 cm below the infraorbital margin; (d) the *incisive fossa* above the incisor teeth; and (e) the *canine fossa* lateral to the canine eminence (see Fig. 1.29).

In addition, three out of four processes of the maxilla are also seen in this norma. (a) The *frontal process of the maxilla* is directed upwards. It articulates anteriorly with the nasal bone, posteriorly with the lacrimal bone, and superiorly with the frontal bone. (b) The *zygomatic process of the maxilla* is short but stout and articulates with the zygomatic bone. (c) The *alveolar process of the maxilla* bears sockets for the upper teeth.

Zygomatic Bone

Zygomatic bone forms the prominence of the cheek. The *zygomaticofacial foramen* is seen on its surface.

Mandible

Mandible forms the lower jaw. The *upper border* or *alveolar arch* lodges the lower teeth. The *lower border* or *base* is rounded. The middle point of the base is called the *mental point or gnathion*. The *anterior surface* of the body of the mandible presents: (a) The *symphysis menti*, the *mental protuberance* and the *mental tubercles* anteriorly; (b) the *mental foramen* below the interval between the two premolar teeth, transmitting the *mental nerve and vessels*; and (c) the *oblique line* which runs upwards and backwards from the mental tubercle to the anterior border of the ramus of the mandible.

Sutures of the Norma Frontalis

1. Internasal
2. Frontonasal
3. Nasomaxillary
4. Lacrimomaxillary
5. Frontomaxillary
6. Intermaxillary
7. Zygomaticomaxillary
8. Zygomaticofrontal

Attachments

1. The medial part of the superciliary arch gives origin to the *corrugator supercilii* muscle (Fig. 2.6).

2. The *procerus* muscle arises from the nasal bone near the median plane (Fig. 1.6).

3. The orbital part of the *orbicularis oculi* arises from the frontal process of the maxilla and from the nasal part of the frontal bone (Fig. 2.6).

4. The *medial palpebral ligament* is attached to the frontal process of the maxilla between the frontal and maxillary origins of the orbicularis oculi.

5. The *levator labii superior alaeque nasi* arises from the frontal process of the maxilla in front of the orbicularis oculi (Fig. 2.8).

6. The *levator labii superioris* arises from the maxilla between the infraorbital margin and the infraorbital foramen (Fig. 2.6).

7. The *levator anguli oris* arises from the canine fossa.

8. The *nasalis* and the *depressor septi* arise from the surface of the maxilla bordering the nasal notch.

9. The *incisive* muscle arises from an area just below the depressor septi (Fig. 1.7). It forms part of orbicularis oris.

10. The *zygomaticus major and minor* arise from the surface of the zygomatic bone (Fig. 2.7).

The *zygomaticus minor* muscle arises below the zygomaticofacial foramen. The *zygomaticus major* arises lateral to the minor muscle.

11. *Buccinator* arises from maxilla and mandible opposite molar teeth and from *pterygomandibular raphe* (Fig. 1.7). It also forms part of orbicularis oris.

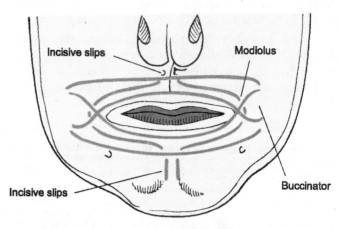

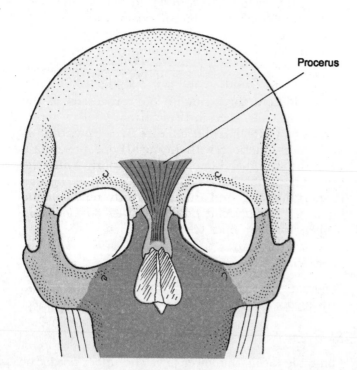

Fig. 1.6: *Procerus.*

Fig. 1.7: *Fibres of orbicularis oris.*

Structures Passing through Foramina

1. The *supraorbital notch or foramen* transmits the *supraorbital nerves and vessels* (Fig. 2.5).

2. The *external nasal nerve* emerges between the nasal bone and the upper nasal cartilage.

3. The *infraorbital foramen* transmits the *infraorbital nerve and vessels* (Fig. 2.19).

4. The *zygomaticofacial foramen* transmits the nerve of the same name, a branch of *maxillary nerve*.

5. The *mental foramen* on the mandible transmits the mental nerve and vessels.

NORMA LATERALIS

Bones

1. Frontal; 2. parietal; 3. occipital; 4. temporal; 5. sphenoid; 6. zygomatic; 7. mandible; 8. maxilla; 9. nasal (Fig. 1.8).

Features

1. The *temporal lines* have been studied in the norma verticalis. The inferior temporal line, in its posterior part, turns downwards and forwards and becomes continuous with the *supramastoid crest* on the squamous temporal bone near its junction with the mastoid temporal. This crest is continuous anteriorly with the posterior root of the zygoma.

2. The *zygomatic arch* is a horizontal bar on the side of the head, in front of the ear, a little above the tragus. It is formed by the temporal process of the zygomatic bone in anterior one-third and the zygomatic process of the temporal bone in posterior two-thirds. The *zygomatico-temporal suture* crosses the arch obliquely downwards and backwards.

The arch is separated from the side of the skull by a gap which is deeper in front than behind. Its *lateral surface* is subcutaneous. The anterior end of the upper border is called the *jugal point*. The posterior end of the zygoma is attached to the squamous temporal bone by *anterior* and *posterior roots*. The *articular tubercle* of the root of the zygoma lies on its lower border, at the junction of the anterior and

posterior roots. The anterior root passes medially in front of the *articular fossa*. The posterior root passes backwards along the lateral margin of the mandibular fossa, then above the external acoustic meatus to become continuous with the supramastoid crest. Two projections are visible in relation to these roots. One is articular tubercle or tubercle of the root of zygoma at its lower border. The other is visible just behind the mandibular or articular fossa and is known as postglenoid tubercle.

3. The *external acoustic meatus* opens just below the posterior part of the posterior root of the zygoma. Its anterior and inferior margins and the lower part of the posterior margin are formed by the tympanic plate; and the posterosuperior margin is formed by the squamous temporal bone. The margins are roughened for the attachment of the auricular cartilage.

The *suprameatal triangle* is a small depression posterosuperior to the meatus. It is *bounded* above by the supramastoid crest; in front by the posterosuperior margin of the external meatus; and behind by a vertical tangent to the posterior margin of the meatus. The *suprameatal spine* may be present on the anteroinferior margin of the triangle. The triangle forms the lateral wall of the tympanic or mastoid antrum.

4. The *mastoid part of the temporal bone* lies just behind the external acoustic meatus. It is continuous anterosuperiorly with the squamous temporal bone. A partially obliterated *squiamomastoid suture* may be

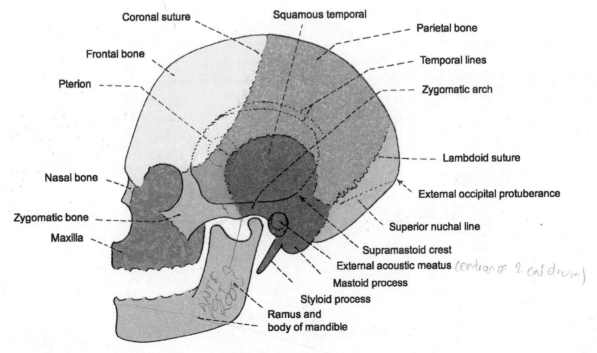

Fig. 1.8: *Norma lateralis*

visible just in front of and parallel to the roughened area for muscular insertions.

The mastoid temporal bone articulates posterosuperiorly with the posteroinferior part of the parietal bone at the horizontal *parietomastoid suture;* and posteriorly with the squamous occipital bone at the *occipitomastoid suture.* These two sutures meet at the lateral end of the lambdoid suture. The *asterion* is the point where the parietomastoid, occipitomastoid and lambdoid sutures meet. In infants the asterion is the site of the *posterolateral* or *mastoid fontanelle,* which closes at the end of the first year (Figs 1.2, 1.3).

The *mastoid process* is a nipple-like large projection from the lower part of the mastoid temporal bone, posteroinferior to the external acoustic meatus. It appears during the second year of life. The *tympanomastoid fissure* is placed on the anterior aspect of the base of the mastoid process (Fig. 1.3). The *mastoid foramen* lies at or near the occipito-mastoid suture.

5. The *styloid process* is a needle like thin, long projection from the norma basalis situated anteromedial to the mastoid process. It is directed downwards, forwards and slightly medially. Its base is partly ensheathed by the tympanic plate. The apex or tip is usually hidden from view by the posterior border of the ramus of the mandible (Fig. 1.14).

6. The *temporal fossa. Boundaries:* (a) *Above,* by the temporal line of the frontal bone. (b) *Below,* by the upper border of the zygomatic arch laterally; and by the infratemporal crest of the greater wing of the sphenoid bone medially. Through the gap deep to the zygomatic arch, the temporal fossa communicates with the infratemporal fossa. (c) The *anterior wall* is formed, by the zygomatic bone and by parts of the frontal and sphenoid bones. This wall separates the fossa from the orbit (Figs 10.1, 10.2).

Floor: The anterior part of the floor is crossed by an H-shaped suture where four bones; frontal, parietal, sphenoid and temporal adjoin each other; This area is termed the *pterion.* It lies 4 cm above the midpoint of the zygomatic arch or 4 cm above the zygoma and 2.5 cm behind the frontozygomatic suture. Deep to the pterion there lie the *middle meningeal vein,* the *anterior division of the middle meningeal artery,* and *the stem of the lateral sulcus of the brain* (Fig. 1.9).

On the temporal surface of the zygomatic bone forming the anterior wall of the fossa there is the *zygomatico-temporal foramen.*

7. *Infratemporal fossa. Boundaries:* (a) The *roof* is formed medially by the infratemporal surface of the greater wing of the sphenoid and by a small part of the squamous temporal bone. Laterally, the roof is incomplete where the infratemporal fossa communicates with the temporal fossa through the gap deep to the zygomatic arch. The roof formed by greater wing is pierced by the *foramen ovale* and by the *foramen spinosum.* (b) The *floor* is open. (c) The *medial wall* is formed by the lateral pterygoid plate and the pyramidal process of the palatine bone. (d) The *lateral wall* is formed by the ramus of the

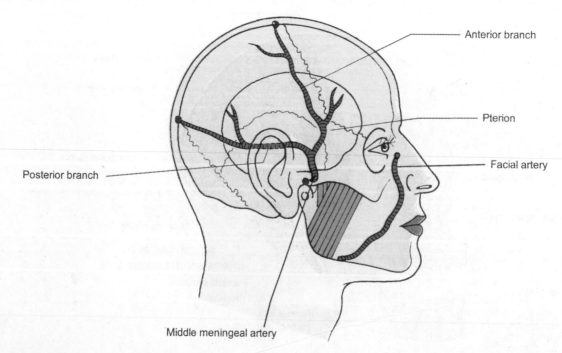

Fig. 1.9: Surface marking of facial artery and middle meningeal artery with its anterior and posterior branches.

mandible. (e) The *anterior wall* is formed by the infratemporal or posterior surface of the maxilla and by the medial surface of the zygomatic bone. The anterior and medial walls are separated in their upper parts by the pterygomaxillary fissure through which the infratemporal fossa communicates with the pterygopalatine fossa. The upper end of the pterygomaxillary fissure is continuous with the anterior part of the inferior orbital fissure through which the infratemporal fossa communicates with the orbit. (f) The *posterior wall* is open (Fig. 15.11).

The contents of the fossa are described in Chapter 10.

8. *Pterygopalatine fossa:* It is described in Chapter 15.

Attachments

1. The *temporal fascia* is attached to the superior temporal line and to the area between the two temporal lines. Inferiorly, it is attached to the outer and inner lips of the upper border of the zygomatic arch.

2. The *temporalis muscle* arises from the whole of the temporal fossa, except the part formed by the zygomatic bone. Beneath the muscle there lie the *deep temporal vessels* and *nerves*. The *middle temporal vessels* produce vascular markings on the temporal bone just above the external acoustic meatus (Fig. 1.10).

3. The medial surface and lower border of the zygomatic arch give origin to the *masseter* (Fig. 1.10).

4. The *lateral ligament* of the *temporomandibular joint* is attached to the tubercle of the root of the zygoma (Fig. 10.9).

5. The *sternocleidomastoid, splenius capitis and longissimus capitis* are inserted in that order from before backwards on the posterior part of the lateral surface of the mastoid process (Fig. 1.15).

6. The *gap* between the zygomatic arch and the side of the skull transmits: (a) The tendon of the temporalis muscle; (b) the deep temporal vessels; and (c) the deep temporal nerves.

Structures Passing Through Foramina

1. The *tympanomastoid fissure* on the anterior aspect of the base of the mastoid process transmits the *auricular branch* of the *vagus nerve*.

2. The mastoid foramen transmits: (a) An *emissary vein* connecting the *sigmoid sinus* with the *posterior auricular vein;* and (b) a meningeal branch of the occipital artery (Table 1.1).

3. The *zygomaticotemporal foramen* transmits the nerve of the same name and a minute artery.

NORMA BASALIS

For convenience of study, the norma basalis is divided arbitrarily into anterior, middle and posterior

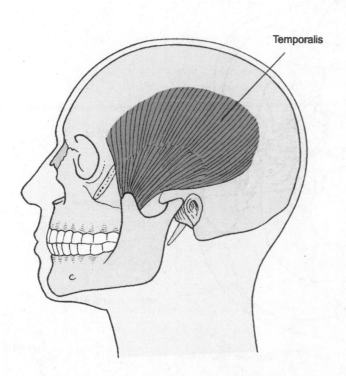
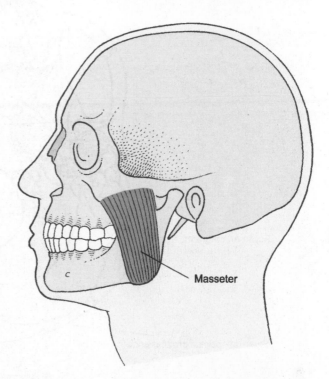

Fig. 1.10: Temporalis and masseter muscles.

Table 1.1: The emissary veins of the skull

Name	Foramen of skull	Veins outside skull	Venous sinus
1. Parietal emissary vein	Parietal foramen	Veins of scalp	Superior sagittal
2. Mastoid emissary vein	Mastoid foramen	Veins of scalp	Transverse sinus
3. Emissary vein	Hypoglossal canal	Internal jugular vein	Sigmoid sinus
4. Condylar emissary vein	Posterior condylar foramen	Suboccipital venous plexus	Sigmoid sinus
5. 2-3 emissary veins	Foramen lacerum	Pharyngeal venous plexus	Cavernous sinus
6. Emissary vein	Foramen ovale	Pterygoid venous plexus	Cavernous sinus
7. Emissary vein	Foramen caecum	Veins of roof of nose	Superior sagittal sinus

parts. The *anterior part* is formed by the hard palate and the alveolar arches. The *middle and posterior parts* are separated by an imaginary transverse line passing through the anterior margin of the foramen magnum (Fig. 1.11).

Anterior Part of Norma Basalis

Alveolar Arch

Alveolar arch bears sockets for the roots of the upper teeth.

Hard Palate

1. *Formation:* (a) Anterior two-thirds, by the palatine processes of the maxillae and (b) posterior one-third by the horizontal plates of the palatine bones.

2. *Sutures:* The palate is crossed by a cruciform suture made up of intermaxillary, interpalatine and palatomaxillary sutures.

3. *Dome:* (a) It is arched in all directions, and (b) shows pits for the palatine glands.

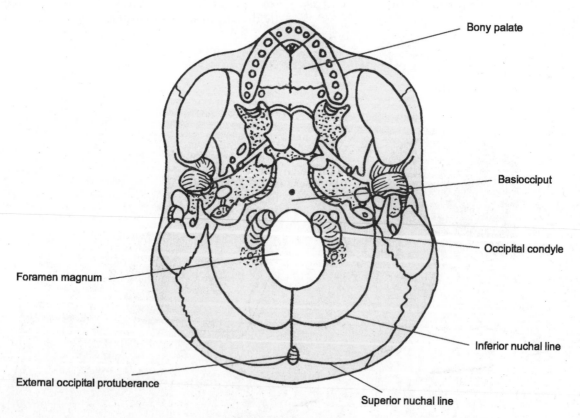

Fig. 1.11: Norma basalis.

4. The *incisive fossa* is a deep fossa situated anteriorly in the median plane (Fig. 1.12). Two *incisive* canals, right and left, pierce the walls of the incisive fossa, usually one on each side, but occasionally in the median plane, the left being anterior and the right, posterior.

5. The *greater palatine foramen*, one on each side, is situated just behind the lateral part of the palatomaxillary suture. A groove leads from the foramen towards the incisive fossa.

6. The *lesser palatine foramina*, two or three in number on each side, lie behind the greater palatine foramen, and perforate the pyramidal process of the palatine bone (Fig. 15.11).

7. The *posterior border* of the hard palate is free and presents the *posterior nasal spine* in the median plane.

8. The *palatine crest* is a curved ridge near the posterior border. It begins behind the greater palatine foramen and runs medially (Fig. 1.12).

Middle Part of Norma Basalis

The middle part extends from the posterior border of the hard palate to the arbitrary transverse line passing through the anterior margin of the foramen magnum.

Median Area

1. The median area shows: (a) The posterior border of the *vomer;* and (b) a *broad bar of bone* formed by fusion of the posterior part of the body of the sphenoid and the basilar part of the occipital bone (Fig. 1.13).

2. The vomer separates the two posterior nasal apertures. Its inferior border articulates with the bony palate. The superior border splits into two *alae* and articulates with the *rostrum* of the *sphenoid bone.*

3. The *palatinovaginal canal.* The inferior surface of the vaginal process of the medial pterygoid plate is marked by an anteroposterior groove which is converted into the palatinovaginal canal by the upper

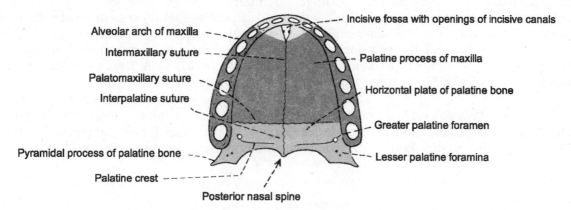

Fig. 1.12: *Anterior part of the norma basalis.*

Labels:
Alveolar arch of maxilla
Intermaxillary suture
Palatomaxillary suture
Interpalatine suture
Pyramidal process of palatine bone
Palatine crest
Posterior nasal spine
Incisive fossa with openings of incisive canals
Palatine process of maxilla
Horizontal plate of palatine bone
Greater palatine foramen
Lesser palatine foramina

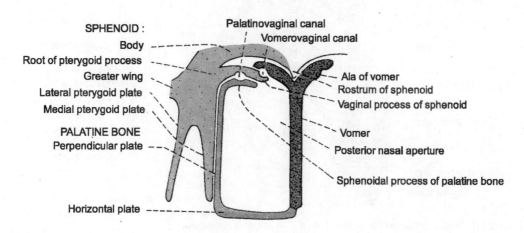

Fig. 1.13: *Posterior view of a coronal section through the posterior nasal aperture showing the formation of the palatinovaginal and vomerovaginal canals.*

Labels:
SPHENOID:
Body
Root of pterygoid process
Greater wing
Lateral pterygoid plate
Medial pterygoid plate
PALATINE BONE
Perpendicular plate
Horizontal plate
Palatinovaginal canal
Vomerovaginal canal
Ala of vomer
Rostrum of sphenoid
Vaginal process of sphenoid
Vomer
Posterior nasal aperture
Sphenoidal process of palatine bone

surface of the sphenoidal process of the palatine bone. The canal opens anteriorly into the posterior wall of the pterygopalatine fossa (Fig. 15.11).

4. The *vomerovaginal canal.* The lateral border of each ala of the vomer comes into relationship with the vaginal process of the medial pterygoid plate, and may overlap it from above to enclose the vomerovaginal canal.

5. The broad bar of bone is marked in the median plane by the *pharyngeal tubercle* a little in front of the foramen magnum.

Lateral Area

1. The lateral area shows two parts of the sphenoid bone—pterygoid process and greater wing. Also seen are three parts of the temporal bone; petrous temporal, tympanic plate and squamous temporal.

2. The *pterygoid process* projects downwards from the junction of the greater wing and the body of the sphenoid behind the third molar tooth. Inferiorly it divides into the *medial and lateral pterygoid plates* which are fused together anteriorly, but are separated posteriorly by the V-shaped *pterygoid fossa.* The fused anterior borders of the two plates articulate medially with the perpendicular plate of the palatine bone, and are separated laterally from the posterior surface of the body of the maxilla by the pterygo-maxillary fissure.

The *medial pterygoid plate* is directed backwards. It has medial and lateral surfaces and a free posterior border. The upper end of this border divides to

enclose a triangular depression called the *scaphoid fossa.* Medial to this fossa there is a small *pterygoid tubercle* which projects into the *foramen lacerum.* It hides from view the posterior opening of the pterygoid canal. The lower end of the posterior border is prolonged downwards and laterally to form the *pterygoid hamulus* (Fig. 1.13).

The *lateral pterygoid plate* is directed backwards and laterally. It has medial and lateral surfaces and a free posterior border. The lateral surface forms the medial wall of the infratemporal fossa. The lateral and medial surfaces give origin to muscles. The posterior border sometimes has a projection called the *pterygospinous process* which projects towards the spine of the sphenoid (Fig. 1.13).

3. The *infratemporal surface of the greater wing of the sphenoid* is pentagonal: (a) Its *anterior margin* forms the posterior border of the inferior orbital fissure; (b) its *anterolateral margin* forms the infratemporal crest; (c) its *posterolateral margin* articulates with the squamous temporal; (d) its *posteromedial margin* articulates with petrous temporal; and (e) *anteromedially* it is continuous with the pterygoid process and with the body of the sphenoid bone. The posteriormost point between the posterolateral and posteromedial margins projects downwards to form the *spine* of the sphenoid (Fig. 1.14).

Along the posteromedial margin, the surface is pierced by the following foramina: (a) The *foramen ovale* is large and oval in shape. It is situated posterolateral to the upper end of the posterior

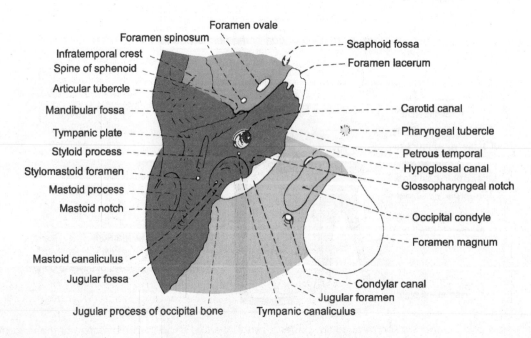

Fig. 1.14: *Middle part of norma basalis.*

border of the lateral pterygoid plate. (b) The *foramen spinosum* is small and circular in shape. It is situated posterolateral to the foramen ovale, and is limited posterolaterally by the spine of the sphenoid (Fig. 1.14). (c) Sometimes there is the *emissary sphenoidal foramen or foramen of Vesalius*. It is situated between the foramen ovale and the scaphoid fossa. Internally, it opens between the foramen ovale and the foramen rotundum. (d) At times there is a *canaliculus innominatus* situated between the foramen ovale and the foramen spinosum.

The *spine* of the sphenoid may be sharply pointed or blunt.

The *sulcus tubae* is the groove between the posteromedial margin of the greater wing of the sphenoid and the petrous temporal bone. It lodges the *cartilaginous part of the auditory tube*. Posteriorly, the groove leads to the bony part of the auditory tube which lies within the petrous temporal bone (Figs 14.18, 14.19, 18.10).

4. The inferior surface of the petrous part of the temporal bone is triangular in shape with its apex directed forwards and medially. It lies between the greater wing of the sphenoid and the basiocciput. Its *apex* is perforated by the upper end of the carotid canal, and is separated from the sphenoid by the foramen lacerum. The *inferior surface* is perforated by the lower end of the *carotid canal* posteriorly.

The *carotid canal* runs forwards and medially within the petrous temporal bone.

The *foramen lacerum* is a short, wide canal, 1 cm long. Its lower end is bounded posterolaterally by the apex of the petrous temporal, medially by the basiocciput and the body of the sphenoid, and anteriorly by the root of the pterygoid process and the greater wing of the sphenoid bone.

A part of the petrous temporal bone, called the *tegmen tympani* is present in the middle cranial fossa. It has a downturned edge which is seen in the *squamotympanic fissure* and divides it into the *petrotympanic* and *petrosquamous* fissures.

5. *The tympanic part of the temporal bone also called as the tympanic plate* is a triangular curved plate which lies in the angle between the petrous and squamous parts. Its apex is directed medially and lies close to the spine of the sphenoid. The *base or border* is curved, free and roughened. Its *anterior surface* forms the posterior wall of the mandibular fossa. The *posterior surface* is concave and forms the anterior wall, floor, and lower part of the posterior wall of the bony external acoustic meatus. Its *upper border* bounds the petrotympanic fissure. The *lower border* is sharp and free. *Medially* it passes along the anterolateral margin of the lower end of the carotid canal; and *laterally* it forms the anterolateral

part of the *sheath of the styloid process. Internally,* the tympanic plate is fused to the petrous temporal bone (Fig. 1.14).

6. *The squamous part of the temporal bone* forms: (a) The anterior part of the mandibular articular fossa which articulates with the head of the mandible to form the temporomandibular joint; (b) the articular tubercle which is continuous with the anterior root of the zygoma; and (c) a small posterolateral part of the roof of the infratemporal fossa (Fig. 10.8).

Posterior Part of Norma Basalis

Median Area

1. The median area shows from before backwards: (a) The foramen magnum, (b) the external occipital crest; and (c) the external occipital protuberance.

2. The *foramen magnum* is the largest foramen of the skull. It opens upwards into the posterior cranial fossa, and downwards into the vertebral canal. It is oval in shape, being wider behind than in front where it is overlapped on each side by the occipital condyles (Fig. 1.14).

3. The *external occipital crest* begins at the posterior margin of the foramen magnum and ends posteriorly and above at the external occipital protuberance.

4. The *external occipital protuberance* is a projection located at the posterior end of the crest. It is easily felt in the living, in the midline, at the point where the back of the neck becomes continuous with the scalp.

The superior nuchal lines begin at the external occipital protuberance and the inferior nuchal lines at the middle of the crest. Both of them curve laterally and backwards and then laterally and forwards.

Lateral Area

1. The lateral area shows: (a) The condylar part of the occipital bone; (b) the squamous part of the occipital bone; (c) the jugular foramen between the occipital and petrous temporal bones; (d) the styloid process of the temporal bone; and (e) the mastoid part of the temporal bone.

2. The *condylar or lateral part of the occipital bone* presents the following. (a) The *occipital condyles* are oval in shape and are situated on each side of the anterior part of the foramen magnum. Their long axis is directed forwards and medially. They articulate with the superior articular facets of the atlas vertebra to form the atlanto-occipital joints. (b) The *hypoglossal* or *anterior condylar canal* pierces the bone anterosuperior to the occipital condyle, and is directed laterally and slightly forwards. (c) The *condylar*

or *posterior condylar canal* is occasionally present in the floor of a condylar fossa present behind the occipital condyle. Superiorly it opens into the sigmoid sulcus. (d) The *jugular process of the occipital bone* lies lateral to the occipital condyle and forms the posterior boundary of the jugular foramen (Fig. 1.14).

3. *Squamous pat of occipital bone.* This is marked by the superior and inferior nuchal lines mentioned above.

4. The *jugular foramen* is large and elongated, with its long axis directed forwards and medially. It is placed at the posterior end of the petro-occipital suture (Fig. 1.14).

At the posterior end of the foramen, its anterior wall (petrous temporal) is hollowed out to form the *jugular fossa* which lodges the superior bulb of the internal jugular vein. The fossa is larger on the right side than on the left.

The lateral wall of the jugular fossa is pierced by a minute canal, the *mastoid canaliculus.* Near the medial end of the jugular foramen there is the *jugular notch.* At the apex of the notch there is an opening that leads into the *cochlear canaliculus* (Fig. 1.14).

The *tympanic canaliculus* opens on or near the thin edge of bone between the jugular fossa and the lower end of the carotid canal.

5. The *styloid process* will be described in Chapter 12.

The *stylomastoid foramen* is situated posterior to the root of the styloid process, at the anterior end of the mastoid notch.

6. The *mastoid process* is a large conical projection located posterolateral to the stylomastoid foramen. It is directed downwards and forwards. It forms the lateral wall of the *mastoid notch* (Fig. 1.3).

Attachments on Exterior of Skull

1. The posterior border of the hard palate provides attachment to the palatine aponeurosis. The posterior nasal spine gives origin to the musculus uvulae (Fig. 1.15).

2. The palatine crest provides attachment to a part of the tendon of the tensor veli palatini muscle.

3. The attachments on the inferior surface of the basioccipital are as follows:

The *pharyngeal tubercle* gives attachment to the raphe which provides insertion to the upper fibres of the *superior constrictor* muscle of the pharynx (Fig. 14.17). The area in front of the tubercle forms the *roof* of the *nasopharynx* and supports the *pharyngeal tonsil.* The *longus capitis* is inserted lateral to the pharyngeal tubercle. The *rectus capitis anterior* is inserted a little posterior and medial to the hypoglossal canal (Fig. 1.15).

4. The attachments on the medial pterygoid plate are as follows:

(a) The *pharyngobasilar fascia* is attached to the whole length of its posterior border (Fig. 14.17).

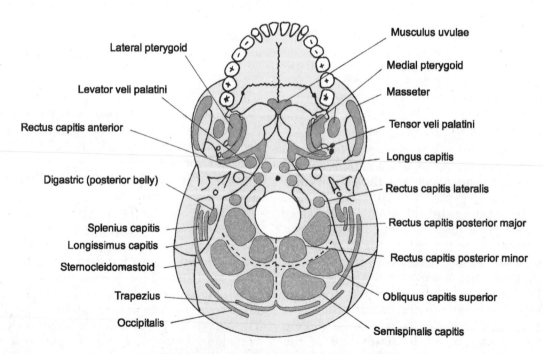

Fig. 1.15: Muscles attached to the base of skull.

(b) The lower part of the posterior border, and the pterygoid hamulus, give origin to the superior constrictor of the pharynx.

(c) The upper part of the posterior border is notched by the *auditory* tube.

(d) The *pterygomandibular raphe* is attached to the tip of the pterygoid hamulus.

5. The attachments on the lateral pterygoid plate are as follows:

(a) Its lateral surface gives origin to the *lower head* of the *lateral pterygoid muscle* (Fig. 1.16).

(b) Its medial surface gives origin to the *deep head of the medial pterygoid*. The small, superficial head of this muscles arises from the *maxillary tuberosity* and the adjoining part of the pyramidal process of the palatine bone.

(c) The pterygospinous process gives attachment to the ligament of the same name.

6. The infratemporal surface of the greater wing of the sphenoid gives origin to the *upper head* of the *lateral pterygoid muscle*, and is crossed by the deep temporal and masseteric nerves.

7. The *spine* of the *sphenoid is related laterally to* the *auriculotemporal nerve*, and *medially to the chorda tympani nerve* and *auditory tube*. Its *tip* provides attachment to the *sphenomandibular ligament*. Its

anterior aspect gives origin to the most posterior fibres of the *tensor veli palatini muscle*.

8. The inferior surface of the petrous temporal bone gives origin to the *levator veli palatini*.

9. The margins of the foramen magnum provide attachment to: (a) The *anterior atlanto-occipital membrane* anteriorly; (b) the *posterior atlanto-occipital membrane* posteriorly; and (c) the *alar ligaments* on the roughened medial surface of each occipital condyle (Figs 13.3, 13.4).

10. The *ligamentum nuchae* is attached to the external occipital protuberance and crest.

11. The *rectus capitis lateralis* is inserted into the inferior surface of the jugular process of the occipital bone (Fig. 1.15).

12. The following are attached to the squamous part of the occipital bone. The area between the superior and inferior nuchal lines provides insertion medially to the *semispinalis capitis*, and laterally to the *superior oblique* muscle. The area below the inferior nuchal line provides insertion medially to the *rectus capitis posterior minor*, and laterally to the *rectus capitis posterior major* (Fig. 4.5).

13. The *mastoid notch* gives origin to the *posterior belly of the digastric muscle* (Fig. 11.1).

Structures Passing Through Foramina

1. Each *incisive foramen* transmits: (a) The terminal parts of the *greater palatine vessels* from the palate to the nose; and (b) the terminal part of the *nasopalatine nerve* from the nose to the palate (Figs 15.5, 15.8).

2. The *greater palatine foramen* transmits: (a) The *greater palatine vessels*, and (b) the *anterior palatine nerve*, both of which run forwards in the groove that passes forwards from the foramen (Fig. 15.12).

3. The *lesser palatine foramina* transmit the *middle* and *posterior palatine nerves*.

4. The *palatinovaginal canal* transmits: (a) A *pharyngeal branch* from the *pterygopalatine ganglion*; and (b) a small *pharyngeal branch* of the *maxillary artery*.

5. The *vomerovaginal canal* (if patent) transmits branches of the *pharyngeal nerve* from pterygo palatine ganglion and vessels.

6. The *foramen ovale* transmits the *mandibular nerve*, the *lesser petrosal nerve*, the *accessory meningeal artery*, an *emissary vein* connecting the cavernous sinus with the pterygoid plexus of veins, and occasionally the anterior trunk of the middle meningeal vein (MALE).

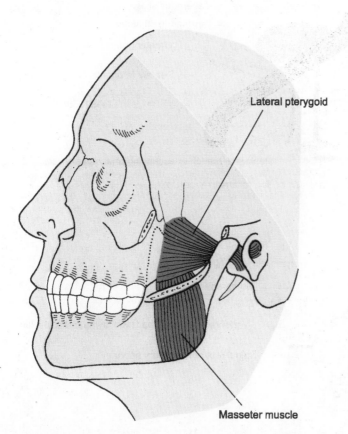

Fig. 1.16: *Masseter and lateral pterygoid muscles.*

Lateral pterygoid

Masseter muscle

7. The *foramen spinosum* transmits the *middle meningeal artery*, the meningeal branch of the mandibular nerve or nervus spinosus, and the posterior trunk of the middle meningeal vein.

8. The *emissary sphenoidal foramen* transmits an *emissary vein* connecting the cavernous sinus with the pterygoid plexus of veins.

9. When present the *canalis innominatus* transmits the lesser petrosal nerve.

10. The *carotid canal* transmits the *internal carotid artery*, and the *venous* and *sympathetic plexuses* around the artery (Fig. 1.17).

11. The structures passing through the *foramen lacerum* are as follows. During life the lower part of the foramen is filled with cartilage, and no significant structure passes through the whole length of the canal, except for the meningeal branch of the ascending pharyngeal artery and an emissary vein from the cavernous sinus. However, the upper part of the foramen is traversed by the internal carotid artery with venous and sympathetic plexuses around it. In the anterior part of the foramen, the *greater petrosal nerve* unites with *the deep petrosal nerve* to form the *nerve of the pterygoid canal* which leaves the

foramen by entering the pterygoid canal in the anterior wall of the foramen lacerum (Fig. 1.17).

12. The medial end of the *petrotympanic fissure* transmits the chorda tympani nerve and the anterior tympanic artery.

13. The *foramen magnum* transmits the following (Fig. 1.18).

Through wider posterior part

   a. Lowest part of medulla oblongata

   b. Three meninges.

Through the subarachnoid space

   a. Spinal accessory nerves.

   b. Vertebral arteries.

   c. Sympathetic plexus around the vertebral arteries.

   d. Posterior spinal arteries.

   e. Anterior spinal artery.

Through the narrow anterior part

   a. Apical ligament of dens.

   b. Vertical brand of cruciate ligament.

   c. Membrana tectoria (Fig. 13.3).

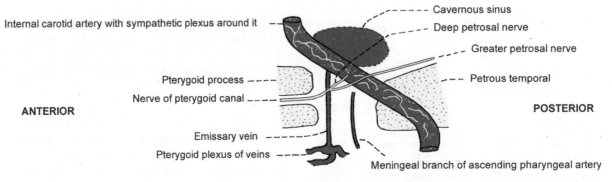

Fig. 1.17: *Diagram showing some relationships of the foramen lacerum.*

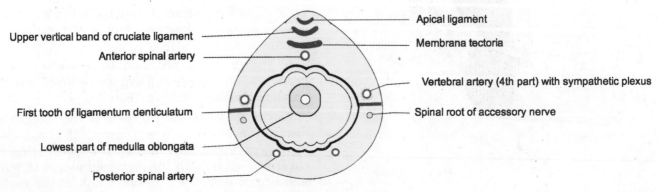

Fig. 1.18: *Structures passing through foramen magnum.*

14. The *hypoglossal* or *anterior condylar* canal transmits the *hypoglossal nerve*, the *meningeal branch* of the hypoglossal nerve, the *meningeal branch* of the ascending pharyngeal artery, and an *emissary vein* connecting the sigmoid sinus with the internal jugular vein.

15. The *posterior condylar canal* transmits an emissary vein connecting the sigmoid sinus with the suboccipital venous plexus (Table 1.1).

16. The *jugular foramen* transmits the following structures.

Through the anterior part

a. Inferior petrosal sinus

b. Meningeal branch of the ascending pharyngeal artery.

Through the middle part

IXth, Xth and XIth cranial nerves.

Through the posterior part

a. Internal jugular vein.

b. Meningeal branch of the occipital artery.

The glossopharyngeal notch near the medial end of the jugular foramen lodges the inferior ganglion of the glossopharyngeal nerve.

17. The mastoid canaliculus in the lateral wall of the jugular fossa transmits the auricular branch of the vagus. The nerve passes laterally through the bone, crosses the facial canal, and emerges at the tympanomastoid fissure. The nerve is extracranial at birth, but becomes surrounded by bone as the tympanic plate and mastoid process develop.

18. The *tympanic canaliculus* on the thin edge of the partition between the jugular fossa and the carotid canal transmits the tympanic branch of the glossopharyngeal nerve to the middle ear cavity.

19. The *stylomastoid foramen* transmits the facial nerve and the stylomastoid branch of the posterior auricular artery.

INTERIOR OF THE SKULL

Before beginning a systematic study of the interior, the following general points may be noted.

1. The cranium is lined internally by *endocranium* which is continuous with the pericranium through the foramina and sutures.

2. The *thickness* of the cranial vault is variable. The bones covered with muscles, i.e. temporal and posterior cranial fossae are thinner than those covered with scalp. Further, the bones are thinner in females than in males, and in children than in adults.

3. Most of the cranial bones consist of: (a) An *outer table* of compact bone which is thick, resilient and tough; (b) an *inner table* of compact bone which is thin and brittle; and (c) the *diploe* which consists of spongy bone filled with red marrow, in between the two tables.

The skull bones derive their blood supply mostly from the meningeal arteries from inside and very little from the arteries of the scalp. Blood supply from the outside is rich in those areas where muscles are attached, e.g. the temporal fossa and the suboccipital region. The blood from the diploe is drained by four diploic veins on each side draining into venous sinuses (Table 1.2).

Many bones like vomer, pterygoid plates do not have any diploe.

Internal Surface of Cranial Vault

The shape, the bones present, and the sutures uniting them have been described with the norma verticalis.

The following features may be noted.

1. The *inner table* is thin and brittle. It presents *markings* produced by meningeal vessels, venous sinuses, arachnoid granulations, and to some extent by cerebral gyri. It also presents raised ridges formed by the attachments of the dural folds.

	Table 1.2: Diploic veins		
1.	Frontal diploic vein	Supraorbital foramen	Drain into supraorbital vein
2.	Anterior temporal or parietal diploic vein	In the greater wing of sphenoid	Sphenoparietal sinus or in anterior deep temporal vein
3.	Posterior temporal or parietal diploic vein	Mastoid foramen	Transverse sinus
4.	Occipital diploic vein (largest)	Foramen in occipital bone	Occipital vein or confluence of sinuses
5.	Small unnamed diploic veins	Pierce inner table of skull close to the margins of superior sagittal sinus	Venous lacunae

2. The *frontal crest* lies anteriorly in the median plane. It projects backwards.

3. The *sagittal sulcus* runs from before backwards in the median plane. It becomes progressively wider posteriorly. It lodges the superior sagittal sinus.

4. The *granular foveolae* are deep, irregular, large, pits situated on each side of the sagittal sulcus. They are formed by arachnoid granulations. They are larger and more numerous in aged persons.

5. The *vascular markings.* The groove for the anterior branch of the middle meningeal artery, and the accompanying vein runs upwards 1 cm behind the coronal suture. Smaller grooves for the branches from the anterior and posterior branches of the middle meningeal vessels run upwards and backwards over the parietal bone (Fig. 1.9).

6. The *parietal foramina* open near the sagittal sulcus 2.5 to 3.75 cm in front of the lambdoid suture.

7. The *impressions for cerebral gyri* are less distinct. These become very prominent in cases of raised intracranial tension.

Internal Surface of the Base of the Skull

The interior of the base of the skull presents natural subdivisions into the anterior, middle and posterior cranial fossae. The dura mater is firmly adherent to the floor of the fossae and is continuous with the pericranium through the foramina and fissures (Fig. 1.19).

Anterior Cranial Fossa

Boundaries

Anteriorly and on the sides, by the frontal bone (Fig. 1.20).

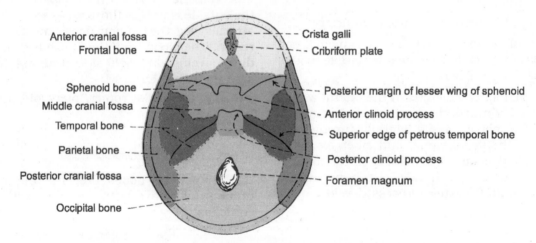

Fig. 1.19: *The cranial fossae. The boundaries of the bones present in the floor of the fossae are shown in interrupted lines.*

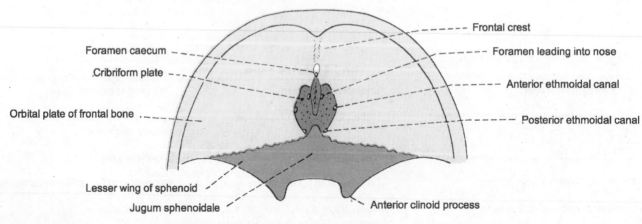

Fig. 1.20: *Some features to be seen in the anterior cranial fossa.*

Posteriorly, it is separated from the middle cranial fossa by the free *posterior border* of the *lesser wing of the sphenoid,* the *anterior clinoid process,* and the *anterior margin of the sulcus chiasmaticus.*

Floor

In the median plane, it is formed anteriorly by the *cribriform plate of the ethmoid bone,* and posteriorly by the superior surface of the anterior part of the body of the sphenoid or *jugum sphenoidale.*

On each side, the floor is formed mostly by the *orbital plate of the frontal bone,* and is completed posteriorly by the lesser wing of the sphenoid.

Other Features

1. The *cribriform plate of the ethmoid bone* separates the anterior cranial fossa from the nasal cavity. It is quadrilateral in shape. (a) The *anterior* margin articulates with the frontal bone at the *frontoethmoidal suture* which is marked in the median plane by the *foramen caecum.* This foramen is usually blind, but is occasionally patent. (b) The *posterior margin* articulates with the jugum sphenoidale. At the posterolateral corners we see the *posterior ethmoidal canals.* (c) Its *lateral margins* articulate with the orbital plate of the frontal bone: the suture between them presents the *anterior ethmoidal canal* placed behind the crista galli (Fig. 1.20).

Anteriorly, the cribriform plate has a midline projection called the *crista galli.* On each side of the crista galli there are foramina through which the anterior *ethmoidal nerve and vessels* pass to the nasal cavity. The plate is also perforated by *numerous foramina* for the passage of olfactory nerve rootlets.

2. The *jugum sphenoidale* separates the anterior cranial fossa from the sphenoidal sinuses.

3. The *orbital plate of the frontal bone* separates the anterior cranial fossa from the orbit. It supports the orbital surface of the frontal lobe of the brain, and presents reciprocal impressions. The *frontal air sinus* may extend into its anteromedial part. The *medial margin* of the plate covers the labyrinth of the ethmoid; and the *posterior margin* articulates with the lesser wing of the sphenoid.

4. The *lesser wing of the sphenoid* is broad medially where it is continuous with the jugum sphenoidale and tapers laterally. The free *posterior border* fits into the *stem of the lateral sulcus of the brain.* It ends medially as a prominent projection, the *anterior clinoid process.* Inferiorly, the posterior border forms the upper boundary of the *superior orbital fissure.* Medially, the lesser wing is connected to the body of the sphenoid by *anterior and posterior roots,* which enclose the *optic canal* (Fig 1.21).

CLINICAL ANATOMY

Fracture of the anterior cranial fossa may cause bleeding and discharge of cerebrospinal fluid through the nose. It may also cause a condition called *black eye* which is produced by seepage of blood into the eyelid.

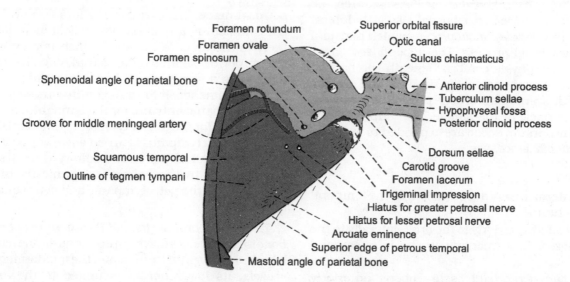

Fig. 1.21: *Some features to be seen in the middle cranial fossa.*

Middle Cranial Fossa

It is deeper than the anterior cranial fossa, and is shaped like a butterfly, being narrow and shallow in the middle; and wide and deep on each side.

Boundaries

Anterior: (a) Posterior border of the lesser wing of the sphenoid; (b) anterior clinoid process; and (c) anterior margin of the sulcus chiasmaticus (Fig. 1.21).

Posterior: (a) Superior border of the petrous temporal bone; and (b) the dorsum sellae of the sphenoid.

Lateral: (a) Greater wing of the sphenoid; (b) anteroinferior angle of the parietal bone; and (c) the squamous temporal bone in the middle.

Floor: Floor is formed by body of sphenoid in the median region and by greater wing of sphenoid, squamous temporal and anterior surface of petrous temporal on each side.

Other Features

Median Area

The body of the sphenoid presents the following features.

(a) The *sulcus chiasmaticus* or *optic groove* leads, on each side, to the optic canal. The optic chiasma does not occupy the sulcus; it lies at a higher level well behind the sulcus.

(b) The *optic canal* leads to the orbit. It is bounded laterally by the lesser wing of the sphenoid, in front and behind by the two roots of the lesser wing, and medially by the body of the sphenoid.

(c) The *sella turcica.* The upper surface of the body of the sphenoid is hollowed out in the form of a Turkish saddle, and is known as the sella turcica. It consists of the tuberculum sellae in front, the hypophyseal fossa in the middle and the *dorsum sellae* behind. The *tuberculum sellae* separates the optic groove from the *hypophyseal fossa.* Its lateral ends form the *middle clinoid process* which may join the anterior clinoid process. The *hypophyseal fossa* lodges the hypophysis cerebri. Beneath the floor of the fossa lie the sphenoidal air sinuses. The *dorsum sellae* is a transverse plate of bone projecting upwards; it forms the back of the saddle. The superolateral angles of the dorsum sellae are expanded to form the *posterior clinoid processes.*

Lateral Area

1. The lateral area is deep and lodges the temporal lobe of the brain.

2. It is related anteriorly to the orbit, laterally to the temporal fossa, and inferiorly to the infratemporal fossa.

3. The *superior orbital fissure* opens anteriorly into the orbit. It is *bounded* above by the lesser wing, below by the greater wing, and medially by the body of the sphenoid. The medial end is wider than the lateral. The long axis of the fissure is directed laterally, upwards and forwards. The lower border is marked by a small projection, which provides attachment to the *common tendinous ring of Zinn.* The ring divides the fissure into three parts.

4. The *greater wing of the sphenoid* presents the following features: (a) The *foramen rotundum* lies posteroinferior to the medial end of the superior orbital fissure. It leads anteriorly to the pterygopalatine fossa containing pterygopalatine ganglia (Table 1.3). (b) The *foramen ovale* lies posterolateral to the foramen rotundum and lateral to the lingula. It leads inferiorly to the infratemporal fossa. (c) The *foramen spinosum* lies posterolateral to the foramen ovale. It also leads, inferiorly, to the infratemporal fossa. (d) The *emissary sphenoidal foramen* or foramen of Vesalius. These foramina have been seen on the base of the skull. (e) The *groove for the middle meningeal* vessels leads forwards from the foramen spinosum (Fig. 1.21).

5. The *foramen lacerum* lies at the posterior end of the carotid groove and posteromedial to the foramen ovale. Its upper end is bounded posterolaterally by the apex of the petrous temporal bone, and anteromedially by the body of the sphenoid and by the posteromedial margin of the greater wing.

6. The *anterior surface of the petrous temporal bone* presents the following features: (a) The *trigeminal impression* lies near the apex, behind the foramen lacerum. It lodges the trigeminal ganglion within its dural cave (Figs 6.11, 6.12). (b) The *hiatus and groove for the greater petrosal nerve* are present lateral to the trigeminal impression. They lead to the foramen lacerum. (c) The *hiatus and groove for the lesser petrosal nerve,* lie lateral to the hiatus for the greater petrosal nerve. They lead to the foramen ovale or to the canaliculus innominatus. (d) Still more laterally there is the *arcuate eminence* which is produced by the superior semicircular canal. (e) The *tegmen tympani* is a thin plate of bone anterolateral to the arcuate eminence. It forms a continuous sloping roof for the tympanic antrum, for the tympanic cavity and for the canal for the tensor tympani. The lateral margin of the tegmen tympani is turned downwards; it forms the lateral wall of the bony auditory tube. Its lower edge is seen in the squamotympanic fissure and divides it into the petrotympanic and petrosquamous fissures.

7. The *cerebral surface of the squamous temporal bone* is concave. It shows impressions for the temporal lobe and grooves for branches of the middle meningeal vessels. Its lower border is united to the anterior surface of the petrous temporal, but traces of the

Table 1.3: Connections of parasympathetic ganglia

Ganglia	Sensory root	Sympathetic root	Secretomotor root	Motor root	Distribution
Ciliary	From nasociliary nerve.	Plexus along ophthalmic artery.	—	Edinger-Westphal nucleus → oculomotor nerve → nerve to inferior oblique.	i) Ciliaris muscles and ii) Sphincter pupillae
Otic	Branch from auriculotemporal nerve.	Plexus along middle meningeal artery.	Inferior salivatory nucleus → glossopharyngeal nerve → tympanic branch → tympanic plexus → lesser petrosal nerve.	Branch from nerve to medial pterygoid.	i) Secretomotor to parotid gland via auriculotemporal nerve. ii) Tensor veli palatini and tensor tympani via nerve to med. pterygoid (unrelayed).
Pterygopalatine	2 branches from maxillary nerve.	Deep petrosal from plexus around internal carotid artery.	Superior salivatory nucleus, and lacrimatory nucleus → nervus intermedius → facial nerve → geniculate ganglion → greater petrosal nerve. + deep petrosal nerve = nerve of pterygoid canal.		i) Mucous glands of nose, paranasal sinuses, palate, nasopharynx. ii) Some fibres pass through zygomatic nerve - zytemp. nerve - communicating br. to lacrimal nerve - lacrimal gland.
Submandibular	2 branches from lingual nerve.	Branch from plexus around facial art.	Superior salivatory nucleus → facial nerve → chorda tympani-joins the lingual nerve.	—	i) Submandibular, ii) Sublingual and iii) Anterior lingual glands.

petrosquamosal suture are often seen even in the adult.

CLINICAL ANATOMY

Fracture of the middle cranial fossa produces:

(a) Bleeding and discharge of CSF through the ear; (b) bleeding through the nose or mouth may occur due to involvement of the sphenoid bone; and (c) the seventh and eighth cranial nerves may be damaged if the fracture also passes through the internal acoustic meatus. If a semicircular canal is damaged, vertigo may occur.

The middle cranial fossa is most commonly fractured. The fracture line usually follows a definite course. It begins at the parietal tuber which is usually the site of injury and passes through the parietal bone, the squamous temporal, and the petrous temporal bones usually involving the tegmen tympani, and frequently involving the internal acoustic meatus and the foramen ovale.

Posterior Cranial Fossa

This is the largest and deepest of the three cranial fossae. The posterior cranial fossa contains the *hindbrain* which consists of the *cerebellum behind and the pons and medulla in front.*

Boundaries

Anterior: (a) Superior border of the petrous temporal bone; and (b) the dorsum sellae of the sphenoid bone (Fig. 1.22).

Posterior: Squamous part of the occipital bone.

On each side: (a) Mastoid part of the temporal bone and (b) the mastoid angle of the parietal bone.

Floor

Median area: (a) Sloping area behind the dorsum sellae or clivus in front; (b) the foramen magnum in the middle; and (c) the squamous occipital behind.

Lateral area: (a) Condylar or lateral part of occipital bone; (b) posterior surface of the petrous temporal

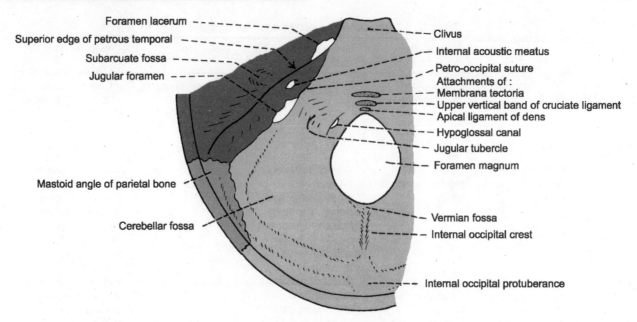

Fig. 1.22: *Some features to be seen in the posterior cranial fossa.*

bone; (c) mastoid temporal bone; and (d) mastoid angle of the parietal bone.

Other Features

I. Median Area

1. The *clivus* is the sloping surface in front of the foramen magnum. It is formed by fusion of the posterior part of the body of the sphenoid including the dorsum sellae with the basilar part of the occipital bone or basiocciput. It is related to the *basilar plexus of veins*, and supports the pons and medulla (Fig. 1.22).

On each side, the clivus is separated from the petrous temporal bone by the *petro-occipital fissure* which is grooved by the inferior petrosal sinus, and is continuous behind with the jugular foramen.

2. The *foramen magnum* lies in the floor of the fossa. It is *bounded* anteriorly by the basiocciput, posteriorly by the squamous part of the occipital bone, and on each side by the condylar part of the occipital bone. The anterior part of the foramen is narrow because it is *overlapped* by the medial surfaces of the occipital condyles.

3. The *squamous part of the occipital bone* shows the following features. (a) The *internal occipital crest* runs in the median plane from the internal occipital protuberance to the foramen magnum where it forms a shallow depression, the *vermian fossa*. (b) The *internal occipital protuberance* lies opposite the external occipital protuberance. It is related to the confluence of sinuses, and is grooved on each side by the beginning of the transverse sinuses. (c) The

transverse sulcus is quite wide and runs laterally from the internal occipital protuberance to the mastoid angle of the parietal bone where it becomes continuous with the sigmoid sulcus. The transverse sulcus lodges the *transverse sinus*. The right transverse sulcus is usually wider than the left and is continuous medially with the superior sagittal sulcus. (d) On each side of the internal occipital crest there are *deep fossae* which lodge the cerebellar hemispheres.

II. Lateral Area

1. The *condylar part of the occipital bone* is marked by the following: (a) The *jugular tubercle* lies over the occipital condyle. (b) The *hypoglossal canal* pierces the bone posteroanterior to the jugular tubercle and runs obliquely forwards and laterally along the line of fusion between the basilar and the condylar parts of the occipital bone. (c) The *condylar canal* opens in the lower part of the sigmoid sulcus which indents the jugular process of the occipital bone (Fig. 1.22).

2. The *posterior surface of the petrous part of the temporal bone* forms the anterolateral wall of the posterior cranial fossa. The following features may be noted: (a) The *internal acoustic meatus* opens above the anterior part of the jugular foramen. It is about one cm long and runs transversely in a lateral direction. It is closed laterally by a perforated plate of bone known as *lamina cribrosa* which separates it from the internal ear. (b) The orifice of the *aqueduct of the vestibule* is a narrow slit lying behind the internal acoustic meatus. (c) The *subarcuate fossa*

lies below the arcuate eminence, lateral to the internal acoustic meatus.

3. The *jugular foramen* lies at the posterior end of the petro-occipital fissure between the deep jugular notch of the petrous temporal bone above and the shallow jugular notch of the occipital bone below. The upper margin is sharp and irregular, and presents the *glossopharyngeal notch*. The lower margin is smooth and regular.

4. The *mastoid part of the temporal bone* forms the lateral wall of the posterior cranial fossa just behind the petrous part of the bone. Anteriorly, it is marked by the *sigmoid sulcus* which begins as a downward continuation of the transverse sulcus at the mastoid angle of the parietal bone, and ends at the jugular foramen. The sigmoid sulcus lodges the *sigmoid sinus* which become the internal jugular vein at the jugular foramen. The sulcus is related anteriorly to the *tympanic antrum*. The *mastoid foramen* opens into the upper part of the sulcus.

CLINICAL ANATOMY

Fracture of the posterior cranial fossa causes bruising over the mastoid region extending down over the sternocleidomastoid muscle.

Attachments and Relations of the Interior of the Skull

Attachment on Vault

1. The frontal crest gives attachment to the falx cerebri (Fig. 1.20).

2. The lips of the sagittal sulcus give attachment to the falx cerebri (Fig. 6.2).

Anterior Cranial Fossa

1. The crista galli gives attachment to the falx cerebri.

2. The orbital surface of the frontal bone supports the frontal lobe of the brain.

3. The anterior clinoid processes give attachment to the free margin of the tentorium cerebelli (Fig. 6.3).

Middle Cranial Fossa

1. The middle cranial fossa lodges the *temporal lobe of the cerebral hemisphere*.

2. The tuberculum sellae provides attachment to the *diaphragma sellae* (Fig. 6.5).

3. The hypophyseal fossa lodges the *hypophysis cerebri*.

4. The upper margin of the dorsum sellae provides attachment to the diaphragma sellae; and the posterior clinoid process to the anterior end of the attached margin of the tentorium cerebelli, and to the petrosphenoidal ligament (Fig. 6.3).

5. One *cavernous sinus* lies on each side of the body of the sphenoid. The internal carotid artery passes through the cavernous sinus (Fig. 6.6).

6. The superior border of the petrous temporal bone is grooved by the *superior petrosal sinus* and provides attachment to the *attached margin of the tentorium cerebelli*. It is grooved in its medial part by the *trigeminal nerve*.

Posterior Cranial Fossa

1. The posterior cranial fossa contains the hindbrain which consists of the cerebellum behind, and the pons and medulla in front.

2. The lower part of the clivus provides attachment to the *apical ligament of the dens* near the foramen magnum, upper vertical band of cruciate ligament and to the *membrana tectoria* just above the apical ligament (Fig. 1.22).

3. The internal occipital crest gives attachment to the *falx cerebelli*.

4. The jugular tubercle is grooved by the *ninth, tenth and eleventh cranial nerves* as they pass to the jugular foramen.

5. The subarcuate fossa on the posterior surface of the petrous temporal bone lodges the *flocculus of the cerebellum*.

Structures Passing Through Foramina

The following foramina seen in the cranial fossae have been dealt with under the normal basalis: foramen ovale, foramen spinosum, emissary sphenoidal foramen, foramen lacerum, foramen magnum, jugular foramen, hypoglossal canal, and posterior condylar canal. Additional foramina seen in the cranial fossae are as follows.

1. The *foramen caecum* in the anterior cranial fossa is usually blind, but occasionally it transmits a vein from the upper part of the nose to the superior sagittal sinus.

2. The *posterior ethmoidal canals* transmit the vessels of the same name. Note that the nerves do not pass through the canals as they terminate earlier.

3. The *anterior ethmoidal canals* transmit the corresponding nerves and vessels.

4. The *optic canal* transmits the optic nerve and the ophthalmic artery.

5. The three parts of the *superior orbital fissure* (Fig. 7.4) transmit the following structures:

Lateral part: (a) Lacrimal nerve; (b) frontal nerve; (c) trochlear nerve; (d) superior ophthalmic vein;

(e) meningeal branch of the lacrimal artery; and (f) anastomotic branch of the middle meningeal artery which anastomoses with the recurrent branch of the lacrimal artery.

Middle part: (a) Upper and lower divisions of the oculomotor nerve; (b) nasociliary nerve in between the two divisions of the oculomotor; and (c) the abducent nerve, inferolateral to the foregoing nerves.

Medial part: (a) Inferior ophthalmic vein and (b) sympathetic nerves from the plexus around the internal carotid artery.

6. The *foramen rotundum* transmits the maxillary nerve (Fig. 15.13).

7. The *internal acoustic meatus* transmits the *seventh and eighth cranial nerves* and the *labyrinthine vessels* (Fig. 9.7).

Principles Governing Fractures of the Skull

1. Fractures of the skull are prevented by: (a) Its elasticity; (b) rounded shape; (c) construction from a number of secondary elastic arches, each made up of a single bone; and (d) the muscles covering the thin areas.

2. Since the skull is an elastic sphere filled with the semifluid brain, a violent blow on the skull produces a *splitting effect* commencing at the site of the blow and tending to pass along the lines of least resistance.

3. The *base of the skull is more fragile* than the vault, and is more commonly involved in such fractures, particularly along the foramina.

4. The *inner table is more brittle* than the outer table. Therefore, fractures are more extensive on the inner table, causing considerable damage to the brain. Occasionally only the inner table is fractured and the outer table remains intact.

5. The *common sites* of fracture in the skull are: (a) The *parietal area* of the vault; and (b) the *middle cranial fossa* of the base. This fossa is weakened by numerous foramina and canals.

The facial bones commonly fractured are: (a) The *nasal bone* and (b) the *mandible*.

THE ORBIT

The orbits are pyramidal bony cavities, situated one on each side of the root of the nose. They provide sockets for rotatory movements of the eyeballs. They also protect the eyeballs.

Shape and Disposition

Each orbit resembles a four-sided pyramid on one side. Thus it has: (a) *An apex* situated at the posterior

end of the orbit at the medial end of superior orbital fissure; (b) *a base* the orbital opening on the face; and (c) *four walls*: roof, floor, lateral and medial walls (Fig. 1.5).

The long axis of the orbit passes backwards and medially. The medial walls of the two orbits are parallel and the lateral walls are set at right angles to each other (Fig. 1.23).

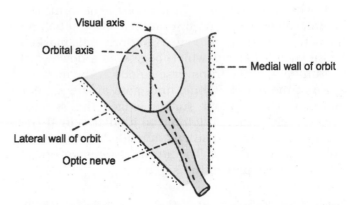

Fig. 1.23: *Diagram comparing the orientation of the orbital axis and the visual axis.*

Roof

It is concave from side to side. It is formed (a) mainly by the orbital plate of the frontal bone; and (b) is completed posteriorly by the lesser wing of the sphenoid (Fig. 1.24).

Relations

(a) It separates the orbit from the anterior cranial fossa. (b) The frontal air sinus may extend into its anteromedial part.

Named Features

(a) The *lacrimal fossa,* placed anterolaterally, lodges the lacrimal gland, (b) the *optic canal lies* posteriorly, at the junction of the roof and medial wall, (c) the *trochlear fossa,* lies anteromedially. It provides attachment to the fibrous pulley or trochlea for the tendon of the *superior oblique muscle.*

Lateral Wall

This is the thickest and strongest of all the walls of the orbit. It is formed: (a) By the anterior surface of the greater wing of the sphenoid bone posteriorly; and (b) the orbital surface of the frontal process of the zygomatic bone anteriorly.

Relations

(a) The greater wing of the sphenoid separates the orbit from the middle cranial fossa. (b) The zygomatic bone separates it from the temporal fossa.

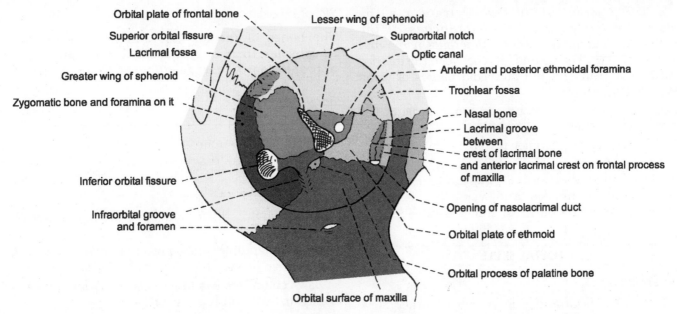

Orbital plate of frontal bone
Superior orbital fissure
Lacrimal fossa
Greater wing of sphenoid
Zygomatic bone and foramina on it
Inferior orbital fissure
Infraorbital groove and foramen
Orbital surface of maxilla

Lesser wing of sphenoid
Supraorbital notch
Optic canal
Anterior and posterior ethmoidal foramina
Trochlear fossa
Nasal bone
Lacrimal groove between crest of lacrimal bone and anterior lacrimal crest on frontal process of maxilla
Opening of nasolacrimal duct
Orbital plate of ethmoid
Orbital process of palatine bone

Fig. 1.24: The orbit seen from the front. All the features shown cannot be seen from any particular direction.

Named Features

(a) The *superior orbital fissure* occupies the posterior part of the junction between the roof and lateral wall. (b) The *foramen for the zygomatic nerve* is seen in the zygomatic bone. (c) *Whitnall's* or *zygomatic tubercle* is a palpable elevation on the zygomatic bone just within the orbital margin. It provides attachment to the lateral check ligament of the eyeball.

Floor

It slopes upwards and medially to join the medial wall. It is formed: (a) Mainly by the orbital surface of the maxilla; (b) by the lower part of the orbital surface of the zygomatic bone, anterolaterally; and (c) the orbital process of the palatine bone, at the posterior angle.

Relation

It separates the orbit from the maxillary sinus.

Named Features

(a) The *inferior orbital fissure* occupies the posterior part of the junction between the lateral wall and floor. Through this fissure the orbit communicates with the infratemporal fossa anteriorly and with the pterygopalatine fossa posteriorly. (b) The *infraorbital groove* runs forwards in relation to the floor. (c) A small depression on the anteromedial part of the floor gives origin to the *inferior oblique muscle*.

Medial Wall

It is very thin. From before backwards it is formed by: (a) The frontal process of the maxilla; (b) the lacrimal bone; (c) the orbital plate of the ethmoid; and (d) the body of the sphenoid bone.

Relations

(a) The *lacrimal groove,* formed by the maxilla and the lacrimal bone, separates the orbit from the nasal cavity. (b) The orbital plate of the ethmoid separates the orbit from the ethmoidal air sinuses. (c) The sphenoidal sinuses, are separated from the orbit only by a thin layer of bone.

Named Features

(a) The lacrimal groove lies anteriorly on the medial wall. It is bounded anteriorly by the lacrimal crest of the frontal process of the maxilla, and posteriorly by the crest of the lacrimal bone. The floor of the groove is formed by the maxilla in front and by the lacrimal bone behind. The groove lodges the lacrimal sac which lies deep to the lacrimal fascia bridging the lacrimal groove. The groove leads inferiorly, through the nasolacrimal canal, to the inferior meatus of the nose. (b) The *anterior and posterior ethmoidal foramina* lie on the frontoethmoidal suture, at the junction of the roof and medial wall.

Foramina in Relation to the Orbit

1. The structures passing through the optic canal and through the superior orbital fissure have been described in cranial fossae (Fig. 7.4).

2. The *inferior orbital fissure* transmits the *zygomatic nerve*, the *orbital branches of the pterygopalatine ganglion*, the *infraorbital nerve and vessels*, and the communication between the inferior ophthalmic vein and the pterygoid plexus of veins (Fig. 15.12).

3. The *infraorbital groove and canal* transmit the corresponding nerve and vessels.

4. The *zygomatic foramen* transmits the zygomatic nerve.

5. The *anterior ethmoidal foramina* transmit the corresponding nerves and vessels. Posterior ethmoidal foramina only transmit vessels.

FOETAL SKULL

Dimensions

1 . Skull is large in proportion to the other parts of skeleton.

2. *Foetal skeleton* is small as compared to calvaria. In foetal skull, the facial skeleton is 1/8th of calvaria; in adults, it is half of calvaria. The foetal skeleton is small due to rudimentary mandible and maxillae, non-eruption of teeth, and small size of maxillary sinus and nasal cavity. The large size of calvaria is due to precocious growth of brain.

3. *Base of the skull* is short and narrow, though internal ear is almost of adult size the petrous temporal has not reached the adult length.

Structure of Bones

The bones of the cranial vault are smooth and unilamellar; there is no diploe. The tables and diploe appear by fourth year of age (Fig. 1.25) and Table 1.2.

Bony Prominences

1. Frontal and parietal tubera are prominent.

2. Glabella, superciliary arches and mastoid processes are not developed.

Ossification of Bones

1. Two halves of frontal bone are separated by metopic suture.

2. The mandible is also present in two halves. It is a derivative of the first branchial arch (Table 1.4).

3. Occipital bone is in four parts (squamous one, condylar two, and basilar one).

4. The four bony elements of temporal bone are separate, except for the commencing union of the tympanic part with the squamous and petrous parts. The second centre for styloid process has not appeared.

5. Unossified membranous gaps a total of 6 fontanelles at the angles of the parietal bones are present (Fig. 1.2).

Paranasal Air Sinuses

These are rudimentary or absent.

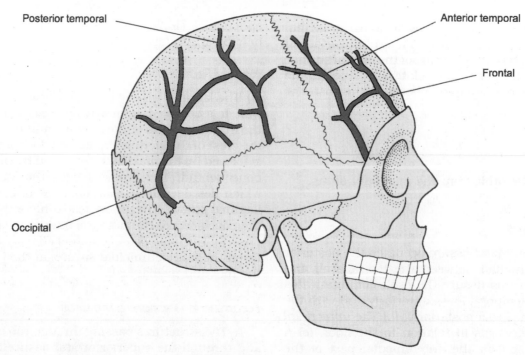

Fig. 1.25: Diploic veins.

Table 1.4: Mesodermal derivatives of pharyngeal/branchial arches

The bones, cartilages, ligaments of arches are formed from neural crest derived mesenchyme. Mesoderm giving origin to the muscles is derived from unsegmented para-axial mesenchyme of head, the somatomeres

Arch	Skeletal elements	Muscles	Nerve
I Arch (a) Maxillary swelling palatopterygo-quadrate cartilage (b) Mandibular swelling (Meckel's cartilage)	Incus Malleus, anterior ligament of malleus and sphenomandibular ligament. Most of the mandible (intramembranous ossification)	Muscles of mastication, i.e. temporalis, masseter, lateral and medial pterygoid, tensor veli palatini, levator veli palatini, mylohyoid and anterior belly of digastric	Mandibular division of V nerve

Note: By intramembranous ossification of mesenchyme of I arch, maxilla, zygomatic, squamous part of temporal are developed

II Arch Reichert's cartilage	Stapes, styloid process, stylo-hyoid ligament, lesser cornua and upper half of body of hyoid	Muscles of facial expression and occipitofrontalis, auricular muscles, platysma, stylohyoid and posterior belly of digastric	Facial nerve (VII)
III Arch	Greater cornua of hyoid and lower half of hyoid bone	Stylopharyngeus	Glossopharyngeal nerve (IX nerve)
IV and VI Arch	Thyroid, cricoid, arytenoid, cuneiform and corniculate cartilages	Cricothyroid, constrictors of pharynx and other muscles of larynx	External laryngeal and recurrent laryngeal branches of vago-accessory complex

Temporal Bone

1. The internal ear, tympanic cavity, tympanic antrum, and ear ossicles are of adult size (Table 1.5).

2. The tympanic part is represented by an incomplete tympanic ring.

3. Mastoid process is absent, it appears during the later part of second year.

4. External acoustic meatus is short and straight. Its bony part is unossified and represented by a fibrocartilaginous plate.

5. Tympanic membrane faces more downwards than laterally due to the absence of mastoid process (Table 1.6).

6. Stylomastoid foramen is exposed on the lateral surface of the skull because mastoid portion is flat.

7. Styloid process lies immediately behind the tympanic ring and has not fused with the remainder of the temporal bone.

8. Mandibular fossa is flat and placed more laterally, and the articular tubercle has not developed.

Table 1.5: Derivatives of endodermal pouches

Pharyngeal pouch	Derivatives
Dorsal ends of I and II pouches form — Tubotympanic recess	Proximal part of tubotympanic recess gives rise to auditory tube Distal part gives rise to tympanic cavity and mastoid antrum. Mastoid cells develop at about two years of age
Ventral part of II pharyngeal pouch	Epithelium covering the palatine tonsil and tonsillar crypts, lymphoid tissue is mesodermal in origin
III Pharyngeal pouch	Thymus and inferior parathyroid gland or parathyroid III. Thymic epithelial reticular cells and Hassall's corpuscles are endodermal. Lymphocytes are derived from haemopoietic stem cells during 12th week
IV Pharyngeal pouch	Superior parathyroid or parathyroid IV
V Pharyngeal pouch (ultimobranchial body)	Parafollicular or 'C' cells of the thyroid gland

Table 1.6: Derivatives of ectodermal clefts	
Dorsal part of I ectodermal cleft —	Epithelium of external auditory meatus
Auricle	Six auricular hillocks; three from I arch and three from II arch
Rest of ectodermal clefts obliterated by the overgrowth of II pharyngeal arch. The closing membrane of the first cleft is the tympanic membrane	

9. The subarcuate fossa is very deep and prominent.

10. Facial canal is short.

Orbits

These are large. The germs of developing teeth lies close to the orbital floor.

POSTNATAL GROWTH OF SKULL

The growth of calvaria and facial skeleton proceeds at different rates and over different periods. Growth of calvaria is related to growth of brain, whereas that of the facial skeleton is related to the development of dentition, muscles of mastication, and of the tongue. The rates of growth of the base and vault are also different.

Growth of the Vault

1. *Rate:* Rapid during first year, and then slow up to the seventh year when it is almost of adult size.

2. *Growth in breadth:* This growth occurs at the sagittal suture, sutures bordering greater wings, occipitomastoid suture, and the petro-occipital suture at the base.

3. *Growth in height:* This growth occurs at the frontozygomatic suture, pterion, squamosal suture, and asterion.

4. *Growth in anteroposterior diameter:* This growth occurs at the coronal and lambdoid sutures.

Growth of the Base

The base grows in anteroposterior diameter at the three cartilaginous plates situated between the occipital and sphenoid bones, between the pre- and postsphenoids, and between the sphenoid and ethmoid.

Growth of the Face

1. Growth of orbits and ethmoid is complete by seventh year.

2. In the face, the growth occurs mostly during first year, although it continues till puberty and even later.

Closure of Fontanelles

Anterior fontanelle by 18 months: posterior fontanelle by 2–3 months; sphenoidal fontanelle by 2–3 months; and mastoid fontanelle by 12 months (Fig. 1.2).

Thickening of Bones

1. Two tables and diploe appear by fourth year. Differentiation reaches maximum by about thirty-five years, when the diploic veins produce characteristic marking in the radiographs (Fig. 1.25).

2. Mastoid process appears during second year, and the mastoid air cells during 6th year.

Obliteration of Sutures of the Vault

1. Obliteration begins on the inner surface between thirty and forty years, and on the outer surface between forty and fifty years.

2. The timings are variable, but it usually takes place first in the lower part of the coronal suture, next in the posterior part of the sagittal suture, and then in the lambdoid suture.

In Old Age

The skull generally becomes thinner and lighter but in small proportion of cases it increases in thickness and weight. The most striking feature is reduction in the size of mandible and maxillae due to loss of teeth and absorption of alveolar processes. This causes decrease in the vertical height of the face and a change in the angles of the mandible which become more obtuse.

SEX DIFFERENCES IN THE SKULL

There are no sex differences until puberty. The postpubertal differences are listed in Table 1.7.

Wormian or Sutural Bones

These are small irregular bones found in the region of the fontanelles, and are formed by additional ossification centres.

Table 1.7: Sex differences in the skull

Features	Males	Females
1. Weight	Heavier	Lighter
2. Size	Larger	Smaller
3. Capacity	Greater in males	10% less than males
4. Walls	Thicker	Thinner
5. Muscular ridges, glabella, super-ciliary arches, temporal lines, mastoid processes, superior nuchal lines, and external occipital protuberance	More marked	Less marked
6. Tympanic plate	Larger, and margins roughened	Smaller and margins are less roughened
7. Supraorbital margin	More rounded	Sharp
8. Forehead	Sloping (receding)	Vertical
9. Frontal and parietal tubera	Less prominent	More prominent
10. Vault	Rounded	Somewhat flattened
11. Contour of face	Longer due to greater depth of the jaws (more of the lower jaw). Chin is bigger and projects more forwards. In general, the skull is more rugged due to muscular markings and processes; and zygomatic bones are more massive	Rounded; facial bones are smoother; and mandible and maxillae are smaller

They are most common at the lambda and at the asterion; common at the pterion (epipteric bone); and rare at the bregma (os Kerckring). Wormian bones are common in hydrocephalic skulls.

CRANIOMETRY

1. Cephalic Index

It expresses the shape of the head, and is the proportion of breadth to length of the skull. Thus:

$$\text{Cephalic index} = \frac{\text{breadth} \times 100}{\text{length}}$$

The length or longest diameter is measured from the glabella to the occipital point; the breadth or widest diameter is measured usually a little below the parietal tubera.

Human races may be: (a) *Dolichocephalic* or long-headed when the index is 75 or less; (b) *mesaticephalic* when the index is between 75 and 80; and (c) *brachycephalic* or short-headed or round-headed when the index is above 80. Dolichocephaly is a feature of primitive races like Eskimoes, Negroes, etc. Brachycephaly through mesaticephaly has been a continuous change in the advanced races, like the Europeans.

2. Facial Angle

This is the angle between two lines drawn from the nasion to the basion or anterior margin of foramen magnum and the prosthion or central point on upper incisor alveolus.

Facial angle is a rough index of the degree of development of the brain because it is the angle between facial skeleton, i.e. splanchnocranium, and the calvaria, i.e. neurocranium, which are inversely proportional to each other. The angle is smallest in the most evolved races of man; it is larger in lower races, and still larger in anthropoids.

3. Abnormal Crania

Oxycephaly or acrocephaly, tower-skull, or steeple-skull is a abnormally tall skull. It is due to premature closure of the suture between presphenoid and postsphenoid, and the coronal suture, so that the skull is very short anteroposteriorly. Compensation is done by the upward growth of skull for the enlarging brain.

Scaphocephaly or boat-shaped skull is due to premature synostosis in the sagittal suture, as a result the skull is very narrow from side to side but greatly elongated.

THE MANDIBLE

The *mandible*, or lower jaw, is the largest and strongest bone of the face. It develops from the *first pharyngeal arch*. It has a horseshoe-shaped body which lodges the teeth, and a *pair of rami* which project upwards from the posterior ends of the *body* and provide attachment to muscles.

The Body

Each half of the body has outer and inner surfaces, and upper and lower borders.

The *outer surface* presents the following features.

(1) The *symphysis menti* is the line at which the right and left halves of the bone meet each other. It is marked by a faint ridge.

(2) The *mental protuberance* (*mentum* = chin) is a median triangular projecting area in the lower part of the midline. The inferolateral angles of the protuberance form the mental tubercles.

(3) The *mental foramen* lies below the interval between the premolar teeth (Fig. 1.26).

(4) The *oblique line* is the continuation of the sharp anterior border of the ramus of the mandible. It runs downwards and forwards towards the mental tubercle.

(5) The *incisive fossa* is a depression that lies just below the incisor teeth.

The *inner surface* presents the following features.

(1) The *mylohyoid line* is a prominent ridge that runs obliquely downwards and forwards from below the third molar tooth to the median area below the genial tubercles (see below).

(2) Below the mylohyoid line the surface is slightly hollowed out to form the *submandibular fossa*, which lodges the submandibular gland.

(3) Above the mylohyoid line there is the *sublingual fossa* in which the sublingual gland lies.

(4) The posterior surface of the symphysis menti is marked by four small elevations called the superior and inferior genial tubercles.

(5) The mylohyoid groove (present on the ramus) extends on to the body below the posterior end of the mylohyoid line.

The *upper or alveolar border* bears sockets for the teeth.

The *lower border* of the mandible is also called the *base*. Near the midline the base shows an oval depression called the *digastric fossa*.

The Ramus

The ramus is quadrilateral in shape and has two surfaces, lateral and medial; four borders, upper, lower, anterior and posterior; and the coronoid and condyloid processes.

The *lateral surface* is flat and bears a number of oblique ridges.

The *medial surface* presents the following.

1. The *mandibular foramen* lies a little above the centre of the ramus at the level of the occlusal surfaces of the teeth. It leads into the *mandibular canal* which descends into the body of the mandible and opens at the *mental foramen*.

2. The anterior margin of the mandibular foramen is marked by a sharp tongue-shaped projection called the *lingula*. The lingula is directed towards the head of the mandible.

3. The *mylohyoid groove* begins just below the mandibular foramen, and runs downwards and forwards to be gradually lost over the submandibular fossa.

The *upper border* of the ramus is thin and is curved downwards forming the *mandibular notch*.

The *lower border* is the backward continuation of the base of the mandible. Posteriorly, it ends by becoming continuous with the posterior border at the *angle* of the mandible.

The *anterior border* is thin, while the *posterior border* is thick.

The *coronoid process* is a flattened triangular upward projection from the anterosuperior part of the ramus. Its anterior border is continuous with the anterior border of the ramus. The posterior border bounds the mandibular notch.

The *condyloid process* is a strong upward projection from the posterosuperior part of the ramus. Its upper end is expanded from side to side to form the *head*. The head is covered with fibrocartilage and articulates with the temporal bone to form the temporomandibular joint. The constriction below the head is the *neck*. Its anterior surface presents a depression called the *pterygoid fovea*.

Attachments and Relations of the Mandible

1. The oblique line on the lateral side of the body gives origin to the *buccinator* as far forwards as the anterior border of the first molar tooth. In front of this origin, the *depressor labii inferioris* and the *depressor anguli oris* arise from the oblique line below the mental foramen (Fig. 1.26).

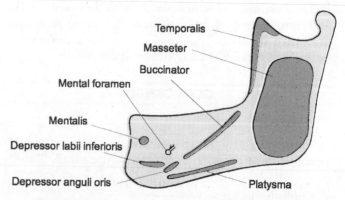

Fig. 1.26: Outer surface of the left half of the mandible.

2. The incisive fossa gives origin to the *mentalis* and the *mental slips of the orbicularis oris* (Fig. 1.7).

3. Parts of both the inner and outer surfaces just below the alveolar margin are covered by the mucous membrane of the mouth.

4. The mylohyoid line gives origin to the *mylohyoid muscle* (Fig. 1.27).

5. The *superior constrictor muscle* of the pharynx arises from an area above the posterior end of the mylohyoid line.

6. The *pterygomandibular raphe* is attached immediately behind the third molar tooth in continuation with the origin of the superior constrictor.

7. The *upper genial tubercle* gives origin to the *genioglossus*, and the *lower tubercle* to the *geniohyoid* (Fig. 1.27).

8. The *anterior belly of the digastric* muscle arises from the digastric fossa.

9. The *deep cervical fascia* (investing layer) is attached to the whole length of the lower border (Fig. 3.2).

10. The *platysma* is inserted into the lower border.

11. The whole of the lateral surface of the ramus except the posterosuperior part provides insertion to the *masseter muscle* (Fig. 1.10).

12. The posterosuperior part of the lateral surface is covered by the *parotid gland* (Fig. 9.1).

13. The *sphenomandibular ligament* is attached to the lingula.

14. The *medial pterygoid muscle* is inserted on the medial surface of the ramus, on the roughened area below and behind the mylohyoid groove. It is in contact with the medial surface in front of the groove (Fig. 1.27).

15. The *temporalis* is inserted into the apex and medial surface of the coronoid process. The insertion extend downwards on the anterior border of the ramus (Fig. 1.10).

16. The *lateral pterygoid muscle* is inserted into the pterygoid fovea on the anterior aspect of the neck. The muscle is related to the medial surface of the ramus, above the mandibular foramen (Fig. 1.16).

17. The lateral surface of the neck provides attachment to the *lateral ligament of the temporomandibular joint* (Fig. 10.9).

Foramina and Relations to Nerves and Vessels

1. The mental foramen transmits the *mental nerve and vessels* (Fig. 2.19).

2. The *inferior alveolar nerve and vessels* enter the mandibular canal through the mandibular foramen, and run forwards within the canal (Fig. 1.27).

3. The *mylohyoid nerve and vessels* lie in the mylohyoid groove.

4. The *lingual nerve* is related to the medial surface of the ramus in front of the mylohyoid groove (Fig. 1.27).

5. The area above and behind the mandibular foramen is related to the *inferior alveolar nerve and vessels* and to the *maxillary artery*.

6. The *masseteric nerve and vessels* pass through the mandibular notch.

7. The *auriculotemporal nerve* is related to the medial side of the neck of the mandible.

Ossification: The mandible is the *second bone, next to the clavicle, to ossify* in the body. Its greater part ossifies *in membrane*. The parts ossifying in *cartilage* include the *incisive part* below the incisor

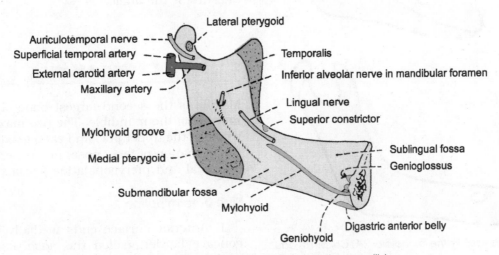

Fig. 1.27: Inner surface of the left half of the mandible.

teeth, the *coronoid and condyloid processes*, and the *upper half of the ramus* above the level of the mandibular foramen.

Each half of the mandible ossifies from only one *centre* which appears at about the *6th week* of intrauterine life in the mesenchymal *sheath of Meckel's cartilage* near the future mental foramen. Meckel's cartilage is the skeletal element of *first pharyngeal arch*.

At birth the mandible consists of two halves connected at the *symphysis menti* by fibrous tissue. Bony union takes place during the first year of life.

Age Changes in the Mandible

In Infants and Children

1. The two halves of the mandible fuse during the first year of life (Fig. 1.28A).

2. At birth the *mental foramen, opens* below the sockets for the two deciduous molar teeth *near the lower border*. This is so because the bone is made up only of the alveolar part with teeth sockets. The *mandibular canal runs near the lower border*. The foramen and canal gradually shift upwards.

3. The angle is *obtuse*. It is 140 degrees or more because the head is in line with the body. The coronoid process is large and projects upwards above the level of the condyle.

In Adults

1. The *mental foramen opens midway between the upper and lower borders* because the alveolar and subalveolar parts of the bone are equally developed. The mandibular canal runs parallel with the mylo-hyoid line.

2. The *angle reduces to about 110 or 120 degrees* because the ramus becomes almost vertical (Fig. 1.28B).

In Old Age

1. Teeth fall out and the alveolar border is absorbed, so that the height of the body is markedly reduced (Fig. 1.28C).

2. The *mental foramen and the mandibular canal are close to the alveolar border*.

3. The *angle again becomes obtuse about 140 degrees* because the ramus is oblique.

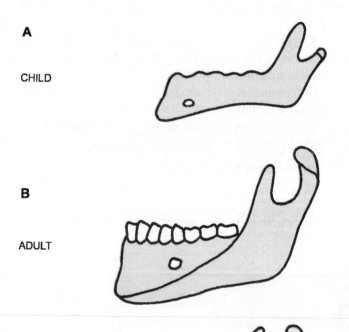
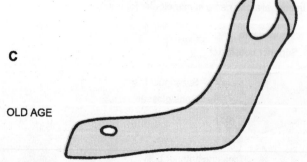

A

CHILD

B

ADULT

C

OLD AGE

Fig. 1.28: *Age changes in the mandible. (A) Child, (B) adult, (C) old age.*

CLINICAL ANATOMY

The mandible is commonly fractured at the canine socket where it is weak. Involvement of the inferior alveolar nerve in the callus may cause neuralgic pain, which may be referred to the areas of distribution of the buccal and auriculotemporal nerves. If the nerve is paralysed, the area supplied by the mental nerve becomes insensitive.

The next common fracture of the mandible occurs at the angle.

THE MAXILLA

Maxilla is the second largest bone of the face, the first being the mandible. The two maxillae form the whole of the upper jaw, and each maxilla enters into the formation of face, nose, mouth, orbit, the infra-temporal and pterygopalatine fossae.

Side Determination

1. Anterior surface ends medially into a deeply concave border, called the *nasal notch*. Posterior surface is convex.

2. Alveolar border with sockets for upper teeth faces downwards with its convexity directed outwards. Frontal process is the longest process which is directed upwards.

3. Medial surface is marked by a large irregular opening, the *maxillary hiatus.*

Features

Each maxilla has a body and four processes, the frontal, zygomatic, alveolar and palatine.

Body of Maxilla

The body of maxilla is pyramidal in shape, with its base directed medially at the nasal surface, and the apex directed laterally at the zygomatic process. It has four surfaces and encloses a large cavity; the *maxillary sinus.* The surfaces are : (1) Anterior or facial; (2) posterior or infratemporal; (3) superior or orbital; and (4) medial or nasal.

Anterior or Facial Surface

1. Anterior surface is directed forwards and laterally.

2. Above the incisor teeth there is a slight depression, the *incisive fossa,* which gives origin to *depressor septi. Incisivus* arises from the alveolar margin below the fossa, and the *nasalis* superolateral to the fossa along the nasal notch.

3. Lateral to canine eminence there is a larger and deeper depression, the *canine fossa,* which gives origin to *levator anguli oris* (Fig. 1.29).

4. Above the canine fossa there is *infraorbital foramen,* which transmits *infraorbital nerve and vessels.*

5. *Levator labii superioris* arises between the infraorbital margin and infraorbital foramen.

6. Medially, the anterior surface ends in a deeply concave border, the *nasal notch,* which terminates below into process which with the corresponding process of opposite maxilla forms the anterior nasal spine. Anterior surface bordering the nasal notch gives origin to *nasalis* and *depressor septi.*

Posterior or Infratemporal Surface

1. Posterior surface is convex and directed backwards and laterally.

2. It forms the anterior wall of *infratemporal fossa,* and is separated from anterior surface by the zygomatic process and a rounded ridge which descends from the process to the first molar tooth.

3. Near the centre of the surface open two or three *alveolar canals* for *posterior superior alveolar nerve and vessels.*

4. Posteroinferiorly, there is a rounded eminence, the *maxillary tuberosity,* which articulates superomedially with pyramidal process of palatine bone, and gives origin laterally to the *superficial head of medial pterygoid muscle.*

5. Above the maxillary tuberosity the smooth surface forms anterior wall of *pterygopalatine fossa,* and is grooved by *maxillary nerve.*

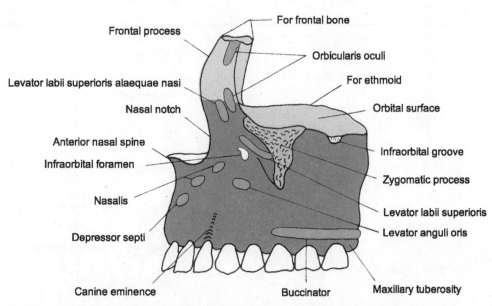

Frontal process
For frontal bone
Orbicularis oculi
Levator labii superioris alaequae nasi
For ethmoid
Nasal notch
Orbital surface
Anterior nasal spine
Infraorbital foramen
Infraorbital groove
Zygomatic process
Nasalis
Levator labii superioris
Levator anguli oris
Depressor septi
Canine eminence
Buccinator
Maxillary tuberosity

Fig. 1.29: *Lateral aspect of maxilla with muscular attachments.*

Superior or Orbital Surface

1. Superior surface is smooth, triangular and slightly concave, and forms the greater part of the *floor of orbit*.

2. *Anterior border* forms a part of infraorbital margin. Medially it is continuous with the lacrimal crest of the frontal process.

3. *Posterior border* is smooth and rounded; it forms most of the anterior margin of inferior orbital fissure. In the middle it is notched by the infraorbital groove.

4. *Medial border* presents anteriorly the lacrimal notch which is converted into *nasolacrimal canal* by the descending process of lacrimal bone. Behind the notch, the border articulates from before backwards with the *lacrimal, labyrinth of ethmoid, and the orbital process of palatine bone.*

5. The surface presents *infraorbital groove* leading forwards to *infraorbital canal* which opens on the anterior surface as *infraorbital foramen.* The groove, canal and foramen transmit the *infraorbital nerve and vessels.* Near the midpoint the canal gives off laterally a branch, the *canalis sinuosus,* for the passage of *anterior superior alveolar nerve and vessels.*

6. *Inferior oblique muscle* of eyeball arises from a depression just lateral to lacrimal notch at the anteromedial angle of the surface.

Medial or Nasal Surface

1. Medial surface forms a part of the *lateral wall of nose.*

2. *Posterosuperiorly* it displays a large irregular opening of the maxillary sinus, the *maxillary hiatus* (Figs 1.30, 1.31).

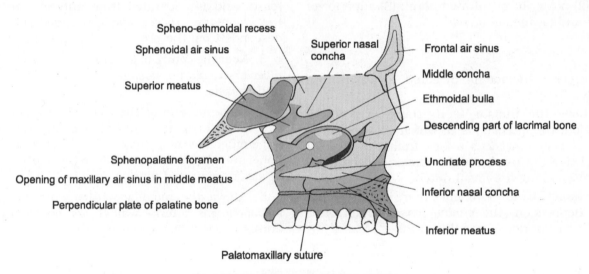

Fig. 1.30: *Medial aspect of intact maxilla.*

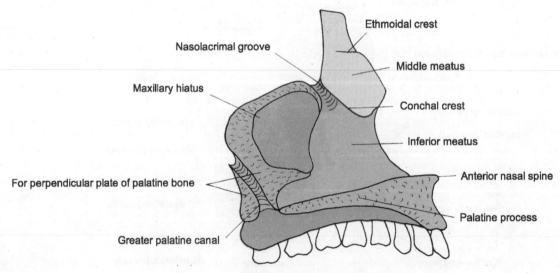

Fig. 1.31: *Medial aspect of disarticulated left maxilla.*

3. Above the hiatus, there are *parts of air sinuses* which are completed by the ethmoid and lacrimal bones.

4. Below the hiatus, the smooth concave surface forms a part of *inferior meatus of nose.*

5. Behind the hiatus, the surface articulates with perpendicular plate of palatine bone, enclosing the *greater palatine canal* which runs downwards and forwards, and transmits *greater palatine vessels and the anterior, middle and posterior palatine nerves* (Fig. 1.31).

6. In front of the hiatus, there is *nasolacrimal groove*, which is converted into the nasolacrimal canal by articulation with the *descending process of lacrimal bone* and the *lacrimal process of inferior nasal concha*. The canal transmits *nasolacrimal duct to the inferior meatus of nose* (Fig 1.31).

7. More anteriorly, an oblique ridge forms the *conchal crest* for articulation with the inferior nasal concha.

8. Above the conchal crest, the shallow depression forms a part of the *atrium of middle meatus* of nose (Fig. 15.6).

Maxillary Sinus

1. The maxillary sinus is a large cavity in the body of maxilla. It is *pyramidal* in shape, with its base directed medially towards the lateral wall of nose, and the apex directed laterally into the zygomatic process of maxilla.

2. The sinus opens into the middle meatus of nose usually by two openings one of which is closed by mucous membrane. The large bony *hiatus of the sinus is reduced* in the articulated skull by following bones: (a) From above, by uncinate process of ethmoid and descending part of lacrimal bone (b) from below, by inferior nasal concha; and (c) from behind, by perpendicular plate of palatine bone (Fig. 1.30).

3. Size is variable. Average measurements are: height 3.7 cm; width, 2.5 cm; and anteroposterior depth, 3.7 cm.

4. Its *roof* is formed by the floor of orbit, and is traversed by the infraorbital canal. The *floor* is formed by the alveolar process of maxilla and lies about 1.2 cm below the level of floor of nose. The floor is marked by several conical elevations produced by the roots of upper molar and premolar teeth; they may even penetrate the bony floor to lie beneath the mucous lining. Canine tooth may project into the anterolateral wall.

5. *Maxillary sinus is first to develop.* It appears as a shallow groove on the medial surface of maxilla during fourth month of intrauterine life, grows rapidly during six to seven years, and reaches full size after the eruption of all permanent teeth. Koranne and Monteiro (1969) noted in 12 human foetuses that the sinus appears in the ninth week of intrauterine life (37 mm CR length) rather than at the fourth month.

6. Carcinoma of maxillary sinus arises from mucosal lining. Thin wall of the sinus may allow extension of the growth upwards into the orbit pushing the eyeball medially into the nasal cavity, forwards on the cheek, or backwards into the infratemporal fossa. Extraction of molar teeth may damage the floor of the sinus.

Four Processes of Maxilla

Zygomatic Process

The zygomatic process is a pyramidal lateral projection on which the anterior, posterior, and superior surfaces or maxilla converge. In front and behind, it is continuous with the corresponding surfaces of the body, but superiorly it is rough for articulation with the zygomatic bone.

Frontal Process

1. The frontal process projects upwards and backwards to *articulate* above with the nasal margin of frontal bone, in front with nasal bone, and behind with lacrimal bone.

2. *Lateral surface* is divided by a vertical ridge, the *anterior lacrimal crest*, into a smooth anterior part and a grooved posterior part. The lacrimal crest gives attachment to *lacrimal fascia* and the *medial palpebral ligament*, and is continuous below with the infraorbital margin. The anterior smooth area gives origin to the *orbital part of orbicularis oculi* and *levator labii superioris alaeque nasi*. The posterior grooved area forms the anterior half of the floor of *lacrimal groove* (Fig. 1.29).

3. *Medial surface* forms a part of the lateral wall of nose. From above downwards the surface presents following features: (a) Uppermost area is rough for articulation with ethmoid to close the anterior ethmoidal sinuses. (b) *Ethmoidal crest* is a horizontal ridge about the middle of the process. Posterior part of the crest articulates with middle nasal concha, and the anterior part lies beneath the agger nasi. (c) The area below the ethmoidal crest is hollowed out to form the atrium of the middle meatus. (d) Below the atrium is the *conchal crest* which articulates with inferior nasal concha. (e) Below the conchal crest there lies the inferior meatus of the nose with nasolacrimal groove ending just behind the crest (Fig. 1.31).

Alveolar Process

1. It alveolar process forms half of the alveolar arch, and bears sockets for the roots of upper teeth.

In adults there are eight *sockets*: *canine socket is deepest*; *molar sockets are widest* and divided into three minor sockets by septa; the *incisor and second premolar sockets are single*; and the *first premolar socket* is sometimes *divided into two*.

2. *Buccinator* arises from the posterior part of its outer surface up to the first molar tooth (Fig. 1.29).

3. A rough ridge, the *maxillary torus*, is sometimes present on the inner surface opposite the molar sockets.

Palatine Process

1. The palatine process is a thick horizontal plate projecting medially from the lowest part of the nasal surface. It forms a large part of the roof of mouth and the floor of nasal cavity (Fig. 1.31).

2. The *inferior surface* is concave, and the two palatine processes form anterior three-fourths of the bony palate. It presents numerous vascular foramina and pits for palatine glands. Posterolaterally, it is marked by two anteroposterior grooves for the greater palatine vessels and anterior palatine nerves.

3. The *superior surface* is concave from side to side, and forms greater part of the floor of nasal cavity.

4. *Medial border* is much thicker in front than behind. It is raised superiorly into the nasal crest. Groove between the nasal crests of two maxillae receives lower border of vomer; anterior part of the ridge is high and is known as *incisor crest* which terminates anteriorly into the anterior nasal spine. Incisive canal traverses near the anterior part of the medial border.

5. *Posterior border* articulates with horizontal plate of palatine bone.

6. *Lateral border* is continuous with the alveolar process.

Articulations of Maxilla

1. Superiorly, it articulates with three bones, the nasal, frontal and lacrimal.

2. Medially, it articulates with five bones, the ethmoid, inferior nasal concha, vomer, palatine and opposite maxilla.

3. Laterally, it articulates with one bone, the zygomatic.

Ossification: Maxilla ossifies in membrane from three centres, one for the maxilla proper, and two for os incisivum or *premaxilla*. The centre for maxilla proper appears above the canine fossa during sixth week of intrauterine life.

Of the two premaxillary centres, the main centre appears above the incisive fossa during seventh week of intrauterine life. The second centre (paraseptal or prevomerine) appears at the ventral margin of nasal septum during tenth week and soon fuses with the palatal process of maxilla. Though premaxilla begins to fuse with alveolar process almost immediately after the ossification begins, the evidence of premaxilla as a separate bone may persist until the middle decades.

Age Changes

1. *At birth* (a) The transverse and anteroposterior diameters are each more than the vertical diameter; (b) frontal process is well marked; (c) body consists of a little more than the alveolar process, the tooth sockets reaching to the floor of orbit; (d) maxillary sinus is a mere furrow on the lateral wall of the nose.

2. *In the adult* Vertical diameter is greatest due to development of the alveolar process and increase in the size of the sinus.

3. *In the old* The bone reverts to infantile condition. Its height is reduced as a result of absorption of the alveolar process.

THE HYOID BONE

The hyoid bone is U-shaped. It develops from second and third branchial arches. It is situated in the anterior midline of the neck between the chin and the thyroid cartilage. At rest it lies at the level of the third cervical vertebra behind and the base of the mandible in front. It is kept suspended in position by muscles and ligaments. The hyoid bone provides attachment to the floor of the mouth and to the tongue above, to the larynx below, and to the epiglottis and pharynx behind (Fig. 14.2).

The bone consists of the central part, called the body, and of two pairs of cornua, greater and lesser.

The Body

It has anterior and posterior surfaces, and upper and lower borders.

The *anterior surface* is convex and is directed forwards and upwards. It is often divided by a median ridge into two lateral halves.

The *posterior surface* is concave and is directed backwards and downwards.

Each lateral end of the body is continuous posteriorly with the greater horn or cornua. However, till middle life the connection between the body and greater cornua is fibrous.

The Greater Cornua

These are flattened from above downwards. Each cornua tapers posteriorly, but ends in a tubercle. It has two surfaces—upper and lower; two borders—medial and lateral and a tubercle.

The Lesser Cornua

These are small conical pieces of bone which project upwards from the junction of the body and greater cornua. The lesser cornua are connected to the body by fibrous tissue. Occasionally they are connected to the greater cornua by synovial joints which usually persist throughout life, but may get ankylosed.

Attachments on the Hyoid Bone

1. The anterior surface of the body provides insertion to the *geniohyoid* and *mylohyoid* muscles and gives origin to a part of the *hyoglossus* which extends to the greater cornua (Fig. 1.32).

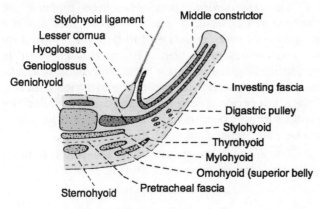

Fig. 1.32: *Anterosuperior view of the left half of hyoid bone showing its attachments.*

2. The *upper border* of the body provides insertion to the lower fibres of the genioglossi and attachment to the *thyrohyoid membrane*.

The *lower border* of the body provides attachment to the *pretracheal fascia*. In front of the fascia, the *sternohyoid* is inserted medially and the *omohyoid* laterally. Below the omohyoid there is the linear attachment of the *thyrohyoid*, extending back to the lower border of the greater cornua (Fig. 1.33).

The *medial border* of the greater cornua provides attachment to the *thyrohyoid membrane, stylohyoid muscle* and *digastric pulley.*

The *lateral border* of the greater cornua provides insertion to the thyrohyoid muscle anteriorly. The *investing fascia* is attached throughout its length.

The lesser cornua provides attachment to the *stylohyoid ligament* at its tip. The *middle constrictor* muscle arises from its posterolateral aspect extending on to the greater cornua (Fig. 1.32).

Development

Upper part of body and lesser cornua develops from second branchial arch, while lower part of body and greater cornua develops from the third arch.

CLINICAL ANATOMY

In a suspected case of murder, fracture of the hyoid bone strongly indicates throttling or strangulation.

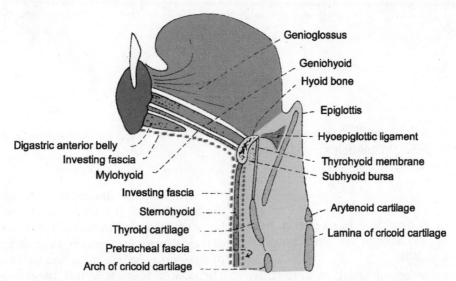

Fig. 1.33: *Sagittal section through the floor of the mouth and larynx showing the attachments to the body of the hyoid bone.*

THE CERVICAL VERTEBRAE

Identification

The cervical vertebrae are identified by the presence of foramina transversaria.

There are seven cervical vertebrae, out of which the third to sixth are typical, while the first, second and seventh are atypical.

TYPICAL CERVICAL VERTEBRA

The Body

(1) The body is *small* and *broader* from side to side than from before backwards. (2) Its *superior surface* is concave transversely with upward projecting lips on each side. The anterior border of this surface may be bevelled. (3) The *inferior surface* is saddle-shaped, being convex from side to side and concave from before backwards. The lateral borders are bevelled and form synovial joints with the projecting lips of the next lower vertebra. The anterior border projects downwards and may hide the intervertebral disc. (4) the *anterior and posterior surfaces* resemble those of other vertebrae (Fig. 1.34).

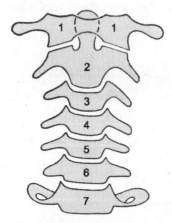

Fig. 1.34: Cervical vertebrae, anterior view.

Vertebral Foramen

Vertebral foramen is larger than the body. It is triangular in shape because the pedicles are directed backwards and laterally.

Vertebral Arch

1. The *pedicles* are directed backwards and laterally. The superior and inferior vertebral notches are of equal size (Fig. 1.35).

2. The *laminae* are relatively long and narrow, being thinner above than below.

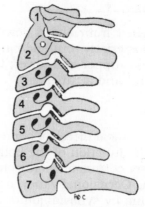

Fig. 1.35: Cervical vertebrae, lateral view.

3. The *superior and inferior articular processes* form articular pillars which project laterally at the junction of pedicle and the lamina. The superior articular facets are flat. They are directed backwards and upwards. The inferior articular facets are also flat but are directed forwards and downwards.

4. The *transverse processes* are pierced by foramina transversaria. Each process has *anterior* and *posterior roots* which end in tubercles joined by the *costotransverse bar*. The *costal element is represented by the anterior root, the costotransverse bar and the posterior tubercle.* The anterior tubercle of the sixth cervical vertebra is large and is called the *carotid tubercle* because the common carotid artery can be compressed against it.

5. The *spine* is short and bifid. The notch is filled up by the ligamentum nuchae (Fig. 1.36).

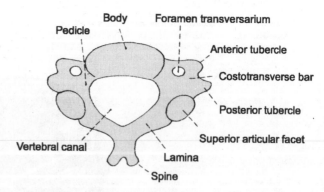

Fig. 1.36: Typical cervical vertebrae seen from above.

Attachments and Relations

1. The *anterior and posterior longitudinal ligaments* are attached to the upper and lower borders of the body in front and behind, respectively. On each side of the anterior longitudinal ligament, the *vertical part of the longus colli* is attached to the anterior surface. The posterior surface has two or more foramina for passage of *basivertebral veins*.

2. The upper borders and lower parts of the anterior surfaces of the laminae provide attachment to the *ligamenta flava*.

3. The *foramen transversarium* transmits the *vertebral artery*, the *vertebral veins* and a *branch from the inferior cervical ganglion*. The *anterior tubercles* give origin to the *scalenus anterior*, the *longus capitis*, and the *oblique part of the longus colli* (Fig. 13.1).

4. The *costotransverse bars* are grooved by the *anterior primary rami* of the corresponding cervical nerves.

5. The *posterior tubercles* give origin to the *scalenus medius, scalenus posterior*, the *levator scapulae*, the *splenius cervicis*, the *longissimus cervicis*, and the *iliocostalis cervicis* (Fig. 4.3).

6. The spine gives origin to the deep muscles of the back of the neck *interspinales, semispinalis thoracis and cervicis, spinalis cervicis, and multifidus* (Fig. 4.4).

Ossification: A typical cervical vertebra ossifies from three primary and six secondary centres. There is one *primary centre* for each half of the neural arch during nine to ten weeks of foetal life and one for the *centrum* in three to four months of foetal life. The two halves of the neural arch fuse posteriorly with each other during the first year. Synostosis at the neurocentral synchondrosis occurs during the third year.

The *secondary centres, two* for the annular epiphyseal discs for the peripheral parts of the upper and lower surfaces of the body, *two* for the tips of the transverse processes, and *two* for the bifid spine appear during puberty, and fuse with the rest of the vertebra by twenty-five years.

FIRST CERVICAL VERTEBRA

It is called the *atlas*. It can be identified by the following features.

It is ring-shaped. It has no body. It also has no spine.

The atlas has a short anterior arch, a long posterior arch, right and left lateral masses, and transverse processes.

The *anterior arch* is marked by a median *anterior tubercle* on its anterior aspect. Its posterior surface bears an *oval facet* which articulates with the *dens* (Fig. 1.37).

The *posterior arch* forms about two-fifths of the ring and is much longer than the anterior arch. Its posterior surface is marked by a median posterior tubercle. The upper surface of the arch is marked behind the lateral mass by a *groove*.

Each *lateral mass* shows the following important features. Its upper surface bears the *superior articular facet*. This facet is elongated (forwards and medially), concave, and is directed upwards and medially. It articulates with the corresponding condyle to form an atlanto-occipital joint. The lower surface is marked by the *inferior articular facet*. This facet is nearly circular, more or less flat, and is directed downwards, medially and backwards. It articulates with the corresponding facet on the axis vertebra to form an atlantoaxial joint. The medial surface of the lateral mass is marked by a small roughened tubercle.

The *transverse process* projects laterally from the lateral mass. It is unusually long and can be felt on the surface of the neck between the angle of the mandible and the mastoid process. Its long length allows it to act as an effective lever for rotatory movements of the head. The transverse process is pierced by the foramen transversarium.

Attachments and Relations

1. The anterior tubercle provides attachment (in the median plane) to the *anterior longitudinal ligament*, and provides insertion on each side to the *upper oblique part of the longus colli*.

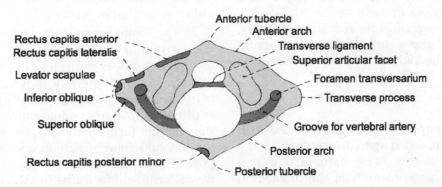

Fig. 1.37: Atlas vertebra seen from above.

2. The upper border of the anterior arch gives attachment to the *anterior atlanto-occipital membrane* (Fig. 13.3).

3. The lower border of the anterior arch gives attachment to the lateral fibres of the *anterior longitudinal ligament.*

4. The posterior tubercle provides attachment to the *ligamentum nuchae* in the median plane and gives origin to the *rectus capitis posterior minor* on each side (Fig. 1.37).

5. The groove on the upper surface of the posterior arch is occupied by the *vertebral artery* and by the *first cervical nerve*. Behind the groove the upper border of the posterior arch gives attachment to the *posterior atlanto-occipital membrane* (Fig. 4.6).

6. The lower border of the posterior arch gives attachment to the highest pair of *ligamenta flava*.

7. The tubercle on the medial side of the lateral mass gives attachment to the *transverse ligament of the atlas* (Fig. 13.4).

8. The anterior surface of the lateral mass gives origin to the *rectus capitis anterior*.

9. The transverse process *gives origin* to the *rectus capitis lateralis* from its upper surface anteriorly, the *superior oblique* from its upper surface posteriorly, the *inferior oblique* from its lower surface of the tip, the *levator scapulae* from its lateral margin and lower border, the *splenius cervicis*, and the *scalenus medius* from the posterior tubercle of transverse process.

Ossification: Atlas ossifies from three centres, one for each lateral mass with half of the posterior arch, one for the anterior arch. The centres for the lateral masses appear during seventh week of intrauterine life and unite posteriorly at about three years. The centre for anterior arch appears at about first year and unites with the lateral mass at about seven years.

SECOND CERVICAL VERTEBRA

This is called the *axis*. It is identified by the presence of the dens or odontoid process which is a strong, tooth-like process projecting upwards from the body. The dens is usually believed to represent the centrum or body of the atlas which has fused with the centrum of the axis.

Body and Dens

1. The *superior surface* of the body is fused with the dens, and is encroached upon on each side by the superior articular facets. The dens articulates anteriorly with the anterior arch of the atlas, and posteriorly with the transverse ligament of the atlas.

CLINICAL ANATOMY

1. Atlas may fuse with the occipital bone. This is called *occipitalization of atlas* and this may at times compress the spinal cord which requires surgical decompression.

2. The pharyngeal and retropharyngeal inflammations may cause decalcification of atlas vertebra. This may lead to loosening of the attachments of transverse ligament which may eventually yield, causing *sudden death* from *dislocation of dens.*

2. The *inferior surface* has a prominent anterior margin which projects downwards.

3. The *anterior surface* presents a median ridge on each side of which there are hollowed out impressions (Fig. 1.38).

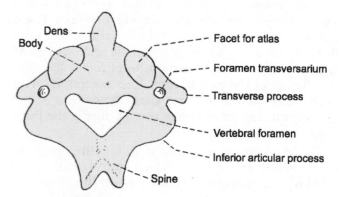

Fig. 1.38: Axis vertebra, posterosuperior view.

Labels: Dens, Body, Facet for atlas, Foramen transversarium, Transverse process, Vertebral foramen, Inferior articular process, Spine

Vertebral Arch

1. The *pedicles* are concealed superiorly by the superior articular processes. The inferior surface presents a deep and wide *inferior vertebral notch*, placed in front of the inferior articular process. The superior vertebral notch is very shallow and is placed on the upper border of the lamina, behind the superior articular process.

2. The *laminae* are thick and strong.

3. Articular facets: Each *superior articular facet* occupies the upper surfaces of the body and of the massive pedicle. Laterally, it overhangs the foramen, transversarium. It is a large, flat, circular facet which is directed upwards and laterally. It articulates with the inferior facet of the atlas vertebra to form the atlantoaxial joint. Each *inferior articular facet* lies posterior to the transverse process and is directed downwards and forwards to articulate with the third cervical vertebra.

4. The *transverse processes* are very small and represent the true posterior tubercles only. The foramen transversarium is directed upwards and laterally (Fig. 1.39).

5. The *spine* is large, thick and very strong. It is deeply grooved inferiorly. Its tip is bifid, terminating in two rough tubercles.

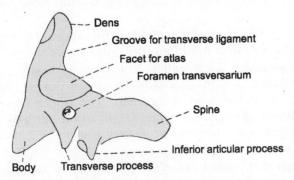

Fig. 1.39: *Axis vertebra, lateral view.*

Attachments

1. The dens provides attachment at its apex to the *apical ligament*, and on each side, below the apex to the *alar ligaments* (Fig. 13.4).

2. The anterior surface of the body receives the insertion of the *longus colli*. The *anterior longitudinal ligament* is also attached to the anterior surface (Fig. 13.1).

3. The posterior surface of the body provides attachment, from below upwards, to the *posterior longitudinal ligament*, the *membrana tectoria* and the *vertical limb* of the *cruciate ligament* (Fig. 13.3).

4. The laminae provide attachment to the *ligamenta flava*.

5. The transverse process gives origin by its tip to the *levator scapulae*, the *sclenus medius* anteriorly and the *splenius cervicis* posteriorly. The *intertransverse muscles* are attached to the upper and lower surfaces of the process.

6. The spine gives attachment to the *ligamentum nuchae*; the *semispinalis cervicis*, the *rectus capitis posterior major*, the *inferior oblique*; the *spinalis cervicis*, the *interspinalis and the multifidus* (Chapter 4).

SEVENTH CERVICAL VERTEBRA

It is also known as the *vertebra prominens* because of its long spinous process, the tip of which can be felt through the skin at the lower end of the nuchal furrow.

Its spine is thick, long and nearly horizontal. It is not bifid, but ends in a tubercle (Fig. 1.40).

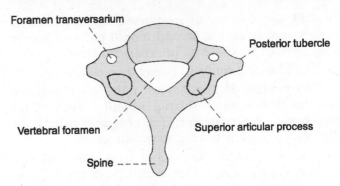

Fig. 1.40: *Seventh cervical vertebra seen from above.*

The transverse processes are comparatively large in size; the posterior root is larger than the anterior. The anterior tubercle is absent. The foramen transversarium is relatively small, sometimes double, or may be entirely absent.

Attachments

1. The tip of the *spine* provides attachment to the *ligamentum* nuchae, the *trapezius*, the *rhomboideus minor*, the *serratus posterior superior*, the *splenius capitis*, the *semispinalis thoracis*, the *spinalis cervicis*, the *interspinales*, and the *multifidus* (Fig. 4.3).

2. *Transverse process.* The *foramen transversarium* usually transmits only an accessory ver tebral vein. The *posterior tubercle* provides attachment to the *suprapleural membrane*. The lower *border* provides attachment to the *levator costarum* (Fig. 4.4).

The anterior root of the transverse process may sometimes be separate. It then forms a *cervical rib* of variable size.

Ossification: Its ossification is similar to that of a typical cervical vertebra. In addition, separate centre for each costal process appears during sixth month of intrauterine life and fuses with the body and transverse process during fifth to sixth years of life.

OSSIFICATION OF CRANIAL BONES

Frontal: It ossifies in membrane. Two primary centres appear during eighth week near frontal eminences. At birth the bone is in two halves, separated by a suture, which soon start to fuse. But remains of metopic suture may be seen in about 9% of adult skulls.

Parietal: It also ossifies in membrane. Two centres appear during seventh week near the parietal eminence and soon fuse with each other.

Occipital: It ossifies partly in membrane and partly in cartilage. The part of the bone above highest nuchal line ossifies in membrane by two centres which appear during second month of foetal life; it may remain separate as interparietal bone.

The following centres appear in cartilage:

Two centres for squamous part below highest nuchal line appear during seventh week. One Kerckring center appears for posterior margin of foramen magnum during sixteenth week.

Two centres one for each lateral parts appear during eighth week. One centre appears for the basilar part during sixth week.

Temporal: Following two parts ossify in membrane:

Squamous part by one center which appears during seventh week. *Tympanic part* from one center which appears during third month. Following two parts ossify in cartilage: *Premastoid part* is ossified by several centres which appear in cartilaginous ear capsule during fifth month. *Styloid process* develops from cranial end of second branchial arch cartilage. Two centres appear in it: Tympanohyal before birth and stylohyal after birth.

Sphenoid: It ossifies in two parts:

A. *Presphenoidal part* which lies in front of tuberculum sellae and lesser wings ossifies from six centers in cartilage: Two for body of sphenoid during ninth week. Two for the two lesser wings during ninth week. Two for the two sphenoidal conchae during fifth month.

B. *Postsphenoidal part* consisting of posterior part of body, greater wings and pterygoid processes ossifies from eight centres:

Two for two greater wings during eighth week forming the root only. Two for postsphenoidal part of body during fourth month. Two centres appear for the two pterygoid hamulus during third month of foetal life. These six centres appear in cartilage. Two centres for medial pterygoid plates appear during ninth week in membrane. The remaining portion of the greater wings and lateral plates ossify in membrane from the centres for the root of greater wing only.

Ethmoid: It ossifies in cartilage. Three centres appear in cartilaginous nasal capsule. One centre appears in perpendicular plate during first year of life.

Two centres one for each labyrinth appear between fourth and fifth months of intrauterine life.

Mandible: Each half of the body is ossified in membrane by one centre which appears during sixth week near the mental foramen. The upper half of ramus ossifies in cartilage. Ossification spreads in condylar and coronoid processes above the level of the mandibular foramen.

Inferior nasal concha: It ossifies in cartilage. One centre appears during fifth month in the lower border of the cartilaginous nasal capsule.

Palatine: One centre appears during eighth week in perpendicular plate. It ossifies in membrane.

Lacrimal: It ossifies in membrane. One centre appears during twelfth week.

Nasal: It also ossifies in membrane from one centre which appears during third month of intrauterine life.

Vomer: It ossifies in membrane. Two centres appear during eighth week on either side of midline. These fuse by twelfth week.

Zygomatic: It ossifies in membrane by one centre which appears during eighth week.

Maxilla: It also ossifies in membrane by three centres. One for main body which appears during sixth week above canine fossa.

Two centres appear for premaxilla during seventh week and fuse soon.

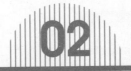

Scalp, Temple and Face

Face is the most prominent part of the body. Facial muscles, being the muscles of facial expression, express a variety of emotions like happiness, joy, sadness, anger, frowning, grinning, etc. The face, therefore, is an *index of mind*. One's innerself is expressed by the face itself as it is controlled by the higher centres.

Facial vein communicates with the cranial venous sinuses. Infection from the face thus can reach the brain. Though the dangerous area of the face is between the nasal openings and the upper lip, the whole of the face is considered dangerous from the infection point of view.

Use of cosmetics should be limited because of their ill-effects and the tendency to cause allergic reactions. Cosmetics try to enhance the external beauty only temporarily. The real beauty of good and helping nature comes from within which no cosmetic can match.

SOME FEATURES THAT CAN BE IDENTIFIED ON THE LIVING FACE

1. The *forehead* is the upper part of the face between the hairline of the scalp and the eyebrows. The superolateral prominence of the forehead is known as the *frontal eminence*.

2. Identify the following in relation to the nose. The prominent ridge separating the right and left halves of the nose is called the *dorsum*. The upper narrow end of the nose just below the forehead, is the root of the nose. The lower end of the dorsum is in the form of a somewhat rounded *tip*. At the lower end of the nose we see the right and left *nostrils* or *anterior nares*. The two nostrils are separated by a soft median partition called the *columella*. This is continuous with the *nasal septum* which separates the two nasal cavities. Each nostril is bounded laterally by the *ala*.

3. The *palpebral fissure* is an elliptical opening between the two eyelids. The lids are joined to each other at the medial and lateral angles or *canthi* of the eye. The free margin of each eyelid has eyelashes or cilia arranged along its outer edge (Fig. 2.1).

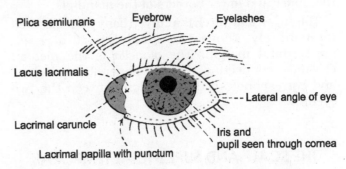

Fig. 2.1: *Some features to be seen on the face around the left eye.*

Through the palpebral fissure are seen: (a) the opaque sclera or white of the eye, (b) the transparent circular *cornea* through which the coloured iris and the dark circular *pupil* can be seen. The eyeballs are lodged in bony sockets, called the *orbits* (Fig. 19.1).

The *conjunctiva* is a moist, transparent membrane. The part which covers the anterior surface of the eyeball is the *bulbar conjunctiva*, and the part lining the posterior surface of the lids is the *palpebral conjunctiva*. The line along which the bulbar conjunctiva becomes the palpebral conjunctiva is known as the *conjunctival fornix*. The space between the two is the *conjunctival* sac (see Fig. 2.28).

4. The *oral fissure* or mouth is the opening between the upper and lower *lips*. It lies opposite the cutting edges of the upper incisor teeth. The angle of the mouth usually lies just in front of the first premolar tooth. Each lip has a *red margin* at mucocutaneous junction and a *black margin*, with a nonhairy thin skin intervening between the two margins. The lips

45

normally close the mouth along their red margins. The *philtrum* is the median vertical groove on the upper lip.

5. The *external ear* is made up of two parts: a superficial projecting part, called the *auricle or pinna*; and a deep canal, called the *external acoustic meatus*. The auricle helps in catching the sound waves, and is a characteristic feature of mammals. Details of the structure of the auricle will be considered later.

Landmarks on the Face

The *supraorbital margin* lies beneath the upper margin of the eyebrow. The supraorbital notch is palpable at the junction of the medial one-third with the lateral two-thirds of the supraorbital margin. A vertical line drawn from the supraorbital notch to the base of the mandible, passing midway between the lower two premolar teeth, crosses the infraorbital foramen five millimetre below the infraorbital margin, and the mental foramen midway between the upper and lower borders of the mandible.

The *superciliary* arch is a curved bony ridge situated immediately above the medial part of each supraorbital margin. The *glabella* is the median elevation connecting the two superciliary arches, and corresponds to the elevation between the two eyebrows.

THE SCALP AND SUPERFICIAL TEMPORAL REGION

The soft tissues covering the cranial vault form the scalp.

Extent of Scalp

Anteriorly, supraorbital margins; posteriorly, external occipital protuberance and superior nuchal lines; and on each side, the superior temporal lines.

Structure

Conventionally, the superficial temporal region is studied with the scalp, and the following description, therefore, will cover both the regions.

The scalp is made up of five layers: (1) Skin, (2) superficial fascia, (3) deep fascia in the form of the epicranial aponeurosis or galea aponeurotica with the occipitofrontalis muscle, (4) loose areolar tissues, and (5) pericranium (Fig. 2.3).

The *skin* is thick and hairy. It is adherent to the epicranial aponeurosis through the dense superficial fascia, as in the palms and soles.

Place 2–3 wooden blocks under the head to raise it about 10–12 cm from the table. Give a median incision in the skin of scalp extending from root of the nose to the prominent external occipital protuberance (Fig. 2.2 line with dashes). Give a coronal incision across the previous incision from root of one auricle to the other. Extend the incision from the auricles to the mastoid process posteriorly and to root of zygoma anteriorly. Reflect the skin in four flaps. Usually the skin is so adherent to the subjacent connective tissue and aponeurotic layers that these all come off together. Dissect the layers, including the nerves, vessels, lymphatics and identify these structures in the cadaver.

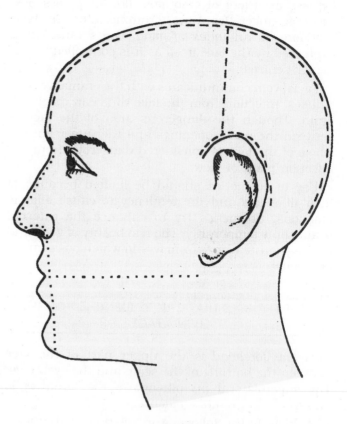

Fig. 2.2: Lines of dissection.

The *superficial fascia* is more fibrous and dense in the centre than at the periphery of the head. It binds the skin to the subjacent aponeurosis, and provides the proper medium for passage of vessels and nerves to the skin.

The *occipitofrontalis muscle* has two bellies, occipital or occipitalis and frontal or frontalis, both of which are inserted into the epicranial aponeurosis. The *occipital bellies* are small and separate. Each

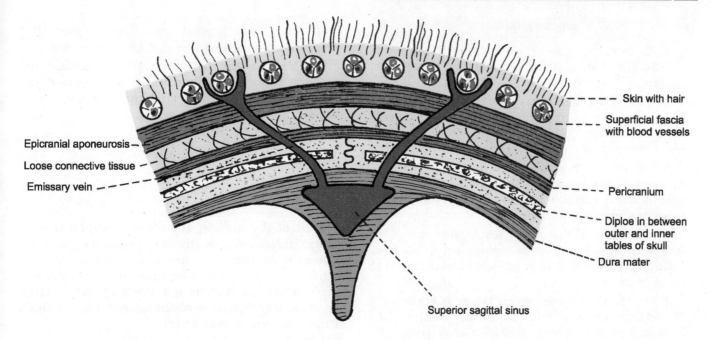

Skin with hair

Superficial fascia with blood vessels

Epicranial aponeurosis

Loose connective tissue

Emissary vein

Pericranium

Diploe in between outer and inner tables of skull

Dura mater

Superior sagittal sinus

Fig. 2.3: Layers of the scalp.

arises from the lateral two-thirds of the superior nuchal line, and is supplied by the *posterior auricular* branch of the *facial nerve*. The *frontal bellies* are longer, wider and partly united in the median plane. Each arises from the skin of the forehead, mingling with the orbicularis oculi and the corrugator supercilli. It is supplied by the *temporal branch* of the facial nerve. The muscle raises the eyebrows and causes horizontal wrinkles in the skin of the forehead (Figs 2.3, 2.4).

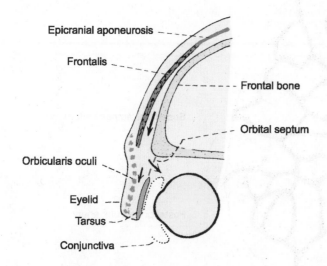

Epicranial aponeurosis

Frontalis

Frontal bone

Orbital septum

Orbicularis oculi

Eyelid

Tarsus

Conjunctiva

Fig. 2.4: Schematic section through the scalp and upper eyelid to show how fluids can pass from the subaponeurotic space of the scalp into the eyelid, and into the subconjunctival area. Note that this is possible because the frontalis muscle has no bony attachment.

The *epicranial aponeurosis*, or galea aponeurotica is freely movable on the pericranium along with the overlying and adherent skin and fascia. Anteriorly, it receives the insertion of the frontalis, posteriorly, it receives the insertion of the occipitalis and is attached to the external occipital protuberance, and to the highest nuchal lines in between the occipital bellies. On each side the aponeurosis is attached to the superior temporal line, but sends down a thin expansion which passes over the temporal fascia and is attached to the zygomatic arch (Fig. 1.4).

The fourth layer of the scalp, is made up of *loose areolar tissue*. It extends anteriorly into the eyelids (Fig 2.4) because the frontalis muscle has no bony attachment; posteriorly to the highest and superior nuchal lines; and on each side to the superior temporal lines.

The fifth layer of the scalp, called the *pericranium*, is loosely attached to the surface of the bones, but is firmly adherent to their sutures where the sutural ligaments bind the pericranium to the endocranium.

Superficial temporal region: It is the area between the superior temporal line and the zygomatic arch. This area contains the following seven layers: 1. Skin, 2. superficial fascia, 3. thin extension of epicranial aponeurosis which gives origin to extrinsic muscles of the auricle, 4. temporal fascia, 5. temporalis muscle, 6. loose areolar tissue and 7. pericranium.

CLINICAL ANATOMY

1. Because of the abundance of sebaceous glands, the scalp is a common site for *sebaceous cysts*.

2. Since the blood supply of scalp and superficial temporal region is very rich; *avulsed portions need not be cut away*. They can be replaced in position and stitched: they usually take up and heal well.

3. *Wounds of the scalp bleed profusely* because the vessels are prevented from retracting by the fibrous fascia. Bleeding can be arrested by applying pressure against the bone.

4. Because of the density of fascia, *subcutaneous haemorrhages are never extensive*, and the *inflammations in this layer cause little swelling but much pain.*

5. The layer of loose areolar tissue is known as the *dangerous area* of the scalp because the emissary veins, which open here may transmit infection from the scalp to the cranial venous sinuses.

6. Collection of blood in the layer of loose connective tissue causes generalised swelling of the scalp. The blood may extend anteriorly into the root of the nose and into the *eyelids*, causing *black eye*. (Fig. 2.4)

7. Wounds of the scalp do not gape unless the epicranial aponeurosis is divided transversely.

8. Because the pericranium is adherent to sutures, collections of fluid deep to the pericranium known as *cephalhaematoma* take the shape of the bone concerned.

Arterial Supply of Scalp and Superficial Temporal Region

In front of the auricle, the scalp is supplied from before backwards by the (1) *Supratrochlear*; (2) *supraorbital*; and (3) *superficial temporal* arteries (Fig. 2.5). The first two are branches of the ophthalmic artery which in turn is a branch of the internal carotid artery. The superficial temporal is a branch of the external carotid artery.

Behind the auricle, the scalp is supplied from before backwards by the (4) *posterior auricular*; and (5) *occipital* arteries, both of which are branches of the external carotid artery.

Thus, the scalp has a *rich blood supply* derived from both the internal and the external carotid arteries, the two systems anastomosing over the temple.

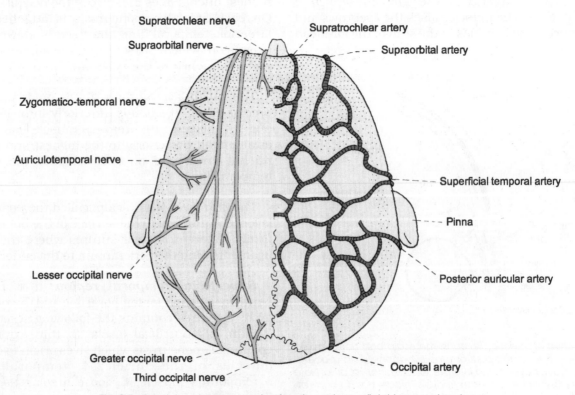

Fig. 2.5: Arterial and nerve supply of scalp and superficial temporal region.

Venous Drainage

The veins of the scalp accompany the arteries and have similar names. The *supratrochlear* and *supraorbital* veins unite at the medial angle of the eye forming the *angular* vein which continues down as the *facial* vein.

The *superficial temporal vein* descends in front of the tragus, enters the parotid gland, and joins the maxillary vein to form the *retromandibular* vein. The anterior division of the retromandibular vein unites with the facial vein to form the common facial vein which drains into the internal jugular vein. The posterior division of the retromandibular vein unites with the *posterior auricular vein* to form the *external jugular vein* which ultimately drains into the subclavian vein. The occipital veins terminate in the suboccipital venous plexus (see Fig. 2.22).

Emissary veins connect the extracranial veins with the intracranial venous sinuses to equalise the pressure. The *parietal emissary vein* passes through the parietal foramen to the superior sagittal sinus. The *mastoid emissary vein* passes through the mastoid foramen to the sigmoid sinus. Remaining emissary veins are put in Table 1.1. Extracranial infections may spread through these veins to intracranial venous sinuses.

The *frontal diploic vein* emerges at the supraorbital notch opens into the supraorbital vein. *Anterior temporal diploic vein* ends in anterior deep temporal vein or sphenoparietal sinus. *Posterior temporal diploic vein* ends in the transverse sinus. The *occipital diploic vein* opens either into the occipital vein, or into the transverse sinus near the median plane (Table 1.2).

Lymphatic Drainage

The anterior part of the scalp drains into the preauricular or parotid lymph nodes, situated on the surface of the parotid gland. The posterior part of the scalp drains into the posterior auricular or mastoid and occipital lymph nodes (see Fig. 2.25).

Nerve Supply

The scalp and temple are supplied by ten nerves on each side. Out of these five nerves (four sensory and one motor) enter the scalp in front of the auricle. The remaining five nerves (again four sensory and one motor) enter the scalp behind the auricle (Fig. 2.5 and Table 2.1).

Table 2.1: Nerves of the scalp and superficial temporal regions

In front of auricle	Behind the auricle
Sensory nerves	*Sensory nerves*
1. Supratrochlear, branch of the frontal (ophthalmic division of trigeminal nerve)	1. Posterior division of great auricular nerve (C2, C3) from cervical plexus
2. Supraorbital, branch of frontal (ophthalmic division of trigeminal nerve)	2. Lesser occipital nerve (C2), from cervical plexus
3. Zygomaticotemporal, branch of zygomatic nerve (maxillary division of trigeminal nerve)	3. Greater occipital nerve (C2, dorsal ramus)
4. Auriculotemporal branch of mandibular division of trigeminal nerve	4. Third occipital nerve (C3, dorsal ramus)
Motor nerve	*Motor nerve*
1. Temporal branch of facial nerve	1. Posterior auricular branch of facial nerve

THE FACE

The face, or countenance, extends superiorly from the adolescent position of hairline, inferiorly to the chin and the base of the mandible, and on each side to the auricle. The forehead is, therefore, common to both the face and the scalp.

Skin

1. The facial skin is *very vascular*. Rich vascularity makes the face blush and blanch. Wounds of the face bleed profusely but heal rapidly. The results of plastic surgery on the face are excellent for the same reason.

2. The facial skin is *rich in sebaceous and sweat glands*. Sebaceous glands keep the face oily, but also cause acne in young adults. Sweat glands help in regulation of the body temperature.

3. *Laxity* of the greater part of the skin facilitates rapid spread of oedema. Renal oedema appears first in the eyelids and face before spreading to other parts of the body.

4. Boils in the nose and ear are acutely painful due to the *fixity* of the skin to the underlying cartilages.

5. Facial skin is very *elastic and thick* because the facial muscles are inserted into it. The wounds of the face, therefore, tend to gape.

Give a median incision from the root of nose, across the dorsum of nose, centre of philtrum of upper lip, to centre of lower lip to the chin. Give a horizontal incision from the angle of the mouth to posterior border of the mandible (Fig. 2.2) line with dots). Reflect the lower flap towards and up to the lower border of mandible. Direct and reflect the upper flap till the auricle. Subjacent to the skin the facial muscles are directly encountered as these are inserted in the skin. Identify the various functional groups of facial muscles.

Trace the various motor branches of facial nerve emerging from the anterior border of parotid gland to supply these muscles. Amongst these motor branches on the face are the sensory branches of the three divisions of the trigeminal nerve. Try to identify all these with the help of their course given in the text (Figs 2.19, 9.5C).

Superficial Fascia

It contains: (1) The facial muscles, all of which are inserted into the skin, (2) the vessels and nerves, on their way to the muscles and to the skin, and (3) a variable amount of fat. Fat is absent from the eyelids, but is well developed in the cheeks, forming the buccal pads that are very prominent in infants in whom they help in sucking.

The *deep fascia is absent* from the face, except over the parotid gland where it forms the parotid fascia, and over the buccinator where it forms the *buccopharyngeal fascia*.

Facial Muscles

The facial muscles, or the muscles of facial expression, are subcutaneous muscles. They bring about different facial expressions.

Embryologically, they develop from the mesoderm of the second branchial arch, and are, therefore, supplied by the facial nerve.

Morphologically, they represent the best remnants of the *panniculus carnosus*, a continuous subcutaneous muscle sheet seen in some animals. All of them are inserted into the skin.

Topographically, the muscles are grouped under the following six heads.

Muscle of the Scalp
1. Occipitofrontalis

Muscles of the Auricle
Situated around the ear

1. Auricularis anterior
2. Auricularis superior
3. Auricularis posterior

Muscles of the Eyelids
1. Orbicularis oculi (Fig. 2.6)
2. Corrugator supercilii (Fig. 2.6)
3. Levator palpebrae superioris (an extraocular muscle, supplied by the third cranial nerve)

Muscles of the Nose
1. Procerus
2. Compressor naris (Fig. 2.6).
3. Dilator naris
4. Depressor septi

Muscles Around the Mouth
1. Orbicularis oris (Fig. 2.6)
2. Levator labii superioris alaequae nasi
3. Zygomaticus major (Fig. 2.7)
4. Levator labii superioris (Fig. 2.8)
5. Levator anguli oris (Fig. 2.7)
6. Zygomaticus minor
7. Depressor anguli oris
8. Depressor labii inferioris
9. Mentalis
10. Risorius
11. Buccinator

Muscles of the Neck
1. Platysma (Fig. 2.7)

Functionally, most of these muscles may be regarded primarily as regulators of the three openings situated on the face, namely the palpebral fissures, the nostrils and the oral fissure. Each opening has a single sphincter, and a variable number of dilators. Sphincters are naturally circular and the dilators radial in their arrangement. These muscles are better developed around the eyes and mouth than around the nose (Table 2.2).

The occipitofrontalis muscle has been described with scalp. Details of the other muscles are given in Table 2.3.

A few of the *common facial expressions* and the muscles producing them are given below.

1. *Smiling and laughing:* Zygomaticus major (Fig. 2.9)

2. *Sadness:* Levator labii superioris and levator anguli oris. (Figs 2.10, 2.11)

3. *Grief:* Depressor anguli oris.

4. *Anger:* Dilator naris and depressor septi.

5. *Frowning:* Corrugator supercilii and procerus. (Figs 2.12, 2.13)

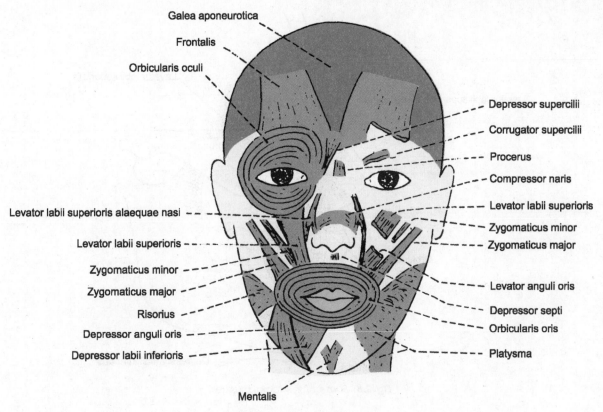

Fig. 2.6: *The facial muscles.*

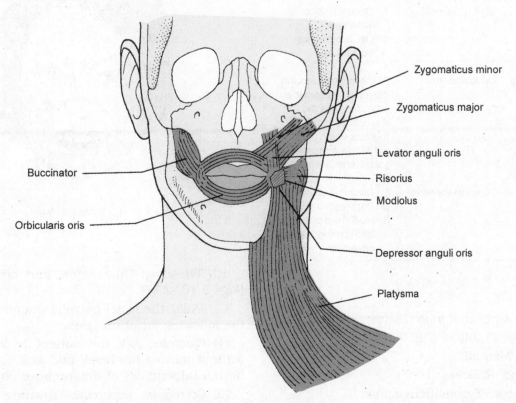

Fig. 2.7: *Some of the facial muscles.*

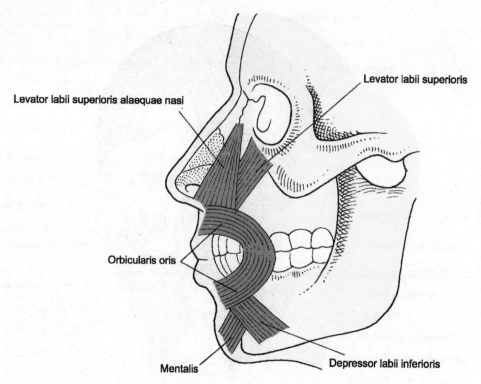

Levator labii superioris alaequae nasi

Levator labii superioris

Orbicularis oris

Mentalis

Depressor labii inferioris

Fig. 2.8: Some of the facial muscles.

Table 2.2: Functional groups of facial muscles

Opening	Sphincter	Dilators
A. Palpebral fissure	Orbicularis oculi	1. Levator palpebrae superioris 2. Occipitofrontalis-frontalis part
B. Oral fissure	Orbicularis oris	All the muscles around the mouth, except the orbicularis oris the sphincter, and the mentalis which does not mingle with orbicularis oris (see above)
C. Nostrils	Compressor naris	1. Dilator naris 2. Depressor septi 3. Medial slip of levator labii superioris alaequae nasi

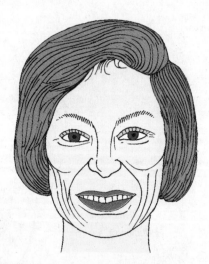

Fig. 2.9: Zygomaticus major—smile.

6. *Horror, terror and fright:* Platysma (Fig. 2.14)
7. *Surprise:* Frontalis (Fig. 2.15)
8. *Doubt:* Mentalis
9. *Grinning:* Risorius
10. *Contempt:* Zygomaticus minor.
11. *Closing the mouth:* Orbicularis oris (Fig. 2.16)

12. *Whistling:* Buccinator, and orbicularis oris (Figs 2.16, 2.17).

Clinically, the facial nerve is examined by testing the following facial muscles.

(1) *Frontalis:* Ask the patient to look upwards without moving his head, and look for the normal horizontal wrinkles of the forehead (Fig. 2.15).

(2) *Corrugator supercilii:* Frowning and making vertical wrinkles of the forehead (Fig. 2.12).

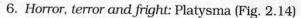

Table 2.3: The facial muscles

Muscle	Origin	Insertion	Action
1. Corrugator supercilii (Fig. 2.12)	Medial end of superciliary arch	Skin of mid-eyebrow	Vertical lines in forehead: frowning
2. Orbicularis oculi (Fig. 2.6) a. Orbital part, on and around the orbital margin	Medial part of medial palpebral ligament and adjoining bone	Concentric rings return to the point of origin	Closes lids tightly; wrinkling; Protects eye from bright light
b. Palpebral part, in the lids	Lateral part of medial palpebral ligament	Lateral palpebral raphe	Closes lids gently; blinking
c. Lacrimal part, lateral and deep to the lacrimal sac	Lacrimal fascia and lacrimal bone	Upper and lower eyelids	Dilates lacrimal sac; directs lacrimal puncta into lacus lacrimalis; supports the lower lid
3. Orbicularis oris a. Intrinsic part, deepest stratum, very thin sheet	Superior incisivus, from maxilla; Inferior incisivus, from mandible	Angle of mouth	Closes and purses the mouth; numerous extrinsic muscles make it most versatile for various types of grimaces
b. Extrinsic part, two strata, formed by converging muscles (Fig. 2.16)	Thickest middle stratum, derived from buccinator; thick superficial stratum, derived from elevators and depressors of lips and their angles	Lips and the angle of the mouth	
4. Buccinator, the muscle of the cheek (Fig. 2.17, 1.7)	1. Upper fibres, from maxilla opposite molar teeth	1. Upper fibres, straight to the upper lip	Flattens cheek against gums and teeth; prevents accumulation of food in the vestibule. This is a whistling muscle
	2. Lower fibres, from mandible, opposite molar teeth	2. Lower fibres, straight to the lower lip	
	3. Middle fibres, from pterygomandibular raphe	3. Middle fibres decussate before passing to the lips	
5. Platysma (Fig. 2.6, 2.14)	Upper parts of pectoral and deltoid fasciae Fibres run upwards and medially	Anterior fibres, to the base of the mandible; posterior fibres to the skin of the lower face and lip, and may be continuous with the risorius	Releases pressure of skin on the subjacent veins; depresses mandible; pulls the angle of the mouth downwards as in horror or surprise

(3) *Orbicularis oculi:* Tight closure of the eyes (Fig. 2.6).

(4) *Orbicularis oris:* Whistling and pursing the mouth. (Fig. 2.16)

(5) *Dilators of mouth:* Showing the teeth.

(6) *Buccinator:* Puffing the mouth and then blowing forcibly as in whistling (Fig. 2.17).

(7) *Platysma:* Forcible pulling of the angles of the mouth downwards and backwards forming prominent vertical folds of skin on the side of the neck. The platysma contracts along with the risorius (Fig. 2.14).

Motor Nerve Supply of the Face

The *facial nerve* is the motor nerve of the face. Its five terminal branches, temporal, zygomatic, buccal, marginal mandibular and cervical emerge from the parotid gland and diverge to supply the various facial muscles as follows.

Temporal—frontalis, auricular muscles, orbicularis oculi (Fig. 2.6).

Zygomatic—orbicularis oculi (Fig. 9.5 C).

Buccal—muscles of the cheek and upper lip (Figs 2.7, 2.8).

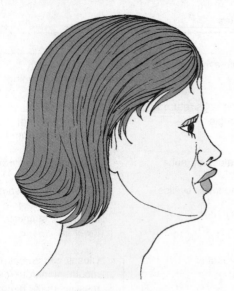

Fig. 2.10: Levator labii superioris — Sadness.

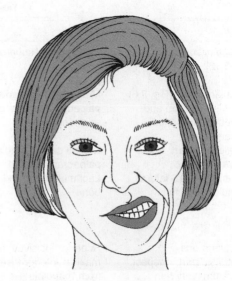

Fig. 2.11: Levator anguli oris—Sadness.

Marginal mandibular—muscles of lower lip. Cervical—platysma.

This can be understood by putting your right wrist on the right ear and spreading five digits; the thumb over the temporal region, the index finger on the zygomatic bone, middle finger on the upper lip, the ring finger on the lower lip and the little finger over the neck.

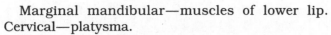

CLINICAL ANATOMY

In *infranuclear lesions* (Fig. 2.18) of the facial nerve, known as Bell's palsy, the whole of the face of the same side gets paralysed. The face becomes asymmetrical and is drawn up to the normal side. The affected side is motionless. Wrinkles disappear from the forehead. The eye cannot be closed. Any attempt to smile draws the mouth to the normal side. During mastication, food accumulates between the teeth and the cheek. Articulation of labials is impaired.

In *supranuclear lesions* of the facial nerve; usually a part of hemiplegia, only the lower part of the opposite side of face is paralysed. The upper part with the frontalis and orbicularis oculi escapes due to its bilateral representation in the cerebral cortex.

Sensory Nerve Supply of the Face

The *trigeminal nerve* through its three branches is the chief sensory nerve of the face (Fig. 2.19; Table

2.4). The skin over the angle of the jaw and over the parotid gland is supplied by the great auricular nerve (C2, C3).

In addition to most of the skin of the face, the sensory distribution of the trigeminal nerve is also to the nasal cavity, the paranasal air sinuses, the eyeball, the mouth cavity, palate, cheeks, gums, teeth and anterior two-thirds of tongue and the supratentorial part of the dura mater, including that lining the anterior and middle cranial fossae (Fig. 2.20; Table 2.4).

CLINICAL ANATOMY

1. The sensory distribution of the trigeminal nerve explains why *headache* is a uniformly common symptom in involvements of the nose (common cold, boils), the paranasal air sinuses (sinusitis), infections and inflammations of teeth and gums, refractive errors of the eyes, glaucoma and infection of the meninges as in meningitis.

2. *Trigeminal neuralgia* may involve one or more of the three divisions of the trigeminal nerve. It causes attacks of very severe burning and scalding pain along the distribution of the affected nerve. Pain is relieved either (a) by *injecting* 90% alcohol into the affected division of the trigeminal ganglion, or (b) by *sectioning* the affected nerve, the main sensory root, or the spinal tract of the trigeminal nerve which is situated superficially in the medulla. The procedure is called medullary tractotomy.

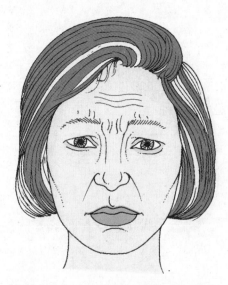

Fig. 2.12: Corrugator supercilii — Frowning.

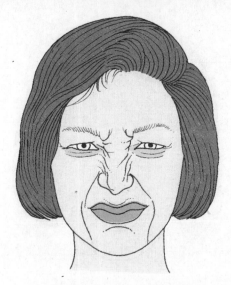

Fig. 2.13: Procerus—Frowning.

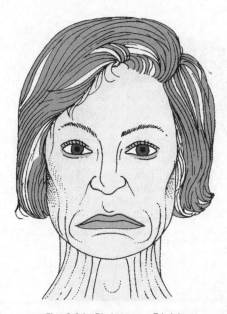

Fig. 2.14: Platysma—Fright.

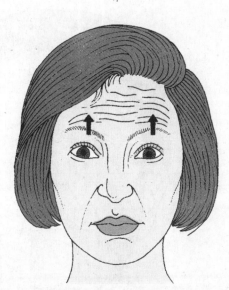

Fig. 2.15: Frontalis—Surprize.

Arteries of the Face

The face is richly vascular. It is supplied by: (1) The facial artery, (2) the transverse facial artery, and (3) arteries that accompany the cutaneous nerves.

DISSECTION

Tortuous facial artery enters the face at the lower border of mandible. Dissect its course from the anteroinferior angle of masseter muscle running to the angle of mouth till the medial angle of eye,

reflecting off some of the facial muscles if necessary. Straight facial vein runs on a posterior plane than the artery. Identify buccopharyngeal fascia on the external surface of buccinator muscle. Clean the deeply placed buccinator muscle situated lateral to the angle of mouth. Identify parotid duct, running across the cheek two centimetre below the zygomatic arch. The duct pierces buccopharyngeal fascia, buccinator muscle, mucous membrane of the mouth to open into its vestibule opposite second upper molar tooth (see Fig. 2.26).

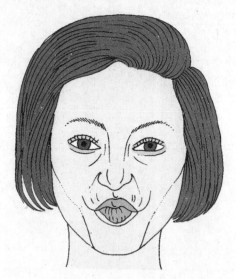

Fig. 2.16: *Orbicularis oris—Pursing the mouth.*

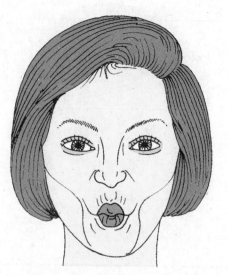

Fig. 2.17: *Buccinator—Whistling.*

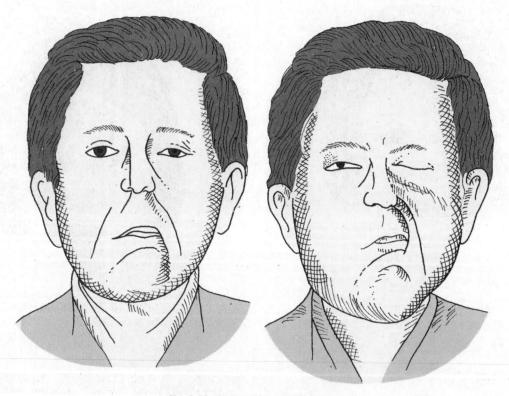

Fig. 2.18: *Bell's palsy on right side.*

Facial Artery (Facial Part)

The facial artery is the chief artery of the face (Fig. 2.21). It is a branch of the external carotid artery given off in the carotid triangle just above the level of the tip of the greater cornua of the hyoid bone. In its cervical course, it passes through the submandibular region, and finally enters the face.

Surface Marking

It is marked on the face by joining the following three points (Fig. 1.9).

(a) A point on the base of the mandible at the anterior border of the masseter muscle.

(b) A second point 1.2 cm lateral to the angle of the mouth.

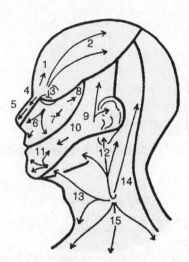

Fig. 2.19: *The sensory nerves of the face. 1. Supratrochlear; 2. Supraorbital; 3 . Palpebral branch of lacrimal; 4. Infratrochlear; 5. External nasal; 6. Infraorbital; 7. Zygomaticofacial; 8. Zygomaticotemporal; 9. Auriculotemporal; 10. Buccal; 11. Mental; 12. Great auricular; 13. Transverse cutaneous nerve of neck; 14. Lesser occipital; 15. Supraclavicular.*

(c) A point at the medial angle of the eye.

The artery is tortuous in its course and is more so between the first two points.

Course

1. It enters the face by winding around the base of the mandible, and by piercing the deep cervical fascia, at the anteroinferior angle of the masseter muscle. It can be palpated here and is called 'anaesthetist's artery'.

2. First it runs upwards and forv
1.25 cm lateral to the angle of the
ascends by the side of the nose up to
of the eye, where it terminates b
lacrimal sac; and by anastomosing
nasal branch of the ophthalmic ar

3. The facial artery is very tortuous. The tortuosity of the artery prevents its walls from being unduly stretched during movements of the mandible, the lips and the cheeks.

4. It lies between the superficial and deep muscles of the face.

The course of the artery in the neck is described in submandibular region.

Branches

The anterior branches on the face are large and named. They are: (1) *Inferior labial*, to the lower lip, (2) *superior labial*, to the upper lip and the anteroinferior part of the nasal septum, and (3) *lateral nasal*, to the ala and dorsum of the nose.

The posterior branches are *small* and unnamed.

Anastomosis

1. The large anterior branches anastomose with similar branches of the opposite side and with the mental artery. In the lips, anastomoses are large, so that cut arteries spurt from both ends.

2. Small posterior branches anastomose with the transverse facial and infraorbital arteries.

	Source		Cutaneous nerve	Area of distribution
A.	Ophthalmic division of trigeminal nerve	1. 2. 3. 4. 5.	Supratrochlear nerve Supraorbital nerve Lacrimal nerve Infratrochlear nerve External nasal nerve	Scalp up to vertex, forehead; upper eyelid; conjunctiva, small part of lower eyelid; and root, dorsum and tip of nose
B.	Maxillary division of trigeminal nerve	1. 2. 3.	Infraorbital nerve Zygomaticofacial nerve Zygomaticotemporal nerve	Upper lip; side and ala of nose; most of the lower eyelid; upper part of cheek; and anterior part of temple
C.	Mandibular division of trigeminal nerve	1. 2. 3.	Auriculotemporal nerve . Buccal nerve Mental nerve	Lower lip; chin; lower part of cheek; lower jaw except over the angle; upper 2/3 of lateral surface of auricle; and side of head
D.	Cervical plexus	1. 2.	Anterior division of great auricular nerve (C2, C3) Upper division of transverse (anterior) cutaneous nerve of neck (C 2, C3)	Skin over the angle of the jaw and over the parotid gland. Lower margin of the lower jaw

Table 2.4: Cutaneous nerves of the face

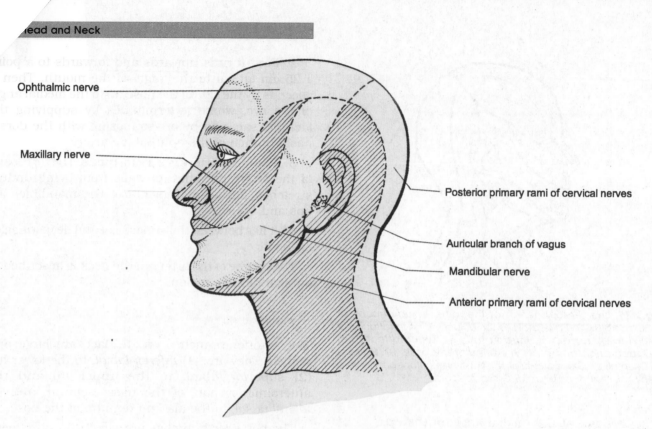

Ophthalmic nerve

Maxillary nerve

Posterior primary rami of cervical nerves

Auricular branch of vagus

Mandibular nerve

Anterior primary rami of cervical nerves

Fig. 2.20: *Distribution of the cutaneous nerves in the head and neck.*

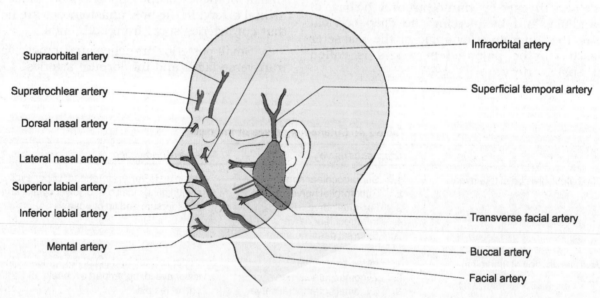

Supraorbital artery

Supratrochlear artery

Dorsal nasal artery

Lateral nasal artery

Superior labial artery

Inferior labial artery

Mental artery

Infraorbital artery

Superficial temporal artery

Transverse facial artery

Buccal artery

Facial artery

Fig. 2.21: *Arteries of the face.*

3. At the medial angle of the eye, terminal branches of the facial artery anastomose with branches of the ophthalmic artery. This is, therefore, a site for anastomosis between the branches of the external and internal carotid arteries.

Transverse Facial Artery

This small artery is a branch of the superficial temporal artery. After emerging from the parotid gland, it runs forwards over the masseter between the parotid duct and the zygomatic arch, accompanied by the upper buccal branch of the facial nerve. It supplies the parotid gland and its duct, masseter and the overlying skin, and ends by anastomosing with neighbouring arteries (Fig. 2.21).

Veins of the Face

1. The veins of the face accompany the arteries and drain into the common facial and retro-mandibular veins. They communicate with the cavernous sinus.

2. The veins on each side form a 'W-shaped' arrangement. Each corner of the 'W' is prolonged upwards into the scalp and downwards into the neck (Figs 2.22, 2.23).

3. The *facial vein* is the largest vein of the face with no valves. It begins as the angular vein at the medial angle of the eye. It is formed by the union of the supratrochlear and supraorbital veins. The angular vein continues as the facial vein, running downwards and backwards behind the facial artery, but with a straighter course. It crosses the anteroinferior angle of the masseter, pierces the deep fascia, crosses the submandibular gland, and joins the anterior division of the retromandibular vein below the angle of the mandible to form the common facial vein. The latter drains into the internal jugular vein. It is represented by a line drawn just behind the facial artery.

The other veins are described with the scalp.

4. *Deep connections* of the facial vein include: (a) A communication between the supraorbital and superior ophthalmic veins, and (b) another with the pterygoid plexus through the *deep facial* vein which passes backwards over the buccinator. The facial vein communicates with the cavernous sinus through these connections. Infections from the face can spread in a retrograde direction and cause *thrombosis* of the cavernous sinus. This is specially likely to occur in the presence of infection in the upper lip and in the lower part of the nose. This area is, therefore, called the *dangerous area of the face* (Fig. 2.24).

Lymphatic Drainage of the Face

The face has three lymphatic territories: (a) The *upper territory*, including the greater part of the forehead, the lateral halves of the eyelids, the conjunctiva, the lateral part of the cheek and the parotid area, drains into the *preauricular parotid nodes*. (b) The *middle territory*, including a strip over the median part of the forehead, the external nose, the upper lip, the lateral part of the lower lip, the medial halves of the eyelids, the medial part of the cheek, and the greater part of the lower jaw, drains into the *submandibular nodes*. (c) The *lower territory*, including the central part of the lower lip and the chin, drains into the *submental nodes* (Fig. 2.25).

Labial, Buccal and Molar Mucous Glands

The labial and buccal mucous glands are numerous. They lie in the submucosa of the lips and cheeks. The molar mucous glands, four or five, lie on the buccopharyngeal fascia around the parotid duct. All these glands open into the vestibule of the mouth (Fig. 2.26).

EYELIDS OR PALPEBRAE

The upper and lower eyelids are movable curtains which protect the eyes from foreign bodies and bright

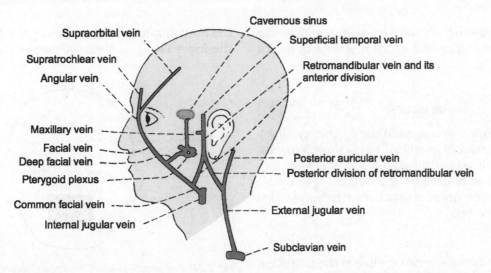

Fig. 2.22: *The veins of the face and their deep connections with the cavernous sinus and the pterygoid plexus of veins.*

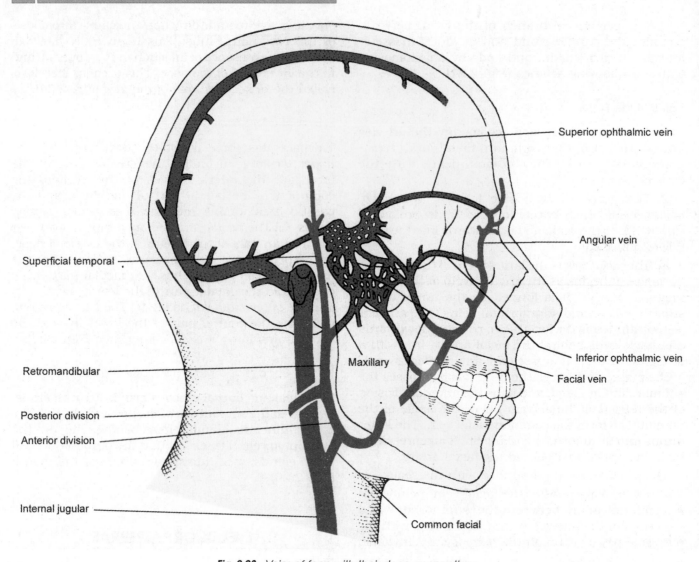

Superior ophthalmic vein

Angular vein

Superficial temporal

Maxillary

Inferior ophthalmic vein

Facial vein

Retromandibular

Posterior division

Anterior division

Internal jugular

Common facial

Fig. 2.23: Veins of face with their deep connections.

light. They keep the cornea clean and moist. The upper eyelid is larger and more movable than the lower eyelid (Fig. 2.27A).

the medial and lateral angles or *canthi* of the eye. At the inner canthus there is a small triangular space,

DISSECTION

Give a circular incision around the roots of eyelids. This will separate the orbital part of orbicularis oculi from the palpebral parts. Carefully reflect the palpebral part towards the palpebral fissure. Identify the structures present beneath the muscle as given in the text.

The space between the two eyelids is the palpebral fissure. The two lids are fused with each other to form

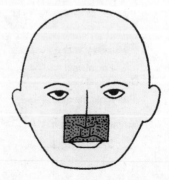

Fig. 2.24: Dangerous area of the face (stippled). Spread of infection from this area can cause thrombosis of the cavernous sinus.

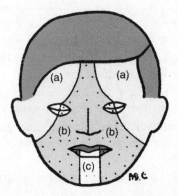

Fig. 2.25: *The lymphatic territories of the face. Area (a) drains into the preauricular nodes; area (b) drains into the submandibular nodes; and area (c) drains into the submental nodes.*

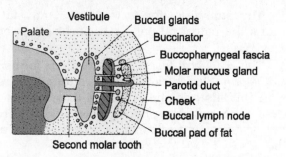

Fig. 2.26: *Scheme of coronal section showing structures in the cheek. The parotid duct pierces buccal pad of fat, buccopharyngeal fascia, buccinator muscle and the mucous membrane to open into the vestibule of mouth opposite the crown of the upper second molar tooth.*

the *lacus lacrimalis*. Within it there is an elevated *lacrimal caruncle*, made up of modified skin and skin glands. Lateral to the caruncle, the bulbar conjunctiva is pinched up to form a vertical fold called the *plica semilunaris* (Fig. 2.1).

Each eyelid is attached to the margins of the orbital opening. Its free edge is broad and has a rounded outer lip and a sharp inner lip. The outer lip presents two or more rows of eyelashes or cilia, except in the boundary of the lacus lacrimalis. At the

point where eyelashes cease, there is a *lacrimal papilla* on the summit of which there is the *lacrimal punctum*. Near the inner lip of the free edge there is a row of openings of the tarsal glands. (Fig. 2.1)

Structure

Each lid is made up of the following layers from without inwards:

1. The *skin* is thin, loose and easily distensible by oedema fluid or blood.

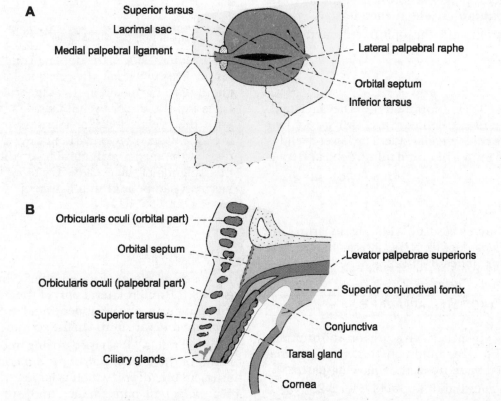

Fig. 2.27: *(A) Orbital septum. (B) Sagittal section of the upper eyelid.*

2. The *superficial fascia* is without any fat. It contains the palpebral part of the orbicularis oculi (Fig. 2.27B).

3. The *palpebral fascia* of the two lids forms the *orbital septum*. Its thickenings form *tarsal plates* or *tarsi* in the lids and the *palpebral ligaments* at the angles. Tarsi are thin plates of condensed fibrous tissue located near the lid margins. They give stiffness to the lids.

The upper tarsus receives two tendinous slips from the *levator palpebrae superioris*. *Tarsal glands* or Meibomian glands are embedded in the posterior surface of the tarsi; their ducts open in a row behind the cilia.

4. The *conjunctiva* lines the posterior surface of the tarsus.

Apart from the usual glands of the skin, and mucous glands in the conjunctiva, the larger glands found in the lids are: (a) Large sebaceous glands also called as *Zeis's glands* at the lid margin associated with cilia; (b) modified sweat glands or *Moll's glands* at the lid margin closely associated with Zeis's glands and cilia, and (c) sebaceous or *tarsal glands*, these are also known as *Meibomian glands*.

Blood Supply

The eyelids are supplied by: (1) The superior and inferior palpebral branches of the ophthalmic artery, and (2) the lateral palpebral branch of the lacrimal artery. They form an arcade in each lid.

The veins drain into the ophthalmic and facial veins.

Nerve Supply

The upper eyelid is supplied by the lacrimal, supraorbital, supratrochlear and infratrochlear nerves from lateral to medial side. The lower eyelid is supplied by the infraorbital and infratrochlear nerves (Fig. 2.19).

Lymphatic Drainage

The medial halves of the lids drain into the submandibular nodes, and the lateral halves into the preauricular nodes (Fig. 2.25).

LACRIMAL APPARATUS

The structures concerned with secretion and drainage of the lacrimal or tear fluid constitute the lacrimal apparatus. It is made up of the following parts:

1. Lacrimal gland and its ducts (Fig. 2.28).
2. Conjunctival sac.

3. Lacrimal puncta and lacrimal canaliculi.
4. Lacrimal sac.
5. Nasolacrimal duct.

Lacrimal Gland

It is a *serous gland* situated chiefly in the lacrimal fossa on the anterolateral part of the roof of the bony orbit and partly on the upper eyelid. Small *accessory lacrimal glands* are found in the conjunctival fornices.

The gland is 'J' shaped, being indented by the tendon of the *levator palpebrae superioris* muscle. It has (a) an *orbital part* which is larger and deeper, and (b) a *palpebral part* smaller and superficial, lying within the eyelid (Fig. 2.28).

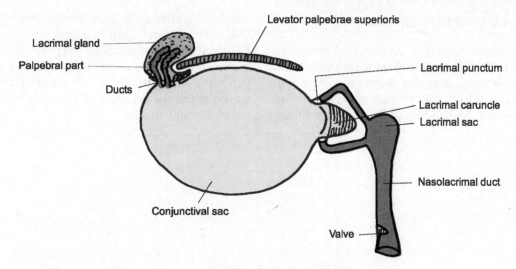

Levator palpebrae superioris

Lacrimal gland

Palpebral part

Ducts

Lacrimal punctum

Lacrimal caruncle

Lacrimal sac

Nasolacrimal duct

Conjunctival sac

Valve

Fig. 2.28: Lacrimal apparatus.

About a dozen of its *ducts* pierce the conjunctiva of the upper lid and open into the conjunctival sac near the superior fornix. Most of the ducts of the orbital part pass through the palpebral part. Removal of the latter is functionally equivalent to removal of the entire gland. After removal, the conjunctiva and cornea are moistened by accessory lacrimal glands.

The gland is supplied by the lacrimal branch of the ophthalmic artery and by the *lacrimal nerve*. The nerve has both sensory and secretomotor fibres.

The secretomotor fibres run as follows: Lacrimatory nucleus—nervus intermedius— geniculate ganglion—greater petrosal nerve—nerve of pterygoid canal—pterygopalatine ganglion—relay—zygomatic nerve—zygomaticotemporal—lacrimal nerve—lacrimal gland (Table 1.3).

The lacrimal fluid secreted by the lacrimal gland flows into the conjunctival sac where it lubricates the front of the eye and the deep surface of the lids. Periodic blinking helps to spread the fluid over the eye. Most of the fluid evaporates. The rest is drained by the lacrimal canaliculi. When excessive, it overflows as *tears*.

Conjunctival Sac

The conjunctiva lining the deep surfaces of the eyelids is called palpebral conjunctiva and that lining the front of the eyeball is bulbar conjunctiva. The potential space between the palpebral and bulbar parts is the *conjunctival sac*. The lines along which the palpebral conjunctiva of the upper and lower eyelids is reflected onto the eyeball are called the superior and inferior *conjunctival fornices*.

The *palpebral conjunctiva* is thick, opaque, highly vascular, and adherent to the tarsal plate. The

bulbar conjunctiva covers the sclera. It is thin, transparent, and loosely attached to the eyeball. Over the cornea it is represented by the anterior epithelium of the cornea.

Lacrimal Puncta and Canaliculi

Each lacrimal canaliculus begins at the *lacrimal punctum*, and is 10 mm long. It has a vertical part which is 2 mm long and a horizontal part which is, 8 mm long. There is a dilated ampulla at the bend. Both canaliculi open close to each other in the lateral wall of the lacrimal sac behind the medial palpebral ligament.

Lacrimal Sac

It is membranous sac 12 mm long and 5 mm wide, situated in the lacrimal groove behind the medial palpebral ligament. Its upper end is blind. The lower end is continuous with the nasolacrimal duct.

The sac is related anteriorly to the medial palpebral ligament and to the orbicularis oculi. Medially, the lacrimal groove separates it from the nose. Laterally, it is related to the lacrimal fascia and the lacrimal part of the orbicularis oculi.

Inflammation of the lacrimal sac is called dacrocystitis.

Nasolacrimal Duct

It is a membranous passage 18 mm long. It begins at the lower end of the lacrimal sac, runs downwards, backwards and laterally, and opens into the inferior meatus of the nose. A fold of mucous membrane called the *valve of Hasner* forms an imperfect valve at the lower end of the duct.

DEVELOPMENT OF FACE

Five processes of face, one frontonasal, two maxillary and, two mandibular processes form the face. Frontonasal process forms the forehead, the nasal septum, philtrum of upper lip and premaxilla bearing upper four incisor teeth. Maxillary process forms whole of upper lip except the philtrum and most of the hard and soft palate except the part formed by the premaxilla. Mandibular process forms the whole lower lip. Cord of ectoderm gets buried at the junction of frontonasal and maxillary processes. Canalisation of ectodermal cord of cells gives rise to nasolacrimal duct.

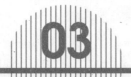

Side of the Neck

The beauty of the neck lies in its deep or cervical fascia. The sternocleidomastoid is an important landmark between the anterior and posterior triangles. The posterior triangle contains the spinal root of accessory nerve deep to its fascial roof and the roots and trunks of brachial plexus deep to its fascial floor. It also contains a part of the subclavian artery, which continues as the axillary artery for the upper limb. Arteries like the rivers are named according to the regions they pass through. Congestive cardiac failure can be seen at a glance by the raised jugular venous pressure. This vein lies in the superficial fascia and if cut, leads to air embolism, unless the deep fascia pierced by the vein is also cut to collapse the vein.

LANDMARKS ON THE SIDE OF THE NECK

1. The *sternocleidomastoid* muscle is seen prominently when the chin is turned to the opposite side. The ridge raised by the muscle extends from the clavicle and sternum to the mastoid process.

2. The *external jugular vein* crosses the sterno-cleidomastoid obliquely, running downwards and backwards from near the auricle to the clavicle. It is better seen in old age.

3. The *greater supraclavicular fossa* lies above and behind the middle one-third of the clavicle. It overlies the cervical part of the brachial plexus and the third part of the subclavian artery.

4. The *lesser supraclavicular fossa* is a small depression between the sternal and clavicular parts of the sternocleidomastoid. It overlies the internal jugular vein.

5. The *mastoid process* is a large bony projection behind the auricle.

6. The *transverse process of the atlas vertebra* can be felt on deep pressure midway between the angle of the mandible and the mastoid process, immediately anteroinferior to the tip of the mastoid process. The *fourth cervical transverse process* is just palpable at the level of the upper border of the thyroid cartilage; and the *sixth cervical transverse process* at the level of the cricoid cartilage. The anterior tubercle of the *transverse process of the sixth cervical vertebra* is the largest of all such processes and is called the *carotid tubercle* of Chassaignac. The common carotid artery can be best pressed against this tubercle, deep to the anterior border of the sternocleidomastoid muscle.

7. The *anterior border of the trapezius muscle* becomes prominent on elevation of the shoulder against resistance.

The side of the neck is roughly quadrilateral in outline. It is *bounded* anteriorly, by the anterior median line; posteriorly, by the anterior border of the trapezius; superiorly, by the base of the mandible, a line joining the angle of the mandible to the mastoid process, and the superior nuchal line; and inferiorly, by the clavicle.

This quadrilateral space is divided obliquely by the sternocleidomastoid muscle into the *anterior and posterior triangles* (Fig. 3.1)

Skin

The skin of the neck is supplied by the second, third and fourth cervical nerves. The anterolateral part is supplied by anterior primary rami through the anterior cutaneous, great auricular, lesser occipital and supraclavicular nerves. A broad band of skin over the posterior part is supplied by dorsal posterior primary rami (Fig. 2.20).

First cervical spinal nerve has no cutaneous distribution. Cervical five, six, seven, eight and thoracic one nerves supply the upper limb through the brachial plexus; and, therefore, do not supply the neck. The territory of fourth cervical nerve extends

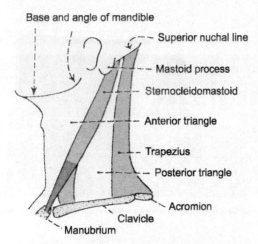

Fig. 3.1: *The triangles of the neck. Lateral view.*

into the pectoral region through the supraclavicular nerves and meets second thoracic dermatome at the level of the second costal cartilage.

DEEP CERVICAL FASCIA (FASCIA COLLI)

The deep fascia of the neck is condensed to form the following layers: (1) Investing layer, (2) pretracheal layer, (3) prevertebral layer, (4) carotid sheath, (5) buccopharyngeal fascia, and (6) pharyngobasilar fascia.

Investing Layer

It lies deep to the platysma, and surrounds the neck like a collar. It forms the roof of the posterior triangle of the neck.

Attachments

Superiorly: (a) External occipital protuberance, (b) superior nuchal line, (c) mastoid process and the, (d) base of the mandible, (e) between the angle of the mandible and the mastoid process, the fascia splits to enclose the parotid gland. The superficial lamina named as *parotid fascia* is thick and dense, and is attached to the zygomatic arch. The deep lamina is thin and is attached to the styloid process, the mandible and the tympanic plate. Between the styloid process and the angle of the mandible the deep lamina is thick and forms the *stylomandibular ligament* which separates the parotid gland from the submandibular gland, and is pierced by the external carotid artery.

Inferiorly: (a) Spine of scapula, (b) acromion process, (c) clavicle, and (d) manubrium. The fascia splits to enclose the suprasternal and supraclavicular spaces, both of which are described below (Fig. 3.2).

Posteriorly: (a) Ligamentum nuchae; and (b) spine of seventh cervical vertebra.

Anteriorly: (a) Symphysis menti; (b) hyoid bone. Both above and below the hyoid bone it is continuous with the fascia of the opposite side.

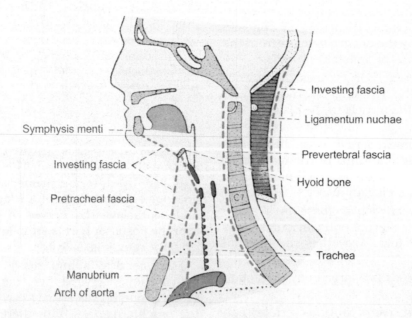

Fig. 3.2: *Vertical extent of the first three layers of the deep cervical fascia. Continuity between the tissue space of the neck and the mediastinum can be seen.*

Other Features

(1) The investing layer of deep cervical fascia *splits* to enclose: (a) *Muscles*—trapezius and sternocleidomastoid; (b) *salivary glands*—parotid and submandibular, and (c) *spaces*—suprasternal and supraclavicular.

(2) It also forms *pulleys* to bind the tendons of the digastric and omohyoid muscles.

The *suprasternal space* contains: (a) The sternal heads of the right and left sternocleidomastoid muscles, (b) the jugular venous arch, (c) a lymph node, and (d) the interclavicular ligament.

The *supraclavicular space* is traversed by: (a) The external jugular vein, (b) the supraclavicular nerves, and (c) cutaneous vessels, including lymphatics.

Pretracheal Fascia

The importance of this fascia is that it encloses and suspends the thyroid gland and forms its false capsule (Fig. 3.3).

Attachments

Superiorly: (a) Hyoid bone in the median plane (b) oblique line of thyroid cartilage, and (c) cricoid cartilage, more laterally.

Inferiorly: Below the thyroid gland it encloses the inferior thyroid veins, passes behind the brachiocephalic veins, and finally blends with the arch of the aorta.

On either side: It fuses with the front of the carotid sheath deep to the sternocleidomastoid (Fig. 12.4).

Other Features

(1) The posterior layer of the thyroid capsule is thick. On either side it forms a *suspensory ligament* for the thyroid gland known as *ligament of Berry* (Fig. 12.4). The ligaments are attached chiefly to the cricoid cartilage, and may extend to the thyroid cartilage. They support the thyroid gland, and do not let it sink into the mediastinum. The capsule of the thyroid is very weak along the posterior borders of the lateral lobes.

(2) The fascia provides a slippery surface for free movements of the trachea during swallowing.

Prevertebral Fascia

It lies in front of the prevertebral muscles, and forms the floor of the posterior triangle of the neck (Fig. 3.3).

Attachments and Relations

Superiorly: It is attached to the base of the skull (Fig. 3.2).

Inferiorly: It extends into the superior mediastinum where it is attached to the anterior longitudinal ligament and to the body of the fourth thoracic vertebra.

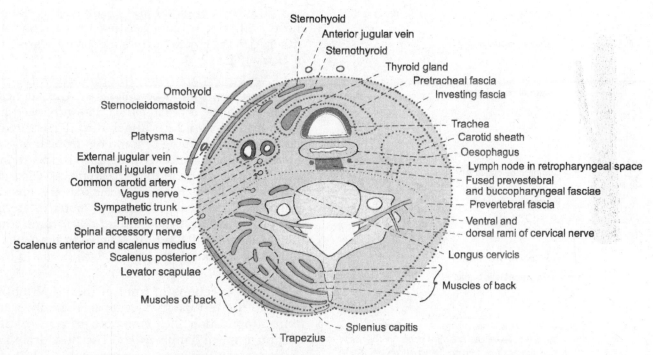

Sternohyoid
Anterior jugular vein
Sternothyroid
Thyroid gland
Pretracheal fascia
Investing fascia
Omohyoid
Sternocleidomastoid
Trachea
Platysma
Carotid sheath
External jugular vein
Oesophagus
Internal jugular vein
Lymph node in retropharyngeal space
Common carotid artery
Fused prevestebral and buccopharyngeal fasciae
Vagus nerve
Sympathetic trunk
Prevertebral fascia
Phrenic nerve
Ventral and
Spinal accessory nerve
dorsal rami of cervical nerve
Scalenus anterior and scalenus medius
Scalenus posterior
Longus cervicis
Levator scapulae
Muscles of back
Muscles of back
Splenius capitis
Trapezius

Fig. 3.3: *Transverse section through the neck at the level of the seventh cervical vertebra.*

Anteriorly: It is separated from the pharynx and buccopharyngeal fascia by the retropharyngeal space containing loose areolar tissue.

Laterally: It is lost deep to the trapezius.

Other Features

1. The cervical and brachial plexuses lie behind the prevertebral fascia. The fascia is pierced by the four cutaneous branches of the cervical plexus (Fig. 12.28).

2. As the trunks of the brachial plexus, and the subclavian artery, pass laterally through the interval between the scalenus anterior and the scalenus medius, they carry with them a covering of the prevertebral fascia known as the *axillary sheath* which extends into the axilla. The subclavian and axillary veins lie outside the sheath and as a result they can dilate during increased venous return from the limb.

3. Fascia provides a fixed base for the movements of the pharynx, the oesophagus and the carotid sheaths during movements of the neck and during swallowing.

Carotid Sheath

It is a condensation of the fibroareolar tissue around the main vessels of the neck. There are the common and internal carotid arteries and internal jugular vein and the vagus nerve. It is thin over the vein (Fig. 3.4A, B).

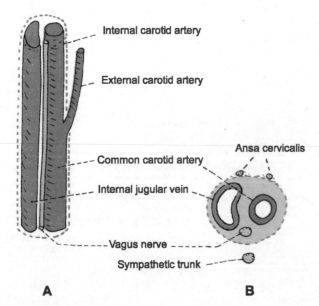

Internal carotid artery

External carotid artery

Ansa cervicalis

Common carotid artery

Internal jugular vein

Vagus nerve

Sympathetic trunk

A **B**

Fig. 3.4: *Right carotid sheath with its contents. (A) Surface view, (B) Sectional view. The ansa cervicalis is embedded in the anterior wall of the sheath, whereas the sympathetic chain lies posterior to the sheath.*

Relations

1. The ansa cervicalis lies embedded in the anterior wall of the carotid sheath.

2. The cervical sympathetic chain lies behind the sheath, plastered to the prevertebral fascia.

3. The sheath is overlapped by the anterior border of the sternocleidomastoid, and is fused to the first three layers of the deep cervical fascia.

Buccopharyngeal Fascia

This fascia covers the superior constrictor muscle externally and extends on to the superficial aspect of the buccinator muscle (Fig. 14.10).

Pharyngobasilar Fascia

This fascia is especially thickened between the upper border of superior constrictor muscle and the base of the skull. It lies deep to the pharyngeal muscles (Figs 14.10, 14.15).

CLINICAL ANATOMY

Cervical Fascia

1. Parotid swellings are very painful due to the unyielding nature of the parotid fascia.

2. While excising the submandibular salivary gland, the external carotid artery should be secured before dividing it, otherwise it may retract through the stylomandibular ligament and cause serious bleeding.

3. The thyroid gland and all thyroid swellings move with deglutition because the thyroid is attached to the larynx by the suspensory ligaments of Berry (Fig. 12.4).

4. *Neck infections behind the prevertebral fascia* arise usually from tuberculosis of the cervical vertebrae or the cervical caries. Pus produced as a result may extend in various directions. It may pass forwards forming a *chronic retropharyngeal abscess* which may form a bulging in the posterior wall of the pharynx, in the median plane. The pus may extend laterally through the axillary sheath and point in the posterior triangle, or in the lateral wall of the axilla. It may extend downwards into the superior mediastinum, where its descent is limited by fusion of the prevertebral fascia to the fourth thoracic vertebra.

5. Neck infections in front of the prevertebral fascia in the retropharyngeal space usually arise from suppuration, i.e. formation of pus in the retropharyngeal lymph nodes. The pus forms an *acute retropharyngeal abscess* which bulges

forwards in the paramedian position due to fusion of the buccopharyngeal fascia to the prevertebral fascia in the median plane. The infection may extend down through the superior mediastinum into the posterior mediastinum (Fig. 3.3).

6. *Neck infections in front of the pretracheal facia* may bulge in the suprasternal area or extend down into the anterior mediastinum.

7. Division of the external jugular vein in the supraclavicular space may cause *air embolism and consequent death* because the cut ends of the vein are prevented from retraction and closure by the fascia, attached firmly to the vein.

POSTERIOR TRIANGLE

The posterior triangle is a space on the side of the neck situated behind the sternocleidomastoid muscle.

Boundaries

Anterior: Posterior border of sternocleidomastoid (Fig. 3.5).

Posterior: Anterior border of trapezius.

Inferior or base: Middle one-third of clavicle.

Apex: Lies on the superior nuchal line where the trapezius and sternocleidomastoid meet.

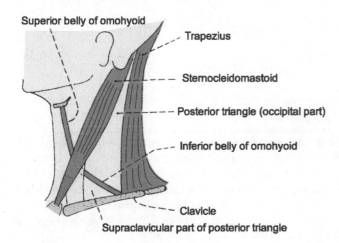

Fig. 3.5: *Boundaries of the posterior triangle. Note that the inferior belly of the omohyoid divides the triangle into upper or occipital and lower or supraclavicular parts.*

DISSECTION

1. Give a median incision from the chin downwards towards the suprasternal notch situated above the manubrium of sternum.

2. Make another incision in the skin of base and along the posterior border of the mandible till the

mastoid process. Reflect only the skin towards the anterior border of trapezius muscle. Platysma, a part of the subcutaneous muscle is visible. Reflect the platysma towards the mandible. Identify the anterior or transverse cutaneous nerve of the neck in the upper part of superficial fascia. Anterior jugular vein running vertically close to the median plane is also encountered. Remove the superficial fascia till the deep fascia of neck is seen (Fig. 3.6).

3. Another incision is given along the upper border of clavicle.

To open up the suprasternal space make a horizontal incision just above the sternum. Extend this incision along the anterior border of sternocleidomastoid muscle for 3-4 cm. Reflect the superficial lamina to expose the suprasternal space and identify its contents.

Define the attachments of investing layer, pretracheal layer, prevertebral layer and carotid sheath.

Try to dissect and clean the cutaneous nerves which pierce the investing layer of fascia at the middle of posterior border of sternocleidomastoid muscle. Demarcate the course of external jugular vein. Cut carefully the deep fascia of posterior border of sternocleidomastoid muscle and reflect it towards trapezius muscle. Identify the accessory nerve lying just deep to the investing layer seen at the middle of the posterior border of sternocleidomastoid muscle and across the posterior triangle to reach the anterior border of trapezius which it supplies (Fig. 3.7).

Define the boundaries, roof, floor, divisions and contents of the posterior triangle.

Identify and clean the inferior belly of omohyoid. Find the transverse cervical artery along the upper border of this muscle. Trace it both ways. Deep to this muscle is the upper or supraclavicular part of brachial plexus. Identify the roots, trunks and their branches carefully. The branches are suprascapular nerve, dorsal scapular nerve, long thoracic nerve, nerve to subclavius. Medial to the brachial plexus locate the third part of subclavian artery. Follow the terminal part of external jugular vein through the deep fascia into the deeply placed subclavian vein. Identify suprascapular artery running just above the clavicle (Fig. 3.7).

Define the attachments and relations of sternocleidomastoid muscle. To expose scalenus anterior muscle cut across the clavicular head of sternocleidomastoid muscle and push it medially. Scalenus anterior muscle covered by well defined prevertebral fascia can be identified. Locate the subclavian artery and upper part of brachial plexus deep to the scalenus anterior muscle.

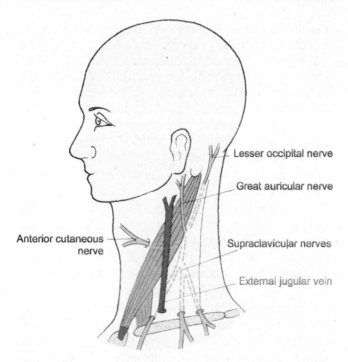

Fig. 3.6: Structures seen in relation to the fascial roof of the posterior triangle.

Labels: Lesser occipital nerve; Great auricular nerve; Anterior cutaneous nerve; Supraclavicular nerves; External jugular vein

Roof

The roof is formed by the *investing layer of deep cervical fascia*. The superficial fascia over the posterior triangle contains: (a) The platysma, (b) the external jugular and posterior external jugular veins; (c) parts of the supraclavicular, great auricular, transverse cutaneous and lesser occipital nerves, (d) unnamed arteries derived from the occipital, transverse cervical and (Fig. 3.8) suprascapular arteries; and (e) lymph vessels which pierce the deep fascia to end, in the supraclavicular nodes.

The *external jugular vein:* It lies deep to the platysma (Fig. 3.6). It is formed by union of the posterior auricular vein with the posterior division of the retromandibular vein. It begins within the lower part of the parotid gland, crosses the sternocleidomastoid obliquely, pierces the anteroinferior angle of the roof of the posterior triangle, and opens into the subclavian vein.

As it pierces the fascia, the margins of the vein get adherent to the fascia. So if the vein gets cut, it cannot close and air enters into it and causes air embolism. To prevent this, the deep fascia has to be cut. Its tributaries are: (a) The posterior external jugular vein, (b) the transverse cervical vein; (c) the suprascapular vein; and (d) the anterior jugular vein. The oblique jugular vein connects the external jugular vein with the internal jugular vein across the middle one-third of the anterior border of the sternocleidomastoid.

Surface Marking of External Jugular Vein

The vein is usually visible through the skin and can be made more prominent by blowing with the mouth and nostrils closed.

It can be marked, if not visible, by joining the following points.

(a) The first point a little below and behind the angle of the mandible.

(b) The second point on the clavicle just lateral to the posterior border of the sternocleidomastoid (Fig. 3.6).

The external jugular vein is *examined to assess the venous pressure;* the right atrial pressure is reflected in it because there are no valves in the entire course of this vein.

Floor

The floor of the posterior triangle is formed by the prevertebral layer of deep cervical fascia, covering the following muscles: (a) Splenius capitis; (b) levator scapulae; (c) scalenus medius (Fig. 3.7) and occasionally scalenus posterior.

Division of the Posterior Triangle

It is subdivided by the inferior belly of the omohyoid into (a) a larger upper part, called the *occipital triangle,* and (b) a smaller lower part, called the *supraclavicular* or the *subclavian triangle* (Fig. 3.7).

Contents of the Posterior Triangle

These are enumerated in Table 3.1. Some of the contents are considered below:

Relevant Features of the Contents of the Posterior Triangle

The *spinal accessory nerve* emerges a little above the middle of the posterior border of the sternocleidomastoid. It runs through a tunnel in the fascia forming the roof of the triangle, passing downwards and laterally, and disappears under the anterior border of the trapezius about 5 cm above the clavicle (Figs 3.7, 3.8).

The four *cutaneous branches of the cervical plexus* pierce the fascia covering the floor of the triangle, pass through the triangle and pierce the deep fascia at different points to become cutaneous (Fig. 3.6).

Muscular branches to the levator scapulae and to the trapezius (C3, C4) appear about the middle of the sternocleidomastoid. Those to the levator soon end in it; those to the trapezius run below and parallel to the accessory nerve across the middle of the triangle. Both nerves lie deep to the fascia of the floor (Fig. 3.9).

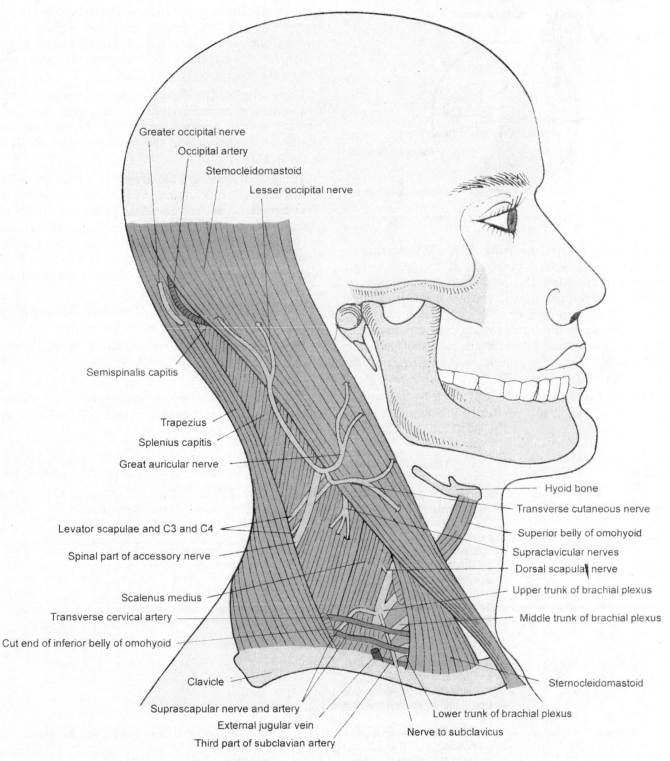

Greater occipital nerve

Occipital artery

Sternocleidomastoid

Lesser occipital nerve

Semispinalis capitis

Trapezius

Splenius capitis

Great auricular nerve

Levator scapulae and C3 and C4

Spinal part of accessory nerve

Scalenus medius

Transverse cervical artery

Cut end of inferior belly of omohyoid

Clavicle

Suprascapular nerve and artery

External jugular vein

Third part of subclavian artery

Hyoid bone

Transverse cutaneous nerve

Superior belly of omohyoid

Supraclavicular nerves

Dorsal scapular nerve

Upper trunk of brachial plexus

Middle trunk of brachial plexus

Sternocleidomastoid

Lower trunk of brachial plexus

Nerve to subclavius

Fig. 3.7: *The posterior triangle of neck.*

The *nerve to the rhomboideus* (C5) pierces the scalenus medius and passes deep to the levator scapulae to reach the back where it lies deep or anterior to the rhomboideus muscles.

The *nerve to the serratus anterior* (C5, C6, C7) arises by three roots. The roots from C5 and C6 pierce the scalenus medius and join the root from C7 over the first digitation of the serratus anterior. The nerve passes behind the brachial plexus. It descends over the serratus anterior in the medial wall of the axilla and gives branches to the digitations of the muscle (Fig. 3.9).

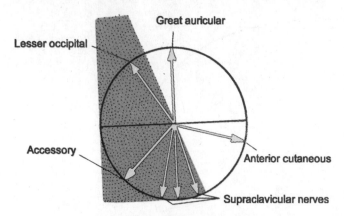

Fig. 3.8: Some nerves of the right posterior triangle.

The *nerve to the subclavius* (C5, C6) descends in front of the brachial plexus and the subclavian vessels, but behind the omohyoid, the transverse cervical and suprascapular vessels and the clavicle to reach the deep surface of the subclavius muscle. As it runs near the lateral margin of the scalenus anterior, it sometimes gives off the *accessory phrenic nerve* which joins the phrenic nerve in front of the scalenus anterior (Fig. 3.7).

The *suprascapular nerve* (C5, C6) (Fig. 3.7) arises from the upper trunk of the brachial plexus and crosses the lower part of the posterior triangle just above and lateral to the brachial plexus, deep to the transverse cervical vessels and the omohyoid. It passes backwards over the shoulder to reach the scapula. It supplies the supraspinatus and infraspinatus muscles (Fig. 3.9).

Three trunks of the *brachial plexus* emerge between the scalenus anterior and medius, and carry the axillary sheath around them. The sheath contains the brachial plexus and the subclavian artery (Figs 3.10, 3.11).

The *transverse cervical artery* is a branch of the thyrocervical trunk. It crosses the scalenus anterior, the phrenic nerve, the upper trunks of the brachial plexus, the nerve to the subclavius, the suprascapular nerve, and the scalenus medius. At the anterior border of the levator scapulae it divides into superficial and deep branches. The inferior belly of the omohyoid crosses the artery.

The *occipital artery* crosses the apex of the posterior triangle superficial to the splenius capitis.

The *suprascapular artery* is also a branch of the thyrocervical trunk. It passes laterally and backwards behind the clavicle.

The *subclavian artery* passes behind the tendon of the scalenus anterior, over the first rib. The subclavian vein passes in front of the tendon.

Table 3.1: Contents of the posterior triangle		
Contents (Figs 3.9–3.11)	*Occipital triangle*	*Subclavian triangle*
A. Nerves	1. Spinal accessory nerve 2. Four cutaneous branches of cervical plexus: 　a. Lesser occipital (C2) 　b. Great auricular (C2, C3) 　c. Anterior cutaneous nerve of neck (C2, C3) 　d. Supraclavicular nerves (C3, C4) 3. Muscular branches: 　a. Two small branches to the levator scapulae (C3, C4) 　b. Two small branches to the trapezius (C3, C4) 　c. Nerve to rhomboideus (C5) 4. Upper part of the brachial plexus	1. Three trunks of brachial plexus 2. Nerve to serratus anterior (long thoracic, C5, C6, C7) 3. Nerve to subclavius (C5, C6) 4. Suprascapular nerve (C5, C6)
B. Vessels	a. Transverse cervical artery and vein b. Occipital artery	a. Third part of subclavian artery and subclavian vein b. Suprascapular artery and vein c. Commencement of transverse cervical artery and termination of the corresponding vein d. Lower part of external jugular vein
C. Lymph nodes	Along the posterior border of the sternocleidomastoid, more in the lower part, the supraclavicular nodes and a few at the upper angle the occipital nodes	A few members of the supraclavicular chain

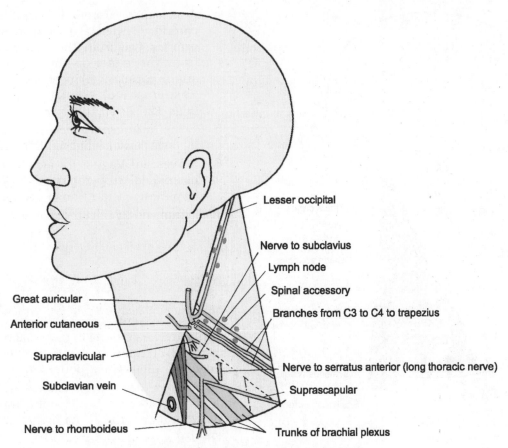

Fig. 3.9: *Nerves seen in the posterior triangle of the neck.*

STERNOCLEIDOMASTOID MUSCLE (Sternomastoid)

The sternocleidomastoid and trapezius are large superficial muscles of the neck. Both of them are supplied by the spinal root of the accessory nerve. The trapezius, because of its main action on the shoulder girdle, is considered with the upper limb. The sternocleidomastoid is described below.

Origin

1. The *sternal head* is tendinous and arises from the superolateral part of the front of the manubrium sterni (Fig. 3.7).

2. The *clavicular head* is musculotendinous and arises from the medial one-third of the superior surface of the clavicle. It passes deep to the sternal head, and the two heads blend below the middle of the neck. Between the two heads there is a small triangular depression of the lesser supraclavicular fossa, overlying the internal jugular vein.

Insertion

It is inserted (a) by a thick tendon into the lateral surface of the *mastoid process*, from its tip to its superior border, and (b) by a thin aponeurosis into the lateral half of the *superior nuchal line* of the occipital bone.

Nerve Supply

(1) The spinal accessory nerve provides the motor supply. It passes through the muscle, (2) branches from the ventral rami of C2, (3) are proprioceptive.

Blood Supply

Arterial supply—one branch each from superior thyroid artery and suprascapular artery and, two branches from the occipital artery veins follow the arteries. Veins follow the arteries.

Actions

(A) When one muscle contracts: (a) It turns the chin to the opposite side. (b) It can also tilt the head towards the shoulder.

(B) When both muscles contract together: (a) They draw the head forwards, as in eating and in lifting the head from a pillow. (b) With the longus colli, they flex the neck against resistance. (c) The reverse action helps in forced inspiration.

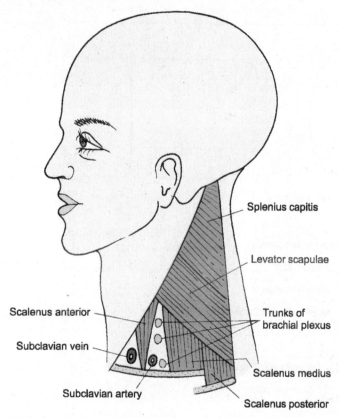

Fig. 3.10: *Structures forming the floor of the posterior triangle. Some related structures are also shown.*

Relations

The sternocleidomastoid is enclosed in the investing layer of deep cervical fascia, and is pierced by the accessory nerve and by the four sternocleidomastoid arteries. It has the following relations:

Superficial

1. Skin
2. (a) Superficial fascia; and (b) superficial lamina of the deep cervical fascia (Fig. 3.3).
3. Platysma.
4. External jugular vein, and superficial cervical lymph nodes lying along the vein.
5. (a) Great auricular, (b) transverse or anterior cutaneous, and (c) medial supraclavicular nerves (Fig. 3.9).
6. The parotid gland overlaps the muscle.

Deep

1. Bones and joints: (a) Mastoid process above, and (b) sternoclavicular joint below.
2. Carotid sheath (Fig. 3.3).
3. Muscles: (a) Sternohyoid, (b) sternothyroid; (c) omohyoid; (d) three scaleni; (e) levator scapulae, (f) splenius capitis, (g) longissimus capitis, and (h) posterior belly of digastric (Fig. 3.7).

4. Arteries: (a) Common carotid, (b) internal carotid, (c) external carotid, (d) sternomastoid arteries two from the occipital artery, one from the superior thyroid, one from the suprascapular, (e) occipital, (f) subclavian, (g) suprascapular, and (h) transverse cervical (Figs 12.15, 12.16).
5. Veins: (a) Internal jugular, (b) anterior jugular, (c) facial and (d) lingual (Fig. 12.12).
6. Nerves: (a) Vagus; (b) accessory (c) cervical plexus, (d) upper part of brachial plexus, (e) phrenic, and (f) ansa cervicalis.
7. Lymph nodes, deep cervical.

CLINICAL ANATOMY

1. The most common *swelling in the posterior triangle* is due to enlargement of the supraclavicular lymph nodes. A swelling in this region may also be caused by a lipoma, cystic hygroma or lymphangioma, pharyngeal pouch, or a cervical rib.

Supraclavicular lymph nodes are commonly enlarged in tuberculosis, Hodgkin's disease, and in malignant growths of the breast, arm or chest.

The *left supraclavicular nodes* or *Virchow's* or *scalene nodes* are also involved in malignant growths of distant organs, e.g. the stomach, the testis and other abdominal organs. They are, therefore, known as *signal nodes*. Scalene node biopsy is very helpful in the early diagnosis of such malignancies. This is to be correlated with the vast territory drained by the thoracic duct.

2. *Torticollis or wry neck* is a deformity in which the head is bent to one side and the chin points to the other side. This is a result of spasm or contracture of the muscles supplied by the spinal accessory nerve, these being the sternocleidomastoid and trapezius. Although there are many varieties of torticollis depending on the causes the common types are :

(a) Rheumatic torticollis due to exposure to cold or draught.

(b) Reflex torticollis due to inflamed or suppurating cervical lymph nodes which irritate the spinal accessory nerve.

(c) Congenital torticollis due to birth injury.

(d) Spasmodic torticollis due to central irritation.

3. *Block dissection* of the neck for malignant diseases is the removal of cervical lymph nodes along with other structures involved in the growth. This procedure does not endanger those nerves of the posterior triangle which lie deep to the

prevertebral fascia, i.e. the brachial and cervical plexuses and their muscular branches.

4. The clinical anatomy of the *arteries of the neck* has been discussed along with the arteries concerned. The following additional points may be noted.

(a) A cervical rib may compress the subclavian artery. In these cases, the radial pulse is diminished or obliterated on turning the patient's head upwards and to the affected side after a deep breath (*Adson's test*) blood.

(b) Dysphagia caused by compression of the oesophagus by an abnormal subclavian artery is called *dysphagia lusoria.*

(c) In *Blalock's operation* for Fallot's tetralogy, the right subclavian artery is anastomosed end to side to short circuit the pulmonary stenosis.

(d) Elective arterial surgery of the common carotid artery is done for aneurysms, AV-fistulae or arteriosclerotic occlusions. It is better to expose the common carotid artery in its upper part where it is superficial. While ligating the artery care should be taken not to include the vagus nerve or the sympathetic chain.

(e) Second part of the subclavian artery may get pressed by the scalenus anterior muscle, resulting in decreased blood supply to the upper limb.

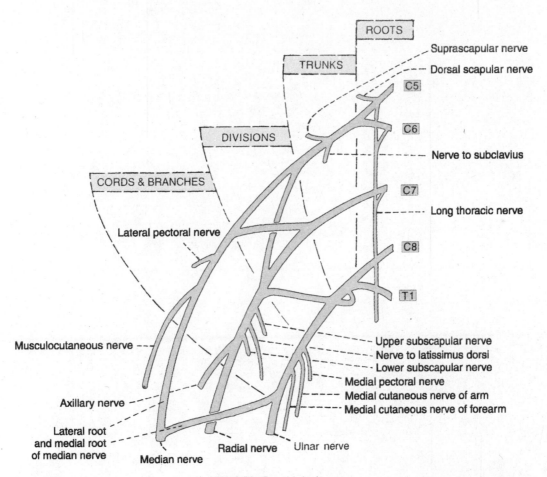

Fig. 3.11: Brachial plexus.

The Back of the Neck

The vertebral column at back provides a median axis for the body. There are big muscles from the sacrum to the skull in different strata which keep the spine straight. As such one must maintain the position of the spine to be gracious and not "spineless". The only triangle of the upper most part here is the suboccipital triangle containing the third part of the vertebral artery, which enters the skull to supply the brain. If it gets pressed, many symptoms appear.

INTRODUCTION

The skin of the nape or back of the neck, and of the back of the scalp is supplied by medial branches of the dorsal rami of C2 the *greater occipital nerve;* C3 the *third occipital nerve* and C4. Each posterior primary ramus divides into a medial and a lateral branch, both of which supply the intrinsic muscles of the back. The medial branch in this region supplies the skin as well. The *dorsal ramus of C1* does not divide into medial and lateral branches, and is distributed only to the muscles bounding the suboccipital triangle.

The *ligamentum nuchae* is a triangular fibrous sheet that separates muscles of the two sides of the neck. It is better developed and is more elastic in quadrupeds in whom it has to support a heavy head.

DISSECTION

Extend the incision from external occipital protuberance to the spine of the seventh cervical spine. Give a horizontal incision from spine of 7th cervical vertebra or vertebra prominens till the acromion. This will expose the upper part and apex of posterior triangle of neck. Look for the occipital artery at its apex (Fig. 4.1).

Close to the median plane in the superficial fascia are seen the greater occipital nerve and occipital artery.

Extend the incision from vertebra prominens to spine of lumbar 5 vertebra. Reflect the skin laterally along a vertical line drawn from the inferior angle of scapula.

Cut through trapezius muscle vertically at a distance of 2 cm from the median plane. Reflect it laterally and identify the accessory nerve, superficial branch of transverse cervical artery and ventral rami of 3rd and 4th cervical nerves.

Latissimus dorsi has already been exposed by the students dissecting the upper limb. Otherwise extend the incision from T12 spine; upwards and laterally across 8th rib to the junction of upper one-third and lower two-thirds of humerus. Reflect the skin and define the margins of broad thin latissimus dorsi.

The second layer comprises splenius muscle, levator scapulae, rhomboideus major, rhomboideus minor, serratus posterior superior and serratus posterior inferior muscles. The splenius is the highest of these muscles. It arises from ligamentum nuchae and spines of C7 and T1–6 vertebrae. It is made up of two parts:

(i) Splenius cervicis which is inserted into the back of C1–C3 transverse processes,(ii) splenius capitis being inserted into the lower part of mastoid process and adjacent superior nuchal line. It is supplied by dorsal rami of C1–C6 nerves.

Levator scapulae forms part of the muscular floor of the posterior triangle. It is positioned between scalenus medius below and splenius capitis above. Follow its nerve and blood supply from dorsal scapular nerve and deep branch of transverse cervical artery respectively.

Rhomboideus minor and major lie on same plane as levator scapulae. Both are supplied by dorsal scapular nerve (C5).

Deep to the two rhomboideus muscles is thin aponeurotic serratus posterior superior muscle from spines of C7 and T1–T2 vertebrae to be inserted into 2–5th ribs. Serratus posterior inferior muscle arises from T11–T12 spines and thoracolumbar fascia and is inserted into 9th-12th ribs.

The third layer is composed of erector spinae or sacrospinalis with its three subdivisions and semispinalis with its three divisions (Fig. 4.2).

Erector spinae arises from the dorsal surface of sacrum and ascends up the lumbar region. There it divides into three subdivisions, the medial one is spinalis, inserted into the spines, the intermediate one is longissimus inserted into the transverse processes and the lateral one is iliocostalis, inserted into the ribs. Each of these divisions are made of short parts, fresh slips arising from the area where the lower slips are inserted.

Deep to erector spinae is the semispinalis again made up of three parts: semispinalis thoracis, semispinalis cervicis and semispinalis capitis.

Both these muscles are innervated by the dorsal rami of cervical, thoracic, lumbar and sacral nerves.

Muscles of fourth layer are the multifidus, rotatores, interspinales, intertransversii and suboccipital muscles.

Suboccipital Triangle

It is deep triangle in the area between the occiput and the spine of second cervical, the axis vertebra. The deepest muscles are the muscles of suboccipital triangle.

Cut the attachments of trapezius from superior nuchal line and reflect it towards the spine of scapula. Cut the splenius capitis from its attachment on the mastoid process and reflect it downwards. Clean the superficial fascia over the semispinalis capitis medially and longissimus capitis laterally. Reflect longissimus capitis downwards from the mastoid process.

Cut through semispinalis capitis and turn it towards lateral side. Define the boundaries and contents of the suboccipital triangle.

MUSCLES OF THE BACK

The *muscles* of the entire back can be grouped into the following four layers from superficial to the deeper plane.

I. Trapezius and latissimus dorsi see Vol. I

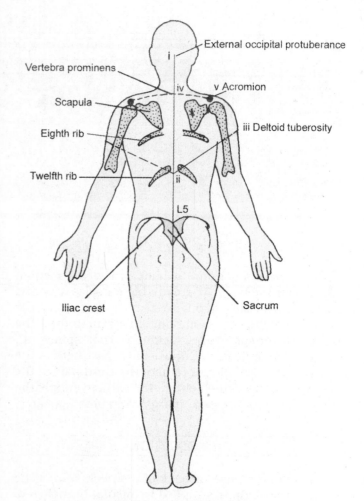

Fig. 4.1: *Lines of dissection.*

II. Levator scapulae, rhomboideus (two), serratus posterior superior have been studied in Volume I, serratus posterior inferior is seen in Volume II. Splenius is described briefly here.

Splenius muscles are two in number. These are splenius cervicis and splenius capitis. These cover the deeper muscles like a bandage (Fig. 4.2).

Origin – from lower half of ligamentum nuchae and spines of upper 6 thoracic vertebrae. These curve in a half spiral fashion and separate into splenius cervicis and splenius capitis.

Splenius cervicis gets inserted into the posterior tubercles of transverse processes of C1-C4 vertebrae. Splenius capitis forms the floor of the posterior triangle and gets inserted into the mastoid process beneath the sternocleidomastoid muscle (Fig. 4.4).

III. a) Erector spinae or sacrospinalis is the true muscle of the back, supplied by posterior rami of the spinal nerves. It extends from the sacrum to the skull (Fig. 4.3).

Origin from the back of sacrum between median and lateral sacral crests, from the dorsal segment of

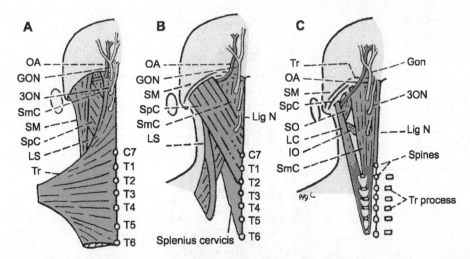

Fig. 4.2: *Three layers of muscles covering the suboccipital triangle. (A) First layer: trapezius (Tr) and sternocleidomastoid (SM). (B) Second layer: splenius capitis (SpC) and levator scapulae (LS). (C) Third layer: semispinalis capitis (SmC) and longissimus capitis (LC), OA=occipital artery, GON=greater occipital nerve, 3ON=third occipital nerve, Lig. N=ligamentum nuchae, SO=superior oblique, and IO=inferior oblique.*

iliac crest and related ligaments. Soon it splits into three columns:

Iliocostalis, longissimus and spinalis –

(i) Iliocostalis is the lateral column and comprised iliocostalis lumborum, Iliocostalis thoracis and iliocostalis cervicis.

These are short slips and are inserted into angles of the ribs and posterior tubercles of cervical transverse process. Origin of the higher slips is medial to the insertion of the lower slips.

(ii) Longissimus is the middle column and is composed of:

Longissimus thoracis – inserted into transverse processes of thoracic vertebrae.

Longissimus cervicis – inserted into transverse process of C2-C6 vertebrae.

Longissimus capitis – inserted into mastoid process (Fig. 4.3).

(iii) Spinalis–is the medial column, extending between lumbar and cervical spines. Its parts are:

Spinalis lumborum

Spinalis thoracis

Spinalis cervicis

b) The other muscle of this layer is semispinalis extending between transverse processes and spines of the vertebrae. It has three parts:

Semispinalis thoracis (Fig. 4.4).

Semispinalis cervicis

Semispinalis capitis

It only lies in the upper half of vertebral column. Semispinalis capitis is its biggest component. It

arises from transverse processes of C3-T4 vertebrae, passes up next to the median plane, and gets inserted into the medial area between superior and inferior nuchal lines of the occipital bone.

(IV) Multifidus, rotatores, interspinales, intertransversii and suboccipital muscles. Multifidus is oblique deep muscles. These arise from mamillary process of lumbar vertebrae to be inserted into 2-3 higher spinous processes. Rotatores are the deepest group. These pass from root of transverse process to the root of the spinous process. These are well developed in thoracic region. Interspinales lie between the adjacent spines of the vertebrae. These are better developed in cervical and lumbar regions. Intertransversii connect the transverse processes of the adjacent vertebrae. Suboccipital muscles are described below in the suboccipital triangle (Fig. 4.4).

In the suboccipital region between the occiput and the spine of the axis vertebra, the four muscular layers are represented by: I. Trapezius; II. splenius capitis; III. semispinalis capitis and longissimus capitis; and IV. the four suboccipital muscles.

The *arteries* found in the back of the neck are: (a) Occipital, (b) deep cervical, (c) third part of the vertebral artery and (d) minute twigs from the second part of the vertebral artery.

The *suboccipital venous plexus* is known for its extensive layout and complex connections.

SUBOCCIPITAL TRIANGLE

The suboccipital triangle is a muscular space situated deep in the suboccipital region.

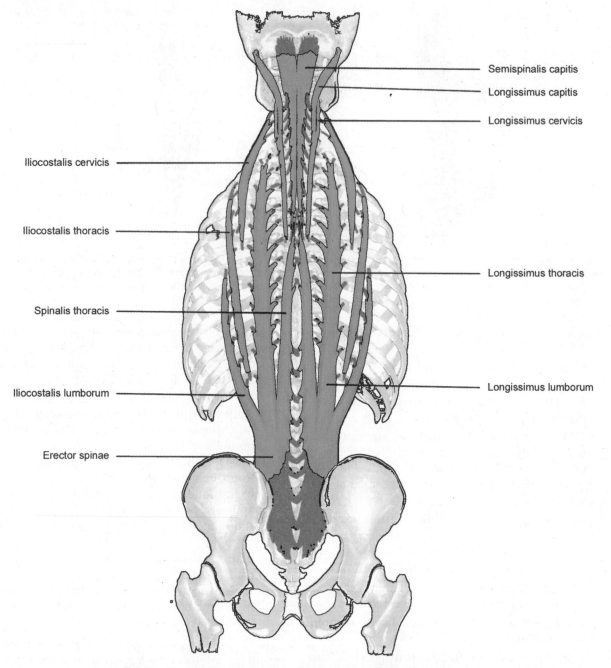

Iliocostalis cervicis

Iliocostalis thoracis

Spinalis thoracis

Iliocostalis lumborum

Erector spinae

Semispinalis capitis

Longissimus capitis

Longissimus cervicis

Longissimus thoracis

Longissimus lumborum

Fig. 4.3: *The erector spinae/sacrospinalis muscle with its three columns.*

Exposure of Suboccipital Triangle

In order to expose the triangle, the following layers are reflected (Fig. 4.2).

1. The *skin* is very thick.

2. The *superficial fascia* is fibrous and dense. It contains: (a) The greater, and third occipital nerves; and (b) the terminal part of the occipital artery, with accompanying veins.

3. The fibres of the *trapezius* run downwards and laterally over the triangle. The sternocleidomastoid overlaps the region laterally.

4. The *splenius capitis* runs upwards and laterally for insertion into the mastoid process deep to the sternocleidomastoid.

5. The *semispinalis capitis* runs vertically upwards for insertion into the medial part of the area between the superior and inferior nuchal lines. In the same plane laterally there lies the *longissimus capitis* which is inserted into the mastoid process deep to the splenius.

Reflection of the semispinalis capitis exposes the *suboccipital triangle*.

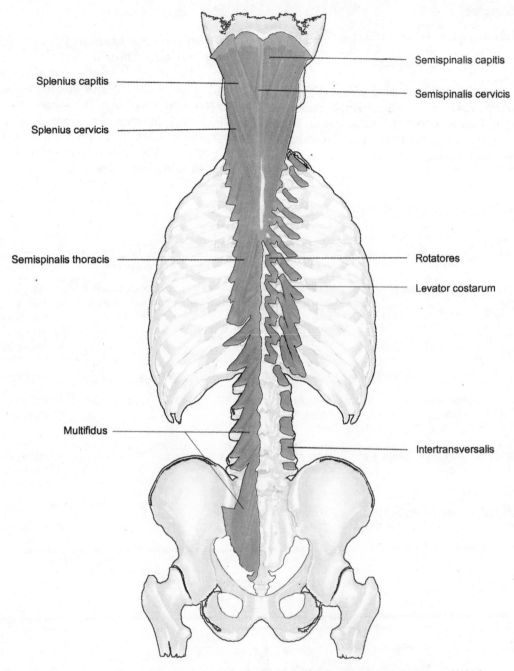

Splenius capitis

Splenius cervicis

Semispinalis thoracis

Multifidus

Semispinalis capitis

Semispinalis cervicis

Rotatores

Levator costarum

Intertransversalis

Fig. 4.4: *Splenius cervicis and capitis; three parts of semispinalis; the multifidus, levator costarum and intertransversalis muscles.*

Boundaries

Superomedially: Rectus capitis posterior major muscle supplemented by the rectus capitis posterior minor (Fig. 4.5).

Superolaterally: Superior oblique muscle.

Inferiorly: Inferior oblique muscle.

Roof

Medially: Dense fibrous tissue covered by the semispinalis capitis.

Laterally: Longissimus capitis and occasionally the splenius capitis.

Floor

1. Posterior arch of atlas, and
2. Posterior atlanto-occipital membrane.

Contents

1. Third part of vertebral artery.
2. Dorsal ramus of nerve C1—suboccipital nerve.
3. Suboccipital plexus of veins.

Suboccipital Muscles

The suboccipital muscles are described in Table 4.1.

Dorsal Ramus of First Cervical Nerve

It emerges between the posterior arch of the atlas and the vertebral artery, and soon breaks up into branches which supply the four suboccipital muscles and the semispinalis capitis. The nerve to the inferior oblique gives off a communicating branch to the greater occipital nerve (Figs 4.5, 4.6).

Greater Occipital Nerve

It is the large medial branch of the dorsal ramus of the second cervical nerve. It is the thickest cutaneous nerve in the body. It winds round the middle of the lower border of the inferior oblique muscle, and runs upwards and medially. It crosses the suboccipital triangle and pierces the semispinalis capitis and trapezius muscles to ramify on the back of the head reaching up to the vertex. It supplies the semispinalis capitis in addition to the scalp.

Table 4.1: The suboccipital muscles

Muscle	Origin	Insertion	Nerve Supply	Actions
1. Rectus capitis posterior major	Spine of axis	Lateral part of the area below the inferior nuchal line	Suboccipital nerve or dorsal ramus C1	1. Mainly postural 2. Acting alone it turns the chin to the same side 3. Acting together the two muscles extend the head
2. Rectus capitis posterior minor	Posterior tubercle of atlas	Medial part of the area below the inferior nuchal line	"	1. Mainly postural 2. Extend the head
3. Obliquus capitis superior (superior oblique)	Transverse process of atlas	Lateral area between the nuchal lines	"	1. Mainly postural 2. Extend the head 3. Flex the head Laterally
4. Obliquus capitis inferior (inferior oblique)	Spine of axis	Transverse process of atlas	"	1. Mainly postural 2. Turns chin to the same side

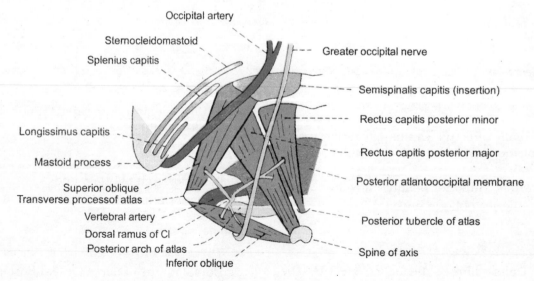

Fig. 4.5: *Left suboccipital triangle; boundaries, floor and contents.*

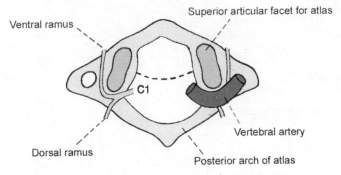

Ventral ramus

Superior articular facet for atlas

C1

Dorsal ramus

Vertebral artery

Posterior arch of atlas

Fig. 4.6: *Relationship of the vertebral artery to the atlas vertebra and to the first cervical nerve, as seen from above.*

Third Occipital Nerve

It is the slender medial branch of the dorsal ramus of the third cervical nerve. After piercing the semispinalis capitis and the trapezius, it ascends medial to the greater occipital nerve. It supplies the skin to the back of the neck up to the external occipital protuberance.

Vertebral Artery

It is the first and largest branch of the first part of the subclavian artery, destined chiefly to supply the brain. Out of its four parts, only the third part appears in the suboccipital triangle. (Figs 4.3, 4.4). This part appears at the foramen transversarium of the atlas, grooves the atlas, and leaves the triangle by passing deep to the lateral edge of the posterior atlanto-occipital membrane. The artery is separated from the posterior arch of the atlas by the first cervical nerve and its dorsal and ventral rami. For complete description of the vertebral artery see Chapter 13.

Occipital Artery

It arises from the external carotid artery, opposite the origin of the facial artery (Figs 4.2, 4.5). It runs backwards and upwards deep to the lower border of the posterior belly of the digastric, crossing the carotid sheath, and the accessory and hypoglossal nerves. Next it runs deep to the mastoid process and to the muscles attached to it; the sternocleidomastoid, digastric, splenius capitis, longissimus capitis. The artery then crosses the rectus capitis lateralis, the superior oblique and the semispinalis capitis muscles at the apex of the posterior triangle. Finally, it pierces the trapezius 2.5 cm from the midline and comes to lie along the greater occipital nerve. In the superficial fascia of the scalp, it has a tortuous course.

Its branches in this region are: (1) *Mastoid*, (2) *meningeal*, and (3) *muscular*. One of the muscular branches is large: it is called the *descending branch* and has superficial and deep branches. The superficial branch anastomoses with the superficial branch of the transverse cervical artery; while the deep branch descends between the semispinalis capitis and cervicis, and anastomoses with the vertebral and deep cervical arteries. It also gives two branches to sternocleidomastoid muscle.

Deep Cervical Artery

It is a branch of the costocervical trunk of the subclavian artery. It passes into the back of the neck just above the neck of the first rib. It ascends deep to the semispinalis capitis and anastomoses with the descending branch of the occipital artery.

Suboccipital Plexus of Veins

It lies in and around the suboccipital triangle, and drains the : (1) Muscular veins, (2) occipital veins, (3) internal vertebral venous plexus, and (4) condylar emissary vein. It itself drains into the deep cervical and vertebral plexus of veins.

CLINICAL ANATOMY

(1) *Neck rigidity*, seen in cases with meningitis, is due to spasm of the extensor muscles. This is caused by irritation of the nerve roots during their passage through the subarachnoid space which is infected.

(2) *Cisternal puncture* is done when lumbar puncture fails. The patient either sits up or lies down in the left lateral position. A needle is introduced in the midline just above the spine of the axis vertebra, and is passed forwards and upwards, parallel to an imaginary line joining the external auditory meatus with the nasion. As the needle pierces the posterior atlanto-occipital membrane at a depth of about 4 to 5 cm in adults, the resistance is suddenly lost and the tip of the needle enters the cisterna magna. In this procedure, there is danger of injury to the medulla which lies 2.5 cm anterior to the posterior atlanto-occipital membrane. Such injury is fatal.

(3) Neurosurgeons approach the posterior cranial fossa through this region.

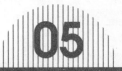

Contents of the Vertebral Canal

When the vertebrae are put in a sequence, their vertebral foramina lie one below the other forming a continuous canal which is called the *vertebral canal.* This canal contains the three meninges with their spaces and the spinal cord including the cauda equina. The intervertebral foramina are a pair of foramina between the pedicles of the adjacent vertebrae. Each foramen contains dorsal and ventral roots, trunk and dorsal and ventral primary rami of the spinal nerve, and spinal vessels. The vertebral canal also lodges quiet, valveless, dangerous vertebral venous plexus connecting veins of the pelvis, abdomen, thorax, neck with those of the brain, providing a route for spread of cancer from any of the viscera to the brain.

CONTENTS

The vertebral canal contains the following structures from without inwards. (Fig. 5.1)

1. Epidural extradural space.
2. Thick dura mater or pachymeninx.
3. Subdural capillary space.
4. Delicate arachnoid mater.
5. Wide subarachnoid space containing cerebro-spinal fluid (CSF).
6. Firm pia mater. The arachnoid and pia together form the leptomeninges.
7. Spinal cord or spinal medulla and the cauda equina.

The spinal cord is considered along with the brain in Chapter 23. The other contents are described below.

Epidural Space

Epidural space lies between the spinal dura mater, and the periosteum and ligaments lining the vertebral canal. It contains: (a) Loose areolar tissue, (b) semiliquid fat, (c) spinal arteries on their way to supply the deeper contents, and (d) the internal vertebral venous plexus.

The *spinal arteries* arise from different sources at different levels; they enter the vertebral canal through the intervertebral foramina, and supply the spinal cord, the spinal nerve roots, the meninges, the periosteum and ligaments.

Venous blood from the spinal cord drains into the epidural or internal vertebral plexus.

DISSECTION
Clean the spines and laminae of the entire vertebral column by removing all the muscles attached to them. Trace the dorsal rami of spinal nerves towards the intervertebral foramina. Saw through the spines and laminae of the vertebrae carefully and detach them so that the spinal medulla/ spinal cord encased in the meninges becomes visible.
Clean the external surface of dura mater enveloping the spinal cord by removing fat and epidural plexus of veins. Carefully cut through a small part of the dura mater by a fine median incision. Extend this incision above and below. See the delicate arachnoid mater. Incise it. Push the spinal cord to one side and try to identify the ligamentum denticulatum. Define the attachments of the dorsal and ventral nerve roots on the surface of spinal cord and their union to form the trunk of the spinal nerve.

Spinal Dura Mater

Spinal dura mater is a thick, tough fibrous membrane which forms a loose sheath around the spinal cord (Fig. 5.1). It is continuous with the meningeal layer of the cerebral dura mater. The spinal dura extends

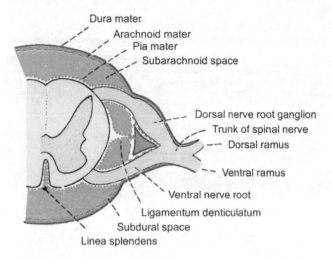

Fig. 5.1: *Schematic transverse section showing the spinal meninges.*

from the foramen magnum to the lower border of the second sacral vertebra; whereas the spinal cord ends at the lower border of first lumbar vertebra. The dura gives tubular prolongations to the dorsal and ventral nerve roots and to the spinal nerves as they pass through the intervertebral foramina.

Subdural Space

Subdural space is a capillary or potential space between the dura and the arachnoid, containing a thin film of serous fluid. This space permits movements of the dura over the arachnoid. The space is continued for a short distance on to the spinal nerves, and is in free communication with the lymph spaces of the nerves.

Arachnoid Mater

Arachnoid mater is a thin, delicate and transparent membrane that loosely invests the entire central

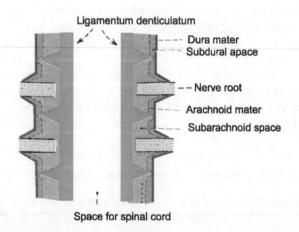

Fig. 5.2: *Ligamentum denticulatum and its relationship to the dura mater and to the arachnoid mater.*

nervous system (Fig. 5.2). Inferiorly, it extends, like the dura, up to the lower border of the second sacral vertebra. It is adherent to the dura only where some structures pierce the membrane, and where the ligamentum denticulata are attached to the dura mater.

Subarachnoid Space

Subarachnoid space is a wide space between the pia and the arachnoid, filled with cerebrospinal fluid (CSF). It surrounds the brain and spinal cord like a water cushion. The spinal subarachnoid space is wider than the space around the brain. It is widest below the lower end of the spinal cord where it encloses the cauda equina. *Lumbar puncture* is usually done in the lower widest part of the space, between third and fourth lumbar vertebrae.

Spinal Pia Mater

Spinal pia mater is thicker, firmer, and less vascular than the cerebral pia, but both are made up of two layers: (a) an outer *epi-pia* containing larger vessels; and (b) An inner *pia-glia or pia-intima* which is in contact with nervous tissue. Between the two layers there are many small blood vessels and also cleft like spaces which communicate with the subarachnoid space. The pia mater closely invests the spinal cord, and is continued below the spinal cord as the filum terminale.

Posteriorly, the pia is adherent to the posterior median septum of the spinal cord, and is also connected to the arachnoid by a fenestrated *subarachnoid septum.*

Anteriorly, the pia is folded into the anterior median fissure of the spinal cord. It thickens at the mouth of the fissure to form a median, longitudinal glistening band, called the *linea splendens* (Fig. 5.1).

On each side between the ventral and dorsal nerve roots, the pia forms a narrow vertical ridge, called the *ligamentum denticulatum.* This is so called because it gives off a series of triangular tooth-like processes which project from its lateral free border (Fig. 5.3). Each ligament has 21 processes; the first at the level of the foramen magnum, and the last between twelfth thoracic and first lumbar spinal nerves. Each process passes through the arachnoid to the dura between two adjacent spinal nerves. The processes suspend the spinal cord in the middle of the subarachnoid space.

The *filum terminale* is a delicate, thread-like structure about 20 cm long. It extends from the apex of the conus medullaris to the dorsum of the first piece of the coccyx. It is composed chiefly of pia mater, although a few nerve fibres rudiments of 2nd

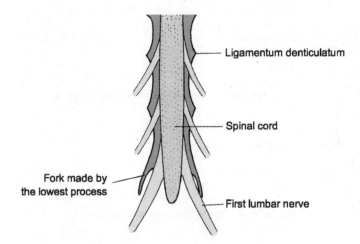

Fig. 5.3: *Ligamentum denticulatum.*

and 3rd coccygeal nerves are found adherent to the upper part of its outer surface. The central canal of the spinal cord extends into it for about 5 mm.

The filum terminale is subdivided into a part lying within the dural sheath (called the filum terminale internum; and a part lying outside the dural sheath, below the level of the second sacral vertebra called the filum terminale externum. The filum terminale internum is 20 cm long, and the externum is 5 cm long.

Pial sheaths surround the nerve roots crossing the subarachnoid space, and the vessels entering the substance of the spinal cord.

Spinal Nerves

The spinal cord gives rise to thirty-one pairs of *spinal nerves:* eight cervical, twelve thoracic, five lumbar, five sacral, and one coccygeal. Each nerve is attached to the cord by two roots, ventral motor and dorsal sensory. Each dorsal nerve root bears a ganglion. The *ventral and dorsal nerve roots* unite in the intervertebral foramen to form the *nerve trunk* which soon divides into ventral and dorsal *rami* (Fig. 5.1).

The uppermost nerve roots pass horizontally from the spinal cord to reach the intervertebral foramina. Lower down they have to pass with increasing obliquity, as the spinal cord is much shorter than the vertebral column. Below the termination of the spinal cord at the level of first lumbar vertebra the obliquity becomes much more marked (Fig. 5.3).

Below the lower end of the spinal cord the roots form a bundle known as the *cauda equina* because of its resemblance to the tail of a horse.

The roots of spinal nerves are surrounded by sheaths derived from the meninges. The *pial and arachnoid sheaths* extend up to the dura mater. The *dural sheath* encloses the terminal parts of the roots, continues over the nerve trunk, and is lost by merging with the epineurium of the nerve.

An intervertebral foramen contains: (a) The ends of the nerve roots, (b) the dorsal root ganglion, (c) the nerve trunk, (d) the beginning of the dorsal and ventral rami, (e) a spinal artery, and (f) an intervertebral vein (Fig. 5.1).

VERTEBRAL SYSTEM OF VEINS

Introduction

The vertebral venous plexus assumes importance in cases of: (1) Carcinoma of the prostate causing secondaries in the vertebral column and the skull; and (2) chronic empyema (collection of pus in the pleural cavity) causing brain abscess by septic emboli.

Anatomy of the Vertebral Venous Plexus

The vertebral venous system is made up of a valveless, complicated network of veins with a longitudinal pattern. It runs parallel to and anastomoses with the superior and inferior venae cavae. This network has three intercommunicating subdivisions (Fig. 5.4).

1. *The epidural plexus:* Lies in the vertebral canal outside the dura mater. The plexus consists of a postcentral and a prelaminar portion. Each portion is drained by two vessels. The plexus drains the structures in the vertebral canal, and is itself drained at regular intervals by segmental veins—vertebral, posterior intercostal, lumbar and lateral sacral.

2. *Plexus within the vertebral bodies:* It drains backwards into the epidural plexus, and anterolaterally into the external vertebral plexus.

3. *External vertebral venous plexus:* It consists of anterior vessels lying in front of the vertebral bodies, and the posterior vessels on the back of the vertebral arches and on adjacent muscles. It is drained by segmental veins.

The suboccipital plexus of veins is a part of the external plexus. It lies in the suboccipital triangle. It receives the occipital veins of the scalp, is connected with the transverse sinus by emissary veins, and drains into the subclavian veins.

Communications and Implications

The valveless vertebral system of veins *communicates:* (1) Above with the intracranial venous sinuses, and (2) below with the pelvic veins, the portal vein, and the caval system of veins.

The veins are *valveless* and the blood can flow in them in either direction. An increase in intrathoracic

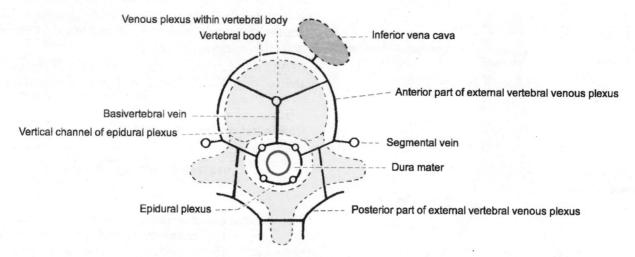

Fig. 5.4: *The vertebral system of veins.*

or intra-abdominal pressure, such as is brought about by coughing and straining, may cause blood to flow in the plexus away from the heart, either upwards or downwards. Such periodic changes in venous pressure are clinically important because they make possible the spread of tumours or infections. For example, cells from pelvic, abdominal, thoracic and breast tumours may enter the venous system, and may ultimately lodge in the vertebrae, the spinal cord, the skull, or the brain.

The common primary sites of tumours causing secondaries in vertebrae are the breast, the prostate, and the kidney. Tubercular infection within the vertebrae-vertebral caries, is similarly explained.

CLINICAL ANATOMY

Leptomeninges

Inflammation due to infection of leptomeninges–pia mater and arachnoid mater is known as meningitis. This is commonly tubercular or pyogenic. It is characterized by fever, marked headache, neck rigidity, often accompanied by delirium and convulsions, and a changed biochemistry of CSF. CSF pressure is raised, its proteins and cell content are increased, and sugars and chloride are selectively diminished.

Vertebral Canal

1. Compression of the spinal cord by a tumour gives rise to paraplegia or quadriplegia, depending on the level of compression.

2. Spinal tumours may arise from dura mater–meningioma; glial cells–glioma, nerve roots–neurofibroma; ependyma–ependymoma; and other tissues. Apart from compression of the spinal cord the tumour causes obstruction of the subarachnoid space so that pressure of CSF is low below the level of lesion. *Froin's syndrome* is seen. There is yellowish discolouration of CSF below the level of obstruction. CSF reveals high level of protein but the cell content is normal *Queckenstedi's test* does not show a sudden rise and a sudden fall of CSF pressure by coughing or by brief pressure over the jugular veins. Spinal block can be confirmed by myelography or CT scan or MRI scan.

3. Compression of the cauda equina gives rise to flaccid paraplegia, saddle anaesthesia and sphincter disturbances. This is called the cauda equina syndrome.

4. Compression of roots of spinal nerves may be caused by prolapse of an intervertebral disc, by osteophytes, formed in osteoarthritis; by a cervical rib, or by an extramedullary tumour. Such compression results in shooting pain along the distribution of the nerve.

The Cranial Cavity

Cranial cavity, the highest placed cavity, contains the brain, meninges, venous sinuses, all cranial nerves, four petrosal nerves, parts of internal carotid artery and a part of the vertebral artery besides the special senses. The anterior branch of middle meningeal artery lies at the pterion and is most likely to be ruptured resulting in extradural haemorrhage.

CRANIAL CAVITY

The convex upper wall of the cranial cavity is called the *vault*. It is uniform and smooth. The base of the cranial cavity is uneven and presents three cranial fossae (anterior, middle and posterior) lodging the uneven base of the brain (Fig. 6.1).

The cranial cavity contains the brain and meninges; the outer dura mater, the middle arachnoid mater, and the inner pia mater. The dura mater is the thickest of the three meninges. It encloses the cranial venous sinuses, and has a distinct blood supply and nerve supply. The dura is separated from the arachnoid by a potential subdural space. The arachnoid is separated from the pia by a wider subarachnoid space filled with cerebrospinal fluid (CSF). The arachnoid, pia, subarachnoid space and CSF are dealt with the brain; the dura is described after dissection.

DISSECTION

Detach the epicranial aponeurosis if not already done laterally till the inferior temporal line. In the region of the temple, detach the temporalis muscle with its overlying fascia and reflect these downwards over the pinna.

Removal of Skull Cap or Calvaria

Draw a horizontal line across the skull one centimetre above the orbital margins and one centimetre above the inion. Saw through the skull. Be careful in the temporal region as skull is rather thin there. Separate the inner table of skull from the fused endosteum and dura mater.

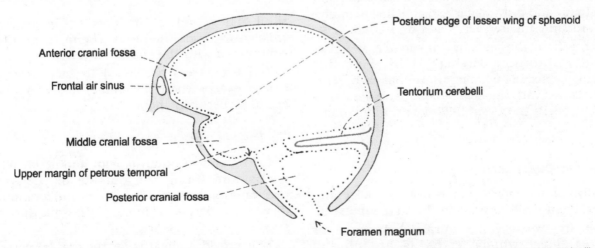

Fig. 6.1: *Parasagittal section through the skull to show the cranial fossae. Note the position of the tentorium cerebelli.*

Removal of the Brain

To remove the brain and its enveloping meninges the structures leaving or entering the brain through various foramina of the skull have to be carefully detached/incised. Start from the anterior aspect by detaching falx cerebri from the crista galli.

Put 2-3 blocks under the shoulders so that head falls backwards. This will expose the olfactory bulb, which may be lifted from the underlying anterior cranial fossa. Identify optic nerve, internal carotid artery, infundibulum passing towards hypophysis cerebri. Divide all three structures. Cut through the oculomotor and trochlear nerves in relation to free margin of tentorium cerebelli (Figs 6.2A, B, C, 6.3). Divide the attachment of tentorium from the petrous temporal bone.

Identify and divide trigeminal, abducent, facial, and vestibulocochlear nerves. Then cut glosso-pharyngeal, vagus, accessory and hypoglossal nerves. All these nerves have to be cut first on one side and then on the other side. Lastly identify the two vertebral arteries entering the skull through foramen magnum on each side of the spinal medulla. With a sharp knife cut through these structures. Thus the whole brain with the meninges can be gently removed from the skull. Preserve it in 5% formaldehyde.

Cut through the dura mater on the ventral aspect of brain till the inferolateral borders along the superciliary margin. Pull upwards the fold of dura mater present between the adjacent medial surfaces of cerebral hemispheres. This will be possible till the occipital lobe of brain. Pull backwards a similar but much smaller fold between two lobes of cerebellum, i.e. falx cerebelli.

Separating the cerebrum from the cerebellum is a double fold of dura mater called tentorium cerebelli. Pull it out in a horizontal plane. Thus the endosteum and dura mater are pulled separately from arachnoid mater, pia mater and brain.

Learn about the folds of dura mater, i.e. falx cerebri, tentorium cerebelli, falx cerebelli, diaphragma sellae including trigeminal cave from the specimen with the help of base of skull. Make a paper model of these dural folds for recapitulation.

The Cerebral Dura Mater

The dura mater is the outermost, thickest and toughest membrane covering the brain (*Dura*=hard).

There are two layers of dura: (a) An outer or *endosteal layer* which serves as an internal periosteum or endosteum or endocranium for the

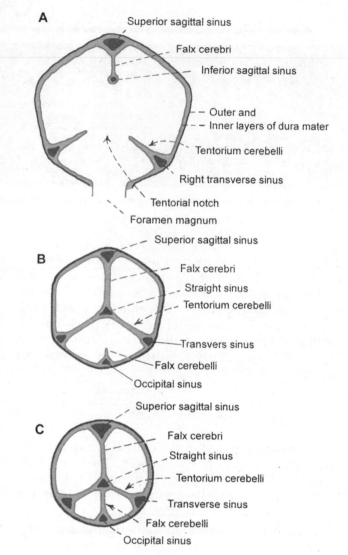

Fig. 6.2: *Coronal sections through the posterior cranial fossa showing folds of dura mater and the venous sinuses enclosed in them. (A) Section through the tentorial notch (anterior part of the fossa); (B) Section through the middle part of the fossa, and (C) Section through the posterior-most part.*

skull bones, and (b) an inner or *meningeal layer* which surrounds the brain. The meningeal layer is continuous with the spinal dura mater.

The two layers are fused to each other at all places, except where the cranial venous sinuses are enclosed between them.

The Endosteal Layer or Endocranium

1. The endocranium is continuous: (a) With the periosteum lining the outside of the skull or pericranium through the sutures and foramina, and (b) with the periosteal lining of the orbit through the superior orbital fissure.

2. It provides sheaths for the cranial nerves: the sheaths fuse with the epineurium outside the skull.

Over the optic nerve, the dura forms a sheath which becomes continuous with the sclera.

3. Its outer surface is adherent to the inner surface of the cranial bones by a number of fine fibrous and vascular processes. The adhesion is most marked at the sutures, on the base of the skull and around the foramen magnum.

The Meningeal Layer

At places, the meningeal layer of dura mater is folded on itself to form partitions which divide the cranial cavity into compartments which lodge different parts of the brain (Fig. 6.2). The folds are the :

A. Falx cerebri   B. Tentorium cerebelli
C   Falx cerebelli   D. Diaphragma sellae

These are described below.

Falx Cerebri

The falx cerebri is a large sickle-shaped fold of dura mater occupying the median longitudinal fissure between the two cerebral hemispheres (Fig. 6.2). It has two ends: (a) The *anterior end* is narrow, and is attached to the crista galli. (b) The *posterior end* is broad, and is attached along the median plane to the upper surface of the tentorium cerebelli.

The falx cerebri has two margins: (a) The *upper margin* is convex and is attached to the lips of the sagittal sulcus; (b) the *lower margin* is concave and free.

The falx cerebri has right and left surfaces each of which is related to the medial surface of the corresponding cerebral hemisphere.

Three important venous sinuses are present in relation to this fold. The *superior sagittal sinus* lies along the upper margin; the *inferior sagittal* sinus along the lower margin; and the *straight sinus* along the line of attachment of the falx to the tentorium cerebelli (Fig. 6.2A, B).

Tentorium Cerebelli

The tentorium cerebelli is a tent-shaped fold of dura mater, forming the roof of the posterior cranial fossa. It separates the cerebellum from the occipital lobes of the cerebrum, and broadly divides the cranial cavity into supratentorial and infratentorial compartments. The infratentorial compartment, in other words, is the posterior cranial fossa containing the hindbrain and the lower part of the midbrain.

The tentorium cerebelli has a free margin and an attached margin (Fig. 6.3). The *anterior free margin* is U-shaped and free. The ends of the 'U' are attached anteriorly to the anterior clinoid processes. This margin bounds the *tentorial notch* which is occupied by the midbrain and the anterior part of the superior vermis. The *outer or attached margin* is convex. Posterolaterally, it is attached to the lips of the transverse sulci on the occipital bone, and on the posteroinferior angle of the parietal bone. Anterolaterally, it is attached to the superior border of the petrous temporal bone and to the posterior clinoid processes. Along the attached margin there are the transverse and superior petrosal venous sinuses. The *trigeminal* or *Meckel's cave* is a recess of dura mater present in relation to the attached margin of the tentorium. It is formed by evagination of the inferior layer of the tentorium over the trigeminal

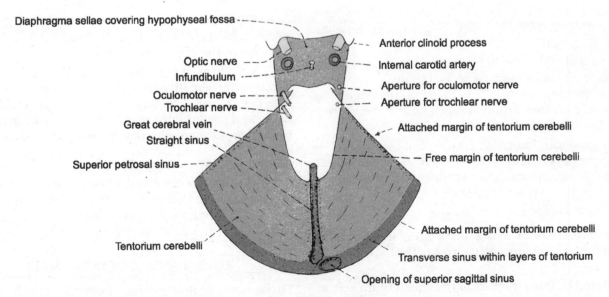

Fig. 6.3: Tentorium cerebelli seen from above.

impression on the petrous temporal bone. It contains the trigeminal ganglion (Fig. 6.4).

The free and attached margins of the tentorium cerebelli cross each other near the apex of the petrous temporal bone. Anterior to the point of crossing there is a triangular area which forms the posterior part of the roof of the cavernous sinus, and is pierced by the third and fourth cranial nerves.

The tentorium cerebelli has two surfaces. The *superior surface* is convex and slopes to either side

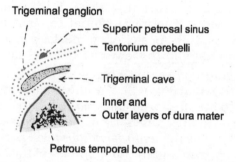

Fig. 6.4: *Parasagittal section through the petrous temporal bone and meninges to show the formation of the trigeminal cave.*

from the median plane. The falx cerebri is attached to this surface, in the midline; the straight sinus lies along the line of this attachment. The superior surface is related to the occipital lobes of the cerebrum. The *inferior surface* is concave and fits the convex superior surface of the cerebellum. The falx cerebelli is attached to its posterior part (Fig. 6.2C).

Falx Cerebelli

The falx cerebelli is a small sickle-shaped fold of dura mater projecting forwards into the posterior cerebellar notch (Fig. 6.2C).

The *base* of the sickle is attached to the posterior part of the inferior surface of the tentorium cerebelli in the median plane. The *apex* of the sickle is frequently divided into two parts which are lost on the sides of the foramen magnum.

The *posterior margin* is convex and is attached to the internal occipital crest. It encloses the occipital sinus. The *anterior margin* is concave and free.

Diaphragma Sellae

The diaphragma sellae is a small circular, horizontal fold of dura mater forming the roof of the hypophyseal fossa.

Anteriorly, it is attached to the tuberculum sellae. Posteriorly, it is attached to the dorsum sellae. On

each side, it is continuous with the dura mater of the middle cranial fossa (Fig. 6.5).

The diaphragma has a central aperture through which the stalk of the hypophysis cerebri passes.

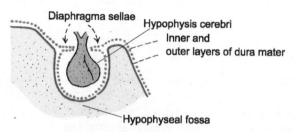

Fig. 6.5: *Diaphragma sellae as seen in a sagittal section through the hypophyseal fossa.*

Blood Supply

The outer layer is richly vascular. The inner meningeal layer is more fibrous and requires little blood supply.

1. The vault or supratentorial space is supplied by the middle meningeal artery.

2. The anterior cranial fossa and the dural lining is supplied by meningeal branches of the anterior ethmoidal, posterior ethmoidal and ophthalmic arteries.

3. The middle cranial fossa is supplied by the middle meningeal, accessory meningeal, and internal carotid arteries; and by meningeal branches of the ascending pharyngeal artery.

4. The posterior cranial fossa is supplied by meningeal branches of the vertebral, occipital and ascending pharyngeal arteries.

Nerve Supply

1. The dura of the *vault* has only a few sensory nerves which are derived mostly from the ophthalmic division of the trigeminal nerve.

2. The dura of the floor has a rich nerve supply and is quite sensitive to pain. (a) The *anterior cranial fossa* is supplied mostly by the anterior ethmoidal nerve and partly by the maxillary nerve, (b) the *middle cranial fossa* is supplied by the maxillary nerve in its anterior half, and by branches of the mandibular nerve and from the trigeminal ganglion in its posterior half, (c) the *posterior cranial fossa* is supplied chiefly by recurrent branches from first, second and third cervical spinal nerves and partly by meningeal branches of the ninth and tenth cranial nerves.

VENOUS SINUSES OF DURA MATER

These are venous spaces, the walls of which are formed by dura mater. They have an inner lining of

1. *Pain sensitive intracranial structures* are:

(a) The large cranial venous sinuses and their tributaries from the surface of the brain;

(b) dural arteries;

(c) the dural floor of the anterior and posterior cranial fossae; and

(d) arteries at the base of the brain.

2. *Headache* may be caused by :

(a) Dilatation of intracranial arteries;

(b) dilatation of extracranial arteries;

(c) traction or distension of intracranial pain sensitive structures;

(d) infection and inflammation of intracranial and extracranial structures supplied by sensory cranial nerves and by cervical nerves.

3. *Extradural and subdural haemorrhages* are both common. An extradural haemorrhage can be distinguished from a subdural haemorrhage because of the following differences.

1. The extradural haemorrhage is arterial due to injury to middle meningeal artery; whereas subdural haemorrhage is venous in nature.

2. Symptoms of cerebral compression are late in extradural haemorrhage.

3. There is no lucid interval in the case of a subdural haemorrhage. In an extradural haemorrhage, a lucid interval is present. This is a temporary phase of consciousness between the earlier unconsciousness of cerebral concussion and the later unconsciousness of cerebral compression.

4. In an extradural haemorrhage, paralysis first appears in the face and then spreads to the lower parts of the body. In a subdural haemorrhage, the progress of paralysis is haphazard.

5. In an extradural haemorrhage, there is no blood in the CSF; while it is a common feature of subdural haemorrhage.

endothelium. There is no muscle in their walls. They have no valves.

Venous sinuses receive venous blood from the brain, the meninges, and bones of the skull. Cerebrospinal fluid is poured into some of them.

Cranial venous sinuses communicate with veins outside the skull through *emissary veins*. These communications help to keep the pressure of blood in the sinuses constant.

There are 23 venous sinuses, of which 8 are paired and 7 are unpaired.

Paired venous sinuses

There is one sinus each on right and left side.

1. Cavernous sinus.
2. Superior petrosal sinus.
3. Inferior petrosal sinus.
4. Transverse sinus.
5. Sigmoid sinus.
6. Sphenoparietal sinus.
7. Petrosquamous sinus.
8. Middle meningeal sinus/veins.

Unpaired venous sinuses

These are median in position.

1. Superior sagittal sinus.
2. Inferior sagittal sinus.
3. Straight sinus.
4. Occipital sinus.
5. Anterior intercavernous sinus.
6. Posterior intercavernous sinus.
7. Basilar plexus of veins.

Cavernous Sinuses

Each cavernous sinus is a large venous space situated in the middle cranial fossa, on either side of the body of the sphenoid bone. Its interior is divided into a number of spaces or caverns by trabeculae. The trabeculae are much less conspicuous in the living than in the dead (Fig. 6.6).

The floor of the sinus is formed by the endosteal dura mater. The lateral wall, roof and medial wall are formed by the meningeal dura mater.

Define the cavernous sinuses situated on each side of the body of the sphenoid bone. Cut through it between the anterior and posterior ends and locate its contents. Define its connections with the other venous sinuses and veins.

Anteriorly, the sinus extends up to the medial end of the superior orbital fissure and *posteriorly*, up to the apex of the petrous temporal bone. It is about 2 cm long, and 1 cm wide.

Relations

Structures outside the sinus:

(a) *Superiorly:* Optic tract, optic chiasma, olfactory tract, internal carotid artery and anterior perforated substance; (b) *inferiorly:* foramen lacerum and the

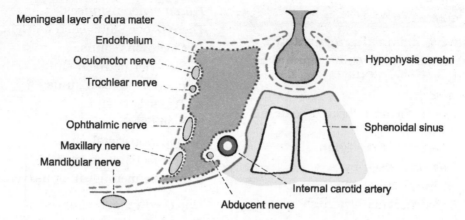

Fig. 6.6: *Coronal section through the middle cranial fossa showing the relations of the cavernous sinus.*

junction of the body and greater wing of the sphenoid bone; (c) *medially:* hypophysis cerebri and sphenoidal air sinus (Fig. 6.6); (d) *laterally:* temporal lobe with uncus; (e) *anteriorly:* superior orbital fissure and the apex of the orbit; (f) *posteriorly:* apex of the petrous temporal and the crus cerebri of the midbrain.

Structures in the Lateral Wall of the Sinus, from above Downwards

(a) *Oculomotor nerve.* In the anterior part of the sinus, it divides into superior and inferior divisions which leave the sinus by passing through the superior orbital fissure; (b) *trochlear nerve.* In the anterior part of the sinus, it crosses superficial to the oculomotor nerve, and enters the orbit through the superior orbital fissure; (c) *ophthalmic nerve.* In the anterior part of the sinus, it divides into the lacrimal, frontal and nasociliary nerves (Figs 7.4, 7.6); (d) *maxillary nerve.* It leaves the sinus by passing through the foramen rotundum on its way to the ptery-

gopalatine fossa; (e) *trigeminal ganglion.* The ganglion and its dural cave project into the posterior part of the lateral wall of the sinus (Fig. 6.4).

Structures Passing through the Centre of the Sinus

(a) *Internal carotid artery* with the venous and sympathetic plexus around it; (b) *abducent nerve,* inferolateral to the internal carotid artery.

The structures in the lateral wall and in the centre of the sinus are separated from blood by the endothelial lining.

Tributaries or Incoming Channels

From the orbit: (a) The superior ophthalmic vein; (b) a branch of the inferior ophthalmic vein or sometimes the vein itself; (c) the central vein of the retina may drain either into the superior ophthalmic vein or into the cavernous sinus (Fig. 6.7).

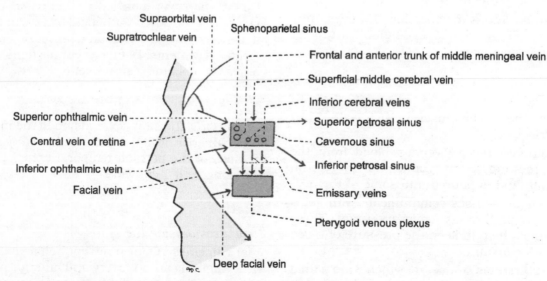

Fig. 6.7: *Side view of the tributaries and communication of the cavernous sinus.*

From the brain: (a) Superficial middle cerebral vein, and (b) inferior cerebral veins from the temporal lobe (Fig. 6.8).

From the meninges: (a) Sphenoparietal sinus; and (b) the frontal trunk of the middle meningeal vein may drain either into the pterygoid plexus through the foramen ovale or into the sphenoparietal or cavernous sinus.

Draining Channels or Communications

The cavernous sinus drains: (a) Into the transverse sinus through the superior petrosal sinus, (b) into the internal jugular vein through the inferior petrosal sinus and through a plexus around the internal carotid artery, (c) into the pterygoid plexus of veins through the emissary veins passing through the foramen ovale, the foramen lacerum and the emissary sphenoidal foramen (Table 1.1), and (d) into the facial vein through the superior ophthalmic vein. (e) The right and left cavernous sinuses communicate with each other through the anterior and posterior intercavernous sinuses and through the basilar plexus of veins (Fig. 6.8).

All these communications are valveless, and blood can flow through them in either direction.

Factors Helping Expulsion of Blood from the Sinus

(a) Expansile pulsations of the internal carotid artery within the sinus, (b) gravity, and (c) position of the head.

Superior Sagittal Sinus

The superior sagittal sinus occupies the upper convex, attached margin of the falx cerebri (Fig. 6.9).

Surface Marking

Superior sagittal sinus is marked by a broad line from the glabella along the sagittal sulcus till the internal occipital protuberance.

It begins anteriorly at the crista galli by the union of tiny meningeal veins. Here it communicates with the veins of the frontal sinus, and occasionally with the veins of the nose, through the foramen caecum. As the sinus runs upwards and backwards, it becomes progressively larger in size. It is triangular on cross-section. It ends near the internal occipital protuberance by turning to one side, usually the right, and becomes continuous with the right transverse sinus (Figs 6.10, 6.11). Sometimes the superior sagittal sinus becomes continuous with the left transverse

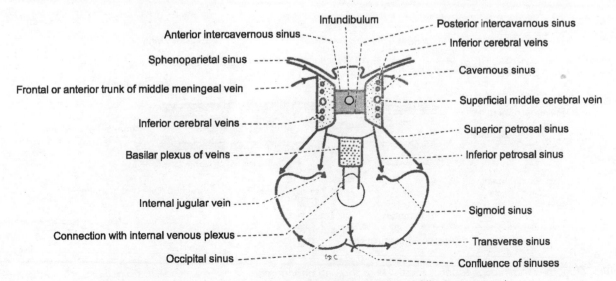

Fig. 6.8: *Superior view of the tributaries and communications of the cavernous sinus.*

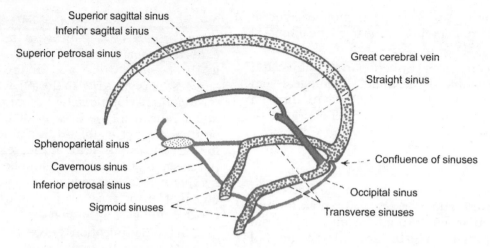

Fig. 6.9: *Scheme to show the intracranial venous sinuses. Lateral view.*

sinus. It generally communicates with the opposite sinus. The junction of all these sinuses is called the *confluence of sinuses*.

The *interior* of the sinus shows: (a) Openings of the superior cerebral veins, (b) openings of venous lacunae, usually three on each side, (c) arachnoid villi and granulations projecting into the lacunae as well as into the sinus, and (d) numerous fibrous bands crossing the inferior angle of the sinus (Fig. 6.10).

Tributaries

The superior sagittal sinus receives these tributaries. (a) Superior cerebral veins which never open into the venous lacunae (Fig. 6.10); (b) parietal emissary veins; (c) venous lacunae, usually three on each side which first, receive the diploic and meningeal veins, and then open into the sinus; (d) occasionally, a vein from the nose opens into the sinus when the foramen caecum is patent.

Inferior Sagittal Sinus

The inferior sagittal sinus, a small channel lies in the posterior two-thirds of the lower, concave free margin of the falx cerebri. It ends by joining the great cerebral vein to form the straight sinus (Fig. 6.9).

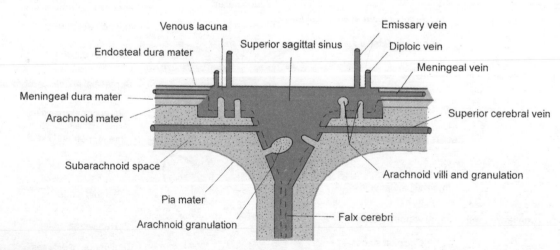

Fig. 6.10: *Coronal section through superior sagittal sinus showing arrangement of the meninges, the arachnoid villi and granulations, and the various (emissary, diploic, meningeal and cerebral) veins in its relation.*

Straight Sinus

The straight sinus lies in the median plane within the junction of falx cerebri and the tentorium cerebelli. It is formed anteriorly by the union of the inferior sagittal sinus with the great cerebral vein, and ends at the internal occipital protuberance by continuing as the transverse sinus usually left (Fig. 6.9). In addition to the veins forming it, it also receives a few of the superior cerebellar veins.

At the termination of the great cerebral vein into the sinus, there exists a ball valve mechanism, formed by a sinusoidal plexus of blood vessels, which regulates the secretion of CSF.

Transverse Sinus

Surface Marking

The transverse sinus is marked by two parallel lines 1.2 cm apart extending between the following two points.

(a) Two points at the inion, situated one above the other and 1.2 cm apart (Fig. 6.11).

(b) Two points at the base of mastoid process, situated one in front of the other 1.2 cm apart.

This sinus is convex upwards, reaching 2 cm above Reid's base line (Chapter 1, Anatomical position of skull).

The transverse sinuses are large sinuses. The right sinus usually larger than the left situated in the posterior part of the attached margin of the tentorium cerebelli. The right transverse sinus is usually a continuation of the superior sagittal sinus, and the left sinus a continuation of the straight sinus. Each sinus extends from the internal occipital protuberance to the posteroinferior angle of the parietal bone at the base of mastoid process where it bends downwards and becomes the sigmoid sinus. Its *tributaries* are: (a) The superior petrosal sinus, (b) the inferior cerebral veins, (c) the inferior cerebellar veins, (d) the diploic (posterior temporal) vein, and (e) the inferior anastomotic vein.

Sigmoid Sinuses

Surface Marking

The sigmoid sinus is marked by two parallel lines situated 1.2 cm apart and extending between the following points:

(a) Two points at the base of the mastoid process, situated one in front of the other 1.2 cm apart (Fig. 6.11).

(b) Two similar points near the posterior border and 1.2 cm above the tip of the mastoid process.

Each sinus right or left is the direct continuation of the transverse sinus. It is S-shaped: hence the name. It extends from the posteroinferior angle of the parietal bone to the posterior part of the jugular foramen where it becomes the superior bulb of the internal jugular vein. It grooves the mastoid part of the temporal bone, where *it is separated anteriorly from the mastoid antrum and mastoid air cells by only*

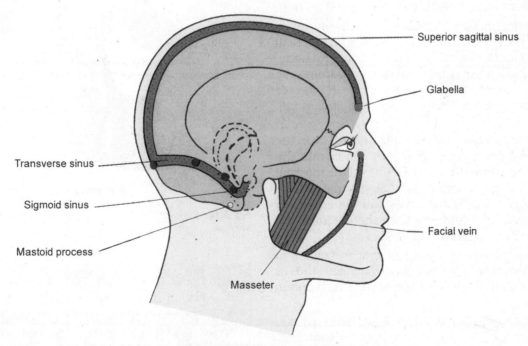

Fig. 6.11: *Venous sinuses and facial vein.*

a thin plate of bone. Its tributaries are: (a) The mastoid and condylar emissary veins, (b) cerebellar veins; and (c) the internal auditory vein.

Other Sinuses

The *occipital sinus* is small, and lies in the attached margin of the falx cerebelli. It begins near the foramen magnum and ends in the confluence of sinuses. (Figs 6.2, 6.9)

The *sphenoparietal sinuses,* right and left lie along the posterior free margin of the lesser wing of the sphenoid bone, and drain into the anterior part of the cavernous sinus. Each sinus may receive the frontal trunk of the middle meningeal vein (Fig. 6.8).

The *superior petrosal sinuses* lie in the anterior part of the attached margin of the tentorium cerebelli along the upper border of the petrous temporal bone. The sinus crosses the trigeminal nerve. It drains the cavernous sinus into the transverse sinus. It receives some inferior cerebral, cerebellar and tympanic veins. (Fig. 6.8).

The *inferior petrosal sinuses* right and left lie in the corresponding petro-occipital fissure, and drain the cavernous sinus into the superior bulb of the internal jugular vein. They receive: (a) Labyrinthine veins through the cochlear canaliculus and the aqueduct of the vestibule; and (b) veins from the medulla, the pons and the cerebellum (Fig. 6.9).

The *basilar plexus of veins* lies over the clivus of the skull. It connects the two inferior petrosal sinuses and communicates with the internal vertebral venous plexus.

The *middle meningeal veins* form two main trunks, one frontal or anterior and one parietal or posterior, which accompany the two branches of the middle meningeal artery. The *frontal trunk* may end either in the pterygoid plexus through the foramen ovale, or in the sphenoparietal or cavernous sinus. The *parietal trunk* usually ends in the pterygoid plexus through the foramen spinosum. The meningeal veins are nearer to the bone than the arteries, and are, therefore, more liable to injury in fractures of the skull.

The *petrosquamous sinus* may or may not be present. It lies in the petrosquamous fissure, and drains into the transverse sinus.

The anterior and posterior *intercavernous sinuses* connect the cavernous sinuses. They pass through the diaphragma sellae, one in front and the other behind the infundibulum. With the cavernous sinuses they form the circular sinus. The irregular venous channels below the hypophysis cerebri drain into the intercavernous sinuses (Fig. 6.8).

Hypophysis Cerebri (Pituitary gland)

Introduction: The hypophysis cerebri is a small endocrine gland situated in relation to the base of the brain. It is often called the master of the endocrine orchestra because it produces a number of hormones which control the secretions of many other endocrine glands of the body (Fig. 6.12).

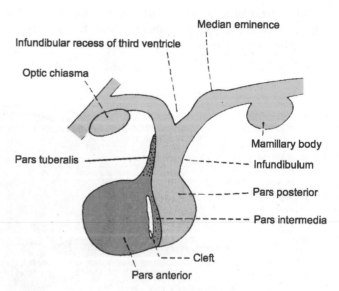

Fig. 6.12: *Parts of the hypophysis cerebri as seen in a sagittal section.*

DISSECTION

Identify diaphragma sellae over the hypophyseal fossa. Incise it radially and locate the hypophysis cerebri lodged in its fossa. Take it out and examine it in detail with the hand lens (Fig. 6.5).

The gland lies in the hypophyseal fossa or sella turcica or pituitary fossa. The fossa is roofed by the diaphragma sellae. The stalk of the hypophysis cerebri pierces the diaphragma sellae and is attached above to the floor of the third ventricle.

The gland is oval in shape, and measures 8 mm anteroposteriorly and 12 mm transversely. It weighs about 500 mg.

Relations

Superiorly: (a) Diaphragma sellae; (b) optic chiasma; (c) tuber cinerium; and (d) infundibular recess of the third ventricle.

Inferiorly: (a) Irregular venous channels between the two layers of dura mater lining the floor of the hypophyseal fossa; (b) hypophyseal fossa; and (c) sphenoidal air sinuses (Figs 6.6, 6.12 and 29.2).

On each side: The cavernous sinus with its contents.

Subdivisions

The gland has two main parts: *Adenohypophysis* and *neurohypophysis* which differ from each other embryologically, morphologically and functionally. The adenohypophysis develops as an upward growth called the Rathke's pouch from the ectodermal roof of the stomodeum. The neurohypophysis develops as a downward growth from the floor of the diencephalon, and is connected to the hypothalamus by neural pathways. Further subdivisions of each part are given below.

Adenohypophysis

a. *Anterior lobe* or *pars anterior, pars distalis,* or *pars glandularis.* This is the largest part of the gland (Fig. 6.12).

b. *Intermediate lobe* or *pars intermedia.* This is in the form of a thin strip which is separated from the anterior lobe by an intraglandular cleft, a remnant of the lumen of Rathke's pouch.

c. *Tuberal lobe* or *pars tuberalis.* It is an upward extension of the anterior lobe that surrounds and forms part of the infundibulum.

Neurohypophysis

a. *Posterior lobe* or *neural lobe, pars posterior.* It is smaller than the anterior lobe and lies in the posterior concavity of the larger anterior lobe.

b. *Infundibular stem,* which contains the neural connections of the posterior lobe with the hypothalamus.

c. *Median eminence* of the tuber cinerium which is continuous with the infundibular stem.

Arterial Supply

The hypophysis cerebri is supplied by the following branches of the internal carotid artery.

1. One superior hypophyseal artery on each side (Fig. 6.13).

2. One inferior hypophyseal artery on each side. Each superior hypophyseal artery supplies: (a) The ventral part of the hypothalamus, (b) the upper part of the infundibulum, and (c) the lower part of the infundibulum through a separate long descending branch, called the trabecular artery.

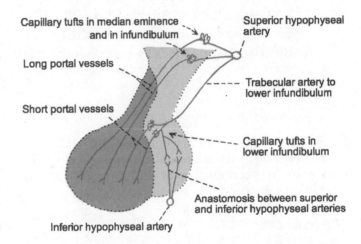

Fig. 6.13: *Arterial supply of the hypophysis cerebri. Note that the neurohypophysis is supplied by the superior and inferior hypophyseal arteries, and the adenohypophysis, exclusively by the portal vessels.*

Each inferior hypophyseal artery divides into medial and lateral branches which join one another to form an arterial ring around the posterior lobe. Branches from this ring supply the posterior lobe and also anastomose with branches from the superior hypophyseal artery.

The anterior lobe or pars distalis is supplied exclusively by *portal vessels* arising from capillary tufts formed by the superior hypophyseal arteries (Fig. 6.13). The long portal vessels drain the median eminence and the upper infundibulum, and the short portal vessels drain the lower infundibulum. The portal vessels are of great functional importance because they carry the *hormone releasing factors* from the hypothalamus to the anterior lobe where they control the secretory cycles of different glandular cells.

Venous Drainage

Short veins emerge on the surface of the gland and drain into neighbouring dural venous sinuses. The hormones pass out of the gland through the venous blood, and are carried to their target cells.

Histology and Hormones

Anterior Lobe

Chromophilic cells (50%)

(a) *Acidophils/alpha-cells;* about 43%
1. Somatotrophs: Secrete growth hormone (STH, GH).
2. Mammotrophs (prolactin cells): Secrete lactogenic hormone.
3. Corticotrophs: Secrete ACTH.

(b) *Basophils/beta-cells,* about 7% of cells
1. Thyrotrophs: Secrete TSH.
2. Gonadotrophs: Secrete FSH.
3. Luteotrophs: Secrete LH or ICSH.

II. *Chromophobic cells 50%* represent the non-secretory phase of the other cell types, or their precursors.

Intermediate Lobe

It is made up of numerous basophil cells, and chromophobe cells surrounding masses of colloid material. It secretes the melanocyte stimulating hormone (MSH).

Posterior Lobe

It is composed of: (a) A large number of nonmyelinated fibres-hypothalamo-hypophyseal tract, and (b) modified neurological cells, called *pituicytes.* They have many dendrites which terminate on or near the sinusoids.

The hypothalamo-hypophyseal tract begins in the preoptic and paraventricular nuclei of the hypothalamus. Its short fibres terminate in relation to capillary tufts of portal vessels, providing the possibility for a neural control of the secretory activity of the anterior lobe. The long fibres of the neurosecretory tract pass to the posterior lobe and terminate near vascular sinusoids.

The hormones related to the posterior lobe are: (a) *Vasopressin (ADH)* which acts on kidney tubules, and (b) *oxytocin* which promotes contraction of the uterine and mammary smooth muscle. These hormones are actually secreted by the hypothalamus, from where these are transported through the hypothalamo-hypophyseal tract to the posterior lobe of the gland.

Trigeminal Ganglion

This is the *sensory ganglion* of the fifth cranial nerve. It is homologous with the dorsal nerve root ganglia of spinal nerves. All such ganglia are made up of pseudounipolar nerve cells, with a 'T'-shaped arrangement of their process; one process arises from

---

CLINICAL ANATOMY

Pituitary tumours give rise to two main categories of symptoms:

A. *General symptoms* due to pressure over surrounding structures: (a) The sella turcica is enlarged in size, (b) pressure over the optic chiasma causes bitemporal hemianopia or bitemporal upper quadrantic hemianopia; (c) pressure over the hypothalamus may cause one of the hypothalamic syndromes like obesity of Frolich's syndrome in cases with Rathke's pouch tumours, and (d) a large tumour may press upon the third ventricle, causing a rise in intracranial pressure.

B. *Specific symptoms* depending on the cell type of the tumour. (a) Acidophil or eosinophil adenoma causes acromegaly in adults and gigantism in younger patients, (b) basophil adenoma causes Cushing's syndrome, (c) chromophobe adenoma causes effects of hypopituitarism, (d) posterior lobe damage causes diabetes insipidus, although the lesion in these cases usually lies in the hypothalamus.

the cell body which then divides into a central and a peripheral process.

The ganglion is crescentic or semilunar in shape, with its convexity directed anterolaterally. The three

DISSECTION

Identify trigeminal ganglion situated on the anterior surface of petrous temporal bone near its apex. Define the three branches emerging from its convex anterior surface.

divisions of the trigeminal nerve emerge from this convexity. The posterior concavity of the ganglion receives the sensory root of the nerve (Fig. 6.14).

Surface Marking

Trigeminal ganglion lies a little in front of the preauricular point at a depth of about 5 cm.

Situation and Meningeal Relations

The ganglion lies on the *trigeminal impression,* on the anterior surface of the petrous temporal bone near its apex. It occupies a special space of dura mater, called the *trigeminal or Meckel's cave.* There are two layers of dura below the ganglion (Fig. 6.14). The cave is lined by pia-arachnoid, so that the ganglion along with the motor root of the trigeminal nerve is surrounded by CSF. The ganglion lies at a depth of about 5 cm from the preauricular point.

Relations

Medially: (a) Internal carotid artery, and (b) posterior part of cavernous sinus.

Laterally: Middle meningeal artery.

Superiorly: Parahippocampal gyrus.

Inferiorly: (a) Motor root of trigeminal nerve, (b) greater petrosal nerve, (c) apex of the petrous temporal bone, and (d) the foramen lacerum (Fig. 6.14).

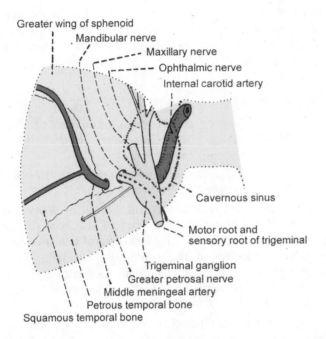

Fig. 6.14: *Superior view of the middle cranial fossa showing some of its contents.*

Associated Root and Branches

The central processes of the ganglion cells form the large *sensory root* of the trigeminal nerve which is attached to pons at its junction with the middle cerebellar peduncle.

The peripheral processes of the ganglion cells form three divisions of the trigeminal nerve, namely the *ophthalmic, maxillary and mandibular.*

The small *motor root* of the trigeminal nerve is attached to the pons superomedial to the sensory root. It passes under the ganglion from its medial to the lateral side, and joins the mandibular nerve at the foramen ovale.

Blood Supply

The ganglion is supplied by twigs from the (a) Internal carotid; (b) middle meningeal; and (c) accessory meningeal arteries and (d) by the meningeal branch of the ascending pharyngeal artery.

Middle Meningeal Artery

The middle meningeal artery is important to the surgeon because this artery is the commonest source of extradural haemorrhage, which is an acute surgical emergency (Fig. 6.14).

Origin: The artery is a branch of the first part of the maxillary artery, given off in the infratemporal fossa. (Chapter 10)

Surface Marking

The artery is marked by joining the following points.

(a) A point immediately above the middle of the zygoma. The artery enters the skull opposite this point (Fig. 1.9); (b) a second point 2 cm above the first point. The artery divides deep to this point; (c) a third point at centre of pterion 3.5 cm behind and 1.5 cm above the frontozygomatic suture. It can also be marked as a point 4 cm above the midpoint of the zygomatic arch; (d) a fourth point midway between the nasion and inion; (e) a fifth point called the lambda 6 cm above the external occipital protuberance.

The line joining points (a) and (b) represents the stem of the middle meningeal artery inside the skull.

The line joining points (b), (c) and (d) represents the anterior or frontal branch. It first runs upwards and forwards (b-c) and then upwards and backwards, towards the point 'd'.

The line joining points (b) and (e) represents the posterior or parietal branch. It runs backwards and upwards, towards the point 'e'.

Course and Relations

1. In the infratemporal fossa, the artery runs upwards and medially deep to the lateral pterygoid muscle and superficial to the sphenomandibular ligament. Here it passes through a loop formed by the two roots of the auriculotemporal nerve (Figs 10.6, 10.10).

2. It enters the middle cranial fossa through the foramen spinosum, (which also transmits the meningeal branch of the mandibular nerve and the parietal trunk of the middle meningeal vein) (Fig. 6.14).

3. In the middle cranial fossa, the artery has an extradural course, but the middle meningeal veins are closer to the bone than the artery. Here the artery runs forwards and laterally for a variable distance, grooving the squamous temporal bone, and divides into a frontal and parietal branch (Fig. 6.14).

4. The *frontal* or *anterior branch* is larger than the parietal branch. First it runs forwards and laterally towards the lateral end of the lesser wing of the sphenoid. Then it runs obliquely upwards and backwards, parallel to, and a little in front of the central sulcus of the cerebral hemisphere. Thus after crossing the pterion the artery is closely related to the motor area of the cerebral cortex.

5. The *parietal* or *posterior branch* runs backwards over, or near, the superior temporal sulcus of the cerebrum, about 4 cm above the level of the zygomatic arch. It ends in front of the posteroinferior angle of the parietal bone by dividing into branches.

Branches

The middle meningeal artery supplies only small branches to the dura mater. It is predominantly a periosteal artery supplying bone and red bone marrow in the diploe.

CLINICAL ANATOMY

The middle meningeal artery is of great surgical importance because it can be torn in head injuries resulting in *extradural haemorrhage. The frontal* or *anterior branch* is commonly involved. The haematoma presses on the motor area, giving rise to hemiplegia of the opposite side. The anterior division can be approached surgically by making a hole in the skull over the pterion, 4 cm above the midpoint of the zygomatic arch.

Rarely, the parietal or posterior branch is implicated, causing contralateral deafness. In this case, the hole is made at a point 4 cm above and 4 cm behind the external acoustic meatus.

Within the cranial cavity it gives off: (1) *Ganglionic branches* to the trigeminal ganglion; (2) a *petrosal branch* to the hiatus for the greater petrosal nerve; (3) a *superior tympanic branch* to the tensor tympani; (4) *temporal branches* to the temporal fossa; and (5) *anastomotic branch* that enters the orbit and anastomoses with the lacrimal artery.

Other Structures Seen in Cranial Fossae after Removal of Brain

The structures seen after removal of the brain are: 12 cranial nerves, cavernous part of internal carotid artery, four petrosal nerves and fourth part of the vertebral artery.

Cranial Nerves

The *first* or *olfactory nerve* is seen in the form of 15 to 20 filaments on each side that pierce the cribriform plate of the ethmoid bone.

The *second* or *optic nerve* passes through the optic canal with the ophthalmic artery.

The *third* or *oculomotor* and *fourth* or *trochlear nerves* pierce the posterior part of the roof of the cavernous sinus formed by crossing of the free and attached margins of the tentorium cerebelli; next they run in the lateral wall of the cavernous sinus. They enter the orbit through the superior orbital fissure (Figs 6.3, 7.4).

The *fifth* or *trigeminal nerve*, has a large sensory root and a small motor root. The roots cross the apex of the petrous temporal bone beneath the superior petrosal sinus, to enter the middle cranial fossa (Fig. 6.14).

The *sixth* or *abducent nerve* pierces the lower part of the posterior wall of the cavernous sinus near the apex of the petrous temporal bone. It runs forwards by the side of the dorsum sellae beneath the petrosphenoidal ligament to reach the centre of the cavernous sinus (Figs 6.6, 7.14).

The *seventh* or *facial* and *eighth* or *stato-acoustic* or vestibulocochlear nerves pass through the internal acoustic meatus with the labyrinthine vessels (Fig. 24.1).

The *ninth* or *glossopharyngeal, tenth* or *vagus and eleventh* or *accessory nerves* pierce the dura mater at the jugular foramen and pass out through it. The spinal part of the accessory nerve first enters the posterior cranial fossa through the foramen magnum, and then passes out through the jugular foramen (Fig. 24.1).

The two parts of the *twelfth* or *hypoglossal nerve* pierce the dura mater separately opposite the hypoglossal canal and then pass out through it.

Internal Carotid Artery (Cavernous Part)

The internal carotid artery begins in the neck as one of the terminal branches of the common carotid artery at the level of the upper border of the thyroid cartilage. Its course is divided into the following four parts.

Cervical part: In the neck it lies within the carotid sheath. This part gives no branches (Fig. 8.12).

Petrous part: Within the petrous part of the temporal bone, in the carotid canal. It will be studied at a later stage.

Cavernous part: Within the cavernous sinus (Fig. 6.6). This part of the artery gives off:

(a) Cavernous branches to the trigeminal ganglion; and (b) the superior and inferior hypophyseal branches to the hypophysis cerebri.

Cerebral part: This part lies at the base of the brain after emerging from the cavernous sinus (Fig. 31.1). It gives off the following arteries: (a) Ophthalmic; (b) anterior cerebral; (c) middle cerebral; (d) posterior communicating; and (e) anterior choroidal. Of these, the ophthalmic artery supplies structures in the orbit; while the others supply the brain.

The curvatures of the petrous, cavernous and cerebral parts of the internal carotid artery together form an 'S'-shaped figure, the carotid siphon of angiograms.

Petrosal Nerves

1. The *greater petrosal nerve* (Fig. 6.14) carries gustatory and parasympathetic fibres. It arises from the geniculate ganglion of the facial nerve, and enters the middle cranial fossa through the hiatus for the greater petrosal nerve on the anterior surface of the petrous temporal bone. It proceeds towards the foramen lacerum, where it joins the deep petrosal nerve which carries sympathetic fibres to form the nerve of the pterygoid canal (Table 1.3).

The nerve of the pterygoid canal passes through the pterygoid canal to reach the pterygopalatine ganglion. The parasympathetic fibres relay in this ganglion. Postganglionic parasympathetic fibres arising in the ganglion ultimately supply the lacrimal gland and the mucosal glands of the nose, palate and pharynx (Fig. 15.13). The gustatory or taste fibres do not relay in the ganglion and are distributed to the palate.

2. The *deep petrosal nerve*, sympathetic in nature is a branch of the sympathetic plexus around the internal carotid artery. It contains postganglionic fibres from the superior cervical sympathetic ganglion. The nerve joins the greater petrosal nerve to form the nerve of the pterygoid canal. The sympathetic fibres in it are distributed through the branches of the pterygopalatine ganglion (Table 1.3).

3. The *lesser petrosal nerve* parasympathetic in nature is a branch of the tympanic plexus, deriving its preganglionic parasympathetic fibres from the tympanic branch of the glossopharyngeal nerve. It emerges through the hiatus for the lesser petrosal nerve, situated just lateral to the hiatus for the greater petrosal nerve, passes out of the skull through the foramen ovale, and ends in the otic ganglion (Fig. 10.15). Postganglionic fibres arising in the ganglion supply the parotid gland through the auriculo-temporal nerve (Table 1.3).

4. The *external petrosal nerve*, sympathetic in nature is an inconstant branch from the sympathetic plexus around the middle meningeal artery to the geniculate ganglion of the facial nerve.

Fourth Part of the Vertebral Artery

It enters the posterior cranial fossa through the foramen magnum after piercing the dura mater near the skull. A small part of this artery has been seen in Chapter 4. Rest will be studied in Chapters 13 and 31.

07

Contents of the Orbit

The orbits are bony cavities lodging the eyeballs, various muscles, nerves, blood vessels and lacrimal gland. Out of 12 pairs of cranial nerves; IInd, IIIrd, IVth, VIth, a part of Vth, and some sympathetic fibres are dedicated to the contents of orbit only. Nature has provided orbit for the safety of the eyeball. We must also try and look after our orbits and their contents.

Introduction

The orbits are pyramidal cavities, situated one on each side of the root of the nose. They provide sockets for rotatory movements of the eyeball. The long axis of the each orbit passes backwards and medially. The medial walls are parallel to each other, but the lateral walls are set at right angles to each other.

DISSECTION

Strip the endosteum from the floor of the anterior cranial fossa. Gently break the orbital plate of frontal bone forming the roof of the orbit and remove it in pieces so that orbital periosteum is clearly visible. Medially the ethmoidal vessels and nerves should be preserved. Posteriorly, identify the optic canal and superior orbital fissure and structures traversing these. Define the orbital fascia and fascial sheath of eyeball.

Divide the orbital periosteum along the middle of the orbit anteroposteriorly. Cut through it horizontally close to anterior margin of orbit.

The *contents* of the orbit are listed below.

1. *Eyeball:* It will be studied in detail separately (Chapter 19).

2. *Fascia:* Orbital and bulbar.

3. *Muscles:* Extraocular.

4. *Vessels:* Ophthalmic artery, superior and inferior ophthalmic veins, and lymphatics.

5. *Nerves:* Optic, oculomotor, trochlear and abducent; branches of ophthalmic and maxillary nerves, and sympathetic nerves.

6. *Lacrimal gland:* It has already been studied in Chapter 2.

7. *Orbital fat.*

Visual Axis and Orbital Axis

Axis passing through centres of anterior and posterior poles of the eyeball is known as visual axis. It makes an angle of 20–25° with the orbital axis (Fig. 1.23), i.e. line passing through optic canal and centre of base of orbit, i.e. opening on the face.

Orbital Fascia or Periorbita

It forms the *periosteum* of the bony orbit. Due to the loose connection to bone, it can be easily stripped. Posteriorly, it is continuous with the dura mater and with the sheath of the optic nerve. Anteriorly, it is continuous with the periosteum lining the bones around the orbital margin (Fig. 7.1).

There is a gap in the periorbita over the inferior orbital fissure. This gap is bridged by connective tissue with some smooth muscle fibres in it. These fibres constitute the orbitalis muscle.

(a) At the upper and lower margins of the orbit the orbital fascia sends off flap-like continuations into the eyelids. These extensions form the *orbital septum;* (b) a process of the fascia holds the fibrous pulley of the tendon of the superior oblique muscle in place; (c) another process forms the *lacrimal fascia* which bridges the lacrimal groove.

Fascial Sheath of Eyeball or Bulbar Fascia

1. *Tenon's capsule* forms a thin, loose membranous sheath around the eyeball, extending from

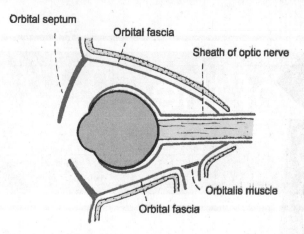

Fig. 7.1: *Orbital fascia and fascial sheath of the eyeball as seen in a parasagittal section.*

the optic nerve to the sclerocorneal junction or limbus. It is separated from the sclera by the episcleral space which is traversed by delicate fibrous bands. The eyeball can freely move within this sheath.

2. The *sheath* is pierced by: (a) The tendons of the various extraocular muscles; and (b) The ciliary vessels and nerves around the entrance of the optic nerve.

3. The sheath gives off a number of expansions. (a) A *tubular sheath* covers each orbital muscle; (b) the *medial check ligament* is a strong triangular expansion from the sheath of the medial rectus muscle; it is attached to the lacrimal bone; (c) the *lateral check ligament* is a strong triangular expansion from the sheath of the lateral rectus muscle; it is attached to the zygomatic bone (Fig. 7.2).

4. The lower part of Tenon's capsule is thickened, and is named the *suspensory ligament of the eye* or the *suspensory ligament of Lockwood* (Fig. 7.3). It is expanded in the centre and narrow at its extremities, and is slung like a hammock below the eyeball. It is formed by union of the margins of the sheaths of the inferior rectus and the inferior oblique muscles with the medial and lateral check ligaments.

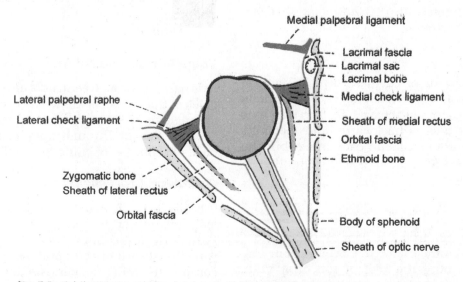

Fig. 7.2: *Orbital fascia and fascial sheath of the eyeball as seen in transverse section.*

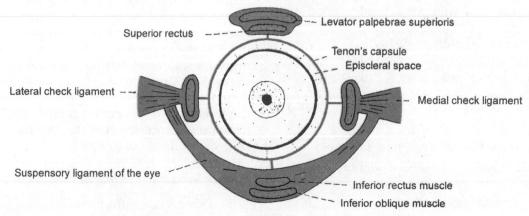

Fig. 7.3: *Fascial sheath of the eyeball as seen in coronal section.*

EXTRAOCULAR MUSCLES

The extraocular muscles are as follows.

Voluntary Muscles

1. Four recti: (a) Superior rectus; (b) inferior rectus; (c) medial rectus; and (d) lateral rectus.

2. Two obliqui: (a) Superior oblique; and (b) inferior oblique.

3. The levator palpebrae superioris elevates the upper eyelid.

Involuntary Muscles

1. The superior tarsal muscle is the deeper portion of the levator palpebrae superioris. It is inserted on the upper margin of the superior tarsus. It elevates the upper eyelid.

2. The inferior tarsal muscle extends from the fascial sheath of the inferior rectus and inferior oblique to the lower margin of the inferior tarsus. It possibly depresses the lower eyelid.

3. The orbitalis bridges the inferior orbital fissure. Its action is uncertain (Fig. 7.1).

DISSECTION

Identify and preserve the trochlear nerve entering the superior oblique muscle in the superomedial angle of the orbit. Find the frontal nerve lying in the midline on the levator palpebrae superioris. It divides into two terminal divisions in the anterior part of orbit.

Beneath the levator palpebrae superioris is the superior rectus muscle. The upper division of oculomotor nerve lies between these two muscles, supplying both of them. Along the lateral wall of the orbit look for lacrimal nerve and artery to reach the superolateral corner of the orbit.

Follow the tendon of superior oblique muscle passing superolaterally beneath the superior rectus to be inserted into sclera behind the equator. After identification, divide frontal nerve, levator palpebrae superioris and superior rectus in the middle of the orbit and reflect them apart. Identify the optic nerve and other structures crossing it. These are nasociliary nerve, ophthalmic artery and superior ophthalmic vein. Along with the optic nerve find two long ciliary nerves and 12–20 short ciliary nerves. Remove the orbital fat and look carefully in the posterior part of the interval between the optic nerve and lateral rectus muscle along the lateral wall of the orbit and identify the pin head sized ciliary ganglion. Trace the roots

connecting it to the nasociliary nerve and nerve to inferior oblique muscle.

Lastly, identify the abducent nerve closely adherent to the medial surface of lateral rectus muscle.

Incise the inferior fornix of conjunctiva and palpebral fascia. Elevate the eyeball and remove the fat and fascia to identify the origin of inferior oblique muscle from the floor of the orbit anteriorly.

Identify the levator palpebrae superioris and superior rectus above the eyeball, superior oblique superomedially, medial rectus medially, lateral rectus laterally, and inferior rectus inferiorly.

The voluntary muscles are miniature ribbon muscles, having short tendons of origin and long tendons of insertion.

Voluntary Muscles

Origin

1. The four recti arise from a *common annular tendon* or *tendinous ring*. This ring is attached to the orbital surface of the apex of the orbit. It encloses the optic canal and the middle part of the superior orbital fissure (Fig. 7.4). The lateral rectus has an additional small tendinous head which arises from the orbital surface of the greater wing of the sphenoid bone lateral to the tendinous ring.

2. The superior oblique arises from the body of the sphenoid, superomedial to the optic canal.

3. The inferior oblique arises from the orbital surface of the maxilla, lateral to the lacrimal groove. The muscle is situated near the anterior margin of the orbit.

4. The levator palpebrae superioris arises from the orbital surface of the lesser wing of the sphenoid bone, anterosuperior to the optic canal and to the origin of the superior rectus.

Insertion

1. The recti are inserted into the sclera, a little posterior to the limbus. The average distances of the insertions from the cornea are: superior 7.7 mm; inferior 6.5 mm, medial 5.5 mm; lateral 6.9 mm (Fig. 7.5).

2. The tendon of the superior oblique passes through a fibrocartilaginous pulley attached to the trochlear fossa of the frontal bone. The tendon then passes laterally, downwards and backward below the superior rectus. It is inserted into the sclera behind the equator of the eyeball, between the superior rectus and the lateral rectus.

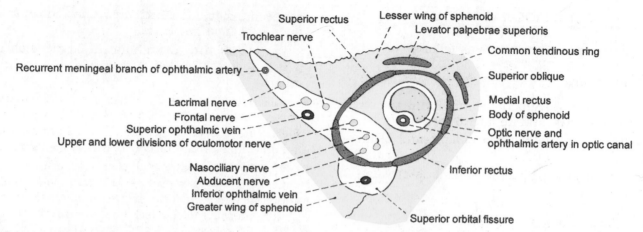

Fig. 7.4: *Apical part of the orbit showing the origins of the extraocular muscles, the common tendinous ring and the structures passing through superior orbital fissure.*

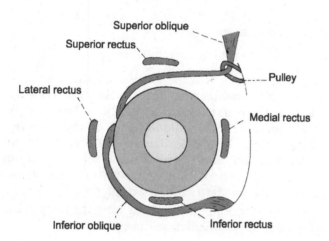

Fig. 7.5: *Scheme to show the insertion of the oblique muscles of the eyeball.*

3. The inferior oblique is fleshy throughout. It passes laterally, upwards and backwards below the inferior rectus and then deep to the lateral rectus. The inferior oblique is inserted close to the superior oblique a little below and posterior to the latter.

4. The flat tendon of the levator splits into a superior or voluntary and an inferior or involuntary lamellae. The superior lamella of the levator is inserted into the anterior surface of the superior tarsus, and into the skin of the upper eyelid. The inferior lamella is inserted into the upper margin of the superior tarsus (Fig. 2.27B).

Nerve Supply

1. The superior oblique is supplied by the IVth cranial or trochlear nerve (SO4) (Fig. 7.6).

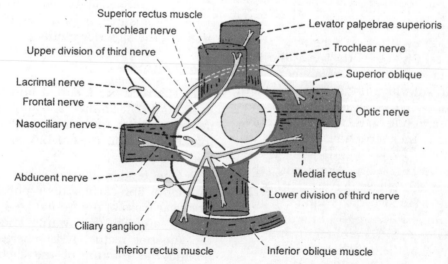

Fig. 7.6: *Scheme to show the nerve supply of the extraocular muscles.*

2. The lateral rectus is supplied by the VIth cranial or abducent nerve (LR6).

3. The remaining five extraocular muscles; superior, inferior and medial recti; inferior oblique and levator palpebrae superioris are all supplied by the IIIrd cranial or oculomotor nerve.

Actions

A. The *movements of the eyeball* are as follows.

I. *Around a transverse axis*

  1. Upward rotation or elevation (33°).

  2. Downwards rotation or depression (33°).

II. *Around a vertical axis*

  1. Medial rotation or adduction (50°).

  2. Lateral rotation or abduction (50°).

III. *Around an anteroposterior axis*

  1. Intortion.

  2. Extortion.

The rotatory movements of the eyeball upwards, downwards, medially or laterally, are defined in terms of the direction of movement of the centre of the pupil. The tortions are defined in terms of the direction of movement of the upper margin of the pupil at 12 O'clock position.

IV. The movements given above can take place in various combinations.

B. *Actions of individual muscles* as shown in Figs 7.7A, 7.7B and Table 7.1.

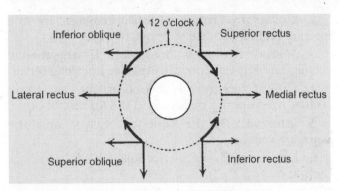

Fig. 7.7A: *Scheme to show the action of the extraocular muscles. Arrows indicates the direction of movement.*

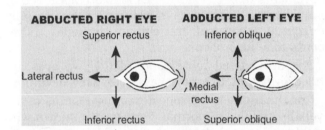

Fig. 7.7B: *The action of extraocular muscles while looking to the right side.*

C. *Single* or *pure movements* are produced by combined actions of muscles. Similar actions get added together, while opposing actions cancel each other enabling pure movements.

1. *Upward rotation or elevation:* By the superior rectus and the inferior oblique.

	Table 7.1: Action of individual muscles		
Muscle	*In primary position*	*Abducted eye*	*Adducted eye*
1. Superior oblique (Fig. 7.7A, B)	Depression Abduction Intortion	Only intortion	Only depression
2. Inferior oblique	Elevation Abduction Extortion	Only extortion	Only elevation
3. Inferior rectus (Fig. 7.7A)	Depression Adduction Extortion	Only depression	Only extortion
4. Superior rectus	Elevation Adduction Intortion	Only elevation	Only intortion
5. Medial rectus	Only adduction	—	—
6. Lateral rectus	Only abduction	—	—

2. *Downward rotation or depression:* By the inferior rectus and the superior oblique.

3. *Medial rotation or adduction:* By the medial rectus, the superior rectus and the inferior rectus.

4. *Lateral rotation or abduction:* By the lateral rectus, the superior oblique and the inferior oblique.

5. *Intortion:* By the superior oblique and the superior rectus.

6. *Extortion:* By the inferior oblique and the inferior rectus.

D. *Combined movements of the eyes*

Normally, movements of the two eyes are harmoniously coordinated. Such coordinated movements of both eyes are called *conjugate ocular movements.* Conjugate movements are usually horizontal or vertical, but oblique conjugate movements may also occur.

The dissociated movements of the two eyes are called as dysjunctive movements, viz., skew deviation.

Conclination or anteroposterior movements of the eyeballs are also abnormal. Persons are known who could squeeze out their eyeballs and take them back at will.

CLINICAL ANATOMY

1. Weakness or paralysis of a muscle causes *squint or strabismus,* which may be concomitant or paralytic. *Concomitant squint* is congenital; there is no limitation of movement, and no diplopia.

In *paralytic squint,* movements are limited, diplopia and vertigo are present, head is turned in the direction of the function of paralysed muscle, and there is a false orientation of the field of vision.

2. *Nystagmus* is characterized by involuntary, rhythmical oscillatory movements of the eyes. This is due to incoordination of the ocular muscles. It may be either vestibular or cerebellar, or even congenital.

3. The *anterior ciliary arteries* arise from the muscular branches of ophthalmic artery. The muscular arteries are important in this respect.

VESSELS OF THE ORBIT

Ophthalmic Artery

Origin

The ophthalmic artery is a branch of the cerebral part of the internal carotid artery, given off medial to the anterior clinoid process close to the optic canal (Figs 7.8, 7.9).

DISSECTION

Trace the ophthalmic artery after it was seen to cross over the optic nerve along with nasociliary nerve and superior ophthalmic vein. Identify its branches especially the central artery of the retina which is an 'end artery'.

Course and Relations

1. The artery enters the orbit through the optic canal, lying inferolateral to the optic nerve. Both the artery and nerve lie in a common dural sheath.

2. In the orbit, the artery pierces the dura mater, ascends over the lateral side of the optic nerve, and crosses above the nerve from lateral to medial side along with the nasociliary nerve. It then runs forwards along the medial wall of the orbit between the superior oblique and the medial rectus muscles, and parallel to the nasociliary nerve.

3. It terminates near the medial angle of the eye by dividing into the supratrochlear and dorsal nasal branches (Fig. 7.8).

Branches

While still within the dural sheath the ophthalmic artery gives off the central artery of the retina. After piercing the dura mater it gives off a large lacrimal branch that runs along the lateral wall of the orbit. The main artery runs towards the medial wall of the orbit giving off a number of branches. The various branches are described below:

1. *Central Artery of Retina*

The central artery of retina (Fig. 7.9) is the first and most important branch of the ophthalmic artery. It first lies below the optic nerve. It pierces the dural sheath of the nerve and runs forwards for a short distance between these two. It then enters the substance of the nerve and runs forwards in its centre to reach the optic disc (Fig. 7.8). Here it divides into branches that supply the retina (Fig. 19.10).

The central artery of the retina is an *end artery*. It does not have effective anastomoses with other arteries. Occlusion of the artery results in blindness. The intraocular part of the artery can be seen, in the living, through an ophthalmoscope.

2. *Branches Arising from the Lacrimal Artery*

(a) Branches are given to the lacrimal gland; (b) two zygomatic branches enter canals in the zygomatic bone. One branch appears on the face through the zygomaticofacial foramen. The other appears on the temporal surface of the bone through the zygomaticotemporal foramen; (c) lateral palpebral branches supply the eyelids; (d) a recurrent meningeal

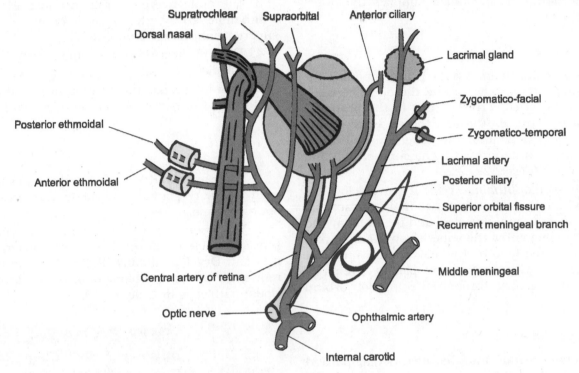

Fig. 7.8: The arteries of the eyeball.

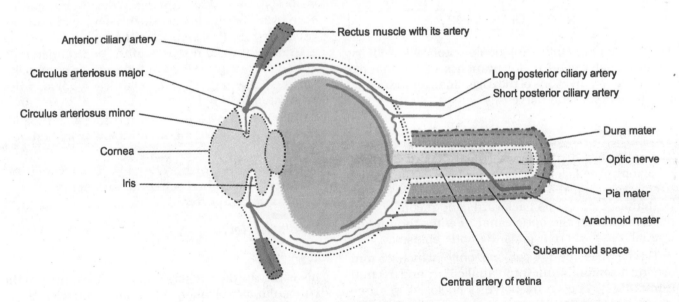

Fig. 7.9: Branches of ophthalmic artery.

branch runs backwards to enter the middle cranial fossa through the superior orbital fissure; (e) muscular branches supply the muscles of the orbit.

3. *Branches Arising from the Main Trunk*

(a) The posterior (long and short) ciliary arteries supply chiefly the choroid and iris. The eyeball is also supplied through anterior ciliary branches which are given off from arteries supplying muscles attached to the eyeball (Fig. 7.9).

(b) The supraorbital and supratrochlear branches supply the skin of the forehead.

(c) The anterior and posterior ethmoidal branches enter foramina in the medial wall of the orbit to supply the ethmoidal air sinuses. They then enter the anterior cranial fossa. The terminal branches of the anterior artery enter the nose and supply part of it.

(d) The medial palpebral branches supply the eyelids.

(e) The dorsal nasal branch supplies the upper part of the nose.

Ophthalmic Veins

The superior ophthalmic vein: It accompanies the ophthalmic artery. It lies above the optic nerve. It receives tributaries corresponding to the branches of the artery, passes through the superior orbital fissure, and drains into the cavernous sinus. It communicates anteriorly with the supraorbital and angular veins (Figs 2.22, 2.23).

The inferior ophthalmic vein: It runs below the optic nerve. It receives tributaries from the lacrimal sac, the lower orbital muscles, and the eyelids, and ends either by joining the superior ophthalmic vein or drains directly into the cavernous sinus. It communicates with the pterygoid plexus of veins by small veins passing through the inferior orbital fissure.

Lymphatics of the Orbit

The lymphatics drain into the preauricular parotid lymph nodes (Fig. 2.25).

NERVES OF THE ORBIT

These are: (a) Optic, (b) oculomotor with ciliary ganglion, (c) trochlear, (d) branches of ophthalmic and maxillary divisions of the trigeminal, (e) abducent, and (f) sympathetic nerves.

Optic Nerve

The optic nerve is the nerve of sight. It is made up of the axons of cells in the ganglionic layer of the retina. It emerges from the eyeball 3 or 4 mm nasal to its posterior pole. It runs backwards and medially, and passes through the optic canal to enter the middle cranial fossa where it joins the optic chiasma.

The nerve is about 4 cm long, out of which 25 mm are intraorbital, 5 mm intracanalicular, and 10 mm intracranial. The entire nerve is enclosed in three meningeal sheaths. The subarachnoid space extends around the nerve up to the eyeball (Fig. 7.9).

Relations in the Orbit

1. At the apex of the orbit the nerve is closely surrounded by the recti muscles. The ciliary ganglion lies between the optic nerve and the lateral rectus (Fig. 7.6).

2. The central artery and vein of the retina pierce the optic nerve inferomedially about 1.25 cm behind the eyeball (Fig. 7.9).

3. The optic nerve is crossed superiorly by the ophthalmic artery, the nasociliary nerve and the superior ophthalmic vein (Fig. 7.8).

4. The optic nerve is crossed inferiorly by the nerve to the medial rectus.

5. Near the eyeball the nerve is surrounded by fat containing the ciliary vessels and nerves (Chapter 19).

Structure

1. There are about 1.2 million myelinated fibres in each optic nerve, out of which about 53% cross in the optic chiasma.

2. The optic nerve is not a nerve in the strict sense. It is actually a tract. It cannot regenerate after it is cut. Developmentally, the optic nerve and the retina are a direct prolongation of the brain. See visual pathways in Chapter 30.

CLINICAL ANATOMY

(a) *Optic neuritis* is characterized by pain in and behind the eye on ocular movements and on pressure. The papilloedema is less but loss of vision is more. When the optic disc is normal as seen by an ophthalmoscopy the same condition is called *retrobulbar neuritis*. The common causes are demyelinating diseases of the central nervous system, any septic focus in the teeth or paranasal sinuses, meningitis, encephalitis, syphilis, and even vitamin B deficiency.

(b) *Optic nerve* has no neurilemma sheath, and has no power of regeneration. It is a tract and not a nerve.

(c) *Optic atrophy* may be caused by a variety of diseases. It may be primary or secondary.

Oculomotor Nerve

Introduction

This is the third cranial nerve. It is distributed to the extraocular as well as the intraocular muscles. Since it is a somatic motor nerve, it is in series with the IVth, VIth and XIIth cranial nerves, and also with the ventral root of spinal nerves.

Functional Components

1. General somatic efferent, for movements of the eyeball (Fig. 25.2).

2. General visceral efferent or parasympathetic, for contraction of the pupil and accommodation.

3. General somatic afferent, for proprioceptive impulses for the muscles of the eyeball. These

impulses are relayed to the mesencephalic nucleus of the trigeminal nerve.

Nucleus

The oculomotor nucleus is situated in the ventromedial part of central grey matter of midbrain at the level of superior colliculus. The fibres for the constrictor pupillae and for the ciliaris arise from the Edinger Westphal nucleus which forms part of the oculomotor nuclear complex.

Ventrolaterally it is closely related to the medial longitudinal bundle (Fig. 24.10).

The nucleus is connected: (a) to the pyramidal tracts of both sides which form the supranuclear pathway of the nerve; (b) to the pretectal nuclei of both sides for the light reflex; (c) to the fourth, sixth and eighth nerve nuclei by medial longitudinal bundle for coordination of the eye movements; and (d) to the tectobulbar tract for visuoprotective reflexes.

Course and Distribution

1. In their *intraneural course,* the fibres arise from the nucleus and pass ventrally through the tegmentum, red nucleus and substantia nigra (Fig. 24.10).

2. *At the base of the brain,* the nerve is attached to the oculomotor sulcus on the medial side of the crus cerebri (Figs 7.10, 24.1).

3. The nerve passes between the superior cerebellar and posterior cerebral arteries, and runs forwards in the interpeduncular cistern, on the lateral side of the posterior communicating artery to reach the cavernous sinus.

4. The nerve *enters the cavernous sinus* by piercing the posterior part of its roof on the lateral side of the posterior clinoid process (Fig. 6.3). it descends to the lateral wall of the sinus where it lies above the trochlear nerve (Fig. 6.6). In the anterior part of the sinus, the nerve divides into a upper and lower division (Fig. 7.11).

5. The two divisions of the nerve *enter the orbit* through the middle part of the superior orbital fissure (Fig. 7.4). In the fissure, the nasociliary nerve lies in between the two divisions while the abducent nerve lies inferolateral to them.

6. *In the orbit,* the smaller upper division ascends on the lateral side of the optic nerve, and supplies the superior rectus and the levator palpebrae superioris. The larger, lower, division divides into three branches for the medial rectus, the inferior rectus and the inferior oblique (Fig. 7.11). The nerve to the inferior oblique is the longest of these. It gives off the motor root to the ciliary ganglion (Fig 7.6).

All branches enter the muscles on their ocular surfaces except that for the inferior oblique which enters its posterior border.

CLINICAL ANATOMY

1. Complete and total *paralysis* of the third nerve results in: (a) ptosis, i.e. drooping of the upper eyelid; (b) lateral squint; (c) dilatation of the pupil; (d) loss of accommodation; (e) slight proptosis, i.e. forward projection of the eye; and (f) diplopia or double vision.

2. A midbrain lesion causing contralateral hemiplegia and ipsilateral paralysis of the third nerve is known as *Weber's syndrome.*

3. *Supranuclear paralysis* of the third nerve causes loss of conjugate movement of the eyes.

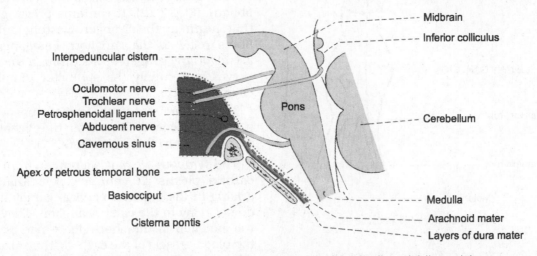

Fig. 7.10: *Scheme to show the precavernous courses of the third, fourth and sixth cranial nerves.*

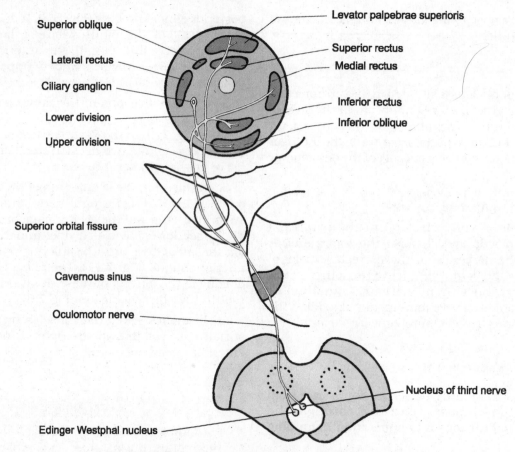

Superior oblique
Lateral rectus
Ciliary ganglion
Lower division
Upper division

Levator palpebrae superioris
Superior rectus
Medial rectus
Inferior rectus
Inferior oblique

Superior orbital fissure

Cavernous sinus

Oculomotor nerve

Nucleus of third nerve

Edinger Westphal nucleus

Fig. 7.11: Origin, course and distribution of oculomotor nerve.

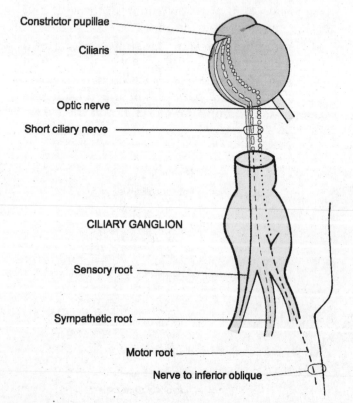

Constrictor pupillae
Ciliaris

Optic nerve
Short ciliary nerve

CILIARY GANGLION

Sensory root

Sympathetic root

Motor root

Nerve to inferior oblique

Fig. 7.12: Roots and branches of ciliary ganglion.

Ciliary Ganglion

Definition

Ciliary ganglion is a peripheral parasympathetic ganglion placed in the course of the oculomotor nerve. It lies near the apex of the orbit between the optic nerve and the tendon of the lateral rectus muscle. It has motor, sensory and sympathetic roots.

The *motor root* arises from the nerve to the inferior oblique (Fig. 7.12). It contains preganglionic fibres that begin in the Edinger Westphal nucleus. The fibres relay in the ganglion. Postganglionic fibres arising in the ganglion pass through the short ciliary nerves and supply the sphincter pupillae and the ciliaris muscle.

The *sensory root* comes from the nasociliary nerve. It contains sensory fibres from the eyeball. The fibres do not relay in the ganglion (7.12).

The *sympathetic root* is a branch from the internal carotid plexus. It contains postganglionic fibres arising in the superior cervical ganglion. The fibres do not relay in the ciliary ganglion. They pass out of the ganglion in the short ciliary nerves and supply the blood vessels of the eyeball. They also supply the dilator pupillae.

Branches. The ganglion gives off 8 to 10 short ciliary nerves which divide into 15 to 20 branches, and then pierce the sclera around the entrance of the optic nerve. They contain fibres from all the three roots of the ganglion.

Trochlear Nerve

This is the fourth cranial nerve. It supplies only the superior oblique muscle of the eyeball (Fig. 7.13).

Functional Components

1. General somatic efferent, for lateral movement of the eyeball.

2. General somatic afferent, for proprioceptive impulses from the superior oblique muscle. These impulses reach the mesencephalic nucleus of the trigeminal nerve.

Nucleus

The trochlear nucleus is situated in the ventromedial part of the central grey matter of midbrain at the level of inferior colliculus. Ventrally, it is closely related to the medial longitudinal bundle (Fig. 24.9).

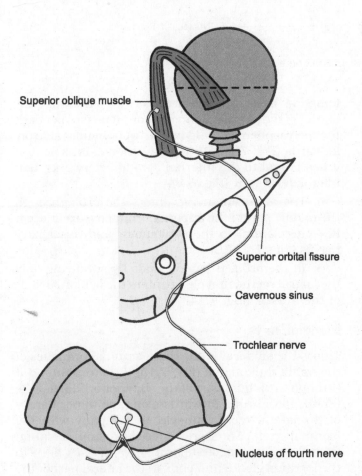

Superior oblique muscle

Superior orbital fissure

Cavernous sinus

Trochlear nerve

Nucleus of fourth nerve

Fig. 7.13: *Origin, course and distribution of the trochlear nerve.*

The connections of the nucleus are similar to those of the oculomotor nucleus, except for the pretectal nuclei.

Course and Distribution

1. In its *intraneural course,* the nerve runs dorsally round the central grey matter to reach the upper part of the superior or anterior medullary velum where it decussates with the opposite nerve to emerge on the opposite side (Figs 7.10, 7.13).

2. *Surface attachment.* Trochlear nerve is attached to the superior medullary velum one on each side of the frenulum veli just below the inferior colliculus. It is the only cranial nerve which emerges on the dorsal aspect of the brainstem (Fig. 24.1).

3. The nerve winds round the superior cerebellar peduncle and the cerebral peduncle just above the pons. It passes between the posterior cerebral and superior cerebellar arteries to appear ventrally between the temporal lobe and upper border of pons.

4. The nerve *enters the cavernous sinus* by piercing the posterior corner of its roof. Next it runs forwards in the lateral wall of the cavernous sinus between the oculomotor and ophthalmic nerves. In the anterior part of the sinus, it crosses over the oculomotor nerve (Figs 6.3, 6.6).

5. Trochlear nerve *enters the orbit* through the lateral part of the superior orbital fissure.

6. *In the orbit,* it passes medially, above the origin of levator palpebrae superioris and ends by supplying the superior oblique muscle on its orbital surface.

CLINICAL ANATOMY

When trochlear nerve is damaged, diplopia occurs on looking downwards; vision is single so long as the eyes look above the horizontal plane.

Abducent Nerve

Introduction

It is the sixth cranial nerve which supplies the lateral rectus muscle of the eyeball (Fig. 7.14). One nerve fibre supplies only six muscle fibres.

Functional Components

1. General somatic efferent, for lateral movement of the eyeball.

2. General somatic afferent, for proprioceptive impulses from the lateral rectus muscle. These impulses are relayed to the mesencephalic nucleus of the trigeminal nerve.

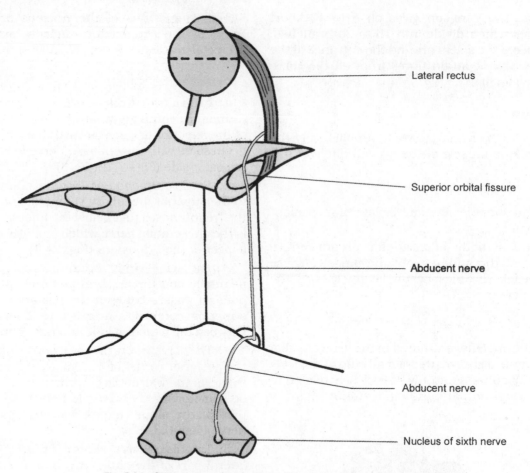

Lateral rectus

Superior orbital fissure

Abducent nerve

Abducent nerve

Nucleus of sixth nerve

Fig. 7.14: Origin, course and distribution of the abducent nerve.

Nucleus

Abducent nucleus is situated in the upper part of the floor of fourth ventricle in the lower pons, beneath the facial colliculus. Ventromedially, it is closely related to the medial longitudinal bundle (Fig. 24.6).

Connections of the nucleus are similar to those of the third nerve, except for the pretectal nuclei.

Course and Distribution

1. In their *intraneural course,* the fibres of the VIth nerve run ventrally and downwards through the trapezoid body, medial lemniscus and basilar part of pons to reach the lower border of the pons (Fig. 24.6).

2. The nerve is attached to the lower border of the pons, opposite the upper end of the pyramid of the medulla (Fig. 24.1).

3. The nerve then runs upwards, forwards and laterally through the cisterna pontis and usually dorsal to the anterior inferior cerebellar artery to reach the cavernous sinus.

4. The abducent nerve *enters the cavernous sinus* by piercing its posterior wall at a point lateral to the dorsum sellae and superior to the apex of the petrous

temporal bone. As the nerve crosses the superior border of the petrous temporal bone it passes beneath the petrosphenoidal ligament, and bends sharply forwards (Fig. 7.10). In the cavernous sinus at first it lies lateral to the internal carotid artery and then inferolateral to it (Fig. 6.6).

5. The abducent nerve *enters the orbit* through the middle part of the superior orbital fissure. Here it lies inferolateral to the oculomotor and nasociliary nerves (Figs 7.4, 7.6).

6. *In the orbit,* the nerve ends by supplying only the lateral rectus muscle. It enters the ocular surface of the muscle (Fig. 7.14).

Lacrimal Nerve

This is the smallest of the three terminal branches of the ophthalmic nerve (Fig. 7.15). It enters the orbit through the lateral part of the superior orbital fissure (Fig. 7.4) and runs forwards along the upper border of the lateral rectus muscle, in company with the lacrimal artery. Anteriorly, it receives communication from the zygomaticotemporal nerve, passes deep to the lacrimal gland, and ends in the lateral part of the upper eyelid.

(i) *Paralysis* of the abducent nerve results in: (a) medial or internal or convergent squint; and (b) diplopia.

(ii) Sixth nerve paralysis is one of the commonest false localizing signs in cases with raised intracranial pressure. Its susceptibility to such damage is due to its long course in the cisterna pontis, to its sharp bend over the superior border of the petrous temporal bone (Fig. 7.10) and the downward shift of the brainstem towards the foramen magnum produced by raised intracranial pressure.

The lacrimal nerve supplies the lacrimal gland, the conjunctiva and the upper eyelid. Its own fibres to the gland are sensory. The secretomotor fibres to the gland come from the greater petrosal nerve through its communication with the zygomaticotemporal nerve (Table 1.3).

Frontal Nerve

This is the largest of the three terminal branches of the ophthalmic nerve (Fig. 7.15). It begins in the lateral wall of the anterior part of the cavernous sinus. It enters the orbit through the lateral part of the superior orbital fissure, and runs forwards on the superior surface of the levator palpebrae superioris. At the middle of the orbit it divides into a small supratrochlear branch and a large supraorbital branch.

The *supratrochlear nerve* emerges from the orbit above the trochlea about one finger breadth from the median plane. It supplies the conjunctiva, the upper eyelid, and a small area of the skin of the forehead above the root of the nose (Figs 2.5, 2.19).

The *supraorbital nerve* emerges from the orbit through the supraorbital notch or foramen about two fingers breadth from the median plane. It divides into medial and lateral branches which runs upwards over the forehead and scalp. It supplies the conjunctiva, the central part of the upper eyelid, the frontal air sinus and the skin of the forehead and scalp up to the vertex, or even up to the lambdoid suture.

Nasociliary Nerve

This is one of the terminal branches of the ophthalmic division of the trigeminal nerve (Fig. 7.15). It begins in the lateral wall of the anterior part of the cavernous sinus. It enters the orbit through the middle part of the superior orbital fissure between the two divisions of the oculomotor nerve (Fig. 7.4). It crosses above the optic nerve from lateral to medial side along with ophthalmic artery and runs along the medial wall of the orbit between the superior oblique and the

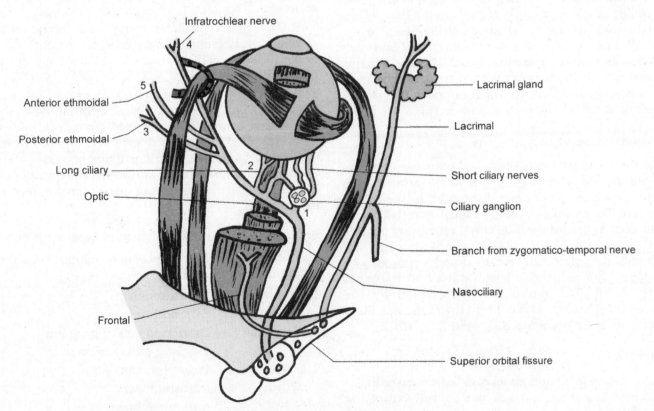

Fig. 7.15: Branches of ophthalmic nerve.

medial rectus. It ends at the anterior ethmoidal foramen by dividing into the infratrochlear and anterior ethmoidal nerves. Its branches are as follows.

1. A *communicating branch to the ciliary ganglion* forms the sensory root of the ganglion. It is often mixed with the sympathetic root (Fig. 7.15).

2. Two or three *long ciliary nerves* run on the medial side of the optic nerve, pierce the sclera, and supply sensory nerves to the cornea, the iris and the ciliary body. They also carry sympathetic nerves to the dilator pupillae (Fig. 7.15).

3. The *posterior ethmoidal nerve* passes through the posterior ethmoidal foramen and supplies the ethmoidal and sphenoidal air sinuses. It is frequently absent (Fig. 7.15).

4. The *infratrochlear nerve* is the smaller terminal branch of the nasociliary nerve given off at the anterior ethmoidal foramen. It emerges from the orbit below the trochlea for the tendon of the superior oblique and appears on the face above the medial angle of the eye. It supplies the conjunctiva, the lacrimal sac and caruncle, the medial ends of the eyelids and the upper half of the external nose (Fig. 2.19).

5. The *anterior ethmoidal nerve* is the larger terminal branch of the nasociliary nerve. It leaves the orbit by passing through the anterior ethmoidal foramen. It appears, for a very short distance, in the anterior cranial fossa, above the cribriform plate of the ethmoid bone. It then descends into the nose through a slit at the side of the anterior part of the crista galli. In the nasal cavity, it lies deep to the nasal bone. It gives off two *internal nasal branches* medial and lateral to the mucosa of the nose. Finally, it emerges at the lower border of the nasal bone as the *external nasal nerve* which supplies the skin of the lower half of the nose (Chapter 15).

Infraorbital Nerve

It is the continuation of the maxillary nerve. It enters the orbit through the inferior orbital fissure. It then runs forwards on the floor of the orbit or the roof of the maxillary sinus, at first in the infraorbital groove and then in the infraorbital canal remaining outside the periosteum of the orbit. It emerges on the face through the infraorbital foramen and terminates by dividing into palpebral, nasal and labial branches (Fig. 2.19). The nerve is accompanied by the infraorbital branch of the third part of the maxillary artery and the accompanying vein (Fig. 10.7).

Branches

1. The *middle superior alveolar nerve* arises in the infraorbital groove, runs in the lateral wall of the maxillary sinus, and supplies the upper premolar teeth. It may be duplicated, or may be absent.

2. The *anterior superior alveolar nerve* arises in the infraorbital canal, and runs in a sinuous canal having a complicated course in the anterior wall of the maxillary sinus. It supplies the upper incisor and canine teeth, the maxillary sinus, and the antero-inferior part of the nasal cavity (Chapter 15).

3. *Terminal branches palpebral, nasal and labial* supply a large area of skin on the face. They also supply the mucous membrane of the upper lip and cheek (Fig. 2.19).

Zygomatic Nerve

It is a branch of the maxillary nerve, given off in the pterygopalatine fossa. It enters the orbit through the lateral end of the inferior orbital fissure, and runs along the lateral wall, outside the periosteum, to enter the zygomatic bone. Just before or after entering the bone it divides into its two terminal branches, the *zygomaticofacial* and *zygomaticotemporal nerves* which supply the skin of the face and of the anterior part of the temple (Fig. 2.19). The communicating branch to the lacrimal nerve, which contains secreto-motor fibres to the lacrimal gland, may arise either from the zygomatic or the zygomaticotemporal nerve, and runs in the lateral wall of the orbit (Chapter 2).

Sympathetic Nerves of the Orbit

Sympathetic nerves arise from the internal carotid plexus and enter the orbit through the following sources.

1. The dilator pupillae of the iris is supplied by sympathetic nerves that pass through the ophthalmic nerve, the nasociliary nerve, and its long ciliary branches.

2. Other sympathetic nerves enter the orbit as follows: (a) A plexus surrounds the ophthalmic artery. (b) A direct branch from the internal carotid plexus passes through the superior orbital fissure and joins the ciliary ganglion. (c) Other filaments pass along the oculomotor, trochlear, abducent, and ophthalmic nerves. All these sympathetic nerves are vasomotor in function.

Branches of Ophthalmic Division of Trigeminal Nerve

Following are the branches of ophthalmic division of trigeminal nerve.

1. Frontal	Supratrochlear
	Supraorbital
2. Nasociliary	Branch to ciliary ganglion
	2–3 long ciliary nerves
	Posterior ethmoidal
	Infratrochlear
	Anterior ethmoidal
3. Lacrimal	

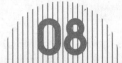

Anterior Triangle of the Neck

The anterior triangle of the neck lies between midline of the neck and sternocleidomastoid muscle. It is subdivided into smaller triangles.

Carotid vessels, their branches and tributaries form the most important contents of the anterior triangle. The external carotid artery gives eight branches which supply thyroid gland, muscles of tongue, face, ear, occiput, pharynx, temporal region and wide area around the maxilla. The carotid body and carotid sinus are situated at the beginning of common carotid artery and act as chemoreceptor and baroreceptor respectively. Parts of glosso-pharyngeal, vagus, spinal root of accessory, hypo-glossal and some of their branches are seen in relation to the branches of the carotid arteries.

Introduction

The anterior triangle of the neck is bounded: (1) *Anteriorly* by the median plane; (2) *posteriorly* by the sternocleidomastoid muscle; (3) *superiorly* by the base of the mandible, and by a line joining the angle of the mandible to the mastoid process. The apex of the triangle lies above the manubrium sterni.

Surface Landmarks

1. The *mandible* forms the lower jaw. The lower border of its horseshoe-shaped body is known as the *base of the mandible.* Anteriorly, this base forms the *chin*, and posteriorly it can be traced to the *angle of the mandible* (Fig. 8.1).

2. The body of the U-shaped *hyoid bone* can be felt in the median plane just below and behind the chin, at the junction of the neck with the floor of the mouth. On each side the body of hyoid bone is continuous posteriorly with the *greater cornua* which is overlapped in its posterior part by the sterno-cleidomastoid muscle.

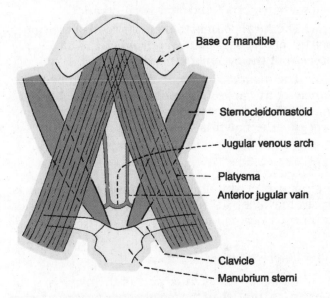

Fig. 8.1: Anterior triangles of the neck showing the platysma and the anterior jugular veins in the superficial fascia.

3. The *thyroid cartilage* of the larynx forms a sharp protuberance in the median plane just below the hyoid bone. This protuberance is called the *laryngeal prominence or Adams apple.* It is more prominent in males.

4. The rounded arch of the *cricoid cartilage* lies below the thyroid cartilage at the upper end of the trachea.

5. The trachea runs downwards and backward from the cricoid cartilage. It is identified by its cartilaginous rings. However, it is partially masked by the *isthmus of the thyroid gland* which lies against second to fourth tracheal rings. The trachea is commonly palpated in the *suprasternal notch* which lies between the tendinous heads of origin of the right and left sternocleidomastoid muscles. In certain diseases, the trachea may shift to one side from the

median plane. This indicates a shift in the mediastinum.

Other Important landmarks

1. The *frontozygomatic suture* can be felt as a
depression in the upper part of the lateral orbital
margin.

2. The *marginal tubercle* lies a short distance
below the frontozygomatic suture along the posterior
border of the frontal process of the zygomatic bone.

3. The *Frankfurt plane* is represented by a
horizontal line joining the infraorbital margin to the
upper margin of the external acoustic meatus.
Posteriorly, the line passes through a point just
below the external occipital protuberance.

4. The *jugal point* is the anterior end of the upper
border of the zygomatic arch where it meets the
process of the zygomatic bone.

5. The *mandibular notch* is represented by a line
concave upwards, extending from the head of
mandible to the posterior border of the coronoid
process. The notch is 1–2 cm deep.

Skin

The skin over the anterior triangle of the neck is
freely movable. Its nerve supply is from anterior
cutaneous nerve of neck (C2, C3).

Superficial Fascia

It contains: (a) The greater part of the platysma; (b)
the cervical branch of the facial nerve; (c) the anterior
jugular vein, and (d) a few lymph nodes.

The platysma is a subcutaneous muscle forming
a wide, thin fleshy sheet running upwards and
medially in the neck from the deltoid and pectoral
fasciae to the base of the mandible. It is supplied by
the cervical branch of the facial nerve, and possibly
helps in releasing pressure of the skin over the
subjacent superficial veins. All superficial nerves
and vessels in this area lie deep to the platysma
(Fig. 8.1).

Anterior Jugular Vein

This is a small vein, beginning in the submental
region below the chin. It descends in the superficial
fascia about 1 cm from the median plane. About 2.5
cm above the sternum, it pierces the investing layer
of deep fascia to enter the suprasternal space where
it is connected to its fellow of the opposite side by a
transverse channel, the *jugular venous arch*. The
vein then turns laterally, runs deep to the sternocleidomastoid just above the clavicle, and *ends in the*

external jugular vein at the posterior border of the
sternocleidomastoid.

The anterior jugular vein is markedly *variable:* (a)
It may be absent on one side; (b) may be represented
by a median vein; or (c) may be large in size when the
common facial vein drains into it.

Lymph Nodes

(a) A few lymph nodes lie alongside the anterior
jugular vein; (b) few submental nodes lie below the
chin; (c) and a few of them lie on the sternocleidomastoid, alongside the external jugular vein.

Structures in the Anterior Median Region of the Neck

This region includes a strip 2 to 3 cm wide extending
from the chin to the sternum. The structures
encountered from are listed below from superficial to
deep.

Skin

It is freely movable over the deeper structures due to
the looseness of the superficial fascia.

DISSECTION

Make median incision in the skin from the chin
to the sternum. Extend the upper end of the
incision along lower border of mandible for 5 cm
on each side. Extend the lower incision upwards
along the anterior border of sternocleidomastoid
muscle by 5 cm. Reflect the skin laterally. Reflect
the platysma upwards. Identify the structures
present in the superficial fascia and the structures
present in the anterior median region of the neck.

Superficial Fascia

It contains: (a) The upper decussating fibres of the
platysma for 1 to 2 cm below the chin; (b) the *anterior
jugular veins* beginning just above the hyoid bone by
the confluence of several superficial veins from the
submandibular region (Fig 8.1); (c) a few small
submental lymph nodes lying on the deep fascia
below the chin (Fig. 12.30); (d) the terminal filaments
of the *transverse or anterior cutaneous nerve* of the
neck may be present in it.

Deep Fascia

Above the hyoid bone, it is a single layer in the median
plane, but splits on each side to enclose the
submandibular salivary gland (Fig. 11.4).

Between the hyoid bone and the cricoid cartilage, it is a single layer extending between the right and left sternocleidomastoid muscles.

Below the cricoid, the fascia splits to enclose the suprasternal space.

Deep Structures Lying above the Hyoid Bone

The *mylohyoid muscle* is overlapped by: (a) The anterior belly of the *digastric;* (b) the superficial part of the *submandibular salivary gland;* (c) the *mylohyoid nerve and vessels;* and (d) the *submental branch of the facial artery* (Figs 8.2, 8.3).

The anteroinferior part of the *hyoglossus muscle* with its superficial relations may also be exposed during dissection. Structures lying in this corner are: (a) The intermediate tendon of the *digastric* muscle with its fibrous pulley; (b) the bifurcated tendon of the *stylohyoid* muscle embracing the digastric tendon; and (c) the *hypoglossal nerve.*

The *subhyoid bursa* lies between the posterior surface of the body of the hyoid bone and the thyrohyoid membrane. It lessens friction between these two structures during the movements of swallowing (Fig. 8.4).

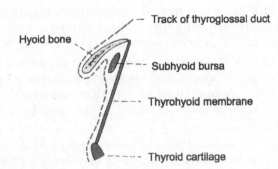

Fig. 8.4: *Sagittal section through the hyoid region of the neck showing the subhyoid bursa and its relations.*

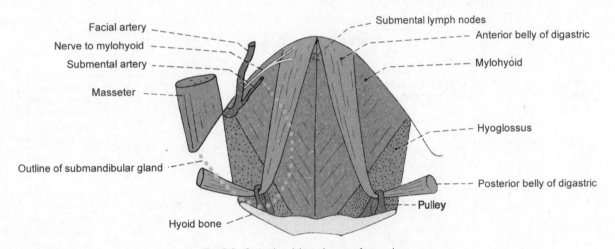

Fig. 8.2: *Suprahyoid region, surface view.*

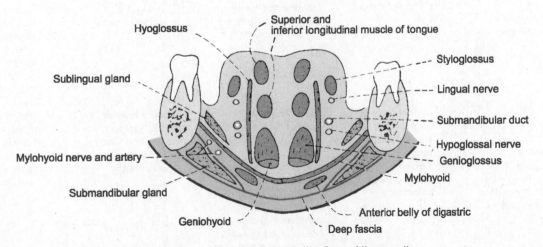

Fig. 8.3: *Coronal section through the floor of the mouth.*

Structures Lying Below the Hyoid Bone

These structures may be grouped into three planes: A superficial plane containing the infrahyoid muscles, a middle plane consisting of the pretracheal fascia and the thyroid gland, and a deep plane containing the larynx, trachea and structures associated with them.

Infrahyoid muscles: (a) Sternohyoid; (b) sternothyroid; (c) thyrohyoid; and (d) superior belly of omohyoid. These are described in Table 8.1 (Fig. 8.5).

Pretracheal fascia: It forms the *false capsule of the thyroid gland* and the *suspensory ligaments* which attach the thyroid gland to the cricoid cartilage. The *inferior thyroid veins* lie within the fascia (Figs 12.2, 12.4).

Deep to the pretracheal fascia there are: (a) The *thyrohyoid membrane* deep to the thyrohyoid muscle: it is pierced by the internal laryngeal nerve and the superior laryngeal vessels (Fig. 8.10); (b) *thyroid cartilage;* (c) *cricothyroid membrane* with the anastomosis of the cricothyroid arteries on its surface;

(d) arch of the *cricoid cartilage;* (e) *cricothyroid muscle* supplied by the external laryngeal nerve; (f) *trachea,* partly covered by the isthmus of the thyroid gland from the second to fourth rings; (g) *carotid sheaths* lie on each side of the trachea; (h) occasionally, the *left brachiocephalic vein* and the *brachiocephalic artery* may lie in front of the trachea in the suprasternal notch (Fig. 8.6).

CLINICAL ANATOMY

1. The common *anterior midline swellings* of the neck are: (a) Enlarged submental lymph nodes and sublingual dermoid in the submental region; (b) thyroglossal cyst and subhyoid bursitis just below the hyoid bone; (c) goitre, carcinoma of larynx and enlarged lymph nodes in the suprasternal region.

2. *Tracheostomy* is an operation in which the trachea is opened and a tube inserted into it to facilitate breathing. It is most commonly done in

Table 8.1: Infrahyoid muscles

Muscle	Origin from	Insertion into	Nerve supply	Actions
1. *Sternohyoid* (Fig. 8.5)	(a) Posterior surface of manubrium sterni (b) Adjoining parts of the clavicle and the posterior sternoclavicular ligament	Medial part of lower border of hyoid bone	Ansa cervicalis	Depresses the hyoid bone following its elevation during swallowing and during vocal movements
2. *Sternothyroid* It lies deep to the sternohyoid	(a) Posterior surface of manubrium sterni (b) Adjoining part of first costal cartilage	Oblique line on the lamina of the thyroid cartilage	Ansa cervicalis	Depresses the larynx after it has been elevated in swallowing and in vocal movements
3. *Thyrohyoid* It lies deep to the sternohyoid	Oblique line of thyroid cartilage	Lower border of the body and the greater cornua of the thyroid cartilage	C1 through hypoglossal nerve	(a) Depresses the hyoid bone: (b) Elevates the larynx when the hyoid is fixed by the suprahyoid muscles
4. *Omohyoid* It has an inferior belly, a common tendon and a superior belly. It arises by the inferior belly; and is inserted through the superior belly	(a) Upper border of scapula near the suprascapular notch (b) Adjoining part of suprascapular ligament	Lower border of body of hyoid bone lateral to the sternohyoid The central tendon lies on the internal jugular vein at the level of the cricoid cartilage and is bound to the clavicle by a fascial pulley	Superior belly by the superior root of the ansa cervicalis; and inferior belly by ansa cervicalis	(a) Depresses the hyoid bone following its elevation during swallowing or in vocal movements

the retrothyroid region after retracting the isthmus of the thyroid gland. A suprathyroid tracheostomy is liable to stricture, and an infrathyroid one is difficult due to the depth of the trachea and is also dangerous because numerous vessels lie anterior to the trachea here.

3. *'Cut throat'* wounds are most commonly situated just above or just below the hyoid bone. The main vessels of the neck usually escape injury because they are pushed backwards to a deeper plane during voluntary extension of the neck.

ANTERIOR TRIANGLE OF NECK

The boundaries of the triangle are:

The anterior median plane of the neck medially; sternocleidomastoid laterally; base of the mandible and a line joining the angle of the mandible to the mastoid process, superiorly (Fig. 8.7).

Subdivisions

The anterior triangle encloses four suprahyoid and four infrahyoid muscles. The suprahyoid muscles

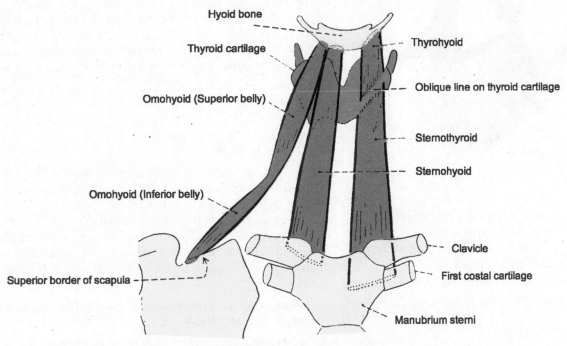

Fig. 8.5: The infrahyoid muscles.

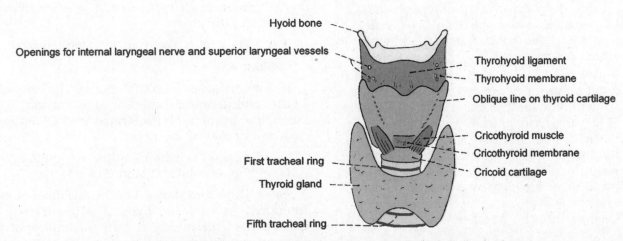

Fig. 8.6: The thyroid gland, the larynx, and the trachea seen from the front.

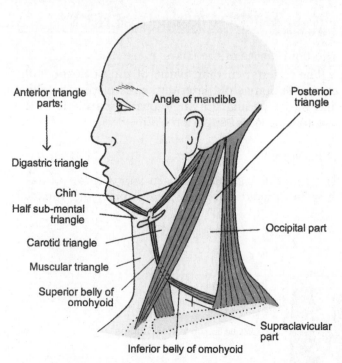

Anterior triangle parts:

Digastric triangle

Chin

Half sub-mental triangle

Carotid triangle

Muscular triangle

Superior belly of omohyoid

Angle of mandible

Posterior triangle

Occipital part

Supraclavicular part

Inferior belly of omohyoid

Fig. 8.7: *The triangles of the neck. Note that the anterior and posterior triangles are subdivided by the digastric and inferior belly of omohyoid muscles respectively.*

are the digastric, the stylohyoid, the mylohyoid and the geniohyoid. The infrahyoid muscles, already examined, are the sternohyoid, the sternothyroid, the thyrohyoid and the omohyoid.

The anterior triangle is subdivided (by the digastric muscle and the superior belly of the omohyoid into: (a) Submental; (b) digastric; (c) carotid; and (d) muscular triangles (Fig. 8.7).

DISSECTION

Remove the deep fascia from anterior bellies of digastric muscles to expose parts of two mylohyoid muscles. Clean the boundaries and contents of the submental triangle.

Cut the deep fascia from the mandible and reflect it downwards to expose the submandibular gland. Identify and clean anterior and posterior bellies of digastric muscles, which form the boundaries of digastric triangle. Identify the intermediate tendon of digastric after pulling the submandibular gland laterally. Clean the stylohyoid muscle which envelops the tendon of digastric and is lying along with the posterior belly of digastric muscle. Identify the contents of digastric triangle.

Submental Triangle

This is a median triangle. It is bounded as follows.

On each side there is the anterior belly of the corresponding digastric muscles. Its base is formed by the body of the hyoid bone. Its apex lies at the chin. The floor of the triangle is formed by the right and left mylohyoid muscles and the median raphe uniting them (Fig. 8.2).

Contents

1. Two to four small *submental lymph nodes* are situated in the superficial fascia between the anterior bellies of the digastric muscles. They drain: (a) Superficial tissues below the chin; (b) central part of the lower lip; (c) the adjoining gum; (d) anterior part of the floor of the mouth; and (e) the tip of the tongue. Their efferents pass to the submandibular nodes.

2. Small submental veins join to form the anterior jugular veins.

Digastric Triangle

The area between the body of the mandible and the hyoid bone is known as the submandibular region. The superificial structures of this region lie in the submental and digastric triangles. The deep structures of the floor of mouth and root of the tongue will be studied separately at a later stage under the heading of Submandibular region (Chapter 11).

Boundaries: The boundaries of the digastric triangle are as follows.

Anteroinferiorly: Anterior belly of digastric.

Posteroinferiorly: Posterior belly of digastric and the stylohyoid.

Superiorly or base: Base of the mandible and a line joining the angle of the mandible to the mastoid process (Fig. 8.7).

Roof : The roof of the triangle is formed by :

1. Skin.

2. Superficial fascia, containing: (a) The platysma; (b) the cervical branch of the facial nerve; and (c) the ascending branch of the transverse or anterior cutaneous nerve of the neck.

3. Deep fascia, which splits to enclose the submandibular salivary gland (Fig. 11.4).

Floor: The *floor* is formed by the mylohoid muscle anteriorly, and by the hyoglossus posteriorly. A small part of the middle constrictor muscle of the pharynx, appears in the floor (Figs 8.8, 8.9).

Contents

Anterior Part of the Triangle

1. *Structures superficial to mylohyoid* are: (a) Superficial part of the submandibular salivary gland (Fig. 8.2). The facial vein and the submandibular lymph nodes are superficial to it and the facial artery is deep to it; (b) submental artery; (c) mylohyoid nerve and vessels.

2. *Structures superficial to the hyoglossus* seen without disturbing the mylohyoid and the submandibular gland are: (a) The submandibular salivary gland: (b) the intermediate tendon of the digastric and the stylohyoid; and (c) the hypoglossal nerve

(Fig. 11.2). Other relations will be studied in the submandibular region.

Posterior Part of the Triangle

1. *Superficial structures* are: (a) Lower part of the parotid gland, and (b) the external carotid artery before it enters the parotid gland.

2. *Deep structures*, passing between the external and internal carotid arteries are: (a) The styloglossus; (b) the stylopharyngeus; (c) the glossopharyngeal nerve; (d) the pharyngeal branch of the vagus nerve; (e) the styloid process; and (f) a part of the parotid gland (Fig. 9.4).

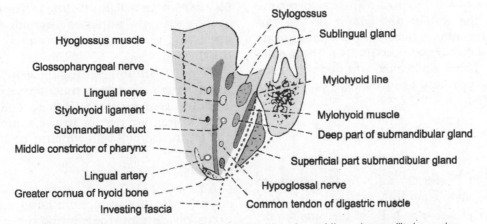

Fig. 8.8: Coronal section through the digastric triangle and the submandibular region.

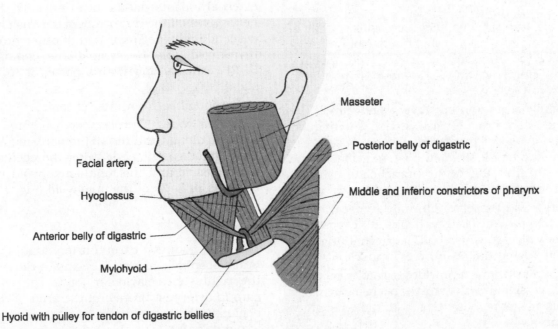

Fig. 8.9: Floor of the digastric triangle.

3. Deepest structures include: (a) The internal carotid artery, (b) the internal jugular vein, and (c) the vagus nerve.

The deep structures will be studied with the submandibular region.

The *submandibular lymph nodes* are clinically very important because of their wide area of drainage. They are very commonly enlarged. The nodes lie beneath the deep cervical fascia on the surface of the submandibular salivary gland. They *drain:* (a) The centre of the forehead; (b) the nose with the frontal, maxillary and ethmoidal air sinuses; (c) the inner canthus of the eye; (d) the upper lip and the anterior part of the cheek with the underlying gum and teeth; (e) the outer part of the lower lip with the lower gum and teeth excluding the incisors; (f) the anterior two-thirds of the tongue excluding the tip, and the floor of the mouth. They also receive efferents from the submental lymph nodes. The *efferents* from the submandibular nodes pass mostly to the jugulo-omohyoid node and partly to the jugulo-digastric node. These nodes are situated along the internal jugular vein and are members of the deep cervical chain (Figs 2.25, 12.29).

Carotid Triangle

Boundaries

Anterosuperiorly: Posterior belly of the digastric muscle; and the stylohyoid (Fig. 8.7).

Anteroinferiorly: Superior belly of the omohyoid.

Posteriorly: Anterior border of the sternocleido-mastoid muscle.

DISSECTION

Clean the area situated between posterior belly of digastric and superior belly of omohyoid muscle, to expose the three carotid arteries with internal jugular vein. Trace IX, X, XI and XII nerves in relation to these vessels.

Carefully clean and preserve superior root, the loop and inferior root of ansa cervicalis in relation to anterior aspect of carotid sheath. Locate the sympathetic trunk situated posteromedial to the carotid sheath. Dissect the branches of external carotid artery.

Identify and preserve internal laryngeal nerve in the thyrohyoid interval. Trace it postero-superiorly till vagus. Also look for external laryngeal nerve supplying the cricothyroid muscle.

The carotid triangle provides a good view of all the large vessels and nerves of the neck, particularly when its posterior boundary is retracted slightly backwards.

Roof

1. Skin.

2. Superficial fascia containing: (a) The plastysma; (b) the cervical branch of the facial nerve; and (c) the transverse cutaneous nerve of the neck.

3. Investing layer of deep cervical fascia.

Floor

It is formed by parts of (a) The thyrohyoid muscle; (b) the hyoglossus; (c) and the middle and inferior constrictors of the pharynx (Fig. 8.10).

Contents

Arteries: (1) The common carotid artery with the carotid sinus and the carotid body at its termination; (2) internal carotid artery; and (3) the external carotid artery with its superior thyroid, lingual, facial, ascending pharyngeal and occipital, branches (Fig. 8.11).

Veins: (1) The internal jugular vein; (2) the common facial vein draining into the internal jugular vein; (3) a pharyngeal vein which may end either in the internal jugular vein or in the common facial vein; and (4) the lingual vein which usually terminates in the internal jugular vein, but may drain into the common facial vein.

Nerves: (1) The vagus running vertically downwards; (2) the superior laryngeal branch of the vagus, dividing into the external and internal laryngeal nerves; (3) the spinal accessory nerve running backwards over the internal jugular vein; and the (4) the hypoglossal nerve running forwards over the external and internal carotid arteries. The hypoglossal nerve gives off the upper root of the ansa cervicalis or descendens hypoglossi, and another branch to the thyrohyoid. (5) The sympathetic chain runs (Fig. 8.12) vertically downwards posterior to the carotid sheath (Fig. 12.4).

Carotid sheath with its contents.

Lymph nodes: The deep cervical lymph nodes are situated along the internal jugular vein, and include the jugulodigastric node below the posterior belly of the digastric and the jugulo-omohyoid node above the inferior belly of the omohyoid (Fig. 12.29).

Common Carotid Artery

The right common carotid artery is a branch of the brachiocephalic artery. It begins in the neck behind the right sternoclavicular joint. The left common carotid artery is branch of the arch of the aorta. It begins in the thorax in front of the trachea opposite a point a little to the left of the centre of the

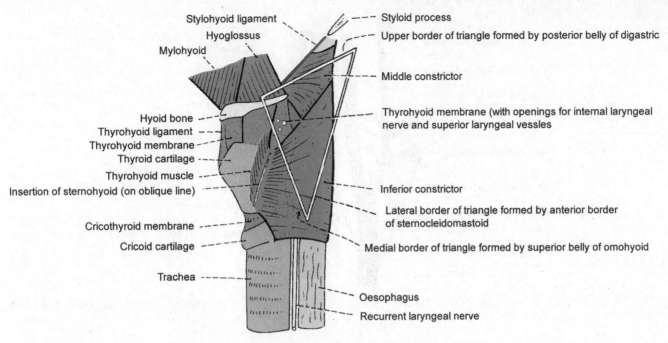

Fig. 8.10: Floor of the carotid triangle.

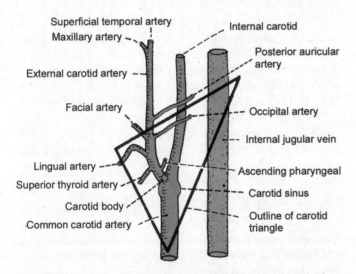

Fig. 8.11: Carotid arteries, branches of the external carotid artery, and the internal jugular vein, in relation to the carotid triangle.

manubrium. It ascends to the back of the left sternoclavicular joint and enters the neck (Fig. 12.11).

In the neck, both arteries have a similar course. Each artery runs upwards within the carotid sheath, under cover of the anterior border of the sternocleidomastoid. It lies in front of the lower four cervical transverse processes. At the level of the upper border of the thyroid cartilage the artery ends by dividing into the <u>external</u> and <u>internal</u> carotid arteries (Fig. 8.12).

Carotid Sinus

The termination of the common carotid artery, or the beginning of the internal carotid artery shows a slight dilatation, known as the carotid sinus. In this region, the tunica media is thin, but the adventitia is relatively thick and receives a rich innervation from the glossopharyngeal and sympathetic nerves. The carotid sinus acts as a *baroreceptor* or *pressure receptor* and regulates blood pressure.

Carotid Body

Carotid body is a small, oval reddish-brown structure situated behind the bifurcation of the common carotid artery. It receives a rich nerve supply mainly from the glossopharyngeal nerve, but also from the vagus and sympathetic nerves. It acts as a <u>chemoreceptor</u> and responds to changes in the oxygen and carbon dioxide and pH content of the blood.

Other *allied chemoreceptors* are found near the arch of the aorta, the ductus arteriosus, and the right subclavian artery. These are supplied by the vagus nerve.

External Carotid Artery

External carotid artery is one of the terminal branches of the common carotid artery. In general, it lies <u>anterior</u> to the <u>internal</u> carotid artery, and is the chief artery of supply to structures in the front of the neck and in the face (Figs 8.11, 8.12).

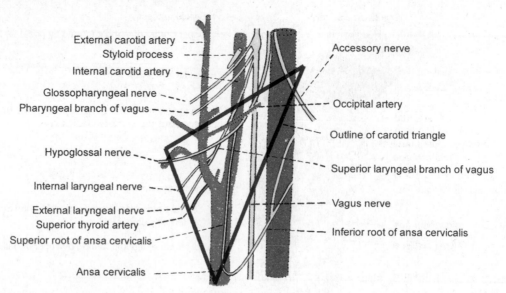

Fig. 8.12: *The ninth, tenth, eleventh and twelfth cranial nerves and their branches related to the carotid arteries and to the internal jugular vein, in and around the carotid triangle.*

Surface Marking

The external carotid artery is marked by joining the following two points.

(a) A point on the anterior border of the sterno-cleidomastoid muscle at the level of the upper border of the thyroid cartilage.

(b) A second point on the posterior border of the neck of the mandible.

The artery is slightly convex forwards in its lower half and slightly concave forwards in its upper half (Fig. 12.10).

Course and Relations

1. The external carotid artery begins in the carotid triangle at the level of the upper border of the thyroid cartilage opposite the disc between the third and fourth cervical vertebrae. It runs upwards and slightly backwards and laterally, and terminates behind the neck of the mandible by dividing into the maxillary and superficial temporal arteries.

2. The external carotid artery has a *slightly curved course,* so that it is anteromedial to the internal carotid artery in its lower part, and anterolateral to the internal carotid artery in its upper part.

3. *In the carotid triangle,* the external carotid artery is comparatively superficial, and lies under cover of the anterior border of the sternocleidomastoid. The artery is crossed superficially by the cervical branch of the facial nerve, the hypoglossal nerve, and the facial, lingual and superior thyroid veins. Deep to the artery there are: (1) The wall of the pharynx; (2) the superior laryngeal nerve which divides into the

external and internal laryngeal nerves; and (3) the ascending pharyngeal artery (Fig. 8.10).

4. *Above the carotid triangle* the external carotid artery lies deep in the substance of the parotid gland. Within the gland, it is related superficially to the retromandibular vein and the facial nerve (Fig. 9.4). Deep to the external carotid artery, there are: (a) The internal carotid artery; (b) structures passing between the external and internal carotid arteries; these being styloglossus, stylopharyngeus, IXth nerve, pharyngeal branch of Xth, and styloid process; and (c) two structures deep to the internal carotid artery, namely the superior laryngeal nerve and the superior cervical sympathetic ganglion (Fig. 8.12).

Branches

The external carotid artery gives off eight branches which may be grouped as follows.

Anterior: (1) Superior thyroid; (2) lingual; and (3) facial.

Posterior: (1) Occipital; and (2) posterior auricular.

Medial: Ascending pharyngeal.

Terminal: (1) Maxillary; and (2) superficial temporal (Fig. 8.12).

Superior Thyroid Artery

The superior thyroid artery arises from the external carotid artery just below the level of the greater cornua of the hyoid bone. It runs downwards and forwards parallel and just superficial to the external laryngeal nerve. It passes deep to the three long infrahyoid muscles to reach the upper pole of the lateral lobe of the thyroid gland. Its relationship to the external laryngeal nerve, which supplies the cricothyroid muscle is important to the surgeon during thyroid surgery. The artery and nerve are close to each other higher up, but diverge slightly near the gland. To avoid injury to the nerve, the superior thyroid artery is ligated as near to the gland as possible (Fig. 12.6).

Apart from its terminal branches to the thyroid gland, it gives one important branch, the *superior laryngeal artery* which pierces the thyrohyoid membrane in company with the internal laryngeal nerve (Fig. 8.6). The superior thyroid artery also gives a sternocleidomastoid branch to that muscle and a cricothyroid branch that anastomoses with the artery of the opposite side in front of the cricovocal membrane (Fig. 12.6).

Lingual Artery

The lingual artery arises from the external carotid artery opposite the tip of the greater cornu of the hyoid bone (Fig. 8.12).

Its course is divided into three parts by the hyoglossus muscle. The *first part* lies in the carotid triangle. It forms a characteristic upward loop which is crossed by the hypoglossal nerve (Fig. 11.2). The lingual loop permits free movements of the hyoid bone. The *second part* lies deep to the hyoglossus along the upper border of hyoid bone. It is superficial to the middle constrictor of the pharynx. The *third part* is called the arteria profunda linguae, or the deep lingual artery. It runs upwards along the anterior border of the hyoglossus, and then horizontally forwards on the undersurface of the tongue as the *fourth part* . In its vertical course, it lies between the genioglossus medially and the inferior longitudinal muscle of the tongue laterally. The horizontal part of the artery is accompanied by the lingual nerve.

During surgical removal of the tongue, the first part of the artery is ligated before it gives any branch to the tongue or to the tonsil.

Facial Artery

The facial artery arises from the external carotid just above the tip of the greater cornua of the hyoid bone.

It runs upwards first in the neck as cervical part and then on the face as facial part. The course of the artery in both places is tortuous. The tortuosity in the neck allows free movements of the pharynx during deglutition. On the face it allows free movements of the mandible, the lips and the cheek during mastication and during various facial expressions. The artery escapes traction and pressure during these movements.

The *cervical part* of the facial artery runs upwards on the superior constrictor of pharynx deep to the posterior belly of the digastric, with the stylohyoid and to the ramus of the mandible. It grooves the posterior border of the submandibular salivary gland. Next the artery makes an S-bend (two loops) first winding down over the submandibular gland, and then up over the base of the mandible (Figs 11.7, 11.8). The course and branches of the *facial part* of the facial artery have been described with the face (Fig. 2.21).

The cervical part of the facial artery gives off the ascending palatine, tonsillar, submental, and glandular branches for the submandibular salivary gland and lymph nodes. The *ascending palatine artery* arises near the origin of the facial artery. It passes upwards between the styloglossus and the stylopharyngeus, crosses over the upper border of the superior constrictor and supplies the tonsil and the root of the tongue. The *submental branch* is a large artery which accompanies the mylohyoid nerve, and supplies the submental triangle and the sublingual salivary gland.

Occipital Artery

The occipital artery arises from the posterior aspect of the external carotid artery, opposite the origin of the facial artery. It is crossed at its origin by the hypoglossal nerve. In the carotid triangle, the artery gives two sternocleidomastoid branches. The upper branch accompanies the accessory nerve, and the lower branch arises near the origin of the occipital artery. The further course of the artery has been described in Chapter 4 (Figs 8.11, 4.2, 4.5).

Posterior Auricular Artery

The posterior auricular artery arises from the posterior aspect of the external carotid just above the posterior belly of the digastric.

It runs upwards and backwards deep to the parotid gland, but superficial to the styloid process. It crosses the base of the mastoid process, and ascends behind the auricle.

It supplies the back of the auricle, the skin over the mastoid process, and over the back of the scalp. It is cut in incisions for mastoid operations. Its *stylomastoid branch* enters the stylomastoid foramen, and supplies the middle ear, the mastoid antrum and air cells, the semicircular canals, and the facial nerve (Fig. 8.11).

Ascending Pharyngeal Artery

This is a small branch that arises from the medial side of the external carotid artery. It arises very close to the lower end of the external carotid artery (Fig. 14.12).

It runs vertically upwards between the side wall of the pharynx, the tonsil, the medial wall of the middle ear and, the auditory tube. It sends meningeal branches into the cranial cavity through the foramen lacerum, the jugular foramen and the hypoglossal canal.

Maxillary Artery

This is the larger terminal branch of the external carotid artery. It begins behind the neck of the mandible under cover of the parotid gland. It runs forwards deep to the neck of the mandible below the auriculotemporal nerve, and enters the infratemporal fossa where it will be studied at a later stage (Chapter 10).

Superficial Temporal Artery

(a) It is the smaller terminal branch of the external carotid artery. It begins, behind the neck of the mandible under cover of the parotid gland (Figs 9.3, 9.5A).

(b) It runs vertically upwards, crossing the root of the zygoma or preauricular point, where its *pulsations* can be easily felt. About 5 cm above the zygoma it divides into anterior and posterior branches which supply the temple and scalp. The anterior branch anastomoses with the supraorbital and supra-trochlear branches of the ophthalmic artery.

(c) In addition to the branches which supply the temple, the scalp, the parotid gland, the auricle and the facial muscles, the superficial temporal artery gives off a *transverse facial artery*, already studied

with the face (Fig. 2.21), and a *middle temporal artery* which runs on the temporal fossa deep to the temporalis muscle.

Ansa Cervicalis or Ansa Hypoglossi

This is a thin nerve loop that lies embedded in the anterior wall of the carotid sheath over the lower part of the larynx. It supplies the infrahyoid muscles (Figs 8.13, 3.4B).

Formation. It is formed by a superior and an inferior root. The *superior root* is the continuation of the descending branch of the hypoglossal nerve. Its fibres are derived from the first cervical nerve. This root descends over the internal carotid artery and the common carotid artery. The *inferior root* or descending cervical nerve is derived from second and third cervical spinal nerves. As this root descends, it winds round the internal jugular vein, and then continues anteroinferiorly to joint the superior root in front of the common carotid artery (Fig. 8.12).

Distribution

Superior root: to the superior belly of the omohyoid.

Ansa cervicalis: to the sternohyoid, the sterno-thyroid and the inferior belly of the omohyoid.

Note that the thyrohyoid and geniohyoid are supplied by separate branches from the first cervical nerve through the hypoglossal nerve (Fig. 8.13).

Muscular Triangle

Boundaries

Anteriorly: anterior median line of the neck from the hyoid bone to the sternum.

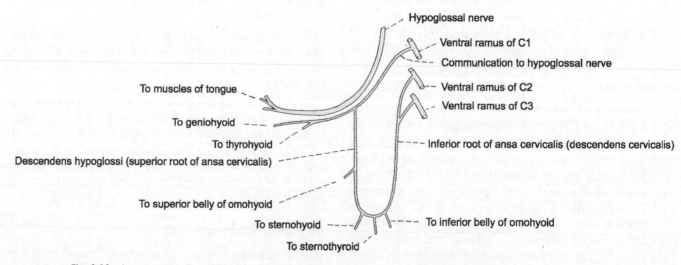

Fig. 8.13: *Ansa cervicalis, and branches of the first cervical nerve distributed through the hypoglossal nerve.*

Posterosuperiorly: superior belly of the omohyoid muscle (Fig. 8.7).

Posteroinferiorly: Anterior border of the sternocleidomastoid muscle.

Contents

The infrahyoid muscles are the chief contents of the triangle. These muscles may also be regarded arbitrarily as forming the floor of the triangle. (Fig. 8.4).

The *infrahyoid muscles* are: (1) The sternohyoid; (2) the sternothyroid; (3) the thyrohyoid; and (4) the omohyoid. These ribbon muscles have the following general features.

(a) They are arranged in two layers, superficial (sternohyoid and omohyoid) and deep (sternothyroid and thyrohyoid) (Fig. 8.5).

DISSECTION

Identify the infrahyoid muscles on each side of the median plane. Cut through the origin of sternocleidomastoid muscle and reflect it upwards. Trace the nerve supply of infrahyoid muscles.

The superficial structures in the infrahyoid region are included in this triangle. The deeper structures (thyroid gland, trachea, oesophagus, etc.) will be studied separately at a later stage.

(b) All of them are supplied by the ventral rami of first, second and third cervical spinal nerves.

(c) Because of their attachment to the hyoid bone and to the thyroid cartilage, they move these structures.

The specific details of infrahyoid muscles are shown in Table 8.1.

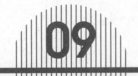

The Parotid Region

Parotid region contains the largest serous salivary gland and the "queen of the face", the facial nerve. Parotid gland contains vertically disposed blood vessels and horizontally situated facial nerve and its various branches. Parotid gland gets affected by virus of mumps, which can extend the territory of its attack up to gonads as well. One must be careful of the branches of facial nerve while incising the parotid abscess by giving horizontal incision.

Facial nerve supplies muscles of the face, scalp, auricle, gives secretomotor branches to the submandibular, sublingual, lacrimal, nasal, palatal, and pharyngeal glands. It indirectly helps in the secretomotor supply to the parotid gland. Even the taste from the most of the anterior two-thirds of tongue is carried by facial nerve. Since it is too much for the facial nerve, so it does not supply the skin of the face which is innervated by trigeminal. To maintain contact with trigeminal nerve, the facial nerve nucleus comes close to trigeminal nerve nucleus. The nucleus of facial nerve can act reflexly in response to sensory impulses from the face. Facial nerve injury causes very typical symptoms.

PAROTID GLAND

(*Para* = around; *otic* = ear)

The Salivary glands

There are three pairs of large salivary glands—the parotid, submandibular and sublingual. In addition there are numerous small glands in the tongue, the palate, the cheeks and the lips. These glands produce saliva which keeps the oral cavity moist, and helps in chewing and swallowing. The saliva also contains enzymes that aid digestion.

Introduction to the Parotid Gland

The parotid is the largest of the salivary glands. It weighs about 15 g. It is situated below the external acoustic meatus, between the ramus of the mandible and the sternocleidomastoid. The gland overlaps these structures. Anteriorly, the gland also overlaps the masseter muscle (Fig. 9.1). A part of this forward extension is often detached, and is known as the *accessory parotid,* and it lies between the zygomatic arch and the parotid duct.

DISSECTION

Carefully cut through the fascial covering of the parotid gland from the zygomatic arch above to the angle of mandible below. While removing tough fascia, dissect the structures emerging at the periphery of the gland.

Trace the duct of the parotid gland anteriorly till the buccinator muscle. Trace one or more of the branches of facial nerve till its trunk in the posterior part of the gland. The trunk can be followed till the stylomastoid foramen. Trace its posterior auricular branch. Trace the course of retromandibular vein and external carotid artery in the gland, removing the glands in pieces. Clean the facial nerve already dissected. Study the entire course of facial nerve from its beginning to the end. Facial nerve is like the queen of the face, supplying all the muscles of facial expression, carrying secretomotor fibres to submandibular, sublingual salivary glands, including those in tongue and floor of mouth. It is also secretomotor to glands in the nasal cavity, palate and the lacrimal gland. It is responsible enough for carrying the taste fibres from anterior two-thirds of tongue also except from the vallate papillae.

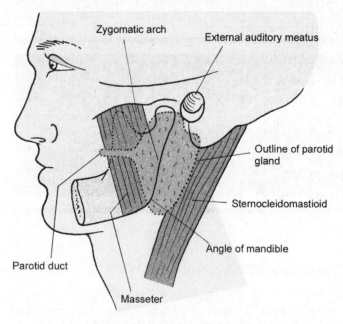

Fig. 9.1: *Position of parotid gland.*

Parotid Capsule

The investing layer of the deep cervical fascia forms a capsule for the gland. The fascia splits (between the angle of the mandible and the mastoid process) to enclose the gland. The superficial lamina, thick and adherent to the gland, is attached above to the zygomatic arch. The deep lamina is thin and is attached to the styloid process, the mandible and the tympanic plate. A portion of the deep lamina, extending between the styloid process and the mandible, is thickened to form the *stylomandibular ligament* which separates the parotid gland from the submandibular salivary gland.

Surface Marking

The parotid gland is marked by joining the following four points with each other (Fig. 9.2).

(a) The first point at the upper border of the head of the mandible.

(b) The second point just above the centre of the masseter muscle.

(c) The third point posteroinferior to the angle of the mandible.

(d) The fourth point on the upper part of the anterior border of the mastoid process.

The anterior border of the gland is obtained by joining the points a–b–c; the posterior border, by joining the points c–d; and the superior curved border with its concavity directed upwards and backwards, by joining the points a-d across the lobule of the ear.

Parotid Duct

To mark this duct first draw a line joining the following two points.

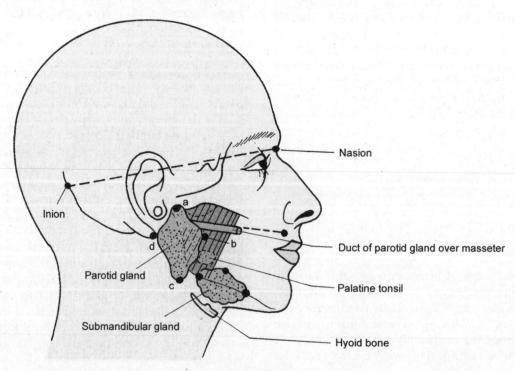

Fig. 9.2: *Surface marking of parotid, submandibular salivary glands and palatine tonsil.*

(a) One point at the lower border of the tragus.

(b) A second point midway between the ala of the nose and the red margin of the upper lip.

The middle-third of this line represents the parotid duct.

External Features

The gland resembles a three sided pyramid. The apex of the pyramid is directed downwards. The gland has four surfaces: (1) Superior (base of the pyramid); (2) superficial; (3) anteromedial; and (4) posteromedial. The surfaces are separated by three borders: (1) Anterior; (2) posterior; and (3) medial.

Relations

The *apex* (Fig. 9.3) overlaps the posterior belly of the digastric and the adjoining part of the carotid triangle. The cervical branch of the facial nerve and the two divisions of the retromandibular vein emerge through it.

The *superior surface* or base forms the upper end of the gland which is small and concave. It is related to: (a) The cartilaginous part of the external acoustic meatus; (b) the posterior surface of the temporomandibular joint; (c) the superficial temporal vessels; and (d) the auriculotemporal nerve (Fig. 9.3).

Surfaces: The *superficial surface* is the largest of the four surfaces. It is covered with: (a) Skin; (b) superficial fascia containing the anterior branches of the great auricular nerve, the preauricular or superficial parotid lymph nodes and the posterior fibres of the platysma and risorius; (c) the parotid fascia which is thick and adherent to the gland; and (d) a few deep parotid lymph nodes embedded in the gland.

The *anteromedial surface* (Fig. 9.4) is grooved by the posterior border of the ramus of the mandible. It is related to: (a) The masseter; (b) the lateral surface

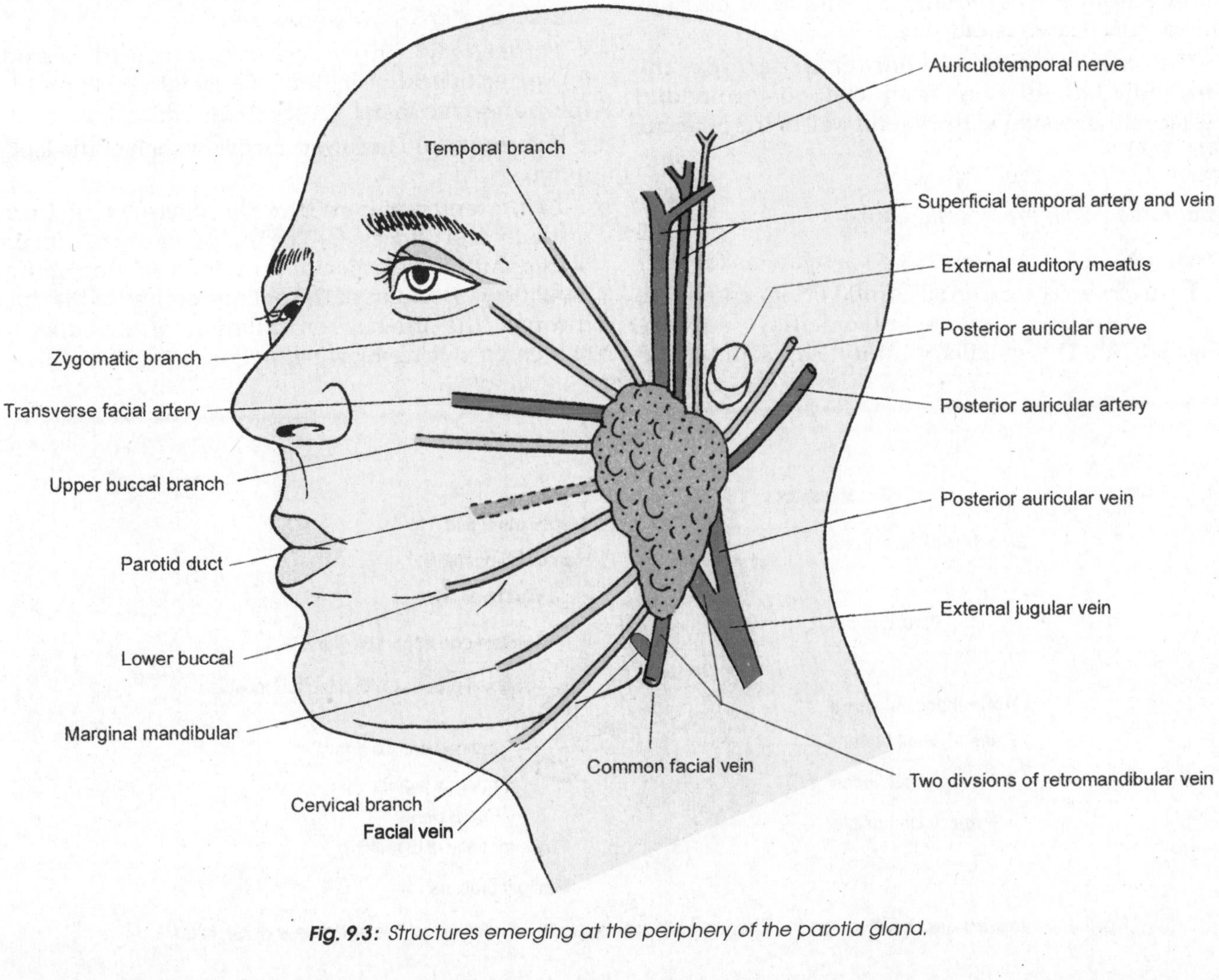
Auriculotemporal nerve
Temporal branch
Superficial temporal artery and vein
External auditory meatus
Posterior auricular nerve
Zygomatic branch
Transverse facial artery
Posterior auricular artery
Upper buccal branch
Posterior auricular vein
Parotid duct
External jugular vein
Lower buccal
Marginal mandibular
Common facial vein
Two divsions of retromandibular vein
Cervical branch
Facial vein

Fig. 9.3: Structures emerging at the periphery of the parotid gland.

of the temporomandibular joint; (c) the posterior border of the ramus of the mandible; (d) the medial pterygoid; and (e) the emerging branches of the facial nerve.

The *posteromedial surface* is moulded to the mastoid and the styloid processes and the structures attached to them. Thus it is related to: (a) The mastoid process, with the sternocleidomastoid and the posterior belly of the digastric; and (b) the styloid process, with structures attached to it. The external carotid artery enters the gland through this surface and the internal carotid artery lies deep to the styloid process (Fig. 9.4).

Borders: The *anterior border* separates the superficial surface from the anteromedial surface. It extends from the anterior part of the superior surface to the apex. The following structures emerge at this border: (a) The parotid duct; (b) most of the terminal branches of the facial nerve; and (c) the transverse facial vessels. In addition, the accessory parotid gland lies on the parotid duct close to this border (Fig. 9.3).

The *posterior border* separates the superficial surface from the posteromedial surface. It overlaps the sternocleidomastoid (Fig. 9.1).

The *medial edge* or *border* separates the anteromedial surface from the posteromedial surface. It is related to the lateral wall of the pharynx (Fig. 9.4).

Structures within the Parotid Gland

From medial to the lateral side these are as follows.

1. *Arteries:* The external carotid artery enters the gland through its posteromedial surface (Fig. 9.5 A). The maxillary artery leaves the gland through its anteromedial surface. The superficial temporal vessels emerge at the anterior part of the superior surface. The posterior auricular artery may arise within the gland.

2. *Veins:* The retromandibular vein is formed within the gland by the union of the superficial temporal and maxillary veins. In the lower part of the gland, the vein divides into anterior and posterior divisions which emerge at the apex (lower pole) of the gland (Fig. 9.5 B).

3. The *facial nerve* enters the gland through the upper part of its posteromedial surface, and divides into its terminal branches within the gland. The branches leave the gland through its anteromedial surface, and appear on the surface at the anterior border (Fig. 9.5 C).

4. Parotid lymph nodes.

Parotid Duct

It is thick walled and is about 5 cm long. It emerges from the middle of the anterior border of the gland. It runs forwards and slightly downwards on the masseter. Here its relations are:

Superiorly: (a) Accessory parotid gland; (b) upper buccal branch of the facial nerve; and (c) the transverse facial vessels (Fig. 9.3).

Inferiorly: (a) The lower buccal branch of the facial nerve.

At the anterior border of the masseter, it turns medially and pierces: (a) The buccal pad of fat, (b) the buccopharyngeal fascia and (c) the buccinator (obliquely). Because of the oblique course of the duct through the buccinator inflation of the duct is prevented during blowing.

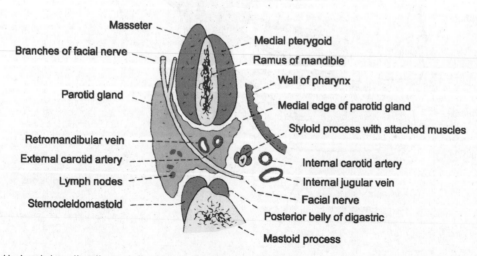

Fig. 9.4: *Horizontal section through the parotid gland showing its relations and the structures passing through it.*

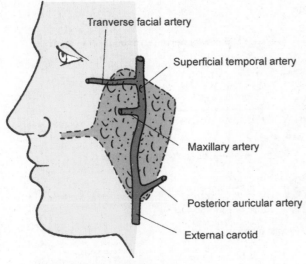

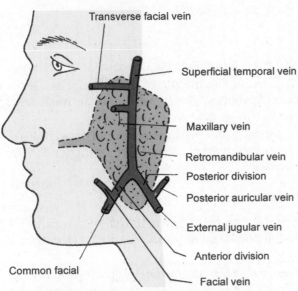

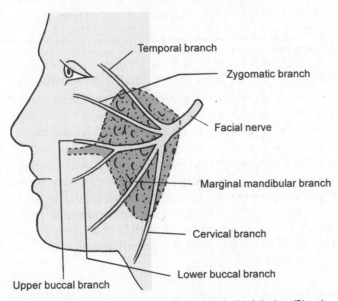

Fig. 9.5: *Structures within the parotid gland. (A) Arteries, (B) veins, (C) nerves.*

The duct runs forwards for a short distance between the buccinator and the oral mucosa. Finally, the duct turns medially and opens into the vestibule of the mouth (gingivo-buccal vestibule) opposite the crown of the upper second molar tooth. (Fig. 2.26).

Blood Supply

The parotid gland is supplied by the external carotid artery and its branches that arise near the gland. The veins drain into the external jugular vein.

Nerve Supply

1. Parasympathetic nerves are secretomotor (Fig. 9.6). They reach the gland through the auriculotemporal nerve. The preganglionic fibres begin in the inferior salivatory nucleus; pass through the glossopharyngeal nerve, its tympanic branch, the tympanic plexus and the lesser petrosal nerve; and relay in the otic ganglion. The postganglionic fibres pass through the auriculotemporal nerve and reach the gland.

2. Sympathetic nerves are vasomotor, and are derived from the plexus around the external carotid artery.

3. Sensory nerves to the gland come from the auriculotemporal nerve, but the parotid fascia is innervated by the sensory fibres of the great auricular nerve (C2).

Lymphatic Drainage

Lymph drains first to the parotid nodes and from there to the upper deep cervical nodes.

Development

The parotid gland is ectodermal in origin. It develops from the buccal epithelium just lateral to the angle of mouth. The outgrowth branches repeatedly to form the duct system and acini.

Parotid Lymph Nodes

The parotid lymph nodes lie partly in the superficial fascia and partly deep to the deep fascia over the parotid gland (Fig. 9.4). They drain: (a) The temple, (b) the side of the scalp, (c) the lateral surface of the auricle, (d) the external acoustic meatus, (e) the middle car, (f) the parotid gland, (g) the upper part of the cheek, (h) parts of the eyelids, and (i) the orbit. Efferents from these nodes pass to the upper group of deep cervical nodes.

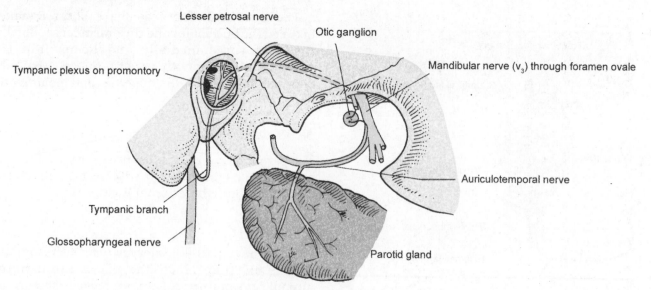

Fig. 9.6: *Parasympathetic nerve supply to the parotid gland.*

CLINICAL ANATOMY

1. *Parotid swellings* are very painful due to the unyielding nature of the parotid fascia.

2. *Mumps* is an infectious disease of the salivary glands (usually the parotid) caused by a specific virus.

3. A *parotid abscess* may be caused by spread of infection from the mouth cavity. An abscess may also form due to suppuration of the parotid lymph nodes draining an infected area.

4. During surgical removal of the parotid gland or parotidectomy, the facial nerve is preserved by removing the gland in two parts, superficial and deep separately. The plane of cleavage is defined by tracing the nerve from behind forwards.

5. Viral parotitis or mumps characteristically does not suppurate. Its complications are orchitis and pancreatitis.

6. A parotid abscess is best drained by horizontal incisions known as Hilton's method.

7. *Mixed parotid tumour* is a slowly growing lobulated painless tumour without any involvement of the facial nerve. Malignant change of such a tumour is indicated by pain, rapid growth, fixity with hardness, involvement of the facial nerve, and enlargement of cervical lymph nodes.

FACIAL NERVE

This is the seventh cranial nerve. It is the nerve of the second branchial arch.

Surface Marking

It is marked by a short horizontal line which joins the following two points (Fig. 10.12).

(a) A point at the middle of the anterior border of the mastoid process. The stylomastoid foramen lies 2 cm deep to this point.

(b) A second point behind the neck of the mandible. Here the nerve divides into its five branches for the facial muscles.

Functional Components

1. Special visceral or *branchial efferent*, to muscles responsible for facial expression and for elevation of the hyoid bone.

2. *General visceral efferent* or parasympathetic. These fibres are secretomotor to the submandibular and sublingual salivary glands, the lacrimal gland, and glands of the nose, the palate and the pharynx (Fig. 25.2).

3. *General visceral afferent* component carries afferent impulses from the above mentioned glands.

4. *Special visceral afferent* fibres carry taste sensations from the anterior two-thirds of the tongue except from vallate papillae and from the palate.

5. *General somatic afferent* fibres probably innervate a part of the skin of the ear. The nerve does not give any direct branches to the ear, but some fibres may reach it through communications with the vagus nerve. Proprioceptive impulses from muscles of the face travel through branches of the trigeminal nerve to reach the mesencephalic nucleus of the nerve.

Nuclei

The fibres of the nerve arise from four nuclei situated

in the lower pons (Fig. 25.2).

1. Motor nucleus or branchiomotor (Fig. 24.6).

2. Superior salivatory nucleus or parasympathetic.

3. Lacrimatory nucleus is also parasympathetic.

4. Nucleus of the tractus solitarius which is gustatory and also receives afferent fibres from the glands.

The motor nucleus lies deep in the reticular formation of the lower pons. The part of the nucleus that supplies muscles of the upper part of the face receives corticonuclear fibres from the motor cortex of both the right and left sides. In contrast, the part of the nucleus that supplies muscles of the lower part of the face receive corticonuclear fibres only from the opposite cerebral hemisphere.

Course and Relations

The facial nerve is attached to the brainstem by two roots, motor and sensory. The sensory root is also called the *nervus intermedius.* (Fig. 24.1).

The two roots of the facial nerve are attached to the lateral part of the lower border of the pons just medial to the eighth cranial nerve. The two roots run laterally and forwards, with the eighth nerve to reach the internal acoustic meatus. *In the meatus*, the motor root lies in a groove on the eighth nerve, with the sensory root intervening (Fig. 9.7). Here the seventh and eighth nerves are accompanied by the labyrinthine vessels. At the bottom or fundus of the meatus, the two roots, sensory and motor fuse to form a single trunk, which lies in the petrous temporal bone (Fig. 9.8). Within the canal, the course of the nerve can be divided into three parts by two bends (Fig. 9.9). The first part is directed laterally above the vestibule; the second part runs backwards in relation to the medial wall of the middle ear, above the promontory (Fig. 18.12). The third part is directed vertically downwards behind the promontory. The first bend at the junction of the first and second parts is sharp. It lies over the anterosuperior part of the promontory, and is also called the *genu*. The geniculate ganglion of the nerve is so called because it lies on the genu. The second bend is gradual, and lies between the promontory and the aditus to the mastoid antrum.

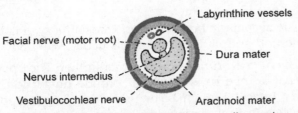

Fig. 9.7: *Structures in the left internal acoustic meatus.*

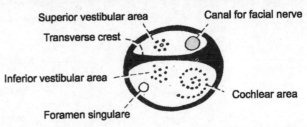

Fig. 9.8: *Some features seen on the fundus of the left internal acoustic meatus.*

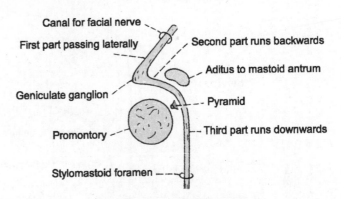

Fig. 9.9: *Course of facial nerve.*

The facial nerve leaves the skull by passing through the stylomastoid foramen.

In its *extracranial course*, the facial nerve crosses the lateral side of the base of the styloid process. It enters the posteromedial surface of the parotid gland, runs forwards through the gland crossing the retromandibular vein and the external carotid artery. Behind the neck of the mandible it divides into its five terminal branches which emerge along the anterior border of the parotid gland (Fig. 9.5C).

Branches and Distribution

A. Within the facial canal: (1) Greater petrosal nerve; (2) the nerve to the stapedius; and (3) the chorda tympani (Fig. 9.10).

B. At its exit from the stylomastoid foramen: (1) Posterior auricular; (2) digastric; and (3) stylohyoid.

C. Terminal branches within the parotid gland: (1) Temporal; (2) zygomatic; (3) buccal; (4) marginal mandibular; and (5) cervical.

D. Communicating branches with adjacent cranial and spinal nerves.

Greater petrosal nerve (see Chapters 6 and 15).

The *nerve to the stapedius* arises opposite the pyramid of the middle ear, and supplies the stapedius muscle. The muscle damps excessive vibrations of the stapes caused by high-pitched sounds. In paralysis of the muscle even normal sounds appear too loud

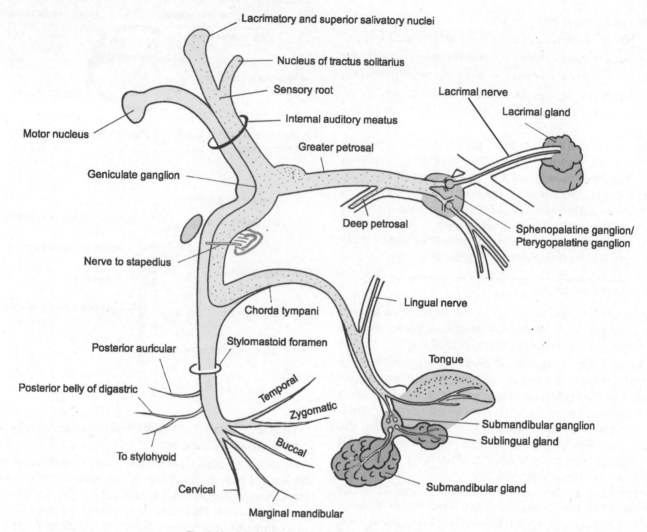

Fig. 9.10: *Components and distribution of facial nerve.*

and is known as hyperacusis.

The *chorda tympani* arises in the vertical part of the facial canal about 6 mm above the stylomastoid foramen. It runs upwards and forwards in a bony canal. It enters the middle ear and runs forwards in close relation to the tympanic membrane (Fig. 18.3). It leaves the middle ear by passing through the petrotympanic fissure. It then passes medial to the spine of the sphenoid and enters the infratemporal fossa. Here it joins the lingual nerve through which it is distributed (Fig. 10.14).

It carries: (a) Preganglionic secretomotor fibres to the submandibular ganglion for supply of the submandibular and sublingual salivary glands and taste fibres from the anterior two-thirds of the tongue.

The *posterior auricular nerve* arises just below the stylomastoid foramen. It ascends between the mastoid process and the external acoustic meatus, and supplies: (a) The auricularis posterior, (b) the occipitalis, and (c) the intrinsic muscles on the back

of the auricle.

The *digastric branch*, arises close to the previous nerve. It is short and supplies the posterior belly of the digastric.

The *stylohyoid branch*, which may arise with the digastric branch, is long and supplies the stylohyoid muscle.

The *temporal branches* cross the zygomatic arch and supply: (a) The auricularis anterior, (b) the auricularis superior, (c) the intrinsic muscles on the lateral side of the ear, (d) the frontalis, (e) the orbicularis oculi, and (f) the corrugator supercilii (Fig. 9.5C).

The *zygomatic branches* run across the zygomatic bone and supply the orbicularis oculi.

The *buccal branches* are two in number. The upper buccal branch runs above the parotid duct and the lower buccal branch below the duct. They supply muscles in that vicinity (see Chapter 2).

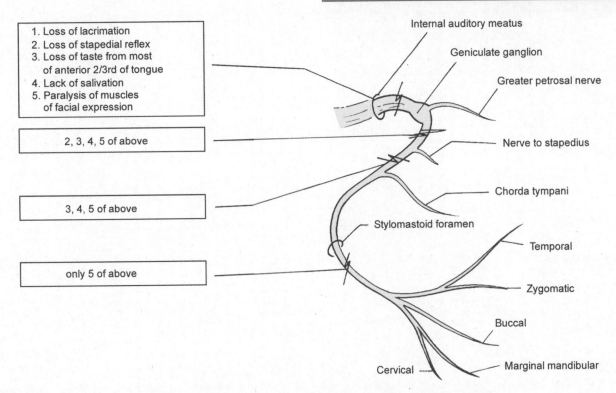

Fig. 9.11: *Symptoms according to the level of injury to cranial nerve VII.*

The *marginal mandibular branch* runs below the angle of the mandible deep to the platysma. It crosses the body of the mandible and supplies muscles of the lower lip and chin (Fig. 2.6).

The *cervical branch* emerges from the apex of the parotid gland, and runs downwards and forwards in the neck to supply the platysma (Fig. 2.7).

Communicating branches. For effective coordination between the movements of the muscles of the first, second and third branchial arches, the motor nerves of the three arches communicate with each other. The facial nerve also communicates with the sensory nerves distributed over its motor territory.

Ganglia

The ganglia associated with the facial nerve are as follows.

1. The geniculate ganglion is located on the first bend of the facial nerve, in relation to the medial wall of the middle ear. It is a *sensory ganglion.* The taste fibres present in the nerve are peripheral processes

CLINICAL ANATOMY

For clinical testing of the facial nerve, and for different types of facial paralysis (supranuclear and infranuclear), (see Fig. 2.18).

Figure 9.11 shows the symptoms according to level of injury of facial nerve.

of pseudounipolar neurons present in the geniculate ganglion (Fig. 9.9).

2. The submandibular ganglion is a *parasympathetic ganglion* for relay of secretomotor fibres to the submandibular and sublingual glands. It is described in Chapter 11 and in Table 1.3 (Fig. 11.11).

3. The pterygopalatine ganglion is also a parasympathetic ganglion. Secretomotor fibres meant for the lacrimal gland relay in this ganglion. It is described in Chapter 15 and in Table 1.3.

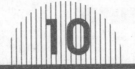

The Temporal and Infratemporal Regions

Temporal and infratemporal regions include muscles of mastication, which develop from mesoderm of first branchial arch. Only one joint, the temporomandibular joint, is present to allow movements during speech and mastication. The parasympathetic ganglion is the otic ganglion, the only ganglion with four roots, i.e. sensory, sympathetic, motor and secretomotor. The motor root from the branch to medial pterygoid supplies two muscles, the tensor veli palatini and tensor veli tympani. The blood supply of this region is through the maxillary artery. Middle meningeal artery is its most important branch, as its injury results in extradural haemorrhage.

Osteology: in order to understand these regions, the osteology of the temporal fossa, the infratemporal fossa and the pterygopalatine fossa should be studied. The *temporal fossa* lies on the side of the skull, and is bounded by the superior temporal line and the zygomatic arch. The pterion lies in the anterior part of its floor where four bones (frontal, parietal, squamous temporal and greater wing of sphenoid) meet at an H-shaped suture. The temporal fossa communicates with the infratemporal fossa through a gap deep to the zygomatic arch. The *infratemporal fossa* lies below the skull (middle cranial fossa), behind the body of the maxilla and lateral to the lateral pterygoid plate. It communicates with the pterygopalatine fossa through the pterygomaxillary fissure. The *pterygopalatine fossa* is a small space which lies between the body of the maxilla and the root of the pterygoid process (of the sphenoid bone) lateral to the perpendicular plate of the palatine bone (Fig. 10.1).

LANDMARKS ON THE LATERAL SIDE OF THE HEAD

The external ear or pinna is a prominent feature on the lateral aspect of the head. The named features on

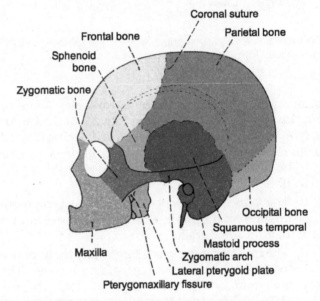

Fig. 10.1: *Some features to be seen on the lateral side of the skull.*

the pinna are shown in Fig. 18.1. Other landmarks on the lateral side of the head are as follows.

1. The *zygomatic bone* forms the prominence of the cheek at the inferolateral corner of the orbit. The *zygomatic arch* bridges the gap between the eye and the ear. It is formed anteriorly by the temporal process of the zygomatic bone, and posteriorly by the zygomatic process or zygoma of the temporal bone. The *preauricular point* lies on the posterior root of the zygoma immediately in front of the upper part of the tragus.

2. The head of the mandible lies in front of the tragus. It is felt best during movements of the lower jaw. The *coronoid process* of the mandible can be felt below the lowest part of the zygomatic bone when the mouth is opened (Fig. 10.2). The process can be traced downwards into the anterior border of the *ramus* of the mandible. The posterior border of the

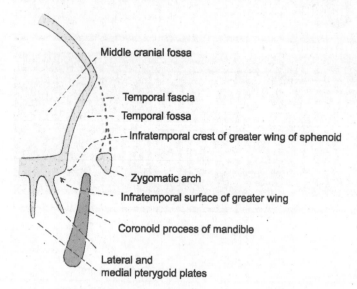

Middle cranial fossa

Temporal fascia

Temporal fossa

Infratemporal crest of greater wing of sphenoid

Zygomatic arch

Infratemporal surface of greater wing

Coronoid process of mandible

Lateral and medial pterygoid plates

Fig. 10.2: *Scheme to show the outline of the temporal and infratemporal fossae in a coronal section.*

ramus, though masked by the parotid gland, can be felt through the skin. The outer surface of the ramus is covered by the masseter which can be felt when the teeth are clenched. The lower border of the mandible can be traced posteriorly into the *angle* of the mandible.

3. The *parietal eminence* is the most prominent part of the parietal bone situated far above and a little behind the auricle.

4. The *mastoid process* is a large bony prominence situated behind the lower part of the auricle. The *supramastoid crest,* about 2.5 cm long, begins immediately above the external acoustic meatus and soon curves upwards and backwards. The crest is continuous anteriorly with the posterior root of the zygoma, and posterosuperiorly with the temporal line.

5. The inferior *temporal line* forms the upper boundary of the temporal fossa which is filled up by the temporalis muscle. The upper margin of the contracting temporalis helps in defining this line which begins at the zygomatic process of the frontal bone, arches posterosuperiorly across the coronal suture, passes a little below the parietal eminence, and turns downwards to become continuous with the supramastoid crest. The area of the temporal fossa on the side of the head, above the zygomatic arch, is called the temple or temporal region.

6. The *pterion* is the area in the temporal fossa where four bones (frontal, parietal, temporal and sphenoid) adjoin each other across an H-shaped suture. The centre of the pterion is marked by a point 4 cm above the midpoint of the zygomatic arch, falling 3.5 cm behind the frontozygomatic

suture. Deep to the pterion lie the anterior branch of the middle meningeal artery, the middle meningeal vein, and deeper still the stem of the lateral sulcus of the cerebral hemisphere (at the *Sylvian point*) dividing into three rami. The pterion is a common site for trephining (making hole in) the skull during operation.

7. The junction of the back of the head with the neck is indicated by the external occipital protuberance and the superior nuchal lines. The *external occipital protuberance* is a bony projection felt in the median plane on the back of the head at the upper end of the nuchal furrow. The *superior nuchal lines* are indistinct curved ridges which extend from the protuberance to the mastoid processes. The back of the head is called the *occiput*. The most prominent median point situated on the external occipital protuberance is known as the *inion* (not onion). However, the posteriormost point on the occiput lies a little above the protuberance.

MUSCLES OF MASTICATION

Introduction: The muscles of mastication move the mandible during mastication and speech. They are the masseter, the temporalis, the lateral pterygoid and the medial pterygoid. They develop from the mesoderm of the first branchial arch, and are supplied by the mandibular nerve which is the nerve of that arch. The muscles are enumerated in Table 10.1. Temporal fascia and relations of lateral and medial pterygoid muscles are described.

DISSECTION

Identify the masseter muscle extending from the zygomatic arch to the ramus of the mandible. Cut the zygomatic arch in front of and behind the attachment of masseter muscle and reflect it downwards. Divide the nerve and blood vessels to the muscle. Clean the ramus of mandible by stripping off the masseter muscle from it.

Give an oblique cut from the centre of mandibular notch to the lower end of anterior border of ramus of mandible. Turn this part of the bone including the insertion of temporalis muscle upwards. Strip the muscle from the skull and identify deep temporal nerves and vessels.

Make one cut through the neck of the mandible. Give another cut through the ramus at a distance of 4 cm from the neck. Remove the bone carefully in between these two cuts, avoiding injury to the underlying structures. The lateral pterygoid is exposed in the upper part and medial pterygoid in the lower part of the dissection.

Table 10.1: Muscles of mastication

Muscle	Origin	Fibres	Insertion	Nerve supply	Actions
1. *Masseter* quadrilateral, covers lateral surface of ramus of mandible, has three layers (Fig. 10.3)	(a) *Superficial layer* (largest): from anterior 2/3 of lower border of zygomatic arch and adjoining zygomatic process of maxilla (b) *Middle layer:* from anterior 2/3 of deep surface and posterior 1/3 of lower border of zygomatic arch (c) *Deep layer:* from deep surface of zygomatic arch	(a) Superficial fibres pass downwards and backwards at 45 degrees (b) Middle and deep fibres pass vertically downwards (c) Three layers are separated posteroinferiorly by an artery and a nerve	(a) Superficial layer: into lower part of lateral surface of ramus of mandible (b) Middle layer: into middle part of ramus (c) Deep layer: into upper part of ramus and coronoid process of the mandible	Masseteric nerve, a branch of anterior division of mandibular nerve	Elevates mandible to close the mouth to bite
2. *Temporalis* Fan-shaped, fills the temporal fossa (Fig. 10.4)	(a) Temporal fossa, excluding zygomatic bone (b) Temporal fascia	Converge and pass through gap deep to zygomatic arch	(a) Margins and deep surface of coronoid process. (b) Anterior border of ramus of mandible	Two deep temporal branches from anterior division of mandibular nerve	(a) Elevates mandible (b) Posterior fibres retract the protruded mandible (c) Helps in side to side grinding movement
3. *Lateral pterygoid* Short, conical, has upper and lower heads (Fig. 10.5)	(a) *Upper head* (small): from infratemporal surface and crest of greater wing of sphenoid bone (b) *Lower head* (larger): from lateral surface of lateral pterygoid plate	Fibres run backwards and laterally and converge for insertion	(a) Pterygoid fovea on the anterior surface of neck of mandible (b) Anterior margin of articular disc and capsule of temporomandibular joint. Insertion is posterolateral and at a slightly higher level than origin	A branch from anterior division of mandibular nerve	(a) Depress mandible to open mouth, with suprahyoid muscle (b) Lateral and medial pterygoid protrude mandible (c) Left lateral pterygoid and right medial pterygoid turn the chin to left side as part of grinding movements
4. *Medial pterygoid* Quadrilateral, has a small superficial and a large deep head (Fig. 10.5)	(a) *Superficial head* (small slip): from tuberosity of maxilla and adjoining bone (b) *Deep head* (quite large): from medial surface of lateral pterygoid plate and adjoining process of palatine bone	Fibres run downwards, backwards and laterally	Roughened area on the medial surface of angle and adjoining ramus of mandible, below and behind the mandibular foramen and mylohyoid groove	Nerve to medial pterygoid, branch of the main trunk of mandibular nerve	(a) Elevates mandible (b) Helps protrude mandible (c) Right medial pterygoid with left lateral pterygoid turn the chin to left side

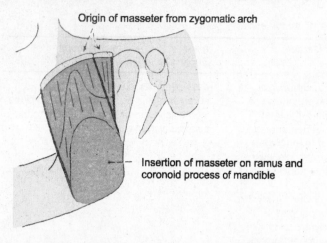

Origin of masseter from zygomatic arch

Insertion of masseter on ramus and coronoid process of mandible

Fig. 10.3: *Origin and insertion of the masseter muscle.*

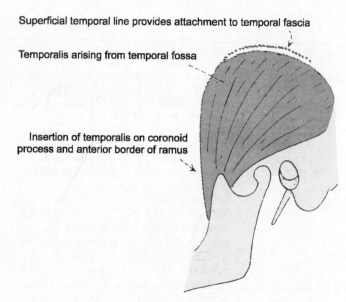

Superficial temporal line provides attachment to temporal fascia

Temporalis arising from temporal fossa

Insertion of temporalis on coronoid process and anterior border of ramus

Fig. 10.4: *Origin and insertion of the temporalis muscle.*

Temporal Fascia

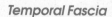

The temporal fascia is a thick aponeurotic sheet that roofs over the temporal fossa and covers the temporalis muscle. Superiorly, the fascia is single layered and is attached to the superior temporal line. Inferiorly, it splits into two layers which are attached to the inner and outer lips of the upper border of the zygomatic arch (Fig. 10.2). The small gap between the two layers contains fat, a branch from the superficial temporal artery and the zygomatico-temporal nerve.

The superficial surface of the temporal fascia receives an expansion from the epicranial aponeurosis. This surface gives origin to the auricularis anterior and superior, and is related to the superficial temporal vessels, the auriculotemporal nerve, and the temporal branches of the facial nerve. The deep surface of the temporal fascia gives origin to some fibres of the temporalis muscle.

The fascia is extremely dense. In some species (e.g., tortoise), the temporal fascia is replaced by bone.

Relations of Lateral Pterygoid

The lateral pterygoid may be regarded as the key muscle of this region because its relations provide a fair idea about the layout of structures in the infratemporal fossa. The relations are as follows:

Superficial: (a) Masseter; (b) ramus of the mandible; (c) tendon of the temporalis; and (d) the maxillary artery.

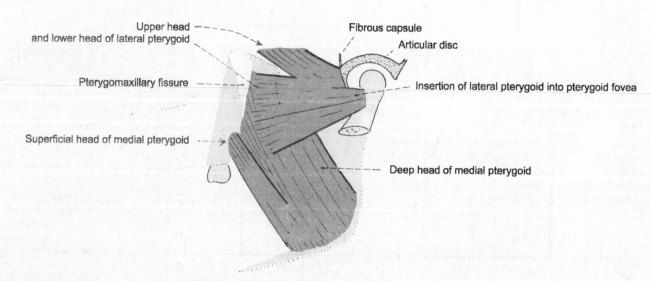

Upper head and lower head of lateral pterygoid

Fibrous capsule

Articular disc

Pterygomaxillary fissure

Insertion of lateral pterygoid into pterygoid fovea

Superficial head of medial pterygoid

Deep head of medial pterygoid

Fig. 10.5: *The lateral and medial pterygoid muscles.*

Deep: (a) Mandibular nerve; (b) middle meningeal artery; (c) sphenomandibular ligament; and (d) deep head of the medial pterygoid.

Structures emerging at the upper border: (a) Deep temporal nerves: (b) masseteric nerve.

Structures emerging at the lower border: (a) Lingual nerve; (b) inferior alveolar nerve; (c) the middle meningeal artery passes upwards deep to it (Fig. 10.6).

Structures passing through the gap between the two heads: (a) The maxillary artery enters the gap and (b) the buccal branch of the mandibular nerve comes out through the gap.

The pterygoid plexus of veins surrounds the lateral pterygoid.

Relations of Medial Pterygoid

Superficial Relations

The upper part of the muscle is separated from the lateral pterygoid muscle by: (a) The lateral pterygoid plate; (b) the lingual nerve; (c) the inferior alveolar nerve (Figs 10.5, 10.6).

Lower down the muscle is separated from the ramus of the mandible by the same nerves, the maxillary artery, and the sphenomandibular ligament.

Deep Relations

The relations are: (a) Tensor veli palatini; (b) superior constrictor of pharynx; (c) styloglossus and (e) stylopharyngeus attached to the styloid process (Fig. 9.4).

MAXILLARY ARTERY

Introduction: This is the larger terminal branch of the external carotid artery, given off behind the neck of the mandible (Fig. 10.6). It has a wide territory of distribution, and supplies: (a) The external and middle ears, and the auditory tube; (b) the dura mater; (c) the upper and lower jaws; (d) the muscles of the temporal and infratemporal regions; (e) the nose and paranasal air sinuses; (f) the palate and (g) the root of the pharynx (Fig. 10.7).

Course and Relations

For descriptive purposes the maxillary artery is divided into three parts (by the lateral pterygoid) (Fig. 10.6).

1. The *first (mandibular) part* runs horizontally forwards, first between the neck of the mandible and the sphenomandibular ligament, below the auriculo-

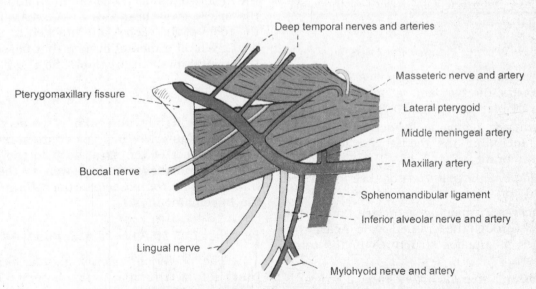

Fig. 10.6: *Some relations of the lateral pterygoid muscle.*

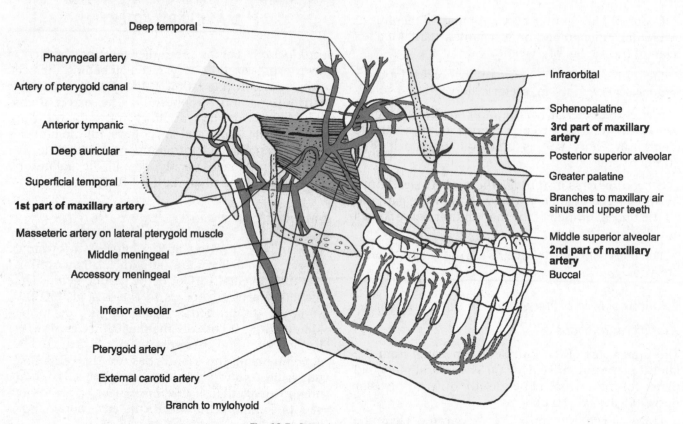

Deep temporal

Pharyngeal artery

Artery of pterygoid canal

Anterior tympanic

Deep auricular

Superficial temporal

1st part of maxillary artery

Masseteric artery on lateral pterygoid muscle

Middle meningeal

Accessory meningeal

Inferior alveolar

Pterygoid artery

External carotid artery

Branch to mylohyoid

Infraorbital

Sphenopalatine

3rd part of maxillary artery

Posterior superior alveolar

Greater palatine

Branches to maxillary air sinus and upper teeth

Middle superior alveolar

2nd part of maxillary artery

Buccal

Fig. 10.7: *Branches of maxillary artery.*

temporal nerve, and then along the lower border of the lateral pterygoid.

2. The *second (pterygoid) part* runs upwards and forwards superficial to the lower head of the lateral pterygoid.

3. The *third (pterygopalatine) part* passes between the two heads of the lateral pterygoid and through the pterygomaxillary fissure, to enter the pterygopalatine fossa where it lies in front of the pterygopalatine ganglion.

Branches of First Part of the Maxillary Artery

1. The *deep auricular artery* supplies the external acoustic meatus, the tympanic membrane and the temporomandibular joint (Fig. 10.7).

2. The *anterior tympanic* branch supplies the middle ear including the medial surface of the tympanic membrane.

3. The *middle meningeal artery* has been described in Chapter 6 and Table 10.2.

4. The *accessory meningeal artery* enters the cranial cavity through the foramen ovale. Apart from the meninges it supplies structures in the infratemporal fossa.

5. The *inferior alveolar artery* runs downwards and forwards medial to the ramus of the mandible to reach the mandibular foramen. Passing through this foramen the artery enters the mandibular canal (within the body of the mandible) in which it runs downwards and then forwards. Before entering the mandibular canal the artery gives off a lingual branch to the tongue; and a mylohyoid branch that descends in the mylohyoid groove (on the medial aspect of the mandible) and runs forwards above the mylohyoid muscle. Within the mandibular canal the artery gives branches to the mandible and to the roots of the each tooth attached to the bone. It also gives off a mental branch that passes through the mental foramen to supply the chin.

Branches of Second Part of the Maxillary Artery

These are mainly muscular. The *deep temporal* branches (anterior and posterior) ascend on the lateral aspect of the skull deep to the temporalis muscle. Branches are also given *to the pterygoid muscles* and *to the masseter. A buccal branch* supplies the buccinator muscle.

Branches of Third Part of the Maxillary Artery

1. The *posterior superior alveolar artery* arises just before the maxillary artery enters the pterygomaxillary fissure. It descends on the posterior

Table 10.2: Branches of maxillary artery

Branches	Foramina transmitting	Distribution
A. *Of first part* (Fig. 10.7)		
1. Deep auricular	Foramen in the floor (cartilage or bone) of external acoustic meatus	Skin of external acoustic meatus, and outer surface of tympanic membrane
2. Anterior tympanic	Petrotympanic fissure	Inner surface of tympanic membrane
3. Middle meningeal	Foramen spinosum	Supplies more of bone and less of meninges; also 5th and 7th nerves, middle ear and tensor tympani
4. Accessory meningeal	Foramen ovale	Main distribution is extracranial to pterygoids
5. Inferior alveolar	Mandibular foramen	Lower teeth and mylohyoid muscle
B. *Of second part*		
1. Deep temporal	—	Temporalis
2. Pterygoid	—	Lateral and medial pterygoids
3. Masseteric	—	Masseter
4. Buccal	—	Buccinator
C. *Of third part* (Fig. 10.2)		
1. Posterior superior alveolar	Alveolar canals in body of maxilla	Upper molar and premolar teeth and gums; maxillary sinus
2. Infraorbital	Inferior orbital fissure	Lower orbital muscles; lacrimal sac; maxillary sinus; upper incisor and canine teeth
3. Greater palatine	Greater palatine canal	Soft palate; tonsil; palatine glands and mucosa; upper gums
4. Pharyngeal	Pharyngeal (palatovaginal) canal	Roof of nose and pharynx; auditory tube; sphenoidal sinus
5. Artery of pterygoid canal	Pterygoid canal	Auditory tube; upper pharynx; and middle ear
6. Sphenopalatine (terminal part)	Sphenopalatine foramen	Lateral and medial walls of nose and various air sinuses

surface of the maxilla and gives branches that enter canals in the bone to supply the molar and premolar teeth, and the maxillary air sinus.

2. The *infraorbital artery* also arises just before the maxillary artery enters the pterygomaxillary fissure. It enters the orbit through the inferior orbital fissure. It then runs forwards in relation to the floor of the orbit, first in the infraorbital groove and then in the infraorbital canal to emerge on the face through the infraorbital foramen. It gives off some orbital branches to structures in the orbit, and the *anterior superior alveolar* branches that enter apertures in the maxilla to reach the incisor and canine teeth attached to the bone. After emerging on the face, the infraorbital artery gives branches to the lacrimal sac, the nose and the upper lip.

The remaining branches of the third part arise within the pterygopalatine fossa (Fig. 10.7).

3. The *greater palatine artery* runs downwards in the greater palatine canal to emerge on the posterolateral part of the hard palate through the greater palatine foramen. It then runs forwards near the lateral margin of the palate to reach the incisive canal (near the midline) through which some terminal branches enter the nasal cavity. Branches of the artery supply the palate and gums. While still within the greater palatine canal it gives off the *lesser palatine arteries* that emerge on the palate through

the lesser palatine foramina, and run backwards into the soft palate and tonsil.

4. The *pharyngeal branch* runs backwards through a canal related to the inferior aspect of the body of the sphenoid bone (pharyngeal or palatovaginal canal). It supplies part of the nasopharynx, the auditory tube and the sphenoidal air sinus.

5. The *artery of the pterygoid canal* runs backwards in the canal of the same name and helps to supply the pharynx, the auditory tube and the tympanic cavity.

6. The *sphenopalatine artery* passes medially through the sphenopalatine foramen to enter the cavity of the nose. It gives off *posterolateral nasal* branches to the lateral wall of the nose and to the paranasal sinuses; and *posterior septal branches* to the nasal septum.

Pterygoid Plexus of Veins

It lies around and within the lateral pterygoid muscle. The tributaries of the plexus correspond to the branches of the maxillary artery. The plexus is drained by the maxillary vein which begins at the posterior end of the plexus and unites with the superficial temporal vein to form the retromandibular vein. Thus the maxillary vein accompanies only the first part of the maxillary artery.

mandibular foramen → mylohyoid branch of inf. alveolar artery & mylohyoid nerve

The plexus communicates: (a) With the inferior ophthalmic vein through the inferior orbital fissure; (b) with the cavernous sinus through the emissary veins; and (c) with the facial vein through the deep facial vein.

TEMPOROMANDIBULAR JOINT

This is a synovial joint of the condylar variety.

Articular Surfaces

The upper articular surface is formed by the following parts of the temporal bone: (a) Articular eminence; and (b) anterior part of the mandibular fossa (Fig. 10.8).

The inferior articular surface is formed by the head of the mandible.

The articular surfaces are covered with fibrocartilage. The joint cavity is divided into upper and lower parts by an intra-articular disc.

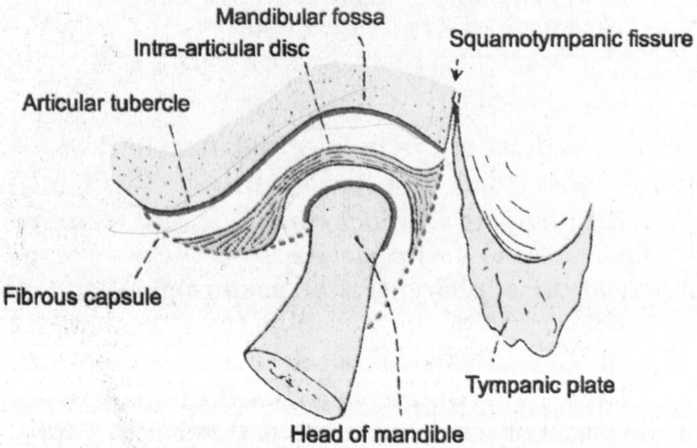

Fig. 10.8: Articular surfaces of the left temporomandibular joint.

DISSECTION

Cut the lateral pterygoid muscle close to its insertion. Dislodge the head of mandible from the articular disc. Locate the articular cartilages covering the head of the mandible and the mandibular fossa. Take out the articular disc as well and study its shape and its role in increasing the varieties of movements.

Ligaments

The ligaments are the fibrous capsule; the lateral ligament; the sphenomandibular ligament; and the stylomandibular ligament.

1. The *fibrous capsule* is attached *above* to the articular tubercle, the circumference of the mandibular fossa and the squamotympanic fissure; and *below* to the neck of the mandible. The capsule is loose above the intra-articular disc, and tight below it. The synovial membrane lines the fibrous capsule and the neck of the mandible (Fig. 10.9).

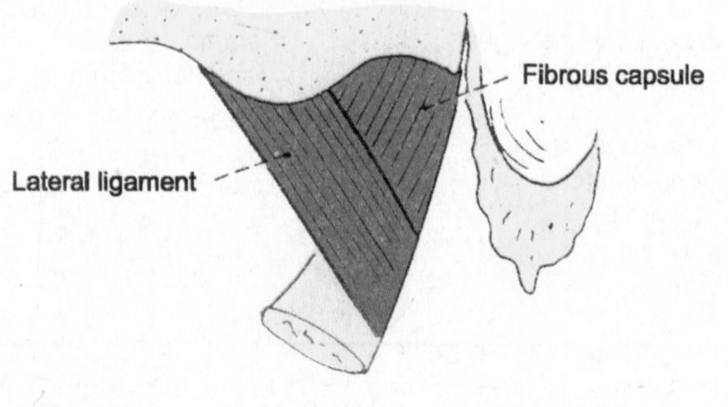

Fig. 10.9: Fibrous capsule and lateral ligament of the temporomandibular joint.

← limits movement of mandible post. Protects ext. acoustic meatus

2. The *lateral* or *temporomandibular ligament* reinforces and strengthens the lateral part of the capsular ligament. Its fibres are directed downwards and backwards. It is attached above to the articular tubercle, and below to the posterolateral aspect of the neck of the mandible.

3. The *sphenomandibular ligament* is an accessory ligament, that lies on a deep plane away from the fibrous capsule. It is attached superiorly to the spine of the sphenoid, and inferiorly to the lingula of the mandibular foramen. It is a remnant of the dorsal part of Meckel's cartilage.

The ligament is related *laterally* to: (a) The lateral pterygoid; (b) the auriculotemporal nerve; (c) the maxillary artery (Figs 10.10, 10.11); and (d) the

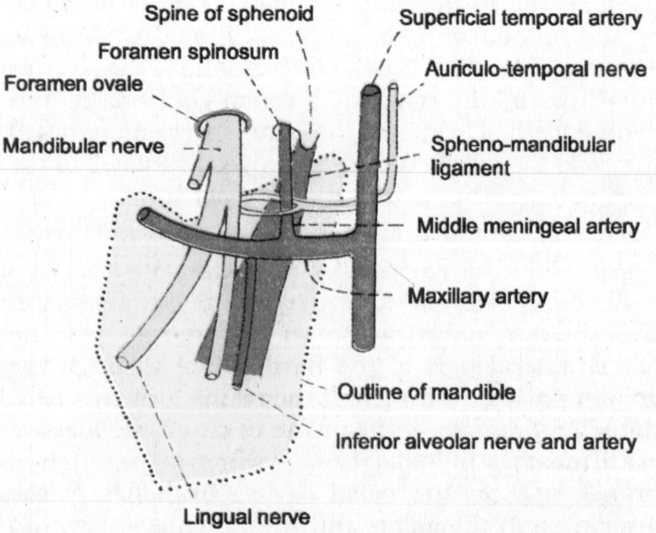

Fig. 10.10: Superficial relations of the sphenomandibular ligament seen after removal of the lateral pterygoid.

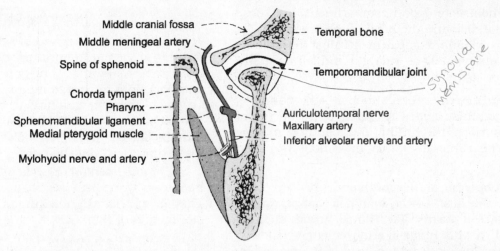

Fig. 10.11: Oblique coronal section through the infratemporal fossa showing relations of the sphenomandibular ligament.

chorda tympani nerve; and (c) the wall of the pharynx. Near its lower end, it is pierced by the mylohyoid nerve and vessels.

4. The *stylomandibular ligament* is another accessory ligament of the joint. It represents a thickened part of the deep cervical fascia which separates the parotid and submandibular salivary glands. It is attached above to the lateral surface of the styloid process, and below to the angle and posterior border of the ramus of the mandible.

Articular Disc

The *articular disc* is an oval fibrous plate that divides the joint into an upper and a lower compartments. The upper compartment permits *gliding* movements, and the lower, *rotatory* as well as *gliding* movements. The disc has a concavoconvex superior surface, and a concave inferior surface. The periphery of the disc is attached to the fibrous capsule. The disc is composed of an anterior extension, anterior thick band, intermediate zone, posterior thick band and bilamellar region (Fig. 10.12). The disc represents the degenerated primitive insertion of lateral pterygoid.

Relations of Temporomandibular Joint

Lateral: (a) Skin and fasciae; (b) parotid gland; and (c) temporal branches of the facial nerve.

Medial: (a) The tympanic plate separates the joint from the internal carotid artery; (b) spine of the sphenoid, with the upper end of the spheno-mandibular ligament attached to it; (c) the auriculotemporal and chorda tympani nerves; (d) middle meningeal artery (Fig. 10.11).

Anterior: (a) Lateral pterygoid; (b) masseteric nerve and vessels.

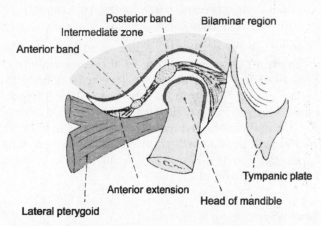

Fig. 10.12: Subdivision and attachment of the articular disc of the temporomandibular joint.

Posterior: (a) The parotid gland separates the joint from the external auditory meatus; (b) superficial temporal vessels; and (c) auriculotemporal nerve (Figs 9.1, 9.3).

Superior: (a) Middle cranial fossa, and (d) middle meningeal vessels.

Inferior: Maxillary artery and vein.

Blood Supply

Branches from superficial temporal and maxillary arteries. Veins follow the arteries.

Nerve Supply
(Both branches of mandibular nerve)
Auriculotemporal nerve and masseteric nerve.

Movements

The movements at the joint can be divided into those between the upper articular surface and the articular disc, i.e. meniscotemporal compartment and those between the disc and the head of the mandible, i.e. meniscomandibular compartment. Most movements occur simultaneously at the right and left temporomandibular joints.

In forward movement or protraction of the mandible, the articular disc glides forwards over the upper articular surface, the head of the mandible moving with it. The reversal of this movement is called retraction.

In slight opening of the mouth or depression of the mandible, the head of the mandible moves on the undersurface of the disc like a hinge. In wide opening of the mouth, this hinge-like movement is followed by gliding of the disc and the head of the mandible, as in protraction. At the end of this movement, the head comes to lie under the articular tubercle. These movements are reversed in closing the mouth or elevation of the mandible.

Chewing movements involve side to side movements of the mandible. In these movements, the head of (say) right side glides forwards along with the disc as in protraction, but the head of the left side merely rotates on a vertical axis. As a result of this the chin moves forwards and to left side (the side on which no gliding has occurred). Alternate movements of this kind on the two sides result in side to side movements of the jaw.

Muscles Producing Movements

Depression is brought about mainly by the lateral pterygoid. The digastric, geniohyoid and mylohyoid muscles help when the mouth is opened wide or against resistance: The origin of only lateral pterygoid is anterior, slightly lower and medial to its insertion. During contraction, it rotates the head mandible and opens the mouth. During wide opening, it pulls the articular disc forwards. So movement occurs in both the compartments. It is also done passively by gravity.

Elevation is brought about by the masseter, the temporalis, and the medial pterygoid muscles of both sides. These are antigravity muscles.

Protrusion is done by the lateral and medial pterygoids.

Retraction is produced by the posterior fibres of the temporalis. It may be resisted by the middle and deep fibres of the masseter, the digastric and geniohyoid muscles.

Lateral or side to side movements, e.g. turning the chin to left side produced by left lateral pterygoid and right medial pterygoid and vice versa.

MANDIBULAR NERVE

This is the largest of the three divisions of the trigeminal nerve. It has both sensory and motor fibres. It is the nerve of the first branchial arch and supplies all structures derived from the mandibular or first branchial arch.

Surface Marking

1. Mandibular Nerve

Mandibular nerve is marked by a short vertical line in the posterior part of the mandibular notch just in front of the head of the mandible.

2. Auriculotemporal Nerve

Auriculotemporal nerve is marked by a line drawn first backwards from the posterior part of the mandibular notch (site of mandibular nerve) across the neck of the mandible, and then upwards across the preauricular point (Fig. 10.13).

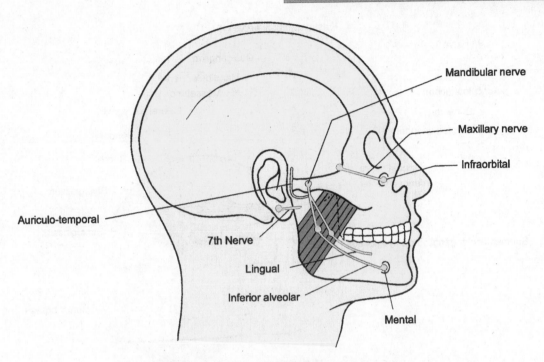

Fig. 10.13: *Surface marking of some nerves on face.*

3. Lingual Nerve

Lingual nerve is marked by a curved line running downwards and forwards by joining the following points (Fig. 10.13).

(a) The first point on the posterior part of the mandibular notch, in line with the mandibular nerve.

(b) The second point a little below and behind the last lower molar tooth.

(c) The third point opposite the first lower molar tooth.

The concavity in the course of the nerve is more marked between points b and c and is directed upwards.

4. Inferior Alveolar

Inferior alveolar is little below and parallel to the lingual nerve.

Course and Relations

Mandibular nerve begins in the middle cranial fossa through a large sensory root and a small motor root. The sensory root arises from the lateral part of the trigeminal ganglion, and leaves the cranial cavity through the foramen ovale (Fig. 6.14).

The motor root lies deep to the trigeminal ganglion and to the sensory root. It also passes through the foramen ovale to join the sensory root just below the foramen thus forming the main trunk. The main trunk lies in the infratemporal fossa, on the tensor veli palatini, deep to the lateral pterygoid. After a short course, the main trunk divides into a small

anterior trunk and a large posterior trunk (Fig. 10.14).

Branches

From the main trunk: (a) Meningeal branch; and (b) nerve to the medial pterygoid.

From the anterior trunk: (a) A sensory branch, the buccal nerve; and (b) motor branches, the masseteric and deep temporal nerves and the nerve to the lateral pterygoid.

From the posterior trunk: (a) Auriculotemporal; (b) lingual; and (c) inferior alveolar nerves.

Meningeal Branch or Nervus Spinosus

Meningeal branch enters the skull through the foramen spinosum with the middle meningeal artery and supplies the dura mater of the middle cranial fossa.

Nerve to Medial Pterygoid

Nerve to medial pterygoid arises close to the otic ganglion and supplies the medial pterygoid from its deep surface. This nerve gives a motor root to the otic ganglion which does not relay and supplies the tensor veli palatini, and the tensor tympani muscles (Fig. 10.15).

Buccal Nerve

Buccal nerve is the only sensory branch of the anterior division of the mandibular nerve. It passes between the two heads of the lateral pterygoid, runs downwards and forwards, and supplies the skin and mucous membrane related to the buccinator

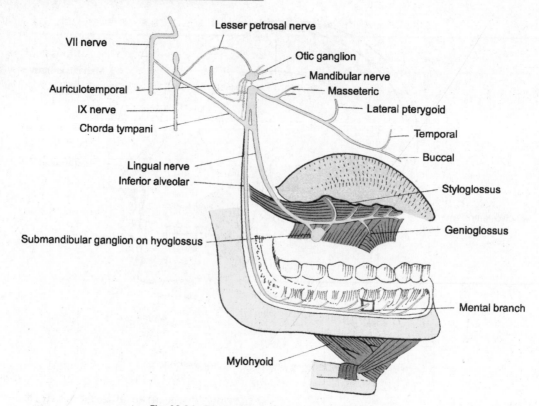

Fig. 10.14: *Distribution of mandibular nerve (V₃).*

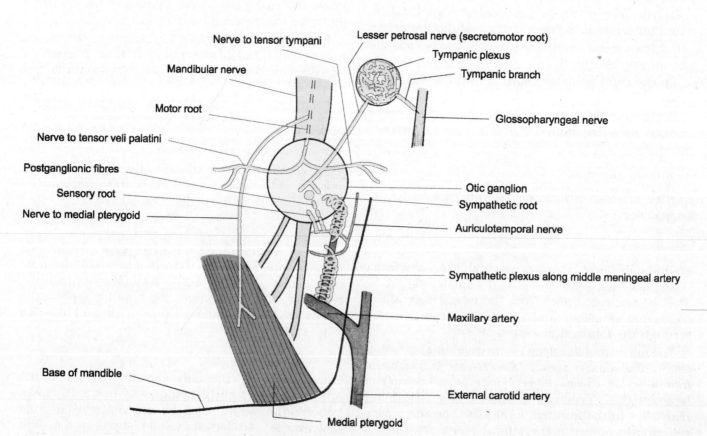

Fig. 10.15: *Right otic ganglion seen from medial side.*

(Fig. 10.6). It also supplies the labial aspect of gums of molar and premolar teeth.

Masseteric Nerve (motor)

Masseteric nerve emerges at the upper border of the lateral pterygoid just in front of the temporomandibular joint, passes laterally through the mandibular notch in company with the masseteric vessels, and enters the deep surface of the masseter. It also supplies the temporomandibular joint (Fig. 10.6).

Deep Temporal Nerves (motor)

Deep temporal nerves are two deep temporal nerves, anterior and posterior. They pass between the skull and the lateral pterygoid, and enter the deep surface of the temporalis. The anterior nerve is often a branch of the buccal nerve. The posterior nerve may arise in common with the masseteric nerve.

Nerve to Lateral Pterygoid (motor)

Nerve to lateral pterygoid enters the deep surface of the muscle. It may be an independent branch or may arise in common with the buccal nerve (Fig. 10.14).

Auriculotemporal Nerve (sensory)

Auriculotemporal nerve arises by two roots which run backwards, encircle the middle meningeal artery, and unite to form a single trunk (Figs 10.10, 10.11). The nerve continues backwards between the neck of the mandible and the sphenomandibular ligament, above the maxillary artery. Behind the neck of the mandible, it turns upwards and ascends on the temple behind the superficial temporal vessels.

The *auricular part* of the nerve supplies the skin of the tragus; and the upper parts of the pinna, the external acoustic meatus and the tympanic membrane. (Note that the lower parts of these regions are supplied by the great auricular nerve and the auricular branch of the vagus nerve). The *temporal part* supplies the skin of the temple (Fig. 2.5). *In addition*, the auriculotemporal nerve also supplies the parotid gland (secretomotor and also sensory) and the temporomandibular joint (Table 1.3).

Lingual Nerve

Lingual nerve is one of the two terminal branches of the posterior division of the mandibular nerve (Fig. 10.13). It is sensory to the anterior two-thirds of the tongue and to the floor of the mouth. However, the fibres of the chorda tympani (branch of facial nerve) which is secretomotor to the submandibular and sublingual salivary glands and gustatory to the anterior two-thirds of the tongue, are also distributed through the lingual nerve (Fig. 10.14).

Course and relations. It begins 1 cm below the skull. It runs first between the tensor veli palatini and the lateral pterygoid, and then between the lateral and medial pterygoids. About 2 cm below the skull it is joined by the chorda tympani nerve. Emerging at the lower border of the lateral pterygoid, the nerve runs downwards and forwards between the ramus of the mandible and the medial pterygoid. Next it lies in direct contact with the mandible, medial to the third molar tooth between the origins of the superior constrictor and the mylohyoid muscles (Fig. 1.27). It soon leaves the gum and runs over the hyoglossus deep to the mylohyoid. Finally, it lies on the surface of the genioglossus deep to the mylohyoid. Here it around winds round the submandibular duct and divides into its terminal branches.

Inferior Alveolar Nerve

Inferior alveolar nerve is the larger terminal branch of the posterior division of the mandibular nerve (Fig. 10.13). It runs vertically downwards lateral to the medial pterygoid and to the sphenomandibular ligament. It enters the mandibular foramen and runs in the mandibular canal. It is accompanied by the inferior alveolar artery (Fig. 1.27).

Branches: (a) The *mylohyoid branch* contains all the motor fibres of the posterior division. It arises just before the inferior alveolar nerve enters the mandibular foramen. It pierces the sphenomandibular ligament with the mylohyoid artery, runs in the mylohyoid groove, and supplies the mylohyoid muscle and the anterior belly of the digastric (Fig. 10.11). (b) While running in the mandibular canal the inferior alveolar nerve gives branches that supply the lower teeth and gums. (c) The *mental nerve* emerges at the mental foramen and supplies the skin of the chin, and the skin and mucous membrane of the lower lip (Fig. 10.14). Its incisive branch supplies the labial aspect of gums of canine and incisor teeth.

CLINICAL ANATOMY

1. The motor part of the mandibular nerve is tested clinically by asking the patient to clench her/his teeth and then feeling for the contracting masseter and temporalis muscles on the two sides. If one masseter is paralysed, the jaw deviates to the paralysed side, on opening the mouth by the action of the normal lateral pterygoid of the opposite side. The activity of the pterygoid muscles is tested by asking the patient to move the chin from side to side.

2. *Referred pain.* In cases with cancer of the tongue, pain radiates to the ear and to the temporal fossa, over the distribution of the auriculotemporal

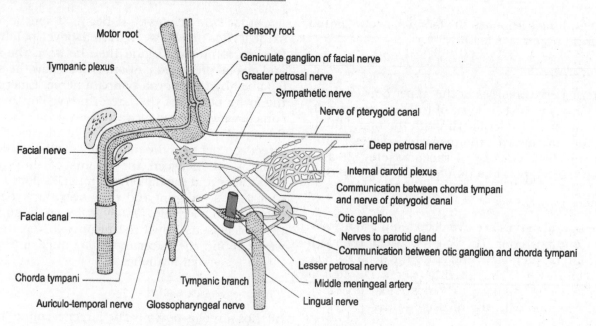

Motor root

Sensory root

Tympanic plexus

Geniculate ganglion of facial nerve

Greater petrosal nerve

Sympathetic nerve

Nerve of pterygoid canal

Facial nerve

Deep petrosal nerve

Internal carotid plexus

Communication between chorda tympani and nerve of pterygoid canal

Facial canal

Otic ganglion

Nerves to parotid gland

Communication between otic ganglion and chorda tympani

Lesser petrosal nerve

Chorda tympani

Tympanic branch

Middle meningeal artery

Auriculo-temporal nerve

Glossopharyngeal nerve

Lingual nerve

Fig. 10.16: Connections of otic ganglion (schematic).

nerve. Sometimes the lingual nerve is divided to relieve intractable pain of this kind. This may be done where the nerve lies in contact with the mandible below and behind the last molar tooth, covered only by mucous membrane.

3. *Mandibular neuralgia.* Trigeminal neuralgia of the mandibular division is often difficult to treat. In such cases, the sensory root of the nerve may be divided behind the ganglion, and this is now the operation of choice when pain is confined to the distribution of the maxillary and mandibular nerves. During division, the ophthalmic fibres that lie in the superomedial part of the root are spared, to preserve the corneal reflex thus avoiding damage to the cornea.

4. Lingual nerve lies in contact with mandible, medial to the third molar tooth. In extraction of malplaced 'wisdom' tooth, care must be taken not to injure the lingual nerve (Fig. 1.27).

OTIC GANGLION

Introduction

It is a peripheral parasympathetic ganglion which relays secretomotor fibres to the parotid gland. Topographically, it is intimately related to the mandibular nerve, but functionally it is a part of the glossopharyngeal nerve (Figs 10.14, 10.15).

Size and Situation

It is 2 to 3 mm in size, and is situated in the infratemporal fossa, just below the foramen ovale. It

lies medial to the mandibular nerve, and lateral to the tensor veli palatini. It surrounds the origin of the nerve to the medial pterygoid (Fig. 10.15).

Connections and Branches

The *motor or parasympathetic root* is formed by the lesser petrosal nerve. The preganglionic fibres are derived from the inferior salivary nucleus – the ninth nerve, its tympanic branch, the tympanic plexus – the lesser petrosal nerve to reach the ganglion. The postganglionic or secretomotor fibres pass through the auriculotemporal nerve to the parotid gland (Table 1.3).

The *sympathetic root* is derived from the plexus on the middle meningeal artery. It contains postganglionic fibres arising in the superior cervical ganglion. The fibres pass through the ganglion without relay and reach the parotid gland via the auriculotemporal nerve. They are vasomotor in function.

The *sensory root* comes from the auriculotemporal nerve and is sensory to the parotid gland.

Other fibres passing through the ganglion are as follows.

(a) The nerve to medial pterygoid gives a motor root to the ganglion which passes through it without relay and supplies medially placed tensor veli palatini and laterally placed tensor tympani muscles.

(b) The chorda tympani nerve is connected to the otic ganglion and also to the nerve of the pterygoid canal (Fig. 10.16). These connections provide an alternative pathway of taste from the anterior two-thirds of the tongue. These fibres do not pass through the middle ear.

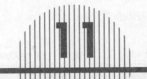

The Submandibular Region

The submandibular region contains the suprahyoid muscles, submandibular and sublingual salivary glands and submandibular ganglion. Chorda tympani from facial nerve provides preganglionic secretomotor fibres to the glands. Chorda tympani also carries fibres of sensation of taste from anterior two-thirds of tongue except from the circumvallate papillae, from where it is carried by the glossopharyngeal nerve.

Introduction

This region includes deeper structures in the area between the mandible and hyoid bone including the floor of the mouth and the root of the tongue.

SUPRAHYOID MUSCLES

The suprahyoid muscles are the digastric, the stylohyoid, the mylohyoid and the geniohyoid. They are described in Table 11.1.

DISSECTION

Cut the facial artery and vein present at the anteroinferior angle of masseter muscle. Separate the origin of anterior belly of digastric muscle from the digastric fossa near the symphysis menti. Push the mandible upwards. Clean and expose the posterior belly of digastric muscle and its accompanying stylohyoid muscle. Identify the digastrics, stylohyoid, mylohyoid, geniohyoid, hyoglossus.

Relations of Posterior Belly of Digastric

Superficial: (a) Mastoid process with the sterno-cleidomastoid, the splenius capitis and the longissimus capitis; (b) the stylohyoid; (c) the parotid gland with retromandibular vein; (d) submandibular salivary gland and lymph nodes; (e) angle of the mandible with the medial pterygoid (Fig. 11.1).

Deep: (a) Transverse process of the atlas with superior oblique and the rectus capitis lateralis; (b) internal carotid, external carotid, lingual, facial and occipital arteries; (c) internal jugular vein; (d) vagus, accessory and hypoglossal cranial nerves; and (e) the hyoglossus muscle.

Its upper border is related to: (a) The posterior auricular artery and (b) the stylohyoid muscle.

Its lower border is related to the occipital artery (Fig. 12.16).

Relations of Mylohyoid

Superficial: (a) Anterior belly of the digastric; (b) superficial part of the submandibular salivary gland; (c) mylohyoid nerve and vessels; and (d) submental branch of the facial artery (Fig. 8.2).

Deep: (a) Hyoglossus with its superficial relations, namely the styloglossus, the lingual nerve, the submandibular ganglion, the deep part of the submandibular salivary gland, the submandibular duct, the hypoglossal nerve, and the vena comitants hypoglossi; and (b) the genioglossus with its superficial relations, namely the sublingual salivary gland, the lingual nerve, submandibular duct, the lingual artery, and the hypoglossal nerve (Figs 11.2, 11.3).

Relations of Hyoglossus

Superficial: Styloglossus, lingual nerve, submandibular ganglion, deep part of the submandibular gland, submandibular duct, hypoglossal nerve and veins accompanying it.

Deep: (a) Inferior longitudinal muscle of the tongue; (b) genioglossus (Fig. 11.3); (c) middle constrictor of

Table 11.1: Suprahyoid muscles

Muscle	Origin	Fibres	Insertion	Nerve supply	Actions
1. Digastric (DG) Has two bellies united by an intermediate tendon (Figs 8.7, 8.9)	(a) Anterior belly (DGA): from digastric fossa of mandible	(a) Anterior belly runs downwards and backwards	Both heads meet at the intermediate tendon which perforates SH and is held by a fibrous pulley to the hyoid bone	(a) Anterior belly by nerve to mylohyoid	(a) Depresses mandible when mouth is opened widely or against resistance; it is secondary to lateral pterygoid
	(b) Posterior belly (DGP): from mastoid notch of temporal bone (Fig. 9.4)	(b) Posterior belly runs downwards and forwards		(b) Facial nerve	(b) Elevates hyoid bone
2. Stylohyoid (SH) small muscle, lies on upper border of DGP (Fig. 11.8)	Posterior surface of styloid process	Tendon is perforated by DGP tendon	Junction of body and greater cornua of hyoid bone	Facial nerve	(a) Pulls hyoid bone upwards and backwards (b) With other hyoid muscles, it fixes the hyoid bone
3. Mylohyoid (MH) Flat, triangular muscle; two mylohyoids form floor of mouth cavity, deep to DGA (Fig. 11.3)	Mylohyoid line of mandible (Fig. 1.27)	Fibres run medially and slightly downwards	(a) Posterior fibres: body of hyoid bone (Fig. 1.32) (b) Middle and anterior fibres; median raphe, between mandible and hyoid bone	Nerve to mylohyoid	(a) Elevates floor of mouth in first stage of deglutition (b) Helps in depression of mandible, and elevation of hyoid bone
4. Geniohyoid (GH) short and narrow muscle; lies above medial part of MH (Fig. 11.2)	Inferior mental spine (genial tubercle)	Runs backwards and downwards	Anterior surface of body of hyoid bone	CI through hypoglossal nerve (Fig. 8.13)	(a) Elevates hyoid bone (b) May depress mandible when hyoid is fixed
5. Hyoglossus. It is a muscle of tongue. It forms important landmark in this region (Fig. 11.2)	Whole length of greater cornua and lateral part of body of hyoid bone	Fibres run upwards and forwards	Side of tongue between styloglossus and inferior longitudinal muscle of tongue (Fig. 11.8)	Hypoglossal (XII) nerve	Depresses tongue makes dorsum convex, retracts the protruded tongue

the pharynx; (d) glossopharyngeal nerve; (e) stylohyoid ligament; and (f) lingual artery.

Structures passing deep to posterior border of hyoglossus, from the above downwards: (a) Glossopharyngeal nerve; (b) stylohyoid ligament; and (c) lingual artery.

SUBMANDIBULAR SALIVARY GLAND

Introduction : This is a large salivary gland, situated in the anterior part of the digastric triangle. The gland is about the size of a walnut. It is roughly J-shaped, being indented by the posterior border of the mylohyoid which divides it into a larger part superficial to the muscle, and a small part lying deep to the muscle (Fig. 11.3).

DISSECTION

Submandibular gland is seen in the digastric triangle. On pushing the superficial part of the gland posteriorly the entire mylohyoid muscle is exposed. The deep part of the gland lies on the

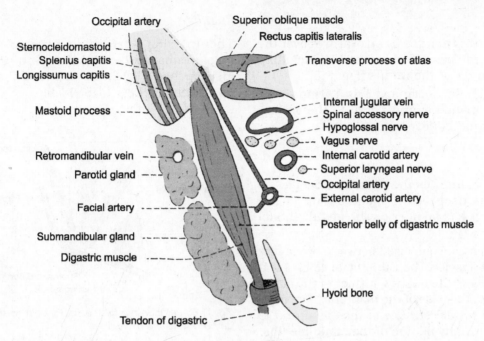

Fig. 11.1: *Posterior belly of the digastric muscle, and structures related to it, seen from below.*

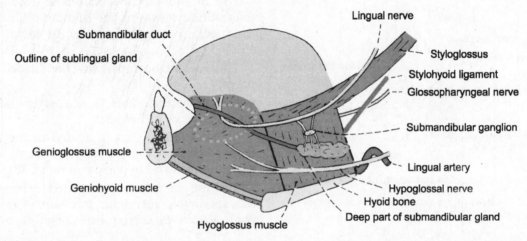

Fig. 11.2: *Submandibular region showing the superficial relations of the hyoglossus and genioglossus muscles.*

superior surface of the muscle. Separate the facial artery from the deep surface of gland and identify its branches in neck. The hyoglossus muscle is recognised as a quadrilateral muscle lying on deeper plane than mylohyoid muscle. Indentify lingual nerve with submandibular ganglion, and hypoglossal nerve running on the hyoglossus muscle from lateral to the medial side. Deep part of gland and its duct are also visible on this surface of hyoglossus muscle (Fig. 11.2).

Carefully release the hyoglossus muscle from the hyoid bone and reflect it towards the tongue. Note the structures deep to the muscle, e.g. genioglossus muscle, lingual artery, vein and middle constrictor of the pharynx.

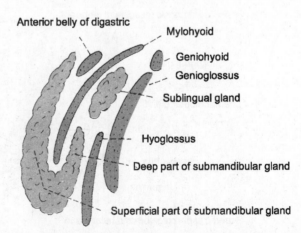

Fig. 11.3: *Horizontal section through the submandibular region showing the location of the submandibular and sublingual glands.*

Surface Marking

This salivary gland is marked by an oval area over the posterior half of the base of the mandible including the posterior border of the ramus (Fig. 9.3).

The submandibular region extends 1.5 cm above the base of the mandible and below to the greater cornua of the hyoid bone.

Superficial Part

This part of the gland fills the digastric triangle. It extends upwards deep to the mandible up to the mylohyoid line. It has (a) inferior; (b) lateral; and (c) medial surfaces.

The gland is partially enclosed between two layers of deep cervical fascia. The superficial (Fig. 11.4) layer of fascia covers the inferior surface of the gland and is attached to the base of the mandible. The deep layer covers the medial surface of the gland and is attached to the mylohyoid line of the mandible (Fig. 11.4).

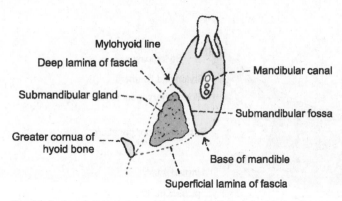

Fig. 11.4: *Fascial covering of the superficial part of the submandibular salivary gland.*

Relations

The inferior surface is covered by: (a) Skin; (b) platysma; (c) cervical branch of the facial nerve; (d) deep fascia; (e) facial vein; and (f) submandibular lymph nodes (Figs 11.5, 11.6).

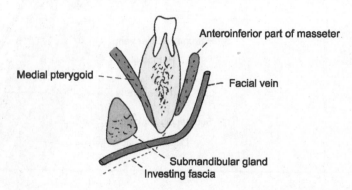

Fig. 11.6: *Relationship of the facial vein to the submandibular gland and to the mandible.*

The lateral surface is related to: (a) The submandibular fossa on the mandible; (b) insertion of the medial pterygoid; and (c) the facial artery (Figs 11.7, 11.8).

The medial surface may be divided into three parts:

(i) The anterior part is related to the mylohyoid muscle, nerve and vessels.

(ii) The middle part is related to the hyoglossus, the styloglossus, the lingual nerve the submandibular ganglion and the hypoglossal nerve (Fig. 11.9).

(iii) The posterior part is related to the styloglossus, the stylohyoid ligament, the ninth nerve, and the wall of the pharynx. Inferiorly, it overlaps the

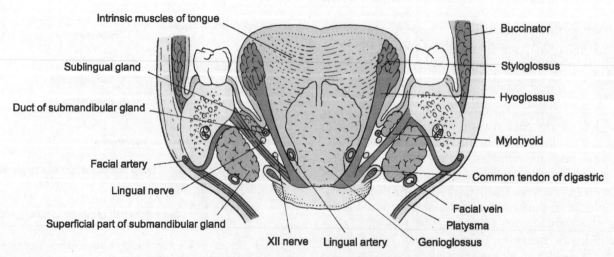

Fig. 11.5: *Coronal section through the mouth posterior to the molar teeth.*

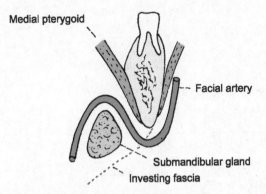

Fig. 11.7: Relationship of the facial artery to the submandibular gland and to the mandible.

Labels: Medial pterygoid, Facial artery, Submandibular gland, Investing fascia

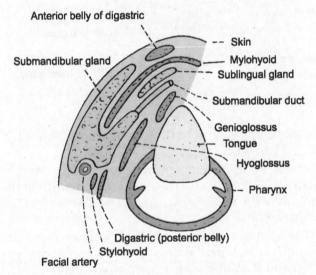

Fig. 11.8: Schematic horizontal section through the submandibular region.

Labels: Anterior belly of digastric, Skin, Submandibular gland, Mylohyoid, Sublingual gland, Submandibular duct, Genioglossus, Tongue, Hyoglossus, Pharynx, Digastric (posterior belly), Stylohyoid, Facial artery

---

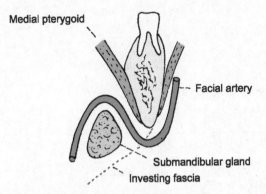

Fig. 11.7: Relationship of the facial artery to the submandibular gland and to the mandible.

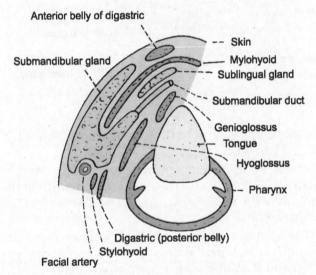

Fig. 11.8: Schematic horizontal section through the submandibular region.

stylohyoid and the posterior belly of the digastric (Figs 11.2, 11.3).

Deep Part

This part is small in size. It lies deep to the mylohyoid, and superficial to the hyoglossus and the styloglossus. Posteriorly, it is continuous with the superficial part round the posterior border of the mylohyoid. Anteriorly, it extends up to the posterior end of the sublingual gland (Fig. 11.3).

Submandibular Duct

It is thin walled, and is about 5 cm long. It emerges at the anterior end of the deep part of the gland and runs forwards on the hyoglossus, between the lingual and hypoglossal nerves. At the anterior border of the hyoglossus the duct is crossed by the lingual nerve (Fig. 11.2). It opens on the floor of the mouth, on the summit of the sublingual papilla, at the side of the frenulum of the tongue (Figs 11.8, 17.2).

Blood Supply and Lymphatic Drainage

It is supplied by the facial artery. The veins drain into the common facial or lingual vein. Lymph passes to submandibular lymph nodes.

Nerve Supply

It is supplied by branches from the submandibular ganglion. These branches convey: (a) Secretomotor fibres; (b) sensory fibres from the lingual nerve, and (c) vasomotor sympathetic fibres from the plexus on the facial artery (Figs 11.10, 11.11).

The secremotor pathway begins in the superior salivary nucleus. Preganglionic fibres pass through the sensory root of the facial nerve, the geniculate

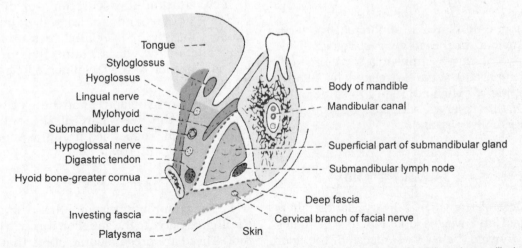

Fig. 11.9: Coronal section of the submandibular region showing the relations of the superficial part of the submandibular salivary gland.

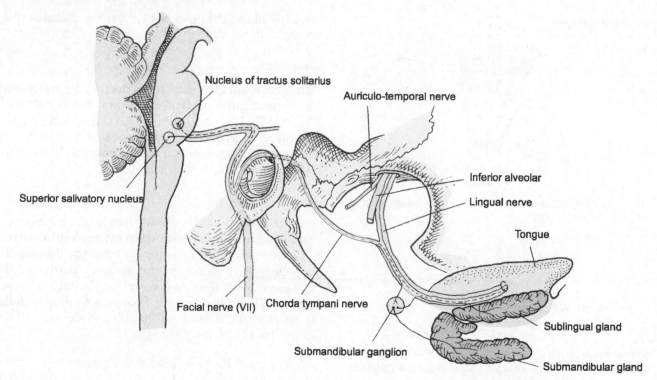

Fig. 11.10: Parasympathetic nerve supply of submandibular and sublingual glands.

ganglion, the facial nerve, the chorda tympani, and the lingual nerve, to reach the submandibular ganglion. Postganglionic fibres emerge from the ganglion and enter the submandibular gland (Table 1.3).

CLINICAL ANATOMY

Excision of the submandibular gland for calculus or tumour is done by an incision below the angle of the jaw. Since the marginal mandibular branch of the facial nerve passes posteroinferior to the angle of the jaw before crossing it, the incision must be placed more than 2.5 cm below the angle to preserve the nerve.

The chorda tympani supplying secretomotor fibres to submandibular and sublingual salivary glands lies medial to the *spine of sphenoid*. The auriculotemporal nerve supplying secretomotor fibres to the parotid gland is related to lateral aspect of spine of sphenoid. Injury to spine may involve both these nerves with loss of secretion from all three salivary glands.

SUBLINGUAL SALIVARY GLAND

This is smallest of the three salivary glands. It is almond-shaped and weighs about 3 to 4 g. It lies above the mylohyoid, below the mucosa of the floor of the mouth, medial to the sublingual fossa of the mandible and lateral to the genioglossus (Figs 11.2, 11.3, 11.5, 11.8, 11.11).

About 15 ducts emerge from the gland. Most of them open directly into the floor of the mouth on the summit of the sublingual fold. A few of them join the submandibular duct.

The gland receives its blood supply from the lingual and submental arteries. The nerve supply is similar to that of the submandibular gland.

SUBMANDIBULAR GANGLION

This is a parasympathetic peripheral ganglion. It is a relay station for secretomotor fibres to the submandibular and sublingual salivary glands. Topographically, it is related to the lingual nerve, but functionally, it is connected to the chorda tympani branch of the facial nerve (chorda tympani) (Table 1.3).

The fusiform ganglion lies on the hyoglossus muscle just above the deep part of the submandibular salivary gland, suspended from the lingual nerve by two roots (Fig. 11.10).

Connections and Branches

1. The motor or parasympathetic fibres pass from the lingual nerve to the ganglion through the posterior root. These are preganglionic fibres that arise in the *superior salivatory nucleus* and pass through the

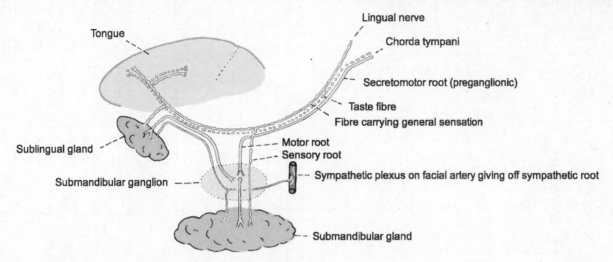

Fig. 11.11: *Connection of the submandibular ganglion.*

facial nerve, the chorda tympani and the lingual nerve to reach the ganglion. The fibres relay in the ganglion. Postganglionic fibres for the submandibular gland reach the gland through five or six branches from the ganglion. Postganglionic fibres for the sublingual and anterior lingual glands re-enter the lingual nerve through the anterior root and travel to the gland through the distal part of the lingual nerve (Fig. 11.10).

2. The sympathetic fibres are derived from the plexus around the facial artery. It contains postganglionic fibres arising in the superior cervical ganglion. They pass through submandibular ganglion without relay, and supply vasomotor fibres to the submandibular and sublingual glands (Fig. 11.11).

3. Sensory fibres reach the ganglion through the lingual nerve.

12

Deep Structures in the Neck

The thyroid gland lies in front of the neck. Skin incision for its surgery should be horizontal, for better healing and for cosmetic reasons. Branches of subclavian artery anastomose with those of axillary around the scapula.

Ninth nerve is the nerve of third branchial arch and supplies the only muscle of that arch, the stylopharyngeus. It carries sensory fibres from the posterior one-third of tongue, tonsil, pharynx, middle ear, taste fibres from posterior one-third of tongue and circumvallate papillae. Lastly, it provides secretomotor fibres to parotid gland.

Vagus in neck gives pharyngeal, carotid sinus and laryngeal branches. These are gracefully borrowed from cranial root of accessory nerve. Vagus gives auricular and cardiac branches as its "own". That is why syringing the ear may cause slowing of the heart rate and even its inhibition. Vagus is the parasympathetic nerve of foregut and midgut. Accessory nerve comprises two roots — cranial root given to vagus and spinal root supplies two muscles of neck, one shrugging muscle, the trapezius, and other, the chin turning muscle, the sternocleidomastoid. Hypoglossal supplies 7 out of 8 muscles of tongue, except palatoglossus. The muscles supplied are 4 intrinsic, i.e. superior longitudinal, inferior longitudinal, transverse and vertical and 3 extrinsic, i.e. styloglossus, genioglossus and hyoglossus.

Scalenus anterior is important. It may compress the subclavian artery to cause "scalenus anterior syndrome". Lymph nodes are clinically important in deciding the prognosis and treatment of malignancies.

Contents: There are numerous deep structures in the neck. For convenience they may be grouped as follows:

A. Glands: thyroid and parathyroid.

B. Thymus.

C. Arteries: subclavian and carotid.

D. Veins: subclavian, internal jugular and brachiocephalic.

E. Nerves: glossopharyngeal, vagus, accessory, hypoglossal, sympathetic chain and cervical plexus.

F. Lymph nodes, and thoracic duct.

G. Viscera: trachea and oesophagus.

H. Scalene muscles.

I. Cervical pleura and suprapleural membrane.

J. Styloid apparatus.

THYROID GLAND
(Thyroid = shield-like)

Introduction

The thyroid is an endocrine gland, situated in the lower part of the front and sides of the neck. It regulates the basal metabolic rate, stimulates somatic and psychic growth, and plays an important role in calcium metabolism.

The gland consists of right and left *lobes* that are joined to each other by the *isthmus.* A third, pyramidal, lobe may project upwards from the isthmus (or from one of the lobes). Sometimes a fibrous or fibromuscular band or *levator of the thyroid gland* descends from the body of the hyoid bone to the isthmus or to the pyramidal lobe.

Accessory thyroid glands are sometimes found as small detached masses of thyroid tissue in the vicinity of the lobes or above the isthmus.

Surface Marking

The isthmus is marked by two transverse parallel lines (each 1.2 cm long) on the trachea, the upper 1.2 cm below and the lower 2.5 cm below the arch of the cricoid cartilage (Fig. 12.1).

Each lobe extends up to the middle of the thyroid cartilage, below till the clavicle, and laterally to be

Sternocleidomastoid muscle has already been reflected laterally from its origin. Cut the sterno-thyroid muscle near its origin and reflect it upwards. Clean the surface of trachea and identify inferior thyroid vein and remains of the thymus gland (darker in colour than fat).

On the tracheal rings 2, 3, 4 lies the isthmus of the thyroid gland. Pyramidal lobe if present projects from the upper border of the isthmus. On each side of isthmus are the lateral lobes of the gland. Clean the lobes and identify the vessels of thyroid gland. Identify the recurrent laryngeal nerves tucked between the lateral surfaces of trachea and oesophagus. Look for beaded thoracic duct present on the left of oesophagus. Trace the superior and inferior thyroid arteries. Identify cricothyroid and inferior constrictor muscles lying medial to the lobes of thyroid gland.

Thyroid Gland

Cut the isthmus of the thyroid gland and turn one of the lobes laterally. Locate an anastomotic artery between the branches of superior thyroid and inferior thyroid arteries supplying the gland. Identify the two parathyroid glands just lateral to this anastomotic vessel.

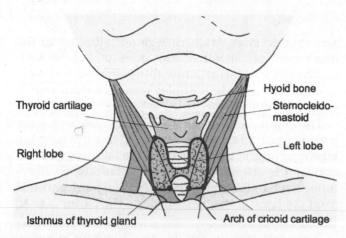

Fig. 12.1: *Surface marking of thyroid gland.*

overlapped by the anterior border of the sterno-cleidomastoid muscle. The upper pole of the gland is pointed, and the lower pole is broad rounded.

Situation and Extent

(a) The gland lies against vertebrae C5, C6, C7 and T1, embracing the upper part of the trachea (Fig. 12.2).

(b) Each lobe extends from the middle of the thyroid cartilage to the fourth or fifth tracheal ring.

(c) The isthmus extends from the second to the fourth tracheal ring.

Dimensions and Weight

Each lobe measures about 5 cm × 2.5 cm × 2.5 cm, and the isthmus 1.2 cm × 1.2 cm. On an average the gland weighs about 25 g. However, it is larger in females than in males, and further increases in size during menstruation and pregnancy.

Capsules of Thyroid

1. The *true capsule* is the peripheral condensation of the connective tissue of the gland.

2. The *false capsule* is derived from the pretracheal layer of the deep cervical fascia (Fig. 12.2). It is thin along the posterior border of the lobes, but thick on the inner surface of the gland where it forms a suspensory ligament (of Berry), which connects the lobe to the cricoid cartilage (see Fig. 12.9).

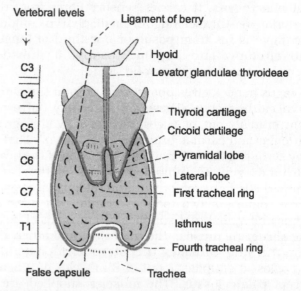

Fig. 12.2: *Scheme to show the location and subdivisions of the thyroid gland including the false capsule.*

A dense capillary plexus is present deep to the true capsule. To avoid haemorrhage during operations the thyroid is removed along with the true capsule. (Compare with the prostate in which the venous plexus lies between the two capsules of the gland; and, therefore, during prostatectomy both capsules are left behind) (Fig. 12.3).

Relations

The lobes are conical in shape having: (a) An apex, (b) a base, (c) three surfaces, lateral, medial and

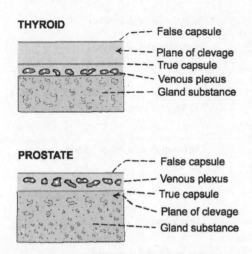

THYROID
- False capsule
- Plane of clevage
- True capsule
- Venous plexus
- Gland substance

PROSTATE
- False capsule
- Venous plexus
- True capsule
- Plane of clevage
- Gland substance

Fig. 12.3: Schemes of comparing the relationship of the venous plexuses related to the thyroid gland and to the prostate, with the true and false capsules around these organs. Note the plane of cleavage along which the organ is separated from neighbouring structures during surgical removal.

posterolateral; and (d) two borders, anterior and posterior.

The *apex* is directed upwards and slightly laterally. It is limited superiorly by the attachment of the sternothyroid to the oblique line of the thyroid cartilage.

The *base* is on level with the 4th or 5th tracheal ring.

The *lateral* or *superficial surface* is convex, and is covered by: (a) The sternohyoid; (b) the superior belly of the omohyoid; (c) the sternothyroid; and (d) the anterior border of the sternocleidomastoid (Fig. 12.4).

The *medial surface* is related to: (a) Two tubes, trachea and oesophagus; (b) two muscles, inferior constrictor and cricothyroid; and (c) two nerves, external laryngeal and recurrent laryngeal (Fig. 12.5).

The *posterolateral* or *posterior surface* is related to the carotid sheath and overlaps the common carotid artery (Fig. 12.4).

The *anterior border* is thin and is related to the anterior branch of the superior thyroid artery (Fig. 12.6).

The *posterior border* is thick and rounded and separates the medial and posterior surfaces. It is related to: (a) The inferior thyroid artery; (b) the anastomosis between the superior and inferior thyroid arteries; (c) the parathyroid glands; and (d) the thoracic duct only on the left side (Fig. 12.7).

The isthmus connects the lower parts of the two lobes. It has: (a) Two surfaces, anterior and posterior; and (b) two borders, superior and inferior. Occasionally the isthmus is absent.

The *anterior surface* is covered by: (a) The right and left sternothyroid and sternohyoid muscles; (b) the anterior jugular veins; (c) fascia and skin (Fig. 12.4).

The *posterior surface* is related to the second to fourth tracheal rings. It may be placed at a higher, or lower level (Fig. 12.2).

The *upper border* is related to the anastomosis between the right and left superior thyroid arteries.

Lower border. Inferior thyroid veins leave the gland at this border.

Arterial Supply

The thyroid gland is supplied by the superior and inferior thyroid arteries.

The *superior thyroid artery* is the first anterior branch of the external carotid artery (Figs 12.6, 12.7). It runs downwards and forwards in intimate relation to the external laryngeal nerve. After giving branches to adjacent structures it pierces the pretracheal fascia to reach the upper pole of the lobe. Here it divides

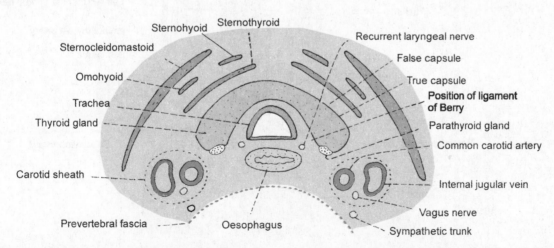

Fig. 12.4: Transverse section through the anterior part of the neck at the level of the isthmus of the thyroid gland.

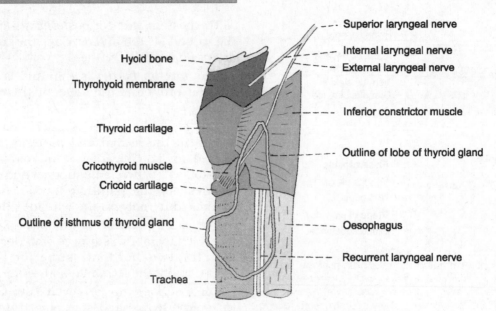

Superior laryngeal nerve

Internal laryngeal nerve

External laryngeal nerve

Hyoid bone

Thyrohyoid membrane

Inferior constrictor muscle

Thyroid cartilage

Outline of lobe of thyroid gland

Cricothyroid muscle

Cricoid cartilage

Outline of isthmus of thyroid gland

Oesophagus

Recurrent laryngeal nerve

Trachea

Fig. 12.5: Deep relations of the thyroid gland.

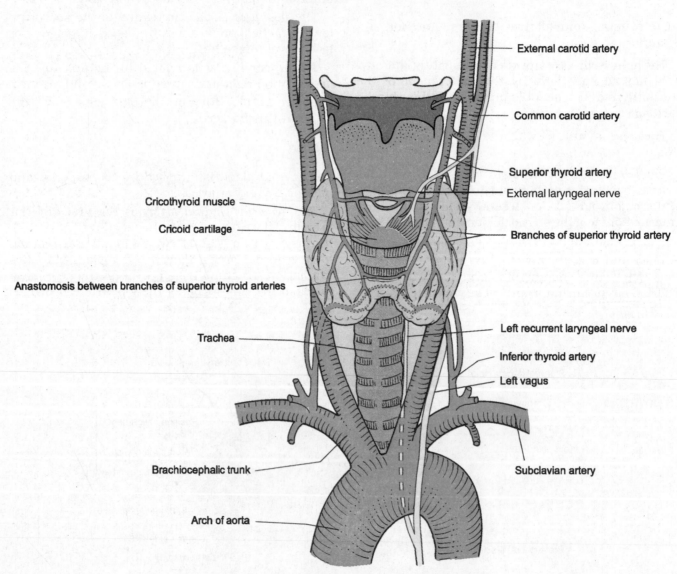

External carotid artery

Common carotid artery

Superior thyroid artery

External laryngeal nerve

Cricothyroid muscle

Cricoid cartilage

Branches of superior thyroid artery

Anastomosis between branches of superior thyroid arteries

Trachea

Left recurrent laryngeal nerve

Inferior thyroid artery

Left vagus

Brachiocephalic trunk

Subclavian artery

Arch of aorta

Fig. 12.6: Arterial supply of anterior aspect of thyroid gland.

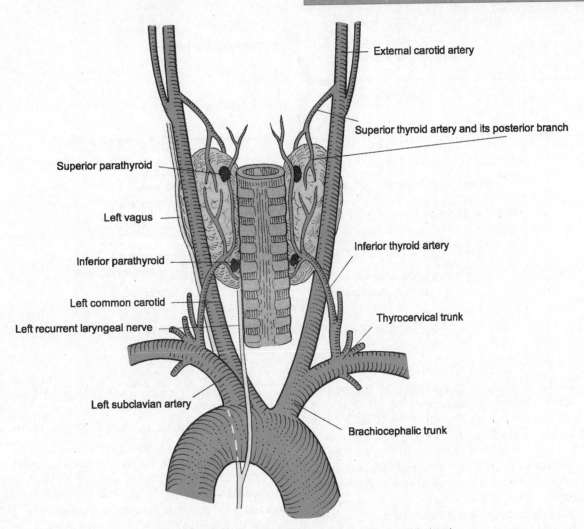

Superior parathyroid

Left vagus

Inferior parathyroid

Left common carotid

Left recurrent laryngeal nerve

Left subclavian artery

External carotid artery

Superior thyroid artery and its posterior branch

Inferior thyroid artery

Thyrocervical trunk

Brachiocephalic trunk

Fig. 12.7: Arterial supply of posterior surface of thyroid gland.

into anterior and posterior branches. The *anterior branch* descends on the anterior border of the lobe and continues along the upper border of the isthmus to anastomose with its fellow of the opposite side. The *posterior branch* descends on the posterior border of the lobe and anastomoses with the ascending branch of the inferior thyroid artery (Fig. 12.7).

The *inferior thyroid artery* is a branch of the thyrocervical trunk (which arises from the subclavian artery). It runs first upwards, then medially, and finally downwards to reach the lower pole of the gland. During its course, it passes behind the carotid sheath and the middle cervical sympathetic ganglion; and in front of the vertebral vessels; and gives off branches to adjacent structures (Fig. 12.8). Its terminal part is intimately related to the recurrent laryngeal nerve. The artery divides into 4 to 5 glandular branches which pierce the fascia separately to reach the lower part of the gland. One *ascending branch* anastomoses with the posterior branch of the superior thyroid artery, and supplies the parathyroid glands.

It is often said that the superior thyroid artery supplies the upper one-third of the lobe and the upper half of the isthmus; and that the inferior thyroid artery supplies the lower two-thirds of the lobe and the lower half of the isthmus. However, the superior and inferior thyroid arteries anastomose freely both on the surface of the gland as well as in its substance; and the territories supplied by the two arteries overlap considerably.

Sometimes (in 3% of individuals), the thyroid is also supplied by the *lowest thyroid artery (thyroidea ima artery)* which arises from the brachiocephalic trunk or directly from the arch of the aorta. It enters the lower part of the isthmus. *Accessory thyroid arteries* arising from tracheal and oesophageal arteries also supply the thyroid.

Venous Drainage

The thyroid is drained by the superior, middle and inferior thyroid veins.

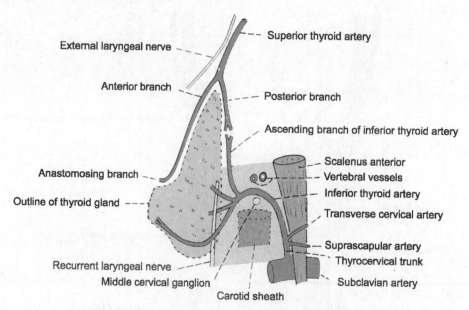

External laryngeal nerve

Anterior branch

Anastomosing branch

Outline of thyroid gland

Recurrent laryngeal nerve

Middle cervical ganglion

Carotid sheath

Superior thyroid artery

Posterior branch

Ascending branch of inferior thyroid artery

Scalenus anterior

Vertebral vessels

Inferior thyroid artery

Transverse cervical artery

Suprascapular artery

Thyrocervical trunk

Subclavian artery

Fig. 12.8: *Arterial supply of the thyroid gland (lateral view).*

The *superior thyroid vein* emerges at the upper pole and accompanies the superior thyroid artery. It ends either in the internal jugular vein or in the common facial vein. The *middle thyroid vein* is a short, wide channel which emerges at the middle of the lobe and soon enters the internal jugular vein. The *inferior thyroid veins* emerge at the lower border of the isthmus. They form a plexus in front of the trachea, and drain into the left brachiocephalic vein. A *fourth thyroid vein* (of Kocher) may emerge between the middle and inferior veins, and drain into the internal jugular vein.

Lymphatic Drainage

Lymph from the upper part of the gland reaches the upper deep cervical lymph nodes either directly or through the prelaryngeal nodes. Lymph from the lower part of the gland drains to the lower deep cervical nodes directly, and also through the pretracheal and paratracheal nodes.

The thyroid is sometimes described as being divided into distinct parts draining in different directions. However, it must be noted that in the thyroid (and for that matter in most other organs) the lymphatics form a plexus through which lymph may pass in any direction.

Nerve Supply

Nerves are derived mainly from the middle cervical ganglion and partly also from the superior and inferior cervical ganglia. These are vasoconstrictor.

HISTOLOGY AND FUNCTION

The thyroid gland is made up of the following two types of secretory cells.

1. *Follicular cells* lining the follicles of the gland secrete triiodothyronin and tetraiodothyronin (thyroxin) which stimulate basal metabolic rate and somatic and psychic growth of the individual. During active phase the lining of the follicles is columnar, while in resting phase, it is cuboidal. Follicles contain the colloid in their lumina.

2. *Parafollicular cells (C cells)* are fewer and light cells lie in between the follicles. They secrete thyrocalcitonin which promotes deposition of calcium salts in skeletal and other tissues, and tends to produce hypocalcaemia. These effects are opposite to those of parathormone.

DEVELOPMENT

The thyroid develops from a *median endodermal thyroid diverticulum* which grows down in front of the neck from the floor of the primitive pharynx, just caudal to the tuberculum impar. The lower end of the diverticulum enlarges to form the gland. The rest of the diverticulum remains narrow and is known as the *thyroglossal duct.* Most of the duct soon disappears. The position of the upper end is marked by the foramen caecum of the tongue, and the lower end often persists as the pyramidal lobe. The gland becomes functional during third month of development.

Remnants of the thyroglossal duct may form thyroglossal cysts, or a thyroglossal fistula. Thyroid tissue may develop at abnormal sites along the course of the duct resulting in lingual or retrosternal thyroids. Accessory thyroids may be present.

PARATHYROID GLANDS

These are two pairs (superior and inferior) of small endocrine glands, that usually lie on the posterior border of the thyroid gland, within the false capsule (Fig. 12.9). The *superior parathyroids* are also referred to as *parathyroid IV* because they develop from the endoderm of the *fourth pharyngeal pouch*. The *inferior parathyroids*, similarly, are also called *parathyroid III* because they develop from the *third pouch*.

The parathyroids secrete the hormone *parathormone* which controls the metabolism of calcium and phosphorus along with thyrocalcitonin.

Each parathyroid gland is oval or lentiform in shape, measuring 6 × 4 × 2 mm (the size of a split pea). Each gland weighs about 50 mg.

Position

The anastomotic artery between the superior and inferior thyroid arteries is usually a good guide to the glands because they usually lie close to it (Fig. 12.9).

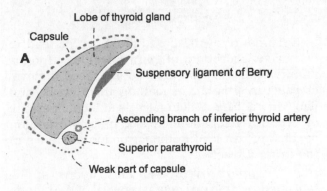
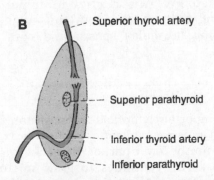

Fig. 12.9: Schemes to show the location of the parathyroid glands. (A) Transverse section through the left lobe of the thyroid gland, (B) posterior view of the left lobe of the thyroid gland.

The *superior parathyroid* is more constant in position and usually lies at the middle of the posterior border of the lobe of the thyroid gland, though it may lie at a higher level. It is usually dorsal to the recurrent laryngeal nerve.

The *inferior parathyroid* is more variable in position. It may lie: (1) Within the thyroid capsule, below the inferior thyroid artery and near the lower pole of the thyroid lobe; (2) behind and outside the thyroid capsule, immediately above the inferior thyroid artery; it (3) within the substance of the lobe near its posterior border. It is usually ventral to the recurrent laryngeal nerve.

Vascular Supply

The parathyroid glands receive a rich blood supply from the inferior thyroid artery and from the anastomosis between the superior and inferior thyroid arteries. The veins and lymphatics of the gland are associated with those of the thyroid and the thymus.

Nerve Supply

Vasomotor nerves are derived from the middle and superior cervical ganglia, directly or through the inferior thyroid plexus. Parathyroid activity is controlled by blood calcium levels; low levels stimulate and high levels inhibit the activity of the glands.

1. Tumours of the parathyroid glands lead to excessive secretion of parathormone (hyper-parathyroidism). This leads to increased removal of calcium from bone making them weak and liable to fracture. Calcium levels in blood increase (hypercalcaemia) and increased urinary excretion of calcium can lead to the formation of stones in the urinary tract.

2. *Hypoparathyroidism* may occur spontaneously or from accidental removal of the glands during thyroidectomy. This results in hypocalcaemia leading to increased neuromuscular irritability causing muscular spasm and convulsions *(tetany).*

THYMUS

The thymus is an important lymphoid organ, situated in the anterior and superior mediastina of the thorax, extending above into the lower part of the neck. It is well developed at birth, continues to grow up to puberty, and thereafter undergoes gradual atrophy and replacement by fat.

The thymus is a bilobed structure, made up of two pyramidal lobes of unequal size which are connected together by areolar tissue. *Each lobe develops from the endoderm of the third pharyngeal pouch.* It lies on the pericardium, the great vessels of the superior mediastinum, and the trachea. Small detached thymic nodules may be found in the neck.

The thymus weighs 10–15 g at birth, 30–40 g at puberty, and only 10 g after mid-adult life. Thus after puberty it becomes inconspicuous due to replacement by fat.

Blood Supply

The thymus is supplied by branches from the internal thoracic and inferior thyroid arteries. Its veins drain into the left brachiocephalic, internal thoracic and inferior thyroid veins.

Nerve Supply

Vasomotor nerves are derived from the stellate ganglion. The capsule is supplied by the phrenic nerve and by the descendens cervicalis.

Functions

1. The thymus controls lymphopoiesis, and maintains an effective pool of circulating lymphocytes, competent to react to innumerable antigenic stimuli.

2. It controls development of the peripheral lymphoid tissues of the body during the neonatal period. By puberty, the main lymphoid tissues are fully developed.

3. The cortical lymphocytes of the thymus arise from stem cells of bone marrow origin. Most (95%) of the lymphocytes (T lymphocytes) produced are autoallergic (act against the host or 'self' antigens), short-lived (3–5 days) and never move out of the organ. They are destroyed within the thymus by phagocytes. Their remnants are seen in Hassall's corpuscles. The remaining 5% of the T lymphocytes are long-lived (3 months or more), and move out of the thymus to join the circulating pool of lymphocytes where they act as immunologically competent but uncommitted cells, i.e. they can react to any unfamiliar, new antigen. On the other hand, the other circulating lymphocytes (from lymph nodes, spleen, etc.) are committed cells, i.e. they can mount an immune response only when exposed to a particular antigen. Thymic lymphopoiesis, lympholysis and involution are all intrinsically controlled.

4. The medullary epithelial cells of the thymus are thought to secrete: (a) *Lymphopoietin,* which stimulates lymphocyte production both in the cortex of the thymus and in peripheral lymphoid organs; and (b) the *competence-inducing factor,* which may be responsible for making new lymphocytes competent to react to antigenic stimuli.

5. Normally there are no germinal centres in the thymic cortex. Such centres appear in autoimmune diseases. This may indicate a defect in the normal function of the thymus.

1. *Involution* of the thymus is enhanced by hypertrophy of the adrenal cortex, injection of cortisone or of androgenic hormone. The involution is delayed by castration and adrenalectomy.

2. Thymic hyperplasia or tumours are often associated with *myasthenia gravis,* characterized by excessive fatiguability of voluntary muscles. The precise role of the thymus in this disease is uncertain; it may influence, directly or indirectly, the transmission at the neuromuscular junction.

3. Thymic tumours may press on the trachea, oesophagus, and the large veins of the neck, causing hoarseness, cough, dysphagia and cyanosis.

SUBCLAVIAN ARTERY

This is the principal artery of the upper limb. It also supplies a considerable part of the neck and brain through its branches.

Origin

On the *right side* it is branch of the brachiocephalic artery. It arises posterior to the sternoclavicular joint. On the *left side* it is a branch of the arch of the aorta. It ascends and enters the neck posterior to the left sternoclavicular joint. Both arteries pursue a similar course in the neck (Fig. 12.7).

Surface Marking

It is marked by a broad curved line, convex upwards, by joining the following two points:

a. A point on the sternoclavicular joint (Fig. 12.10).

b. A second point at the middle of the lower border of the clavicle.

The artery rises about 2 cm above the clavicle.

The thoracic part of the left subclavian artery is marked by a broad vertical line along the left border of the manubrium a little to the left of the left common carotid artery.

Course

1. Each artery arches laterally from the sternoclavicular joint to the outer border of the first rib where it ends by becoming continuous with the axillary artery (Fig. 12.11).

2. The scalenus anterior muscle crosses the artery anteriorly and divides it into three parts. The first part is medial, the second part posterior, and the third part lateral to the scalenus anterior.

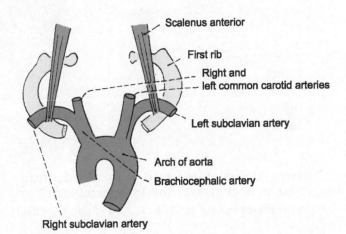

Fig. 12.11: Origin and course of the subclavian arteries.

Relations of the First Part

Anterior: Immediate relations from medial to lateral side are: (1) Common carotid artery; (2) ansa subclavia; (3) cardiac branches of the vagus and of the sympathetic trunk; (4) vagus; (5) vertebral vein; (6) internal jugular vein; (7) left phrenic nerve; and (8) thoracic duct (on left side only). More superficial relations are: (9) The sternothyroid and the sternohyoid muscles; (10) anterior jugular vein; and (11) sternocleidomastoid (Fig. 12.12).

Posterior (posteroinferior): (1) Suprapleural membrane; (2) cervical pleura; (3) apex of lung; (4) ansa subclavia; and (5) right recurrent laryngeal nerve.

Relations of the Second Part

Anterior: (1) Scalenus anterior. Structures in front of the scalenus anterior are: (2) right phrenic nerve deep to the prevertebral fascia: (3) transverse cervical artery; (4) suprascapular artery; (5) subclavian vein; (6) anterior jugular vein; and (7) sternocleidomastoid (Fig. 3.10).

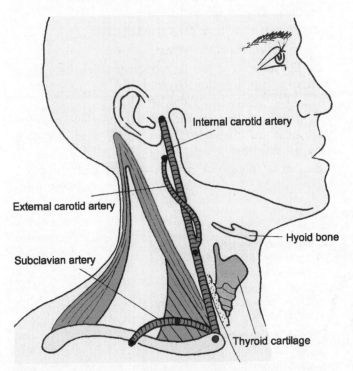

Fig. 12.10: Surface marking of subclavian and carotid arteries.

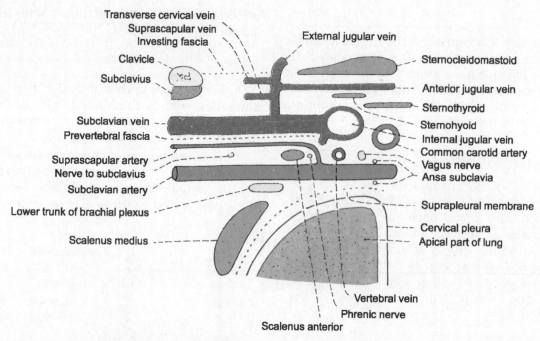

Fig. 12.12: *Schematic transverse section through the lower part of the neck to show the relations of the left subclavian artery.*

Posterior (posteroinferior): (1) Suprapleural membrane; (2) cervical pleura, and (3) apex of lung.

Superior: Upper and middle trunks of the brachial plexus.

Relations of the Third Part

Anterior: (1) Suprascapular vessels; (2) nerve to subcalvius (3) prevertebral fascia; (4) subclavian vein; (5) external jugular vein; (6) anterior jugular vein; (7) transverse cervical vein; (8) suprascapular vein; (9) investing fascia; (10) subclavius; (11) middle one-third of the clavicle, and (12) the posterior border of the sternocleidomastoid (Fig. 3.7).

Posterior (posteroinferior): (1) Scalenus medius; (2) lower trunk of brachial plexus; (3) suprapleural membrane; (4) cervical pleura; and (5) apex of lung.

Superior: (1) Upper and middle trunks of brachial plexus; and (2) inferior belly of omohyoid.

Inferior: First rib.

BRANCHES

The subclavian artery usually gives off four branches. These are as follows:

1. Vertebral artery (Fig. 12.13).

2. Internal thoracic artery.

3. Thyrocervical trunk, which divides into three branches: (a) Inferior thyroid; (b) suprascapular; and (c) transverse cervical arteries.

4. Costocervical trunk, which divides into two branches: (a) Superior intercostal; and (b) deep cervical arteries.

5. Dorsal scapular artery—occasionally.

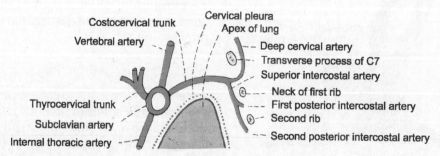

Fig. 12.13: *Branches of the subclavian artery. Note that the branches actually arise at different levels, but are shown at one level schematically.*

Vertebral Artery

Vertebral artery is the first and largest branch of the first part of the subclavian artery. It runs a long course and ends in the cranial cavity by supplying the brain. It is divided into four parts. The *first part* extends from its origin to the foramen transversarium of the sixth cervical vertebra (see Fig. 12.33). This part runs upwards and backwards into the angle between the scalenus anterior and the longus colli muscles, behind the common carotid artery, the vertebral vein and the inferior thyroid artery (Fig. 12.14). Details of all the four parts are described in the section on the prevertebral region (Chapter 13).

Internal Thoracic Artery

Internal thoracic artery arises from the inferior aspect of the first part of the subclavian artery opposite the origin of the thyrocervical trunk. The origin lies near the medial border of the scalenus anterior (Fig. 12.14). The artery runs downwards and medially in front of the cervical pleura. Anteriorly the artery is related to: (1) The sternal end of the clavicle, (2) the internal jugular vein, (3) the brachiocephalic vein, (4) the first costal cartilage, and (5) the phrenic nerve. The artery enters the thorax by passing behind the first costal cartilage. For course of the artery in the thorax see Chapter 14, Volume 2.

Thyrocervical Trunk

Thyrocervical trunk is a short, wide vessel which arises from the front of the first part of the subclavian

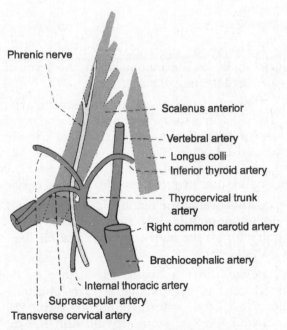

Phrenic nerve

— Scalenus anterior

— Vertebral artery

— Longus colli

— Inferior thyroid artery

— Thyrocervical trunk artery

— Right common carotid artery

— Brachiocephalic artery

— Internal thoracic artery

Suprascapular artery

Transverse cervical artery

Fig. 12.14: *Branches of the right subclavian artery.*

artery, close to the medial border of the scalenus anterior, and between the phrenic and vagus nerves. It almost immediately divides into the inferior thyroid, suprascapular and transverse cervical arteries.

The *inferior thyroid artery* is described with the thyroid gland. In addition to glandular branches (to the thyroid) it gives: (a) The ascending cervical artery which runs upwards in front of the transverse processes of cervical vertebrae; (b) the inferior laryngeal artery which accompanies the recurrent laryngeal nerve, and enters the larynx deep to the lower border of the inferior constrictor; and (c) other branches which supply the pharynx, the trachea, the oesophagus and surrounding muscles (Figs 12.14, 12.7, 12.8).

The *suprascapular artery* runs laterally and downwards, and crosses the scalenus anterior and the phrenic nerve. It lies behind the internal jugular vein and the sternocleidomastoid. It then crosses the trunks of the brachial plexus and runs in the posterior triangle, behind and parallel with the clavicle, to reach the superior border of the scapula. It crosses above the suprascapular ligament and takes part in the anastomosis around the scapula (Chapter 7, Volume 1). In addition to branches to surrounding muscles, the artery also supplies the clavicle, the scapula, and the shoulder and acromioclavicular joints (Fig. 3.11).

The *transverse cervical artery* runs laterally above the suprascapular artery. It crosses the scalenus anterior and the phrenic nerve passing behind the internal jugular vein and the sternocleidomastoid. It then crosses the brachial plexus and the floor of the posterior triangle to reach the anterior border of trapezius, where it divides into a superficial and deep branches. The superficial branch accompanies the spinal root of accessory nerve till the lower end of the muscle. The deep branch passes deep to levator scapulae and takes part in the anastomosis around the scapula. Sometimes the two branches may arise separately; the superficial from thyrocervical trunk and the deep from the third part of subclavian artery. Then these are named as superficial cervical and dorsal scapular arteries.

Dorsal Scapular Artery

Dorsal scapular artery arises occasionally from the third part of subclavian artery. If transverse cervical does not divide into superficial and deep branches but continues as superficial branch, the distribution of deep branch is taken over by dorsal scapular artery.

Costocervical Trunk

Costocervical trunk arises from the posterior surface of the second part of the subclavian artery on the right side; but from the first part of the artery on the left side.

It arches backwards over the cervical pleura, and divides into the superior intercostal and deep cervical arteries at the neck of the first rib (Figs 12.13, 12.14).

The *superior intercostal artery* descends in front of the neck of the first rib, and divides into the first and second posterior intercostal arteries.

The *deep cervical artery* is analogous to the posterior branch of a posterior intercostal artery. It passes backwards between the transverse process of the 7th cervical vertebra and the neck of the first rib. It then ascends between the semipinalis capitis and cervicis up to the axis vertebra. It anastomoses with the occipital and vertebral arteries.

CLINICAL ANATOMY

1. The third part of the subclavian artery can be *effectively compressed* against the first rib after depressing the shoulder. The pressure is applied downwards, backwards, and medially in the angle between the sternocleidomastoid and the clavicle.

2. *A cervical rib* may compress the subclavian artery, diminishing the radial pulse.

3. An *aneurysm* may form in the third part of the subclavian artery. Its pressure on the brachial plexus causes pain, weakness, and numbness in the upper limb.

The right subclavian artery may arise from the descending thoracic aorta. In that case, it passes posterior to the oesophagus which may be compressed and the condition is known as (*dysphagia lusoria*).

COMMON CAROTID ARTERY

Surface Marking

Common Carotid Artery

It is marked by a broad line along the anterior border of the sternocleidomastoid muscle by joining the following two points.

(a) A point on the sternoclavicular joint (Fig. 12.10).

(b) A second point on the anterior border of the sternocleidomastoid muscle at the level of the upper border of the thyroid cartilage.

The thoracic part of the left common carotid artery is marked by a broad line extending from a point a little to the left of the centre of the manubrium to the left sternoclavicular joint.

Internal Carotid Artery

It is marked by a broad line joining the following two points.

(a) A point on the anterior border of the sternocleidomastoid muscle at the level of the upper border of the thyroid cartilage.

(b) A second point on the posterior border of the condyle of the mandible.

The *origin* and *course* of the common carotid arteries has been described in Chapter 8. The relations of the artery in the neck are given:

DISSECTION

The common carotid artery has been exposed in the carotid triangle. Clean it in its entire course. Identify the internal carotid artery and trace it till it leaves the neck.

Veins

Identify the tributaries of subclavian, internal jugular and brachiocephalic veins.

The common carotid artery is enclosed in the *carotid sheath*. The three contents of the sheath are: (1) The common carotid artery medially; (2) the internal jugular vein, laterally; and (3) the vagus in between the artery and the vein, posteriorly (Fig. 3.4A, B).

Anterior Relations

(a) The common carotid artery is crossed by the superior belly of the omohyoid at the level of the cricoid cartilage (Fig. 12.15).

(b) Above the omohyoid (in the carotid triangle) the artery is comparatively superficial, and is related to: (1) The medial (anterior) margin of the sternocleidomastoid, deep to which there are; (2) the descendens hypoglossi nerve; (3) the superior thyroid vein; (4) the sternothyroid; and (5) the ansa cervicalis.

(c) At the level of the omohyoid there are : (1) The sternocleidomastoid; (2) the omohyoid; (3) the sternohyoid; (4) the sternothyroid; and (5) the ansa cervicalis.

(d) Below the omohyoid, the artery is deeply situated, and is covered by: (1) The sternocleidomastoid; (2) the anterior jugular vein; (3) the sternohyoid; (4) The sternothyroid and the middle thyroid vein.

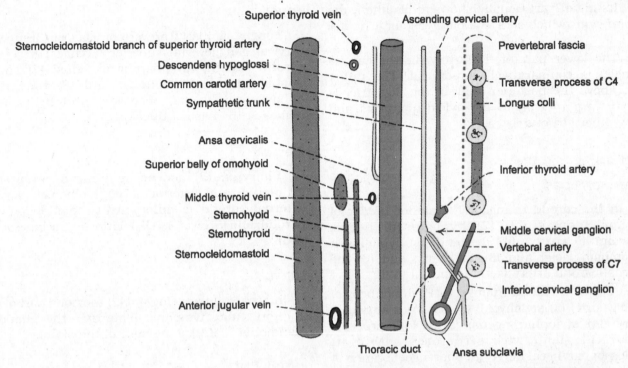

Fig. 12.15: Schematic sagittal section showing anterior and posterior relations of the common carotid artery.

Posterior Relations

(1) Transverse process of vertebrae C4, 5, 6 and 7, and the muscles attached to their anterior tubercles (longus colli, longus capitis, scalenus anterior); (2) the prevertebral fascia covers the muscles; (3) the sympathetic chain descends on the longus colli; (4) the ascending cervical artery ascends in front of the tubercles; (5) the inferior thyroid artery crosses medially at the level of the cricoid cartilage; (6) vertebral artery; (7) on the left side the thoracic duct crosses laterally behind the artery at the level of vertebra C7, in front of the vertebral vessels; (8) on the right side the right recurrent laryngeal nerve crosses medially behind the lower end of the artery (Fig. 12.8).

Medial Relations

(1) Thyroid gland; (2) larynx and pharynx; trachea, oesophagus and recurrent laryngeal nerve (Fig. 12.5).

Lateral relation
Internal jugular vein.

Posterolateral relation
Vagus nerve.

INTERNAL CAROTID ARTERY

The internal carotid artery is one of the two terminal branches of the common carotid artery. It begins at

the level of the upper border of the thyroid cartilage opposite the disc between the third and fourth cervical vertebrae, and ends inside the cranial cavity by supplying the brain. This is the principal artery of the brain and the eye. It also supplies the related bones and meninges.

For convenience of description the course of the artery is divided into four parts: (a) Cervical part, in the neck; (b) petrous part, within the petrous temporal bone; (c) cavernous part, within the cavernous sinus; and (d) cerebral part in relation to the base of the brain.

Cervical Part

1. It ascends vertically in the neck from its origin to the base of the skull to reach the lower end of the carotid canal. This part is enclosed in the carotid sheath (with the internal jugular vein and the vagus).

2. No branches arise from the internal carotid artery in the neck.

3. Its initial part usually shows a dilatation, the *carotid sinus* which acts as a baroreceptor (Chapter 8).

4. The lower part of the artery (in the carotid triangle) is comparatively superficial. The upper part, above the posterior belly of the digastric, is deep to the parotid gland, the styloid apparatus, and many other structures.

Relations

Anterior or Superficial

I. In the carotid triangle: (1) Anterior border of sternocleidomastoid; (2) hypoglossal nerve; (3) occipital artery; (4) descendens hypoglossi; (5) common facial and lingual veins; and (6) the external carotid artery is anteromedial to it.

II. Above the carotid triangle: (1) Posterior belly of the digastric; (2) stylohyoid; (3) posterior auricular artery; (4) stylopharyngeus; (5) styloid process; (6) parotid gland with structures within it; (7) glossopharyngeal nerve; (8) pharyngeal branch of vagus nerve; and (9) the cartilaginous part of the auditory tube and the tensor veli palatini (at the base of the skull) (Fig. 12.16).

Posterior

(1) Longus capitis; (2) prevertebral fascia; (3) superior cervical ganglion; (4) superior laryngeal nerve; (5) carotid sheath; (6) pharyngeal veins; (7) vagus, posterolateral throughout; and (8) the glossopharyngeal, vagus, accessory and hypoglossal nerves at the base of the skull.

Medial

(1) Pharynx; (2) ascending pharyngeal artery; (3) internal and external laryngeal nerves; (4) the external carotid is anteromedial to it below the parotid; and (5) levator veli palatini (at the base of the skull).

Lateral

(1) Internal jugular vein; and (2) the bony part of the auditory tube, tympanic plate and the temporomandibular joint (at the base of the skull).

Petrous Part

1. In the carotid canal, the artery first runs upwards, and then turns forwards and medially at

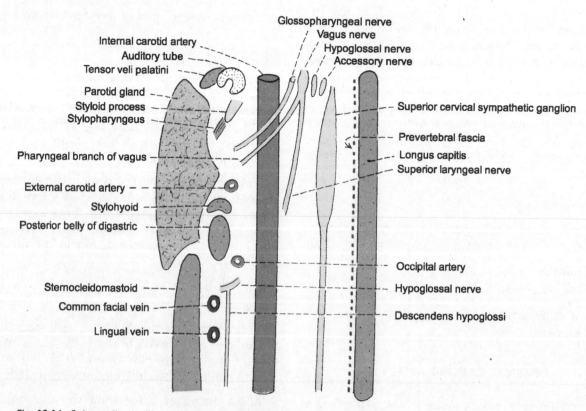

Fig. 12.16: Schematic sagittal section showing the anterior and posterior relations of the internal carotid artery.

right angles. It emerges at the apex of the petrous temporal bone, in the posterior wall of the foramen lacerum where it turns upwards and medially.

2. *Relations:* The artery is surrounded by venous and sympathetic plexuses. It is related to the middle ear and the cochlea (posterosuperiorly); the auditory tube and tensor tympani (anterolaterally); and the trigeminal ganglion (superiorly).

3. *Branches:* (a) *Caroticotympanic* branches enter the middle ear, and anastomose with the anterior and posterior tympanic arteries; and (b) the *pterygoid branch* (small and inconstant) enters the pterygoid canal with the nerve of that canal and anastomoses with the greater palatine artery.

Cavernous and Cerebral Parts of Internal Carotid Artery

See cranial cavity (Chapter 6).

SUBCLAVIAN VEIN

Surface Marking

It is represented by a broad line along the clavicle extending from a little medial to its midpoint to the medial end of the bone (Fig. 12.17).

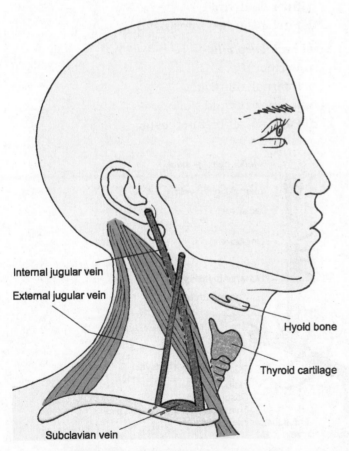

Fig. 12.17: *Surface marking of a few veins.*

Internal jugular vein

External jugular vein

Hyoid bone

Thyroid cartilage

Subclavian vein

Course

It is a continuation of the axillary vein. It begins at the outer border of the first rib, and ends at the medial border of the scalenus anterior by joining the internal jugular vein to form the brachiocephalic vein.

It lies: (a) In front of the subclavian artery, the scalenus anterior and the right phrenic nerve; (b) behind the clavicle and the subclavius; and (c) above the first rib and pleura.

Its tributaries are: (a) The external jugular vein; (b) the dorsal scapular vein (c) the thoracic duct on the left side; and (d) the right lymphatic duct on the right side.

Sometimes, it may also receive: (a) The anterior jugular vein; and (b) a small branch from the cephalic vein which crosses the clavicle to reach the subclavian vein.

INTERNAL JUGULAR VEIN

Surface Marking

It is marked by a broad line by joining the following two points.

a. The first point on the neck medial to the lobule of the ear (Fig. 12.17).

b. The second point at the medial end of the clavicle.

The lower bulb of the vein lies beneath the less supraclavicular fossa between the sternal and clavicular heads of the sternocleidomastoid muscle.

Course

1. It is a direct continuation of the sigmoid sinus. It begins at the jugular foramen, and ends behind the sternal end of the clavicle by joining the subclavian vein to form the brachiocephalic vein.

2. The origin is marked by a dilation, the *superior bulb* which lies in the jugular fossa of the temporal bone, beneath the floor of the middle ear cavity. The termination of the vein is marked by the *inferior bulb* which lies beneath the lesser supraclavicular fossa.

Relations

Superficial: (1) Sternocleidomastoid; (2) posterior belly of digastric; (3) superior belly of omohyoid; (4) parotid gland; (5) styloid process; (6) accessory nerve; (7) posterior auricular artery; (8) occipital artery; (9) sternocleidomastoid arteries; (10) lower root of ansa cervicalis; (11) infrahyoid muscles; (12) anterior jugular vein; (13) deep cervical lymph nodes; and (14) the internal carotid artery, and the glossopharyngeal, vagus, accessory and hypoglossal cranial nerves (at the base of the skull) [see Fig. 12.12].

Posterior: (1) Rectus capitis lateralis; (2) transverse process of atlas; (3) levator scapulae; (4) scalenus medius; (5) cervical plexus; (6) scalenus anterior; (7) phrenic nerve; (8) thyrocervical trunk; (9) inferior thyroid artery; (10) first part of subclavian artery; and (11) thoracic duct (on left side).

Medial: (1) Internal carotid artery; (2) common carotid artery; and (3) vagus nerve.

Tributaries

(1) Inferior petrosal sinus; (2) common facial vein; (3) lingual vein; (4) pharyngeal veins; (5) superior thyroid vein; (6) middle thyroid vein; and (7) sometimes the occipital vein (Fig. 12.18).

The thoracic duct opens into the angle of union between the left internal jugular vein and the left subclavian vein. The right lymphatic duct opens similarly on the right side.

In the middle of the neck, the internal jugular vein may communicate with the external jugular vein through the oblique jugular vein which runs across the anterior border of the sternocleidomastoid.

BRACHIOCEPHALIC VEIN

1. The right brachiocephalic vein (2.5 cm long) is shorter than the left (6 cm long) (Fig. 12.18).

2. Each vein is formed behind the sternoclavicular joint, by the union of the internal jugular vein and the subclavian vein.

3. The right vein runs vertically downwards. The left vein runs obliquely downwards and to the right

behind the upper half of the manubrium sterni. The two brachiocephalic veins unite at the lower border of the right first costal cartilage to form the superior vena cava.

4. The *tributaries* correspond to the branches of the first part of the subclavian artery. These are as follows.

Right brachiocephalic
   a. Vertebral
   b. Internal thoracic
   c. Inferior thyroid
   d. First posterior intercostal.

Left brachiocephalic
   a. Vertebral
   b. Internal thoracic
   c. Inferior thyroid
   d. First posterior intercostal

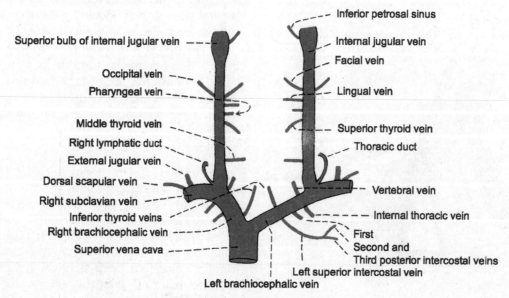

Superior bulb of internal jugular vein
Occipital vein
Pharyngeal vein
Middle thyroid vein
Right lymphatic duct
External jugular vein
Dorsal scapular vein
Right subclavian vein
Inferior thyroid veins
Right brachiocephalic vein
Superior vena cava

Inferior petrosal sinus
Internal jugular vein
Facial vein
Lingual vein
Superior thyroid vein
Thoracic duct
Vertebral vein
Internal thoracic vein
First
Second and
Third posterior intercostal veins
Left superior intercostal vein
Left brachiocephalic vein

Fig. 12.18: The veins of the neck.

e. Left superior intercostal

f. Thymic and pericardial veins

GLOSSOPHARYNGEAL NERVE

Glossopharyngeal is the ninth cranial nerve. It is the nerve of the third branchial arch. It is motor to the stylopharyngeus; secretomotor to the parotid gland; gustatory to the posterior one-third of the tongue including the circumvallate papillae and sensory to the pharynx, the tonsil, the posterior one-third of tongue, carotid body and carotid sinus (Fig. 12.19).

DISSECTION

The course of IX–XII cranial nerves has been seen in different chapters. Now trace these nerves and their branches.

Sympathetic Trunk

The sympathetic trunk has been identified as lying posteromedial to the carotid sheath. Trace it upwards and downwards and locate the three cervical ganglia.

Dissect the formation and branches of the cervical plexus. Identify the phrenic nerve on the surface of scalenus anterior muscle behind the prevertebral fascia.

Functional Components

(a) *Special visceral efferent* fibres arise in the nucleus ambiguus and supply the stylopharyngeus muscle.

(b) *General visceral efferent* fibres (preganglionic) arise in the inferior salivary nucleus and travel to the otic ganglion. Postganglionic fibres arising in the ganglion to supply the parotid gland (Table 1.3).

(c) *General visceral afferent* fibres are peripheral processes of cells in the inferior ganglion of the nerve. They carry general sensations from the pharynx, carotid body and carotid sinus to the ganglion. The central processes convey these sensations to the nucleus of the solitary tract.

(d) *Special visceral afferent* fibres are also peripheral processes of cells in the inferior ganglion. They carry sensations of taste from the posterior one-third of the tongue including circumvallate papillae to the ganglion. The central processes convey these sensations to the nucleus of the solitary tract.

(e) *General somatic afferent* fibres are the peripheral processes of the cells in the inferior ganglion of the nerve. These carry general sensations (pain, touch, temperature) from posterior one-third of tongue, tonsil, pharynx. The central processes carry these sensations to nucleus of spinal tract of trigeminal nerve.

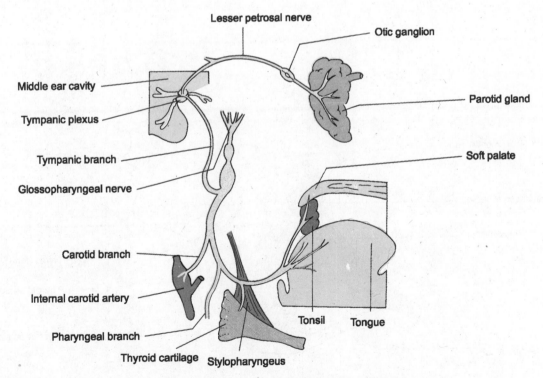

Fig. 12.19: Branches of the glossopharyngeal nerve.

Nuclei

The three nuclei in the upper part of medulla are named below:-

(1) Nucleus ambiguus (branchiomotor) (2) inferior salivary nucleus (parasympathetic) (3) nucleus of tractus solitarius (gustatory).

Surface Marking

Cranial nerve IX is marked by joining the following points.

(a) The first point on the anteroinferior part of the tragus (Fig. 12.20).

(b) The second point anterosuperior to the angle of the mandible.

From point 'b' the nerve runs forwards for a short distance along the lower border of the mandible. The nerve describes a gentle curve in its course.

Course and Relations

1. In their *intraneural course*, the fibres of the nerve pass forwards and laterally, between the olivary nucleus and the inferior cerebellar peduncle, through the reticular formation of the medulla (Chapter 24).

2. At the base of the brain, the nerve is attached by 3 to 4 filaments to the upper part of the postero-lateral sulcus of the medulla, just above the rootlets of the vagus nerve (Fig. 24.1).

3. In their intracranial course the filaments unite to form a single trunk which passes forwards and laterally towards the jugular foramen, crossing and grooving the jugular tubercle of the occipital bone.

4. The nerve *leaves the skull* by passing through the middle part of the *jugular foramen*, anterior to the vagus and accessory nerves. It has a separate sheath of dura mater.

5. In the jugular foramen, the nerve is lodged in a deep groove leading to the cochlear canaliculus, and is separated from the vagus and accessory nerves by the inferior petrosal sinus.

In its *extracranial course*, the nerve descends (i) between the internal jugular vein and the internal carotid artery, deep to the styloid process and the muscles attached to it; (ii) it then turns forwards winding round the lateral aspect of the stylo-pharyngeus, passes between the external and internal carotid arteries, and reaches the side of the pharynx (Fig. 14.11). Here it gives pharyngeal branches. (iii) It enters the submandibular region by passing deep to the hyoglossus (Fig. 11.2), where it breaks up into tonsillar and lingual branches (Fig. 12.19).

6. At the base of skull, ninth nerve presents a superior and an inferior ganglion. Superior ganglion is a detached part of the inferior, and gives no branches. The inferior ganglion is larger, occupies notch on the lower border of petrous temporal, and gives out communicating and tympanic branches.

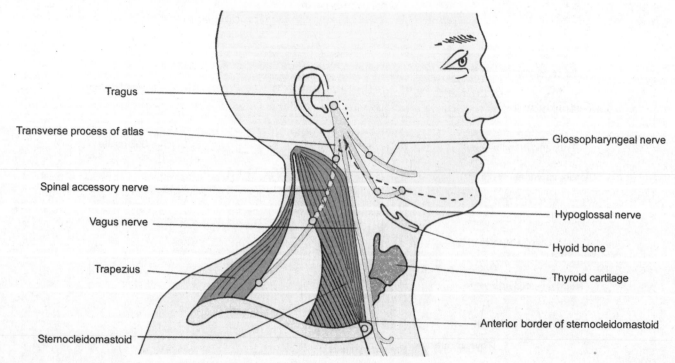

Tragus

Transverse process of atlas

Spinal accessory nerve

Vagus nerve

Trapezius

Sternocleidomastoid

Glossopharyngeal nerve

Hypoglossal nerve

Hyoid bone

Thyroid cartilage

Anterior border of sternocleidomastoid

Fig. 12.20: *Surface marking of cranial nerves IX, X, XI, XII.*

Branches and Distribution

1. The *tympanic nerve* is a branch of the inferior ganglion of the glossopharyngeal nerve. It enters the middle ear through the tympanic canaliculus, takes part in the formation of the tympanic plexus (on the medial wall of the middle ear) and distributes its fibres to the middle ear, the auditory tube, the mastoid antrum and air cells. One branch of the plexus is called the lesser petrosal nerve. It contains preganglionic secretomotor fibres for the parotid gland. For detailed course of these fibres see otic ganglion (Chapter 10).

2. The *carotid branch* descends on the internal carotid artery and supplies the carotid sinus and the carotid body.

3. The *pharyngeal branches* take part in the formation of the pharyngeal plexus, along with vagal and sympathetic fibres. The glossopharyngeal fibres are distributed to the mucous membrane of the pharynx.

4. The *muscular branch* supplies the stylo-pharyngeus (Fig. 14.18).

5. The *tonsillar branches* supply the tonsil and join the lesser palatine nerves to form a plexus from which fibres are distributed to the soft palate and to the palatoglossal arches (Fig. 12.19).

6. The *lingual branches* carry taste and general sensations from the posterior one-third of the tongue including the circumvallate papillae.

CLINICAL ANATOMY

1. The glossopharyngeal nerve is tested clinically in the following way: (a) On tickling the posterior wall of the pharynx, there is reflex contraction of the pharyngeal muscles. No such contraction occurs when the ninth nerve is paralysed. (b) Taste sensibility on the posterior one-third of the tongue can also be tested. It is lost in ninth nerve lesions.

2. Isolated lesions of the ninth nerve are almost unknown. They are usually accompanied by lesions of the vagus nerve.

3. Pharyngitis may cause referred pain in the ear. However, in these cases eustachian catarrh should be excluded.

VAGUS NERVE

Vagus nerve is the tenth cranial nerve. It is so called because of its extensive ('vague') course, through the head, the neck, the thorax and the abdomen. The fibres of the cranial root of the accessory nerve are also distributed through it.

The vagus nerve bears two ganglia, superior and inferior. The *superior ganglion* is rounded and lies in the jugular foramen. The *inferior* ganglion is cylindrical and lies near the base of the skull (Fig. 12.21).

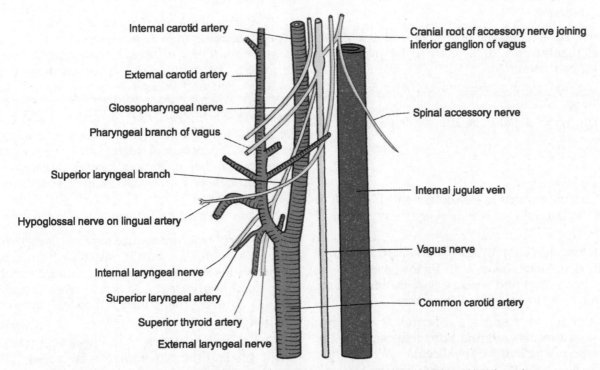

Fig. 12.21: Relation of cranial nerves IX, X, XI, XII to carotid arteries and internal jugular vein.

Functional Components

(a) *Special visceral efferent* fibres arise in the nucleus ambiguus and supply the muscles of the palate, pharynx and larynx.

(b) *General visceral efferent* fibres arise in the dorsal motor nucleus of the vagus. These are preganglionic parasympathetic fibres. They are distributed to thoracic and abdominal viscera. The postganglionic neurons are situated in ganglia lying close to (or within) the viscera to be supplied.

(c) *General visceral afferent* fibres are peripheral processes of cells located in the inferior ganglion of the nerve. They bring sensations from the pharynx, larynx, trachea, oesophagus and from the abdominal and thoracic viscera. These are conveyed by the central processes of the ganglion cells to the nucleus of the tractus solitarius. Some of these fibres terminate in the dorsal nucleus of the vagus.

(d) *Special visceral afferent* fibres are also peripheral processes of neurons in the inferior ganglion. They carry sensations of taste from the posteriormost part of the tongue and from the epiglottis. The central processes of the cells concerned terminate in the upper part of the nucleus of the tractus solitarius.

(e) *General somatic afferent* fibres are peripheral processes of neurons in the superior ganglion and are distributed to the skin of the external ear. The central processes of the ganglion cells terminate in relation to the spinal nucleus of the trigeminal nerve.

Surface Marking

The nerve runs along the posteromedial side of the internal jugular vein. It is marked by joining the following two points.

(a) The first point at the anteroinferior part of the tragus (Fig. 12.20).

(b) The second point at the medial end of the clavicle.

Nuclei

1. Nucleus ambiguus (branchiomotor): mostly a part of the cranial root of accessory nerve; partly of vagus.

2. Dorsal nucleus of vagus (parasympathetic): it is a mixed nucleus, being both motor (visceromotor and secretomotor) and sensory (viscerosensory). Its fibres form the main bulk of the nerve.

3. Nucleus of tractus solitarius (gustatory): distributed through internal laryngeal nerve to the taste buds of epiglottis and vallecula.

4. Nucleus of spinal tract of trigeminal.

Course and Relations in Head and Neck

1. In the *intracranial course*, the fibres run forwards and laterally through the reticular formation of medulla, between the olivary nucleus and inferior cerebellar peduncle (Chapter 24).

2. The nerve is attached, by about ten rootlets, to the posterolateral sulcus of the medulla.

3. In the intracranial course, the rootlets unite to from a large trunk which passes laterally across the jugular tubercle along with the glossopharyngeal and cranial root of accessory nerves, and reaches the jugular foramen.

4. The nerve *leaves the cranial cavity* by passing through the middle part of the jugular foramen, between the sigmoid and inferior petrosal sinuses. In the foramen, it is joined by the cranial root of the accessory nerve.

5. Leaving the skull, the nerve descends within the carotid sheath, in between and posterior to the internal jugular vein (laterally), and the internal and common carotid arteries (medially) (Figs 3.3, 3.4 A, B).

6. At the *root of the neck,* the right vagus enters the thorax by crossing the first part of the subclavian artery, and then inclining medially behind the brachiocephalic vessels, to reach the right side of the trachea. The left vagus enters the thorax by passing between the left common carotid and left subclavian arteries, behind the internal jugular and brachiocephalic veins.

7. Vagus bears two ganglia, superior and inferior. The *superior ganglion* is rounded and lies in the jugular foramen. It gives meningeal and auricular branches of vagus, and is connected to glossopharyngeal and accessory nerves and to superior cervical ganglion of sympathetic chain. The *inferior ganglion* is cylindrical (2.5 cm) and lies near the base of skull. It gives pharyngeal, carotid and superior laryngeal branches of vagus, and is connected to hypoglossal nerve, superior cervical ganglion and the loop between first and second cervical nerves.

Branches in Head and Neck

In the jugular foramen, the superior ganglion gives off: (1) Meningeal, and (2) auricular branches. The ganglion also gives off communicating branches to the glossopharyngeal and cranial root of accessory nerves and to the superior cervical sympathetic ganglion.

The branches arising in the neck are: (1) Pharyngeal; (2) carotid; (3) superior laryngeal; (4) right recurrent laryngeal; and (5) cardiac (Fig. 12.21).

Meningeal branch supplies dura of the posterior cranial fossa. The fibres are derived from sympathetic and upper cervical nerves.

The *auricular branch* arises from the superior ganglion of the vagus. It passes behind the internal jugular vein, and enters the mastoid canaliculus (within the petrous temporal bone). It crosses the facial canal 4 mm above the stylomastoid foramen, emerges through the tympanomastoid fissure, and ends by supplying the concha and root of the auricle, the posterior half of the external auditory meatus, and the tympanic membrane (outer surface).

The *pharyngeal branch* arises from the upper part of the inferior ganglion of the vagus, and contains chiefly the fibres of the cranial root of accessory nerve. It passes between the external and internal carotid arteries, and reaches the upper border of the middle constrictor of the pharynx where it takes part in forming the pharyngeal plexus. Its fibres are ultimately distributed to the muscles of the pharynx and soft palate (except the tensor veli palatini which is supplied by the mandibular nerve).

The *carotid branches* supply the carotid body and carotid sinus.

The *superior laryngeal nerve* arises from the inferior ganglion of the vagus, runs downwards and forwards on the superior constrictor deep to the internal carotid artery, and reaches the middle constrictor where it divides into the external and internal laryngeal nerves. The *external laryngeal nerve* is thin. It accompanies the superior thyroid artery, pierces the inferior constrictor and ends by supplying the cricothyroid muscle. It also gives branches to the inferior constrictor and to the pharyngeal plexus. The *internal laryngeal nerve* is thick. It passes downwards and forwards, pierces the thyrohyoid membrane (above the superior laryngeal vessels) and enters the larynx. It supplies the mucous membrane of the larynx upto the level of the vocal folds (Figs 12.5, 12.6, 12.8).

The *right recurrent laryngeal nerve* arises from the vagus in front of the right subclavian artery, winds backwards below the artery, and they runs upwards and medially behind the subclavian and common carotid arteries to reach the tracheo-oesophageal groove. In the upper part of the groove, it is related to the inferior thyroid artery. It may be superficial or deep to the artery. Occasionally, some branches are in front of the nerve, and some are behind it. The nerve then passes deep to the lower border of the inferior constrictor, and enters the larynx behind the cricothyroid joint. It supplies: (a) All intrinsic muscles of the larynx, except the cricothyroid, (b) sensory nerves to the larynx below the level of the vocal cords; (c) cardiac branches to the deep cardiac plexus;

(d) branches to the trachea and oesophagus; and (e) to the inferior constrictor.

The *left recurrent laryngeal nerve* arises from the vagus in the thorax, as the latter crosses the left side of the arch of the aorta. It loops around the ligamentum arteriosum and reaches the tracheo-oesophageal groove. Its distribution is similar to that of the right nerve. It does not have to pass behind the subclavian and carotid arteries; and usually it is posterior to the inferior thyroid artery (Figs 12.6–12.8).

The *cardiac branches* are superior and inferior. Out of the four cardiac branches of the vagi (two on each side) the left inferior branch goes to the superficial cardiac plexus. The other three cardiac nerves go to the deep cardiac plexus.

CLINICAL ANATOMY

1. The vagus *nerve is tested clinically* by comparing the palatal arches on the two sides. On the paralysed side, there is no arching, and the uvula is pulled to the normal side.

2. *Paralysis of the vagus* nerve produces: (a) Nasal regurgitation of swallowed liquids; (b) nasal twang in voice; (c) hoarseness of voice; (d) flattening of the palatal arch; (e) cadaveric position of the vocal cord; and (f) dysphagia.

3. *Irritation of the auricular branch of the vagus* in the external ear (by ear wax, syringing, etc.) may reflexly cause persistent cough (ear cough), vomiting, or even death due to sudden cardiac inhibition.

4. *Stimulation of the auricular branch* may reflexly produce increased appetite.

5. Irritation of the recurrent laryngeal nerve by enlarged lymph nodes in children may also produce a persistent cough.

6. Some fibres arising in the geniculate ganglion of the facial nerve pass into the vagus through communications between the two nerves. They reach the skin of the auricle through the auricular branch of the vagus. Sometimes a sensory ganglion may have a viral infection (called herpes zoster) and vesicles appear on the area of skin supplied by the ganglion. In herpes zoster of the geniculate ganglion, vesicles appear on the skin of the auricle.

ACCESSORY NERVE

Accessory nerve is the eleventh cranial nerve. It has two roots, cranial and spinal. The cranial root is accessory to the vagus, and is distributed through the branches of the latter. The spinal root has a more independent course (Fig. 12.22).

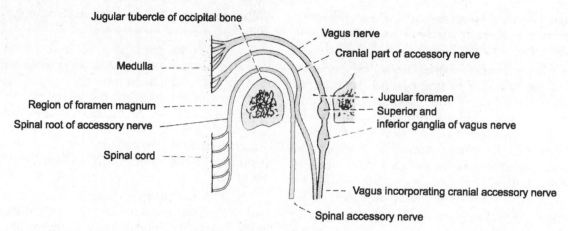

Fig. 12.22: *Course of the accessory nerve.*

Functional Components

1. The cranial root is *special visceral (branchial) efferent.* It arises from the lower part of the nucleus ambiguus. It is distributed through the branches of the vagus to the muscles of the palate, the pharynx, the larynx, and possibly the heart.

2. The spinal root is also special visceral efferent. It arises from a long spinal nucleus situated in the lateral part of the anterior grey column of the spinal cord extending between segments C1 to C5. Its fibres supply the sternocleidomastoid and the trapezius muscles.

Nuclei

The cranial root arises from the lower part of the *nucleus ambiguus.*

The spinal root arises from a long *spinal nucleus* situated on the lateral part of anterior grey column of spinal cord, extending from C1 to C5 segments. It is in line with nucleus ambiguus.

Course and Distribution of the Cranial Root

1. The cranial root emerges in the form of 4 to 5 rootlets which are attached to the posterolateral sulcus of the medulla. Just below, the rootlets soon join together to form a single trunk.

2. It runs laterally with the glossopharyngeal vagus and the spinal accessory nerves, crosses the jugular tubercle, and reaches the jugular foramen.

3. In the jugular foramen, the cranial root unites for a short distance with the spinal root, and again separates from it as it passes out of the foramen.

4. The cranial root finally fuses with the vagus just below its inferior ganglion, and is distributed through the branches of the vagus to the muscles of the palate, the pharynx, the larynx and possibly the heart.

Surface Marking

Accessory nerve is marked by joining the following four points.

(a) The first point at the anteroinferior part of the tragus (Fig. 12.20).

(b) The second point at the tip of the transverse process of the atlas.

(c) The third point at the middle of the posterior border of the sternocleidomastoid muscle.

(d) The fourth point on the anterior border of the trapezius 5 cm above the clavicle.

Course and Distribution of the Spinal Root

1. It arises from the upper five segments of the spinal cord (Fig. 12.22).

2. It emerges in the form of a row of filaments attached to the cord midway between the ventral and dorsal nerve roots.

3. *In the vertebral canal,* the filaments unite to form a single trunk which ascends in front of the dorsal nerve roots and behind the ligamentum denticulatum.

4. The nerve *enters the cranium* through the foramen magnum lying behind the vertebral artery.

5. Within the cranium, the nerve runs upwards and laterally, crosses the jugular tubercle (with the ninth and tenth cranial nerves) and reaches the jugular foramen.

6. The nerve *leaves the skull* through the middle part of the jugular foramen where it fuses with a short length of the cranial root. It soon separates from the latter and passes out of the foramen.

7. In its *extracranial course,* the nerve descends vertically between the internal jugular vein and the internal carotid artery deep to the parotid and to the styloid process (Figs 12.16, 12.21). It reaches a point midway between the angle of the mandible and the

mastoid process. Then it runs downwards and backwards superficial to the internal jugular vein and deep to the sternocleidomastoid. Here it is crossed by the occipital artery, is accompanied by the upper sternocleidomastoid branch of the occipital artery, and is surrounded by lymph nodes.

The nerve pierces the anterior border of the sternocleidomastoid at the junction of its upper one-fourth with the lower three-fourths, and communicates with second and third cervical with spinal nerves within the muscle.

The nerve enters the posterior triangle of the neck by emerging through the posterior border of the sternocleidomastoid a little above its middle. In the triangle (Fig. 12.23), it runs downwards and backwards embedded in the fascial roof of the triangle. Here it lies over the levator scapulae. It is related to the superficial lymph nodes. The nerve leaves the posterior triangle by passing deep to the anterior border of the trapezius 5 cm above the clavicle.

On the deep surface of the trapezius the nerve communicates with spinal nerves C3 and C4, and ends by supplying the trapezius (Chapter 3).

8. *Distribution.* The spinal accessory nerve supplies: (a) The sternocleidomastoid; and (b) the trapezius. Cervical nerves provide a proprioceptive supply to these muscles.

CLINICAL ANATOMY

1. The *accessory nerve is tested clinically:* (a) By asking the patient to shrug his shoulders (trapezius) against resistance and comparing the power on the two sides; and (b) by asking the patient to turn the chin to the opposite side (sternocleidomastoid) against resistance and again comparing the power on the two sides.

2. Lesions of the accessory nerve are usually accompanied by lesions of the glossopharyngeal and vagus nerves because of their close inter-relationship in the cranium.

3. Irritation of the nerve, by enlarged lymph nodes, may produce torticollis or wry neck.

HYPOGLOSSAL NERVE

Hypoglossal is the twelfth cranial nerve. It supplies the muscles of the tongue (Fig. 12.24).

Functional Components/Nuclear Columns

1. General somatic efferent column. The fibres arise from the hypoglossal nucleus which lies in the

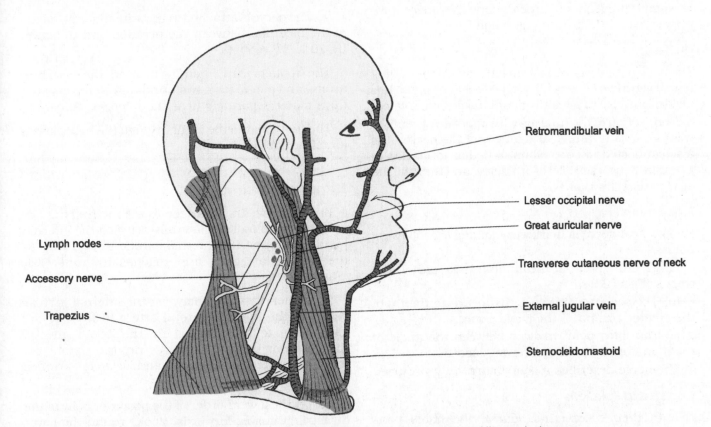

Fig. 12.23: *Accessory nerve with branches of cervical plexus. Veins of the neck also seen.*

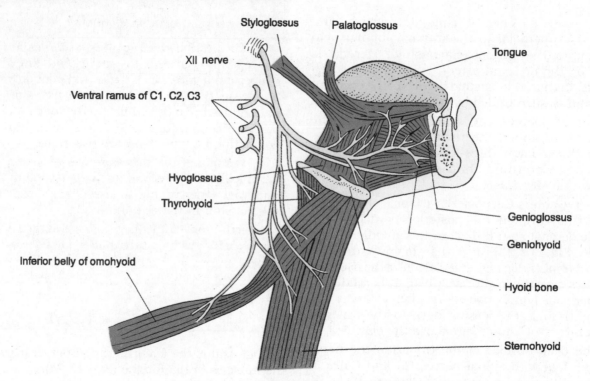

Fig. 12.24: Hypoglossal nerve and ansa cervicalis.

medulla, in the floor of the fourth ventricle deep to the hypoglossal triangle.

2. General somatic afferent column. The nucleus is spinal nucleus of cranial nerve V where proprioceptive fibres from tongue end.

Nucleus

The hypoglossal nucleus, 2 cm long, lies in the floor of fourth ventricle beneath the hypoglossal triangle. It is divided into parts for individual muscles innervated.

Connection of the nucleus with opposite pyramidal tract forms supranuclear pathway of the nerve. It is also connected to cerebellum, reticular formation of medulla, sensory nuclei of 5th nerve, and the nucleus of tractus solitarius.

Surface Marking

Hypoglossal nerve is marked by joining the following points.

(a) The first point at the anteroinferior part of the tragus (Fig. 12.20).

(b) The second point posterosuperior to the tip of the greater cornua of the hyoid bone.

(c) The third point midway between the angle of the mandible and the symphysis menti.

The nerve describes a gentle curve in its course.

Course and Relations

1. In their *intraneural course,* the fibres pass forwards lateral to the medial longitudinal bundle,

medial lemniscus and pyramidal tract, and medial to the reticular formation and olivary nucleus (Chapter 24).

2. The nerve is attached to the anterolateral sulcus of the medulla, between the pyramid and the olive, by 10 to 15 rootlets.

The rootlets run laterally (behind the vertebral artery, and join to form two bundles which pierce the dura mater separately near the hypoglossal canal.

The nerve leaves the skull through the hypoglossal (anterior condylar) canal.

Extracranial Course

(i) The nerve first lies deep to the internal jugular vein, but soon inclines laterally between the internal jugular vein and the internal carotid artery, crosses the vagus (laterally), and reaches in front of it (Fig. 12.21).

(ii) It then descends between the internal jugular vein and the internal carotid artery in front of the vagus, deep to the parotid gland, the styloid process, the posterior belly of the digastric, the stylohyoid, and the posterior auricular and occipital arteries (Fig. 12.16).

(iii) At the lower border of the posterior belly of the digastric it curves forwards, hooks round the lower sternocleidomastoid branch of the occipital artery, crosses the internal and external carotid arteries and the loop of the lingual artery, and passes deep to the posterior belly of the digastric again to enter the submandibular region (Figs 12.24, 11.2).

(iv) The nerve then continues forwards on the hyoglossus and genioglossus, deep to the submandibular gland and the mylohyoid, and enters the substance of the tongue to supply its muscles (Fig. 12.24).

Branches and Distribution

In addition to its own fibres, the nerve also carries some fibres that reach it from spinal nerve C1, and are distributed through it.

Branches containing fibres of the hypoglossal nerve proper. They supply the extrinsic and intrinsic muscles of the tongue, styloglossus, genioglossus, hyoglossus, superior longitudinal, inferior longitudinal, transverse and vertical muscles except the palatoglossus which is supplied by fibres of the cranial accessory nerve through the vagus and the pharyngeal plexus (Fig. 17.3).

Branches of the hypoglossal nerve containing fibres of nerve C1. These fibres join the nerve at the base of the skull.

1. The *meningeal branch* contains sensory and sympathetic fibres. It enters the skull through the hypoglossal canal, and supplies bone and meninges in the anterior part of the posterior cranial fossa.

2. The *descending branch* continues as the descendens hypoglossi or the upper root of the ansa cervicalis.

3. Branches are also given to the thyrohyoid and geniohyoid muscles.

CLINICAL ANATOMY

1. The *hypoglossal nerve is tested clinically* by asking the patient to protrude his/her tongue. Normally, the tongue is protruded straight forwards. If the nerve is paralysed, the tongue deviates to the paralysed side.

2. A *lesion of the hypoglossal nerve* produces paralysis of the tongue on that side. If the lesion is infranuclear there is gradual atrophy of the paralysed half of the tongue. Supranuclear lesions of the hypoglossal nerve causes paralysis without wasting. The tongue moves sluggishly resulting in defective speech. On protrusion, the tongue deviates to opposite side.

CERVICAL PART OF SYMPATHETIC TRUNK

Surface Marking

It is marked by a line joining following points:

(a) Point of the sternoclavicular joint (Fig. 12.25).

(b) A point at the posterior border of the condyle of the mandible.

The *superior cervical ganglion* extends from the transverse process of the atlas to the tip of the greater cornua of the hyoid bone. The *middle cervical ganglion* lies at the level of the cricoid cartilage, and the *inferior cervical ganglion,* at a point 3 cm above the sternoclavicular joint.

Introduction

The cervical parts of the right and left sympathetic trunks are situated one on each side of the cervical part of the vertebral column, behind the carotid sheath (common carotid and internal carotid arteries) and in front of the prevertebral fascia.

Formation

There are no white rami communicans in the neck and this part of the trunk is formed by fibres which emerge from segments T1 to T4 of the spinal cord, and then ascend into the neck.

Relations

Anterior: (a) Internal carotid artery; (b) common carotid artery; (c) carotid sheath; and (d) inferior thyroid artery.

Posterior: (a) Prevertebral fascia; (b) longus capitis and cervicis muscles; and (c) transverse processes of the lower six cervical vertebrae.

Ganglia

Theoretically there should be eight sympathetic ganglia corresponding to the eight cervical nerves, but due to fusion there are only three ganglia, superior, middle and inferior (Fig. 12.26).

Superior Cervical Ganglion

Size and Shape

This is the largest of the three ganglia. It is spindle-shaped, and about 2.5 cm long.

Situation and Formation

It lies just below the skull, opposite the second and third cervical vertebrae, behind the carotid sheath and in front of the prevertebral fascia (longus capitis). It is formed by fusion of the upper 4 cervical ganglia.

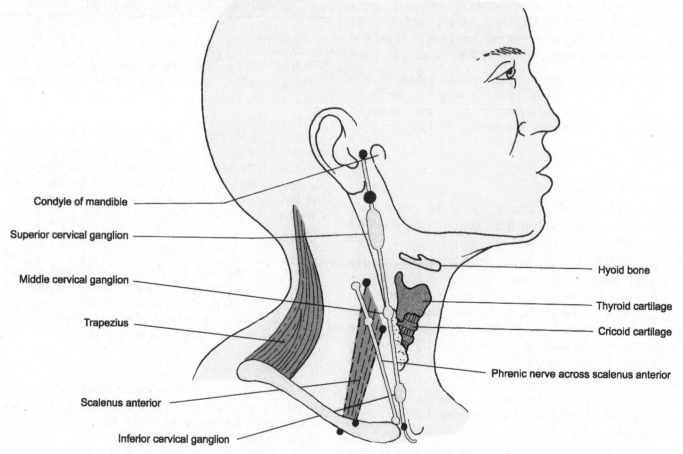

Condyle of mandible

Superior cervical ganglion

Middle cervical ganglion

Trapezius

Scalenus anterior

Inferior cervical ganglion

Hyoid bone

Thyroid cartilage

Cricoid cartilage

Phrenic nerve across scalenus anterior

Fig. 12.25: Surface marking of cervical sympathetic ganglia and phrenic nerve.

Communications. With cranial nerves IX, X and XII, and with the external and recurrent laryngeal nerves.

Branches

1. Grey rami communicans pass to the ventral rami of the upper four cervical nerves (Fig. 12.26).

2. The internal carotid nerve arises from the upper end of the ganglion and forms a plexus around the internal carotid artery. A part of this plexus supplies the dilator pupillae (Chapter 19). Some of these fibres form the deep petrosal nerve for pterygopalatine ganglion; others give fibres along long ciliary nerve for the ciliary ganglion.

3. The external carotid branches form a plexus around the external carotid artery. Some of these fibres form the sympathetic roots of the otic and submandibular ganglia (Table 12.1).

4. Pharyngeal branches take part in the formation of the pharyngeal plexus.

5. The left superior cervical cardiac branch goes to the superficial cardiac plexus while the right branch goes to the deep cardiac plexus.

Middle Cervical Ganglion

Size and Shape

This ganglion is very small. It may be divided into 2 to 3 smaller parts, or may be absent.

Situation

It lies in the lower part of the neck, in front of vertebra C6 just above the inferior thyroid artery, behind the carotid sheath (common carotid artery).

Formation

It is formed by fusion of the fifth and sixth cervical ganglia connections. It is connected with the inferior cervical ganglion directly, and also through a loop that winds round the subclavian artery. This loop is called the *ansa subclavia*.

Branches

1. Grey rami communicans are given to the ventral rami of the 5th and 6th cervical nerves.

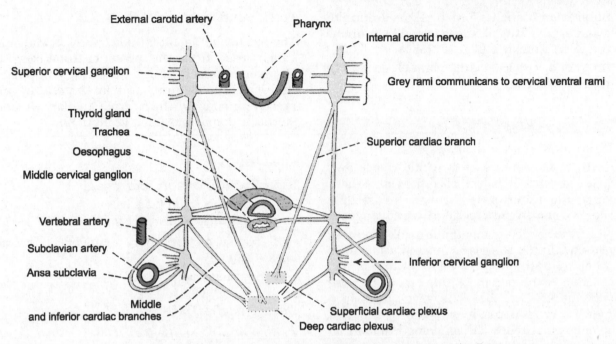

Fig. 12.26: *The cervical sympathetic trunks and their branches.*

Table 12.1: Branches of cervical sympathetic ganglia

			Superior cervical ganglion	Middle cervical ganglion	Inferior cervical ganglion
Arterial branches	(i)		Along Internal carotid artery as internal carotid nerve	Along Inferior thyroid artery	Along subclavian and vertebral arteries
	(ii)		Along common carotid and external carotid arteries		
Grey rami communicans			Along 1–4 cervical nerves	Along 5 and 6 cervical nerves	Along 7 and 8 cervical nerves
Along cranial nerves			Along cranial nerves IX, X, XI and XII	–	–
Visceral branches			Pharynx, cardiac	Thyroid, cardiac	Cardiac

2. Thyroid branches accompany the inferior thyroid artery to the thyroid gland. They also supply the parathyroid glands (Fig. 12.26).

3. Tracheal and oesophageal branches.

4. The middle cervical cardiac branch is the largest of the sympathetic cardiac branches. It goes to the deep cardiac plexus.

Inferior Cervical Ganglion

It is formed by fusion of the 7th and 8th cervical ganglia.

This is often fused with the first thoracic ganglion and is then known as the cervicothoracic ganglion. It is also called the stellate ganglion because it is star-shaped.

It is situated between the transverse process of vertebra C7 and the neck of the first rib. It lies behind the vertebral artery, and in front of ramus of spinal nerve C8. A cervicothoracic ganglion extends in front of the neck of the first rib.

Branches

1. Grey rami communicans are given to the ventral rami of nerves C7 and C8.

2. Vertebral branches form a plexus around the vertebral artery.

3. Subclavian branches form a plexus around the subclavian artery. This plexus is joined by branches from the ansa subclavia (Fig. 12.26).

4. An inferior cervical cardiac branch goes to the deep cardiac plexus.

CLINICAL ANATOMY

1. The head and neck are supplied by sympathetic nerves arising from the upper four thoracic segments of the spinal cord. Most of these preganglionic fibres pass through the stellate ganglion to relay in the superior cervical ganglion.

2. Injury to cervical sympathetic trunk produces *Horner's syndrome*. It is characterized by: (a) Ptosis i.e. drooping of the upper eyelid); (b) miosis (i.e. constriction of the pupil); (c) anhydrosis (i.e. loss of sweating on that side of the face); (d) enophthalmos (i.e. retraction of the eyeball); and (e) loss of the ciliospinal reflex (i.e. pinching the skin on the nape of the neck) does not produce dilatation of the pupil (which normally takes place).

Horner's syndrome can also be caused by a lesion within the central nervous system anywhere at or above the first thoracic segment of the spinal cord involving sympathetic fibres.

CERVICAL PLEXUS

Formation

The cervical plexus is formed by the ventral rami of the upper four cervical nerves. The rami emerge between the anterior and posterior tubercles of the cervical transverse processes, grooving the costo-transverse bars. The four roots are connected with one another to form three loops (Fig. 12.27).

Position and Relations of the Plexus

The plexus is related: (a) *posteriorly,* to the muscles which arise from the posterior tubercles of the transverse processes i.e., the levator scapulae and the scalenus medius; and (b) *anteriorly,* to the prevertebral fascia, the internal jugular vein and the sternocleidomastoid (Fig. 12.28A, B).

Branches

Superficial (Cutaneous) Branches

1. Lesser occipital (C2)
2. Great auricular (C2, C3)
3. Transverse (anterior) cutaneous nerve of the neck (C2, C3)
4. Supraclavicular (C3, C4)

Deep Branches

Communicating Branches

1. Grey rami pass from the superior cervical ganglion to the roots of C1–C4 nerves.

2. A branch from C1 joins the hypoglossal nerve and carries fibres for supply of the thyrohyoid and geniohyoid muscles (directly) and the superior belly of the omohyoid through the ansa cervicalis (Fig. 12.24).

3. A branch from C2 to the sternocleidomastoid and branches from C3 and C4 to the trapezius communicate with the accessory nerve.

Muscular Branches

Muscles supplied solely by cervical plexus:
1. Rectus capitis anterior from C1 (Fig. 12.28B).
2. Rectus capitis lateralis from C1, C2.
3. Longus capitis from C1-C3.

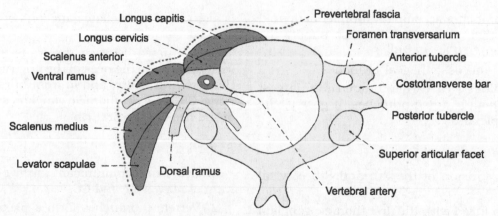

Fig. 12.27: *Scheme to show the position of a cervical nerve relative to the muscles of the region.*

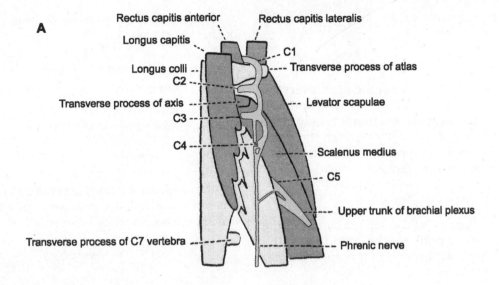

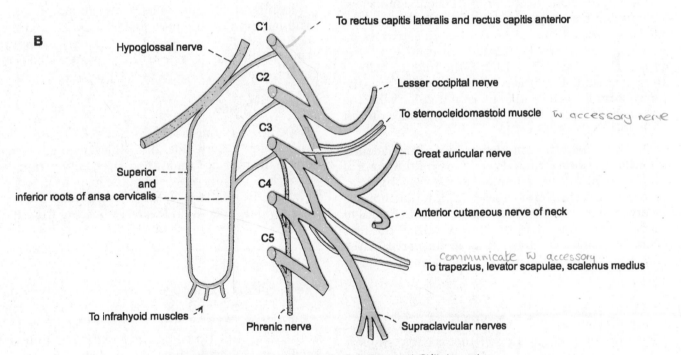

Fig. 12.28: The cervical plexus: (A) Relations and (B) its branches.

4. Lower root of ansa cervicalis (descendens cervicalis) from C2, C3 (to sternohyoid, sternothyroid and inferior belly of omohyoid.

Muscles supplied by cervical plexus along with the brachial plexus or the spinal accessory nerve:

1. Sternocleidomastoid from C2 along with accessory nerve.

2. Trapezius from C3, C4 along with accessory nerve.

3. Levator scapulae from C3, C4 with C5 (dorsal scapular nerve).

4. Phrenic nerve from C3, C4, C5.

5. Longus colli from C3-C8.

6. Scalenus medius from C3-C8.

7. Scalenus anterior from C4-C6.

8. Scalenus posterior from C6-C8.

PHRENIC NERVE

This is a mixed nerve carrying motor fibres to the diaphragm and sensory fibres from the diaphragm, the pleura, the pericardium, and part of the peritoneum.

Origin

Phrenic nerve arises chiefly from the fourth cervical nerve but receives contributions from third and fifth cervical nerves. The contribution from C5 may come directly from the root or indirectly through the nerve to the subclavius. In the latter case, the contribution is known as the *accessory phrenic nerve.*

Course and Relations in the Neck

1. The nerve is formed at the lateral border of the scalenus anterior, opposite the middle of the sternocleidomastoid, at the level of the upper border of the thyroid cartilage.

2. It runs vertically downwards on the anterior surface of the scalenus anterior. Since the muscle is oblique the nerve appears to cross it obliquely from its lateral to its medial border. In this part of its course, the nerve is related anteriorly to the prevertebral fascia (Fig. 12.25), the inferior belly of the omohyoid, the transverse cervical artery, the suprascapular artery, the internal jugular vein, the sternocleidomastoid, and the thoracic duct on left side (Figs 3.7, 12.28A, B).

3. After leaving the anterior surface of the scalenus anterior, the nerve runs downwards on the cervical pleura behind the commencement of the brachiocephalic vein. Here it crosses the internal thoracic artery (either anteriorly or posteriorly) from lateral to medial side, and enters the thorax behind the first costal cartilage. On the left side the nerve leaves (crosses) the medial margin of the scalenus anterior

---

CLINICAL ANATOMY

The phrenic nerve is the sole motor nerve supply to the diaphragm. Before the advent of modern treatments for pulmonary tuberculosis the operation of *"phrenic crush"* used to the done to produce paralysis of the corresponding half of the diaphragm for a few weeks. This gave rest to the diseased lung and promoted healing.

The *accessory phrenic nerve* is commonly a branch from the nerve to the subclavius. It lies lateral to the phrenic nerve and descends behind, or sometimes in front of the subclavian vein. It joins the main nerve usually near the first rib, but occasionally the union may even be below the root of the lung. The accessory phrenic nerve may occasionally arise from spinal nerves C4 or C6 or from the ansa cervicalis.

---

at a higher level and crosses in front of the first part of the subclavian artery.

TRACHEA

The trachea is a noncollapsible, wide tube forming the beginning of the lower respiratory passages. It is kept patent because of the presence of C-shaped cartilaginous 'rings' in its wall. The cartilages are deficient posteriorly, this part of the wall being made up of muscle (trachealis) and fibrous tissue. The soft posterior wall allows expansion of the oesophagus during passage of food.

DISSECTION

Clean and define the cervical parts of the trachea and oesophagus.

Identify the lymph nodes in the submental, the submandibular, the parotid, the mastoid and the occipital regions including the deep cervical nodes. Dissect the main lymph trunk present at the root of the neck.

Scalene Muscle

Scalenus anterior has been seen in relation to subclavian artery. Identify scalenus medius as one of the muscle forming floor of posterior triangle of neck. Scalenus posterior lies deep to the medius. Identify the relations of the cervical pleura. Dissect the styloid process and muscles arising from it.

Dimensions

The trachea is about 10 to 15 cm long. Its upper half lies in the neck and its lower half in the superior mediastinum. The external diameter measures 2 cm in the male and 1.5 cm in the female. The lumen is smaller in the living than in cadavers. It is about 3 mm at 1 year of age, and corresponds to the age in years during childhood, with a maximum of 12 mm at puberty.

Cervical Part of Trachea

1. The trachea begins at the lower border of the cricoid cartilage opposite the lower border of vertebra C6. It runs downwards and slightly backwards in front of the oesophagus, follows the curvature of the spine, and enters the thorax in the median plane.

2. In the neck, the trachea is comparatively superficial and has the following relations.

Anterior: (1) Isthmus of the thyroid gland covering the second and third tracheal rings; (2) inferior thyroid veins below the isthmus; (3) pretracheal fascia enclosing the thyroid and the inferior thyroid veins; (4) sternohyoid and sternothyroid muscles; (5) investing layer of the deep cervical fascia and the suprasternal space; and (6) the skin and superificial fascia. (7) In children, the left brachiocephalic vein extends into the neck and, then, lies in front of the trachea (Fig. 3.3).

Posterior: (1) Oesophagus; (2) longus colli; and (3) recurrent laryngeal nerve in the tracheo-oesophageal groove.

On each side: (1) The corresponding lobe of the thyroid glands; and (2) the common carotid artery within the carotid sheath (Fig. 3.3).

Vessels and Nerves

The trachea is supplied by branches from the inferior thyroid arteries. Its veins drain into the left brachiocephalic vein. Lymphatics drain into the pretracheal and paratracheal nodes.

Parasympathetic nerves (from the vagus through the recurrent laryngeal nerve) are sensory and secretomotor to the mucous membrane, and motor to the trachealis muscle. Sympathetic nerves (from the cervical ganglion) are vasomotor.

CLINICAL ANATOMY

1. The trachea may be compressed by pathological enlargements of the thyroid, the thymus, lymph nodes and the aortic arch. This causes dyspnoea, irritative cough, and often a husky voice.

2. *Tracheostomy* is an emergency operation done in cases of laryngeal obstruction (foreign body, diphtheria, carcinoma, etc.). It is commonly done in the retrothyroid region after retracting the isthmus of the thyroid gland.

3. Please read Chapter 20, Volume 1 in which the thoracic part of the trachea is described.

OESOPHAGUS

The oesophagus is a muscular food passage lying between the trachea and the vertebral column. Normally, its anterior and posterior walls are in contact. The oesophagus expands during the passage of food by pressing into the posterior muscular part of the trachea.

The oesophagus is a downward continuation of the pharynx and begins at the lower border of the cricoid cartilage, opposite the lower border of the body of vertebra C6. It passes downwards behind the trachea, traverses the superior and posterior

mediastina of the thorax, and ends by opening into the cardiac end of the stomach in the abdomen. It is about 25 cm long.

The cervical part of the oesophagus is related;

(a) *Anteriorly,* to the trachea and to the right and left recurrent laryngeal nerves;

(b) *Posteriorly,* to the longus colli muscle and the vertebral column; and

(c) *On each side,* to the corresponding lobe of the thyroid gland; and on the left side, to the thoracic duct (Fig. 3.3).

The cervical part of the oesophagus is supplied by the inferior thyroid arteries. Its veins drain into the left brachiocephalic vein. Its lymphatics pass to the deep cervical lymph nodes.

The oesophagus is narrowest at its junction with the pharynx, the junction being the narrowest part of the gastrointestinal tract, except for the vermiform appendix.

For thoracic part of oesophagus study Chapter 20, Volume 1.

LYMPH NODES OF HEAD AND NECK

The entire lymph from the head and neck drains ultimately into the deep cervical nodes either directly or through the peripheral nodes. The deep cervical nodes form a vertical chain situated along the entire length of the internal jugular vein. For convenience of description these are often grouped as anterosuperior, anteroinferior, posterosuperior and posteroinferior, though there is no clear demarcation between them.

The *jugulodigastric node* (Fig. 12.29) is a member of the anterosuperior group. It lies below the posterior

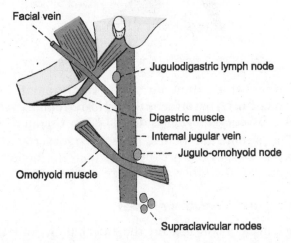

Fig. 12.29: *Some important members of the deep cervical lymph nodes.*

belly of the digastric, between the angle of the mandible and the anterior border of the sternocleidomastoid, in the triangle bounded by the posterior belly of the digastric, the facial vein and the internal jugular vein. It is the main node draining the tonsil.

The *jugulo-omohyoid node* is a member of the posteroinferior group. It lies just above the intermediate tendon of the omohyoid, under cover of the posterior border of the sternocleidomastoid. It is the main lymph node of the tongue.

Efferents of the deep cervical lymph nodes join together to form the jugular lymph trunks, one on each side. The left jugular trunk opens into the thoracic duct. The right trunk may open either into the right lymphatic duct, or directly into the angle of junction between the internal jugular and subclavian veins.

The *peripheral nodes* are arranged in two circles, superficial and deep.

The *superficial circle of cervical lymph nodes* is made up of the following groups: (1) Submental (Fig. 12.30); (2) submandibular; (3) buccal and mandibular (facial); (4) preauricular (parotid); (5) postauricular (mastoid); (6) occipital; (7) anterior cervical; and (8) superficial cervical nodes.

The *deep (inner) circle of cervical lymph nodes*

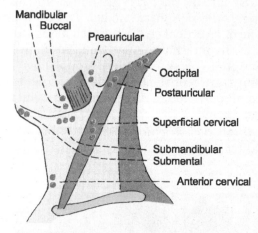

Fig. 12.30: *Superficial lymph nodes of the neck.*

includes the following: (1) Prelaryngeal and pretracheal; (2) paratracheal; and (3) retropharyngeal nodes. Waldeyer's ring is described in Chapter 14.

The submental nodes have been described in Chapter 8, and the preauricular (parotid) nodes in Chapter 9. The other groups are considered below:

Buccal and Mandibular Nodes

The buccal node lies on the buccinator, and the mandibular node at the lower border of the mandible near the anteroinferior angle of the masseter, in close

relation to the mandibular branch of the facial nerve. They drain part of the cheek and the lower eyelid. Their efferents pass to the anterosuperior group of deep cervical nodes.

Postauricular (Mastoid) Nodes

The postauricular nodes lie on the mastoid process superficial to the sternocleidomastoid and deep to the auricularis posterior. They drain a strip of scalp just above and behind the auricle, the upper half of the medial surface and margin of the auricle, and the posterior wall of the external acoustic meatus. Their efferents pass to the posterosuperior group of deep cervical nodes.

Occipital Nodes

The occipital nodes lie at the apex of the posterior triangle superficial to the attachment of the trapezius. They drain the occipital region of the scalp. Their efferents pass to the supraclavicular members of the posteroinferior group of deep cervical nodes.

Anterior Cervical Nodes

The anterior cervical nodes lie along the anterior jugular vein and are unimportant. The suprasternal lymph node is a member of this group. They drain the skin of the anterior part of the neck below the hyoid bone. Their efferents pass to the deep cervical nodes of both sides.

Superficial Cervical Nodes

The superficial cervical nodes lie along the external jugular vein superficial to the sternocleidomastoid. They drain the lobule of the auricle, the floor of the external acoustic meatus, and the skin over the lower parotid region and the angle of the jaw. Their efferents pass round both borders of the muscle to reach the upper and lower deep cervical nodes.

Prelaryngeal and Pretracheal Nodes

The prelaryngeal and pretracheal nodes lie deep to the investing fascia, the prelaryngeal nodes on the cricothyroid membrane, and the pretracheal in front of the trachea below the isthmus of the thyroid gland. They drain the larynx, the trachea and the isthmus of the thyroid. They also receive afferents from the anterior cervical nodes. Their efferents pass to the nearby deep cervical nodes.

Paratracheal Nodes

The paratracheal nodes lie on the sides of the trachea and oesophagus along the recurrent laryngeal nerves. They receive lymph from the oesophagus, the trachea and the larynx, and pass it on to the deep cervical nodes.

Retropharyngeal Nodes

The retropharyngeal nodes lie in front of the prevertebral fascia and behind the buccopharyngeal fascia covering the posterior wall of the pharynx. They extend laterally in front of the lateral mass of the atlas and along the lateral border of the longus capitis. They drain the pharynx, the auditory tube, the soft palate, the posterior part of the hard palate, and the nose. Their efferents pass to the upper deep cervical nodes.

Main Lymph Trunks at the Root of the Neck

1. The *thoracic duct* is the largest lymph trunk of the body. It begins in the abdomen from the upper end of the cisterna chyli, traverses the thorax, and ends on the left side of the root of the neck by opening into the angle of junction between the left internal jugular vein and the left subclavian vein (Fig. 20.8, Vol. 1). Before its termination, it forms an arch at the level of the transverse process of vertebra C7 rising 3 to 4 cm above the clavicle. The relations of the arch are :

Anterior: (1) Left common carotid artery; (2) vagus; and (3) internal jugular vein.

Posterior: (1) Vertebral artery and vein; (2) sympathetic trunk; (3) thyrocervical trunk or its branches; (4) prevertebral fascia; (5) phrenic nerve; and (6) scalenus anterior.

Apart from its tributaries in the abdomen and thorax, the thoracic duct receives (in the neck): (1) The left jugular trunk; (2) the left subclavian trunk; and (3) the left bronchomediastinal trunk. It drains most of the body, except for the right upper limb, the right halves of the head, the neck and the thorax and the superior surface of the liver.

2. The right *jugular trunk* drains half of the head and neck.

3. The right *subclavian trunk* drains the upper limb.

4. The *bronchomediastinal trunk* drains the lung, half of the mediastinum and parts of the anterior walls of the thorax and abdomen.

5. On the right side, the subclavian and jugular trunks may unite to form the *right lymph trunk* which ends in a manner similar to the thoracic duct. Variations in the mode of the termination of the jugular, subclavian and bronchomediastinal trunks are common and are more frequent on the right side (Fig. 12.18).

SCALENE MUSCLES

There are usually three scalene muscles, the scalenus anterior, the scalenus medius and the scalenus posterior. The scalenus medius is the largest, and the scalenus posterior the smallest, of three. These muscles extend from the transverse processes of cervical vertebrae to the first two ribs. They can, therefore, either elevate these ribs or bend the cervical part of the vertebral column laterally (Fig. 12.31).

These muscles are described in Table 12.2.

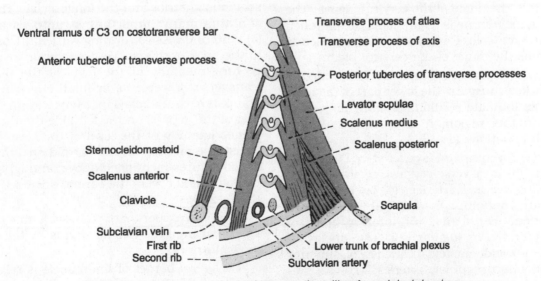

Fig. 12.31: Lateral view of the scalene muscles with a few related structures.

Table 12.2: The scalene muscles

Muscle	Origin from	Insertion into	Nerve supply	Actions
1. *Scalenus anterior* (Fig. 12.31)	Anterior tubercles of transverse processes of cervical vertebrae, 3, 4, 5 and 6	Scalene tubercle and adjoining ridge on the superior surface of the first rib (between subclavian artery and vein)	Ventral rami of nerves C4–C6	1. Anterolateral flexion of cervical spine 2. Rotates cervical spine to opposite side 3. Elevates the first rib during inspiration 4. Stabilizes the neck along with other muscles
2. *Scalenus medius* (Fig. 12.31)	(a) Posterior tubercles of transverse processes of cervical vertebrae 3, 4, 5, 6, 7 (b) Transverse process of axis and sometimes also of the atlas vertebra	Superior surface of the first rib behind the groove for the subclavian artery	Ventral rami of nerves C3-C8	1. Lateral flexion of the cervical spine. 2. Elevation of first rib 3. Stabilizes neck along with other muscles
3. *Scalenus posterior* (Fig. 12.31)	Posterior tubercles of transverse processes of cervical vertebrae, 4, 5, 6	Outer surface of the second rib behind the tubercle for the serratus anterior	Ventral rami of nerves C6-C8	1. Lateral flexion of cervical spine 2. Elevation of the second rib 3. Stabilizes neck along with other muscles

Additional Features of the Scalene Muscles

1. Sometimes a fourth, rudimentary scalene muscle, the *scalenus minimus* is present. It arises from the anterior border of the transverse process of vertebra C7 and is inserted into the inner border of the first rib behind the groove for the subclavian artery and into the dome of the cervical pleura. The *suprapleural membrane* is regarded as the flattened tendon of this muscle. Contraction of the scalenus minimus pulls the dome of the cervical pleura.

2. *Relations of scalenus anterior.* The scalenus anterior is a 'key' muscle of the lower part of the neck because of its intimate relations to many important structures in this region. It is a useful surgical landmark. Its relations are :

Anterior: (1) Phrenic nerve is covered by; (2) prevertebral fascia; (3) transverse cervical, suprascapular and ascending cervical arteries; (4) lateral part of carotid sheath containing the internal jugular vein; (5) descendens cervicalis; (6) inferior belly of omohyoid; (7) anterior jugular vein; (8) subclavian vein; (9) sternocleidomastoid branches of superior thyroid and suprascapular arteries; (10) sternocleidomastoid; and (11) clavicle (Fig. 12.32).

Posterior: (1) Brachial plexus; (2) subclavian artery; (3) scalenus medius; and (4) cervical pleura covered by the suprapleural membrane (Fig. 3.10).

The *medial border* of the muscle is related:

(1) In its lower part to an inverted 'V'-shaped interval, formed by the diverging borders of the scalenus anterior and the longus colli. This interval contains many important structures as follows: (a) Vertebral vessels running vertically from the base to the apex of this space; (b) inferior thyroid artery arching medially at the level of the 6th cervical transverse process; (c) sympathetic trunk; (d) the first part of the subclavian artery traverses the lower part of the gap; (e) on the left side the thoracic duct arches laterally at the level of the seventh cervical transverse process; (f) the carotid sheath covers all the structures mentioned above; and (g) the sternocleidomastoid covers the carotid sheath (Figs 12.33, 13.2, 12.8).

(2) In its upper part, the scalenus anterior is separated from the longus capitis by the ascending cervical artery.

The *lateral border* of the muscle is related to the trunks of the brachial plexus and the subclavian

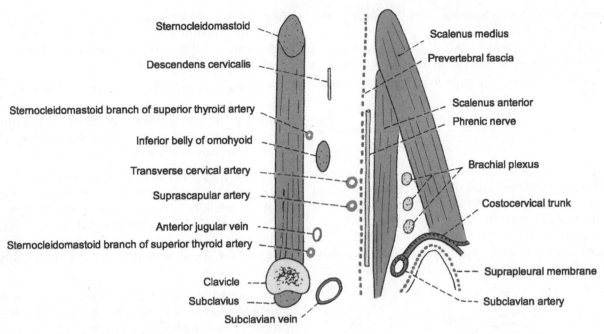

Fig. 12.32: *Schematic sagittal section through the scalenus anterior to show its relations.*

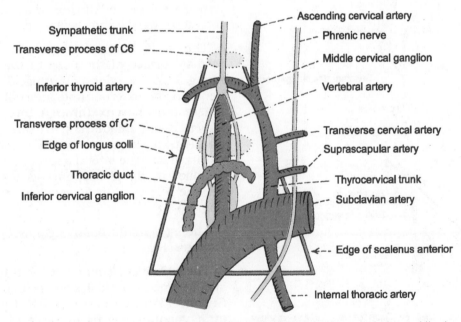

Fig. 12.33: *Structures present in the triangular interval between the scalenus anterior and the longus colli.*

artery which emerges at this border and enter the posterior triangle (Fig. 3.10).

CERVICAL PLEURA

The cervical pleura covers the apex of the lung. It rises into the root of the neck, about 5 cm above the first costal cartilage and 2.5 cm above the medial one-third of the clavicle. The pleural dome is strengthened on its outer surface by the suprapleural membrane so that the root of the neck is not puffed up and down during respiration (Chapter 12, Vol. 2). Relations of the cervical pleura are as follows:

Anterior: (a) Subclavian artery and its branches; and (b) scalenus anterior.

Posterior: Neck of the first rib with the following structures in front of it. (1) Sympathetic trunk; (2) first posterior intercostal vein; (3) superior intercostal artery; and (4) the first thoracic nerve (Fig. 12.12).

Lateral: (a) Scalenus medius; and (b) lower trunk of the brachial plexus.

Medial: (a) Vertebral bodies: (b) oesophagus; (c) trachea; (d) left recurrent laryngeal nerve; (e) thoracic duct (on left side) and (f) large arteries and veins of the neck.

STYLOID APPARATUS

The styloid process with its attached structures is called the styloid apparatus. The structures attached to the process are the stylohyoid, styloglossus and stylopharyngeus muscles; and the stylohyoid and stylomandibular ligaments (Fig. 12.34). The apparatus is of diverse origin. The styloid process, and the stylohyoid ligament and muscle are derived

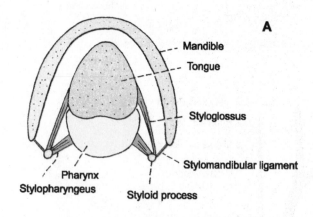

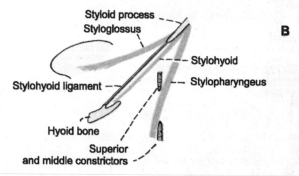

Fig. 12.34: *The styloid apparatus: (A) Superior view, (B) lateral view.*

from the second branchial arch; the stylopharyngeus from the third arch; the styloglossus from occipital myotomes; and the stylomandibular ligament from a part of the deep fascia of the neck.

The *five attachments resemble the reins of a chariot.* Two of these reins (ligaments) are nonadjustable, whereas the other three (muscles) are adjustable and are controlled each by a separate cranial nerve, seventh, ninth and twelfth nerves.

The *styloid process* is a long, slender and pointed bony process projecting downwards, forwards and slightly medially from the temporal bone. It descends between the external and internal carotid arteries to reach the side of the pharynx. It is interposed between the parotid gland laterally and the internal jugular vein medially.

The *styloglossus muscle* arises from the tip and adjacent part of the anterior surface of the styloid process as well as from the upper end of the stylohyoid ligament. It passes downwards and forwards and is inserted into the side of the tongue, intermingling with the fibres of the hyoglossus. It is supplied by the hypoglossal nerve. During swallowing, it pulls the tongue upwards and backwards.

The *stylopharyngeus muscle* arises from the medial surface of the base of the styloid process. Along with the glossopharyngeal nerve it passes between the external and internal carotid arteries, enters the pharynx through the gap between the superior and middle constrictors, and is inserted on the posterior border of the lamina of the thyroid cartilage and the lateral aspect of the epiglottis. It is supplied by the glossopharyngeal nerve. It helps to lift the larynx during swallowing and phonation (Fig. 14.11).

The *stylomandibular ligament* is described in Chapter 10.

The *stylohyoid ligament* extends from the tip of the styloid process to the lesser cornu of the hyoid bone. Stylohyoid muscle is supplied by the facial nerve. Its attachments are given in Table 11.1.

13

The Prevertebral Region

The prevertebral region contains four muscles, vertebral artery and joints of the neck. Vertebral artery, a branch of subclavian artery, comprises four parts — 1st, 2nd and 3rd are in the neck. The fourth part passes through the foramen magnum to reach the subarachnoid space. The vertebral arteries of two sides unite to form a single median basilar artery which gives branches to supply a part of cerebral cortex, cerebellum, internal ear and pons. Congenital or acquired diseases of cervical vertebrae or their joints give rise to lots of symptoms related to branches of vertebral artery.

The apical ligament of dens is a continuation of notochord. Transverse ligament, which is a part of cruciate ligament, keeps the dens of axis in position. If this ligament is injured by disease or in "capital punishment", there is immediate death due to injury to vasomotor centres in medulla oblongata.

PREVERTEBRAL MUSCLES
(Anterior Vertebral Muscles)

The four prevertebral or anterior vertebral muscles are the longus colli (cervicis), the longus capitis, the rectus capitis anterior and the rectus capitis lateralis (Fig. 13.1). These are weak flexors of the head and neck. They extend from the base of the skull to the superior mediastinum. They partially cover the anterior aspect of the vertebral column. They are covered anteriorly by the thick prevertebral fascia. The muscles are described in Table 13.1.

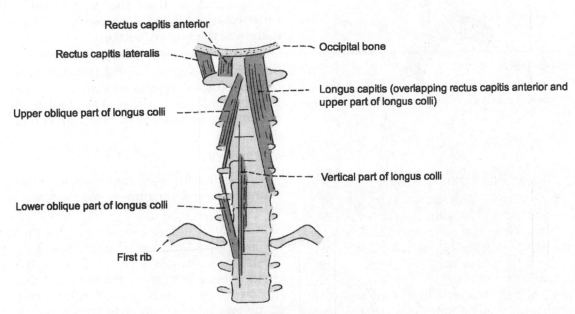

Rectus capitis anterior

Rectus capitis lateralis

Occipital bone

Longus capitis (overlapping rectus capitis anterior and upper part of longus colli)

Upper oblique part of longus colli

Vertical part of longus colli

Lower oblique part of longus colli

First rib

Fig. 13.1: The prevertebral muscles.

VERTEBRAL ARTERY

Introduction

The vertebral artery is one of the two principal arteries which supply the brain. In addition, it also supplies the spinal cord, the meninges, and the surrounding muscles and bones. It arises from the posterosuperior aspect of the first part of the subclavian artery near its commencement. It runs a long course, and ends in the cranial cavity by supplying the brain (Fig. 13.2). The artery is divided into four parts.

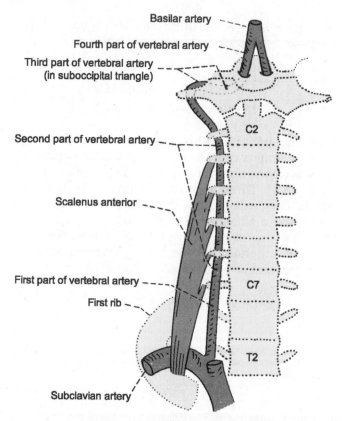

Fig. 13.2: *Scheme showing parts of the vertebral artery, as seen from the front.*

First Part

The first part extends from the origin of the artery (from the subclavian artery) to the transverse process of the sixth cervical vertebra.

This part of the artery runs upwards and backwards in the triangular space between the scalenus anterior and the longus colli muscles called as the vertebral triangle (Figs 12.13, 12.14, 12.33).

Relations. Anterior: (a) Carotid sheath with common carotid artery; (b) vertebral vein; (c) inferior thyroid artery; and (d) thoracic duct on left side (Fig. 12.8).

Posterior: (a) Transverse process of seventh cervical vertebra; (b) inferior cervical ganglion; and (c) ventral rami of nerves C7, C8 (Fig. 12.15).

Second Part

The second part runs through the foramina transversaria of the upper six cervical vertebrae. Its course is vertical up to the axis vertebra. It then runs upwards and laterally to reach the foramen transversarium of the atlas vertebra .

Relations: (a) The ventral rami of second to sixth cervical nerves lie posterior to the vertebral artery (Fig. 12.17). (b) The artery is accompanied by a venous plexus and a large branch from the stellate ganglion (Fig. 12.33).

Third Part

Third part lies in the suboccipital triangle. Emerging from the foramen transversarium of the atlas, the artery winds medially around the posterior aspect of the lateral mass of the atlas. It runs medially lying on the posterior arch of this bone, and enters the vertebral canal by passing deep to the lower arched margin of the posterior atlanto-occipital membrane.

Relations. Anterior: Lateral mass of atlas. *Posterior:* Semispinalis capitis. *Lateral:* Rectus capitis lateralis. *Medial:* Ventral ramus of the first cervical nerve. *Inferior:* (a) Dorsal ramus of the first cervical nerve and (d) the posterior arch of the atlas (Fig. 4.6).

Fourth Part

1. The fourth part extends from the posterior atlanto-occipital membrane to the lower border of the pons.

2. In the vertebral canal, it pierces the dura and the arachnoid, and ascends in front of the roots of the hypoglossal nerve. As it ascends it gradually inclines medially to reach the front of the medulla. At the lower border of the pons, it unites with its fellow of the opposite side to form the basilar artery (Fig. 13.2).

Table 13.1 : The prevertebral muscles (Figs 12.27, 12.28A, 12.33, 13.1)

Muscle	Origin from	Insertion into	Nerve supply	Actions
1. *Longus colli (cervicis).* This muscle extends from the atlas to the third thoracic vertebra. It has upper and lower oblique parts and a middle vertical part	(a) The *upper oblique part:* from the anterior tubercles of the transverse processes of of cervical vertebrae 3, 4, 5 (b) *Lower oblique part:* from bodies of upper 2-3 thoracic vertebrae (c) *Middle vertical part:* from bodies of upper 3 thoracic and lower 3 cervical vertebrae	(a) *Upper oblique part:* into the anterior tubercle of the atlas (b) *Lower oblique part:* into the anterior tubercles of the transverse processes of 5th and 6th cervical vertebrae (c) *Middle vertical part:* into bodies of 2,3,4 cervical vertebrae	Ventral rami of nerves C3-C8	1. Flexes the neck 2. Oblique parts flex the neck laterally 3. Lower oblique part rotates the neck to the opposite side
2. *Longus capitis,* It overlaps the longus colli, It is thick above and narrow below	Anterior tubercles of transverse processes of cervical 3-6 vertebrae	Inferior surface of basilar part of occipital bone	Ventral rami of nerves C1-C3	Flexes the head
3. *Rectus capitis anterior.* This is a very short and flat muscle. It lies deep to the longus capitis	Anterior surface of lateral mass of atlas	Basilar part of the occipital bone in front of the occipital condyle	Ventral ramus of nerve C1	Flexes the head
4. *Rectus capitis lateralis* This is a short, flat muscle	Upper surface of transverse process of atlas	Inferior surface of jugular process of the occipital bone	Ventral rami of nerves C1, C2	Flexes the head laterally

Branches of Vertebral Artery

Cervical Branches

1. Spinal branches enter the vertebral canal through the intervertebral foramina, and supply the spinal cord, the meninges and the vertebrae.

2. Muscular branches arise from the third part and supply the suboccipital muscles.

Cranial Branches

1. *Meningeal* branches arise near the foramen magnum and supply bone and meninges of the posterior cranial fossa.

2. The *posterior spinal* artery is usually a branch from the posterior inferior cerebellar artery, though it may arise from the vertebral artery at the side of the medulla. It descends on the posterolateral aspect of the spinal cord. It is reinforced at lower levels by spinal branches of other arteries. It supplies the posterior one-third of the spinal cord.

3. The *anterior spinal* artery arises near the termination of the vertebral artery. The arteries of the two sides unite (at the level of the lower end of the olive) to form a single anterior spinal artery. It descends in the anterior median fissure of the spinal cord. It is reinforced at lower levels by spinal branches of other arteries. It supplies the anterior two-thirds of the spinal cord. It also supplies part of the medulla.

4. The *posterior inferior cerebellar* artery is the largest branch of the vertebral artery. It arises near the lower end of the olive. The artery first runs backwards and then upwards behind the IX and X cranial nerves to reach the lower border of the pons. It then runs downwards along the inferolateral boundary of the fourth ventricle, and finally laterally into the vallecula of the cerebellum. It *supplies:* (a) Wedge-shaped area on the posterolateral aspect of the medulla; (b) the lower part of the pons; and (c) the cerebellum.

5. Medullary arteries are given off to the medulla.

DEVELOPMENT OF VERTEBRAL ARTERY

Different parts of vertebral artery develop in the following ways.

First part: From a branch of dorsal division of 7th cervical intersegmental artery.

Second part: From postcostal anastomosis.

Third part: From spinal branch of the first cervical intersegmental artery.

Fourth part: From preneural branch of first cervical intersegmental artery.

JOINTS OF THE NECK

Typical Cervical Joints Between the Lower Six Cervical Vertebrae

These correspond in structure to typical intervertebral joints already described in Chapter 13, Vol. I. The only additional point to be noted is that in the cervical region the supraspinous ligaments are replaced by the ligamentum nuchae.

The *ligamentum nuchae* is triangular in shape. Its apex lies at the seventh cervical spine and its base at the external occipital crest. Its anterior border is attached to cervical spines, while the posterior border is free and provides attachment to the investing layer of deep cervical fascia. The ligament gives origin to the splenius, rhomboids and trapezius muscles.

Special Joints Between the Atlas, the Axis and the Occipital Bone

1. The atlanto-occipital and the atlantoaxial joints are designed to permit free movements of the head on the neck (vertebral column).

2. The axis vertebra and the occipital bone are connected together by very strong ligaments. Between these two bones, the atlas is held like a washer. The axis of movement between the atlas and skull is transverse, permitting flexion and extension (nodding), whereas the axis of movement between the axis and the atlas is vertical, permitting rotation of the head (Fig. 13.3).

Atlanto-occipital Joints

Type

These are synovial joints of the ellipsoid variety.

Articular Surfaces

Above :   The occipital condyles, which are convex (Fig. 13.4).

Below :   The superior articular facets of the atlas vertebra. These are concave. The articular surfaces are elongated, and are directed forwards and medially.

Ligaments

1. The *fibrous capsule (capsular ligament)* surrounds the joint. It is thick posterolaterally and thin anteromedially.

2. The *anterior atlanto-occipital membrane* extends from the anterior margin of the foramen magnum above, to the upper border of the anterior arch of the atlas below (Fig. 13.3). Laterally, it is continuous with the anterior part of the capsular ligament, and anteriorly it is strengthened by the cord-like anterior longitudinal ligament.

3. The *posterior atlanto-occipital membrane* extends from the posterior margin of the foramen magnum above, to the upper border of the posterior arch of the

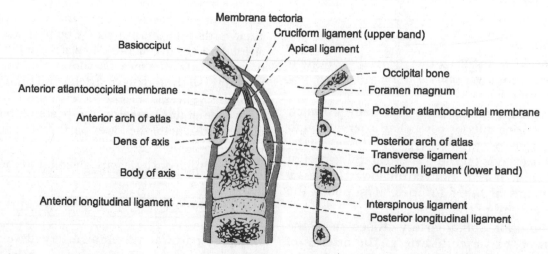

Fig. 13.3: Median section through the foramen magnum and upper two cervical vertebrae showing the ligaments in this region.

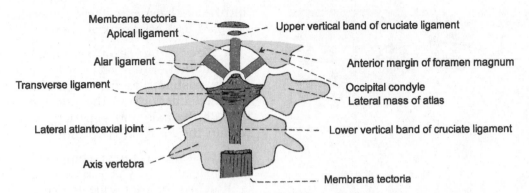

Membrana tectoria

Apical ligament

Upper vertical band of cruciate ligament

Alar ligament

Anterior margin of foramen magnum

Transverse ligament

Occipital condyle

Lateral mass of atlas

Lateral atlantoaxial joint

Lower vertical band of cruciate ligament

Axis vertebra

Membrana tectoria

Fig. 13.4: Posterior view of the ligaments connecting the axis with the occipital bone.

atlas below. Inferolaterally, it has a free margin which arches over the vertebral artery and the first cervical nerve. Laterally, it is continuous with the posterior part of the capsular ligament.

Arterial and Nerve Supply

The joint is supplied by the vertebral artery and by the first cervical nerve.

Movements

Since these are ellipsoid joints, they permit movements around two axes. Flexion and extension (nodding) occur around a transverse axis. Slight lateral flexion is permitted around an anteroposterior axis.

1. *Flexion* is brought about by the longus capitis and the rectus capitis anterior.

2. *Extension* is done by the rectus capitis posterior major and minor, the obliquus capitis superior, the semispinalis capitis, the splenius capitis, and the upper part of the trapezius.

3. *Lateral bending* is produced by the rectus capitis, the semispinalis capitis, the splenius capitis, the sternocleidomastoid, and the trapezius (Fig. 13.5).

Atlantoaxial Joints

Types and Articular Surfaces

These joints comprise:

1. A pair of lateral atlantoaxial joints between the inferior facets of the atlas and the superior facets of the axis. These are plane joints.

2. A median atlantoaxial joint between the dens (odontoid process) and the anterior arch and transverse ligament of the atlas. It is a pivot joint. The joint has two separate synovial cavities, anterior and posterior.

Ligaments

The lateral atlantoaxial joints are supported by: (a) A capsular ligament all around; (b) the lateral part of the anterior longitudinal ligament; and (c) the ligamentum flavum.

The median atlantoaxial joint is strengthened by the following: (a) The anterior smaller part of the joint between the anterior arch of the atlas and the dens is surrounded by a loose capsular ligament. (b) The posterior larger part of the joint between the dens and transverse ligament (often called a bursa) is often continuous with one of the atlanto-occipital joints. Its main support is the transverse ligament which forms a part of the cruciform ligament of the atlas (Fig. 13.3).

The *transverse ligament* (Fig. 13.4) is attached on each side to the medial surface of the lateral mass of the atlas. In the median plane, its fibres are prolonged upwards to the basiocciput and downwards to the body of the axis, thus forming the *cruciform ligament of the atlas vertebra*. The transverse ligament embraces the narrow neck of the dens, and prevents its dislocation.

Movements

Movements at all three joints are rotatory and take place around a vertical axis. The dens forms a pivot around which the atlas rotates (carrying the skull with it). The movement is limited by the alar ligaments (Fig. 13.5).

The rotatory movements are brought about by the obliquus capitis inferior, the rectus capitis posterior major and the splenius capitis of one side, acting with the sternocleidomastoid of the opposite side.

Ligaments Connecting the Axis with the Occipital Bone

These ligaments are the membrana tectoria, the cruciate ligament, the apical ligament of the dens

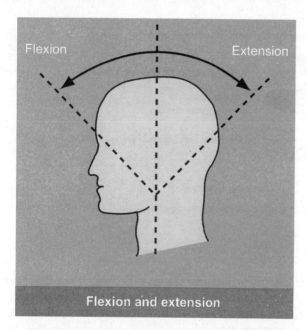

Flexion and extension

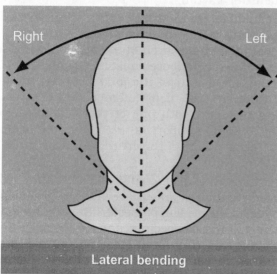

Lateral bending

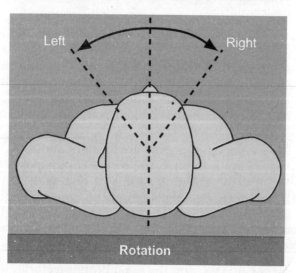

Rotation

Fig. 13.5: *Various movements of the neck.*

and the alar ligaments. They support both the atlanto-occipital and atlantoaxial joints.

1. The *membrana tectoria* is an upward continuation of the posterior longitudinal ligament. It lies posterior to the transverse ligament. It is attached inferiorly to the posterior surface of the body of the axis and superiorly to the basiocciput (within the foramen magnum) (Fig. 13.4).

2. *Cruciate ligament* comprises transverse and vertical ligaments. The *transverse ligament* (Fig. 13.4) is attached on each side to the medial surface of the lateral mass of the atlas. In the median plane, its fibres are prolonged upwards to the basiocciput and downwards to the body of the axis, thus forming the *cruciform ligament of the atlas vertebra.*

3. The *apical ligament of the dens* extends from the apex of the dens close to the anterior margin of the foramen magnum behind of the attachment of the cruciate ligament. It is the continuation of the notochord.

4. The *alar ligament,* one on each side, extends from the upper part of the lateral surface of the dens to the medial surface of the occipital condyles. These are strong ligaments which limit the rotation and flexion of the head. They are relaxed during extension.

CLINICAL ANATOMY

1. Death in execution by hanging is due to dislocation of the dens following rupture of the transverse ligament of the dens, which then crushes the spinal cord and medulla. However, hanging can also cause fracture through the axis, or separation of the axis from the third cervical vertebra.

2. *Cervical spondylosis.* Injury or degenerative changes of old age may rupture the thin postero-lateral parts of the annulus fibrosus (of the inter-vertebral disc) resulting in prolapse of the nucleus pulposus. This is known as disc prolapse or spondylosis. Although it is commonest in the lumbar region, it may occur in the lower cervical region. This causes shooting pain along the distribution of the cervical nerve pressed. A direct posterior prolapse may compress the spinal cord.

3. Cervical vertebrae may be fractured or, more commonly, dislocated by a fall on the head with acute flexion of the neck. In the cervical region, the vertebrae can dislocate without any fracture of the articular processes due to their horizontal position.

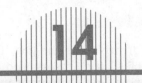

The Mouth
and Pharynx

Vestibule of the mouth lies between the teeth and the cheek. Unconscious patients can be fed through this space. Teeth are of two types – deciduous and permanent. The third molar tooth erupts around 20th year, when one is supposed to be wise and it is rightly called the "wisdom" tooth.

All muscles of soft palate are supplied by vago-accessory complex except tensor veli palatini supplied by mandibular nerve.

Collection of lymphoid tissue at the oropharyngeal junction guards the foreign bodies. Muscles of pharynx are also supplied by vagoaccessory complex except the stylopharyngeus supplied by glossopharyngeal nerve. Inferior constrictor of pharynx receives additional nerve supply from external and recurrent laryngeal nerves. Auditory tube connecting the nasopharynx with the middle ear cavity equalises pressure on the two sides of the tympanic membrane.

Identification

Identify the structures in the oral cavity. Identify the vestibule, lips, cheeks, oral cavity proper and teeth.

The Oral Cavity

The oral or mouth cavity is divided into an outer, smaller portion, the vestibule, and an inner larger part, the oral cavity proper.

Vestibule

1. The vestibule of the mouth is a narrow space *bounded* externally by the lips and cheeks, and internally, by the teeth and gums.

2. It *communicates:* (a) With the exterior through the oral fissure; and (b) with the mouth open it communicates freely with the oral cavity proper. Even when the teeth are occluded a small communication remains behind the third molar tooth.

3. The *parotid duct* opens on the inner surface of the cheek opposite the crown of the upper second molar tooth. Numerous *labial and buccal glands* (mucous) situated in the submucosa of the lips and cheeks open into the vestibule. Four or five *molar glands* (mucous), situated on the buccopharyngeal fascia also open into the vestibule (Fig. 2.26).

4. Except for the teeth, the entire vestibule is lined by mucous membrane. The mucous membrane forms median folds that pass from the lips to the gums, and are called the *frenula of the lips.*

Lips

1. The lips are fleshy folds lined externally by skin and internally by mucous membrane. The *mucocutaneous junction* lines the 'edge' of the lip: part of the mucosal surface is normally seen.

2. Each lip is *composed* of: (a) Skin; (b) superficial fascia; (c) the orbicularis oris muscle; (d) the submucosa, containing mucous labial glands and blood vessels; and (e) mucous membrane.

3. The lips bound the *oral fissure*. They meet laterally at the angles of the mouth. The inner surface of each lip is supported by a *frenulum* which ties it to the gum. The outer surface of the upper lip presents a median vertical groove, the philtrum.

4. *Lymphatics* of the central part of the lower lip drain to the submental nodes; the lymphatics from the rest of the lower lip pass to the submandibular nodes.

Cheeks (Buccae)

1. The cheeks are fleshy flaps, forming a large part of each side of the face. They are continuous in front with the lips, and the junction is indicated by the *nasolabial sulcus* (furrow) which extends from the side of the nose to the angle of the mouth.

2. Each cheek is *composed of:* (a) Skin; (b) superficial fascia containing some facial muscles, the parotid duct, mucous molar glands, vessels and nerves; (c) the buccinator covered by buccopharyngeal fascia and pierced by the parotid duct; (d) submucosa, with mucous buccal glands; and (e) mucous membrane.

3. The *buccal pad of fat* is best developed in infants. It lies on the buccinator partly deep to the masseter and partly in front of it.

4. The *lymphatics* of the cheek drain chiefly into the submandibular and preauricular nodes, and partly also to the buccal and mandibular nodes.

Oral Cavity Proper

1. It is *bounded* anterolaterally by the teeth, the gums and the alveolar arches of the jaws. The roof is formed by the hard and soft palate. The *floor* is occupied by the tongue posteriorly, and presents the sublingual region anteriorly, below the tip of the tongue. Posteriorly, the cavity communicates with the pharynx through the *oropharyngeal isthmus (isthmus of fauces)* which is bounded superiorly by the soft palate, inferiorly by the tongue, and on each side by the palatoglossal arches.

2. The sublingual region presents the following features.

(a) In the median plane there is a fold of mucosa passing from the inferior aspect of the tongue to the floor of the mouth. This is the *frenulum* of the tongue (Fig. 17.2).

(b) One each side of the frenulum there is a *sublingual papilla.* On the summit of this papilla there is the opening of the submandibular duct.

(c) Running laterally and backwards from the *sublingual papilla* there is the sublingual fold which overlies the sublingual gland. A few sublingual ducts open on the edge of this fold.

3. *Lymphatics* from the anterior part of the floor of the mouth pass to the submental nodes. Those from the hard palate and soft palate pass to the retropharyngeal and upper deep cervical nodes. The gums and the rest of the floor drain into the submandibular nodes (Fig. 14.9).

Gums (Gingivae)

1. The gums are the soft tissues which envelop the alveolar processes of the upper and lower jaws and surround the necks of the teeth. These are composed of dense fibrous tissue covered by stratified squamous epithelium.

2. Each gum has two parts: (a) The free part surrounds the neck of the tooth like a collar, (b) The *attached part* is firmly fixed to the alveolar arch of the jaw. The fibrous tissue of the gum is continuous with the periosteum lining the alveoli (periodontal membrane).

3. *Nerve supply:* The upper gums on labial aspect are supplied by posterior, middle and anterior superior alveolar nerves. Their lingual aspects are supplied by anterior or greater palatine and nasopalatine nerves. The lower gums on labial aspect are supplied by buccal branch of mandibular and incisive branch of mental nerves. Their lingual aspect is supplied by the lingual nerve.

4. *Lymphatics* of the upper gum pass to the submandibular nodes. The anterior part of the lower gum drains into the submental nodes, whereas the posterior part drains into the submandibular nodes.

Teeth

The teeth form part of the masticatory apparatus and are fixed to the jaws. In man, the teeth are replaced only once *(diphyodont)* in contrast with non-mammalian vertebrates where teeth are constantly replaced throughout life *(polyphyodont).* The teeth of the first set (dentition) are known as *milk,* or *deciduous teeth,* and the second set, as *permanent teeth.*

The deciduous teeth are twenty in number. In each half of each jaw there are two incisors, one canine, and two molars.

The permanent teeth are thirty two in number, and consist of two incisors, one canine, two premolars, and three molars in each half of each jaw.

Parts of a Tooth

Each tooth has three parts: (1) A *crown*, projecting above or below the gum; (2) a *root*, embedded in the jaw beneath the gum; and (3) a *neck*, between the crown and root and surrounded by the gum (Fig. 14.1).

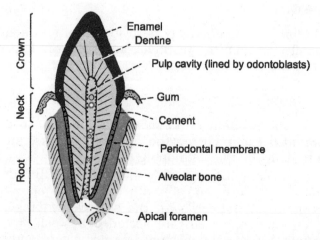

Fig. 14.1: *Parts of a tooth.*

Structure

Structurally, each tooth is composed of : (1) The pulp in the centre; (2) the dentine surrounding the pulp; (3) the enamel covering the projecting part of dentine, or crown; (4) the cementum surrounding the embedded part of the dentine, and (5) the periodontal membrane.

The *pulp* is loose fibrous tissue containing vessels, nerves and lymphatics, all of which enter the pulp cavity through the apical foramen. The pulp is covered by a layer of tall columnar cells, known as odontoblasts which are capable of replacing dentine any time in life.

The *dentine* is a calcified material containing spiral tubules radiating from the pulp cavity. Each tubule is occupied by a protoplasmic process from one of the odontoblasts. The calcium and organic matter are in the same proportion as in bone.

The *enamel* is the hardest substance in the body. It is made up of crystalline prisms lying roughly at right angles to the surface of the tooth.

The *cementum* resembles bone in structure, but like enamel and dentine it has no blood supply, nor any nerve supply. Over the neck, the cementum commonly overlaps the cervical end of enamel; or, less commonly, it may just meet the enamel. Rarely, it stops short of the enamel (10%) leaving the cervical dentine covered only by gum.

The *periodontal membrane (ligament)* holds the root in its socket. This membrane acts as a periosteum to both the cementum as well as the bony socket.

Form and Function (Crowns and Roots)

1. The shape of a tooth is adapted to its function. The *incisors are cutting teeth,* with chisel-like crowns. The upper and lower incisors overlap each other like the blades of a pair of scissors. *The canines are holding and tearing teeth,* with conical and rugged crowns. These are better developed in carnivores. Each *premolar* has two cusps and is, therefore, also called a *bicuspid* tooth. The *molars are grinding teeth,* with square crowns, bearing four or five cusps on their crowns.

2. The incisors, canines and premolars have single roots, with the exception of the first upper premolar which has a bifid root. The upper molars have three roots, of which two are lateral and one is medial. The lower molars have only two roots, an anterior and a posterior.

Eruption of Teeth

The *deciduous teeth* begin to erupt at about the sixth month, and all get erupted by the end of the second year or soon after. The teeth of the lower jaw erupt slightly earlier than those of the upper jaw. The approximate ages of eruption are: Lower central incisors, about 6 months; upper central incisors, 7 months; lateral incisors, 8-9 months; first molar, 1 year; canines, 18 months; and second molars, 2 years.

The *permanent teeth* erupt in the order given below: first molar, about 6 years; medial incisors, 7 years; lateral incisors, 8 years; first premolar, 9 years; second premolar, 10 years; canines, 11 years; second molars, 12 years; and the third molar (wisdom tooth), 17-25 years or even later.

Nerve Supply of Teeth

The pulp and periodontal membrane have the same nerve supply which is different from that of the overlying gum.

The upper teeth are supplied by the posterior superior alveolar, middle superior alveolar, and the anterior superior alveolar nerves (maxillary nerve).

The lower teeth are supplied by the inferior alveolar nerve (mandibular nerve).

Development of Teeth

Teeth are formed in relation to alveolar process. The epithelium thickness to form dental lamina. The cells of dental lamina proliferate at various sites to form enamel organ, which grows into underlying mesenchyme and acquires a cup-shaped appearance, occupied by the mesenchyme. This mesenchyme is of neural crest origin and is called dental papilla. The dental papilla together with enamel organ is known as tooth germ. This stage is called "cap stage". The cells of enamel organ adjacent to dental papilla cells get columnar and are known as ameloblasts.

The mesenchymal cells now arrange themselves along the ameloblasts and are called odontoblasts. The two cell layers are separated by a basement membrane. The rest of the mesenchymal cells form the "pulp of the tooth". This is the "bell stage".

Now ameloblasts lay enamel on the outer aspect, while odontoblasts lay dentine on the inner aspect. Later ameloblasts disappear while odontoblasts remain.

The root of the tooth is formed by laying down of layers of dentine, narrowing the pulp space to a canal for the passage of nerve and blood vessels only. The dentine in the root is covered by mesenchymal cells which differentiate into cementoblasts for laying down the cementum. Outside this is the periodontal ligament connecting root to the socket in the bone.

1. Being the hardest and chemically the most stable tissues in the body, the teeth are selectively preserved after death and may be fossilized. Because of this the teeth are very helpful in medicolegal practice for identification of otherwise unrecognizable dead bodies. The teeth also provide by far the best data to study evolutionary changes and the relationship between ontogeny and phylogeny.

2. In *scurvy* (caused by deficiency of vitamin C), the gums are swollen and spongy, and bleed on touch. In gingivitis, the edges of the gums are red and bleed easily.

3. Improper oral hygiene may cause gingivitis and suppuration with pocket formation between the teeth and gums. This results in a chronic pus discharge at the margin of the gums. The condition is known as *pyorrhoea alveolaris* (chronic periodontitis). Pyorrhoea is common cause of foul breath for which the patient hardly ever consults a dentist because the condition is painless.

4. Decalcification of enamel and dentine with consequent softening and gradual destruction of the tooth is known as dental caries. A carious tooth is tender and mastication painful.

5. Infection of apex of root (*apical abscess*) occurs only when the pulp is dead. The condition can be recognized in a good radiograph.

6. Irregular dentition is common in *rickets* and the upper permanent incisors may be notched, the notching corresponds to a small segment of a large circle. In *congenital syphilis*, also the same teeth are notched, but the notching corresponds to a large segment of a small circle (*Hutchinson's teeth*).

Hard Palate

It is a partition between the nasal and oral cavies. Its anterior two-thirds are formed by the palatine processes of the maxillae; and its posterior one-third by the horizontal plates of the palatine bones (Fig. 14.2).

The *anterolateral margins* of the palate are continuous with the alveolar arches and gums.

The *posterior margin* gives attachment to the soft palate.

The *superior surface* forms the floor of the nose.

The *inferior surface* forms the roof of the oral cavity.

Hard palate: Strip the mucoperiosteum of hard palate.

Soft palate: Remove the mucous membrane of the soft palate in order to identify its muscles. Also remove the mucous membrane over palatoglossal and palatopharyngeal arches and salpingopharyngeal fold to visualise the subjacent muscles.

Vessels and Nerves

Arteries: Greater palatine branch of maxillary artery (Fig. 10.7).

Veins: Drain into the pterygoid plexus of veins.

Nerves: Greater palatine and nasopalatine branches of the pterygopalatine ganglion suspended by the maxillary nerve.

Lymphatics: The lymphatics drain mostly to the upper deep cervical nodes and partly to the retropharyngeal nodes.

SOFT PALATE

Introduction

It is s movable, muscular fold, suspended from the posterior border of the hard palate.

It separates the nasopharynx from the oropharynx, and is often looked upon as traffic controller at the crossroads between the food and air passages (Fig. 14.2).

The soft palate has two surfaces, anterior and posterior; and two borders, superior and inferior.

The *anterior (oral) surface* is concave and is marked by a median raphe.

The posterior surface is convex, and is continuous superiorly with the floor of the nasal cavity.

The *superior border* is attached to the posterior border of the hard palate, blending on each side with the pharynx.

The inferior border is free and bounds the pharyngeal isthmus. From its middle, there hangs a conical projection, called the uvula (Fig. 14.3). From each side of the base of the uvula, two curved folds of mucous membrane extend laterally and downwards. The anterior fold is called the *palatoglossal arch* or anterior pillar of fauces. It contains the palatoglossus muscle and reaches the side of the tongue at the junction of its oral and pharyngeal parts. This fold forms the lateral boundary of the oropharyngeal isthmus or isthmus of fauces. The posterior fold is called the *palatopharyngeal* arch or posterior pillar of fauces. It contains the palatopharyngeus muscle. It forms the posterior boundary

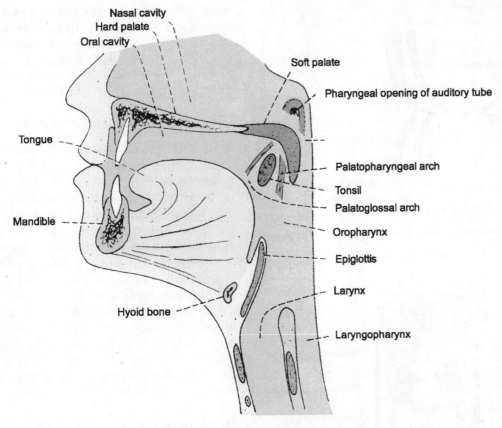

pharyngeal plexus derived from cranial part of accessory nerve thru + vagus nerve

Fig. 14.2: *Sagittal section through the mouth and pharynx.*

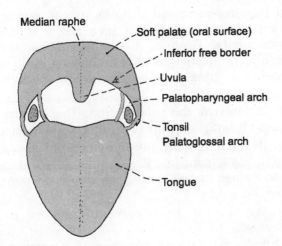

Fig. 14.3: *Anterior view of the soft palate seen after opening the mouth widely.*

of the tonsillar fossa, and merges inferiorly with the lateral wall of the pharynx (Fig. 14.4A).

Structure

The soft palate is a fold of mucous membrane containing the following parts:

The palatine aponeurosis which is the flattened tendon of the tensor veli palatini forms the fibrous basis of the palate. Near the median plane the aponeurosis splits to enclose the musculus uvulae.

The levator veli palatini and the palatopharyngeus lie on the superior surface of the palatine aponeurosis (Fig. 14.4B).

The palatoglossus lies on the inferior surface of the palatine aponeurosis.

Numerous mucous glands, and some taste buds are present.

Muscles of the Soft Palate

They are as follows.

1. Tensor palati (tensor veli palatini) (Fig. 14.5)
2. Levator palati (levator veli palatini)
3. Musculus uvulae
4. Palatoglossus
5. Palatopharyngeus (Fig. 14.4B)

Details of the muscles are given in Table 14.1.

Nerve Supply

1. Motor nerves. All muscles of the soft palate except the tensor veli palatini are supplied by the pharyngeal plexus. The fibres of this plexus are derived from the cranial part of the accessory nerve through the vagus. The tensor veli palatini is supplied by the mandibular nerve.

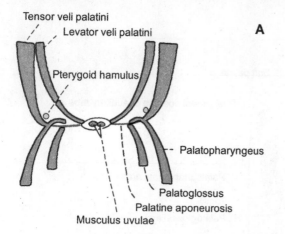

Fig. 14.4A: *Coronal section of the soft palate showing the arrangement of its muscles.*

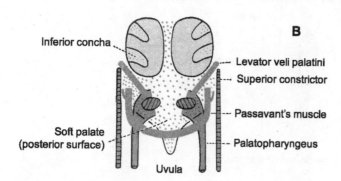

Fig. 14.4B: *Posterior view of the soft palate showing V-sling of levators and U-sling, of the passavant's muscle. The two are interlocked in closure of the nasopharyngeal isthmus.*

2. General sensory nerves are derived from: (a) The middle and posterior lesser palatine nerves, which are branches of the maxillary nerve through the pterygopalatine ganglion (Fig. 15.12) and (b) from the glossopharyngeal nerve (Fig. 12.19).

3. Special sensory or gustatory nerves carrying taste sensations from the oral surface are contained in the lesser palatine nerves. The fibres travel through the greater petrosal nerve to the geniculate ganglion of the facial nerve and from there to the nucleus of the solitary tract (Fig. 12.19).

4. Secretomotor nerves are also contained in the lesser palatine nerves. They are derived from the superior salivatory nucleus and travel through the greater petrosal nerve (Fig. 9.10).

Passavant's Ridge

Some of the upper fibres of the palatopharyngeus pass circularly deep to the mucous membrane of the pharynx, and form a sphincter internal to the superior constrictor. These fibres constitute Passavant's muscle which on contraction raises a ridge called the Passavant's ridge on the posterior wall of the nasopharynx. When the soft palate is elevated it comes in contact with this ridge, the two together closing the pharyngeal isthmus between the nasopharynx and the oropharynx (Fig. 14.4B).

Morphology of Palatopharyngeus

(1) First read paragraph on Passavant's ridge.

(2) In mammals with an acute sense of smell, the epiglottis lies above the level of the soft palate, and is supported by two vertical muscles (stylopharyngeus and salpingopharyngeus) and by a sphincter formed by palatopharyngeus. The palatopharyngeal sphincter clasps the inlet of the larynx.

In man, the larynx descends and pulls the sphincter downwards leading to the formation of the human palatopharyngeus muscle. However, some fibres of the sphincter are left behind and form a sphincter inner to the superior constrictor at the level of the hard palate. These fibres constitute Passavant's muscle. Passavant's muscle is best developed in cases of cleft palate, as this compensates to some extent for the deficiency in the palate.

Movements and Functions of the Soft Palate

The palate controls two gates, the pharyngeal isthmus and the oropharyngeal isthmus. It can completely close them, or can regulate their size according to requirements. Through these movements the soft palate plays an important role in chewing, swallowing, speech, coughing, sneezing, etc. A few specific roles are given below:

1. It isolates the mouth from the oropharynx during chewing, so that breathing is unaffected.

2. It separates the oropharynx from the nasopharynx by locking into Passavant's ridge during the second stage of swallowing, so that food does not enter the nose.

3. By varying the degree of closure of the pharyngeal isthmus, the quality of voice can be modified and various consonants correctly pronounced.

4. During sneezing, the blast of air is appropriately divided and directed through the nasal and oral cavities without damaging the narrow nose. Similarly during coughing it directs air and sputum into the mouth and not into the nose.

Blood Supply

Arteries

(1) Greater palatine branch of maxillary artery;

(2) ascending palatine branch of facial artery; and

Table 14.1: Muscles of the soft palate

Muscle	Origin	Insertion	Actions
1. *Tensor veli palatini* This is a thin, triangular muscle (Fig. 14.5)	(a) Lateral side of auditory tube (b) Adjoining part of the base of the skull (greater wing and scaphoid fossa of sphenoid bone)	Muscle descends, converges to form a delicate tendon which winds round the pterygoid hamulus, passes through the origin of the buccinator, and flattens out to form the palatine aponeurosis Aponeurosis is attached to: (a) Posterior border of hard palate (b) Inferior surface of palate behind the palatine crest	(a) Tightens the soft palate, chiefly the anterior part (b) Opens the auditory tube to equalize air pressure between the middle ear and the nasopharynx
2. *Levator veli palatini* This is a cylindrical muscle that lies deep to the tensor veli palatini	(a) Inferior aspect of auditory tube (b) Adjoining part of inferior surface of petrous temporal bone	Muscle enters the pharynx by passing over the upper concave margin of the superior constrictor, runs downwards and medially and spreads out in the soft palate. It is inserted into the upper surface of the palatine aponeurosis	(a) Elevates soft palate and closes the pharyngeal isthmus (b) Opens the auditory tube, like the tensor veli palatini
3. *Musculus uvulae* This is a longitudinal strip placed on one side of the median plane, within the palatine aponeurosis	(a) Posterior nasal spine (b) Palatine aponeurosis	Mucous membrane of uvula	Pulls up the uvula
4. *Palatoglossus*	Oral surface of palatine aponeurosis	Descends in the palatoglossal arch, to the side of the tongue at the junction of its oral and pharyngeal parts	Pulls up the root of the tongue, approximates the palatoglossal arches, and thus closes the oropharyngeal isthmus
5. *Palatopharyngeus* It consists of two fasciculi that are separated by the levator veli palatini (Also see Passavant's ridge)	(a) Anterior fasciculus: from posterior border of hard palate: (b) Posterior fasciculus: from the palatine aponeurosis	Descends in the palatopharyngeal arch and spreads out to form the greater part of the longitudinal muscle coat of pharynx. It is inserted into: (a) Posterior border of the lamina of the thyroid cartilage (b) Wall of the pharynx and its median raphe	Pulls up the wall of the pharynx and shortens it during swallowing

(3) palatine branch of ascending pharyngeal artery.

Veins: They pass to the pterygoid and tonsillar plexuses of veins.

Lymphatics: Drain into the upper deep cervical and retropharyngeal lymph nodes.

Development of Palate

The premaxilla or primitive palate carrying upper four incisor teeth is formed by the fusion of medial nasal folds, which are folds of frontonasal process.

The rest of the palate is formed by the shelf-like palatine processes of maxilla and horizontal plates of

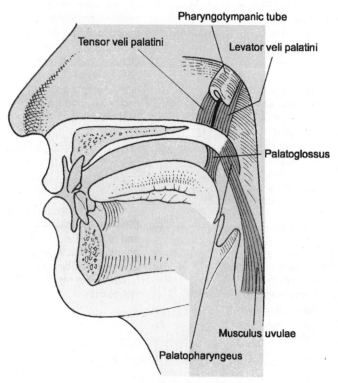

Fig. 14.5: Muscles of the soft palate.

palatine bone. Most of the palate gets ossified to form the hard palate. The unossified posterior part of fused palatal processes forms the soft palate.

Soft palate comprises epithelium, connective tissue and muscles. Epithelium is from the ectoderm of maxillary process. The muscles are derived from 1st, 4th and 6th branchial arches and accordingly are innervated by mandibular and vagoaccessory complex.

CLINICAL ANATOMY

1. Paralysis of the soft palate in lesions of the vagus nerve produces: (a) Nasal regurgitation of liquids; (b) nasal twang in voice, and (c) flattening of the palatal arch.

2. Cleft palate is a congenital defect caused by non-fusion of the right and left palatal processes. It may be of different degrees. In the least severe type, the defect is confined to the soft palate. In the most severe cases, the cleft in the palate is continuous with harelip.

3. Perforation of the hard palate may occur in tertiary syphilis.

4. Epignathus is a teratoma arising specifically from the palate.

PHARYNX

The pharynx is a wide muscular tube, situated behind the nose, the mouth and the larynx. Clinically, it is a part of the upper respiratory passages where infections are common. The upper part of the pharynx transmits only air, the lower part (below the inlet of the larynx), only food, but the middle part is a common passage for both air and food (Fig. 14.6).

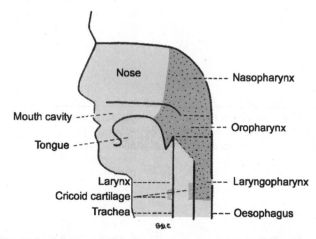

Fig. 14.6: Scheme to show the subdivisions of the pharynx. Also see Fig. 14.2.

DISSECTION

Cut through the centre of the frontal bone, internasal suture, intermaxillary sutures, chin, hyoid bone, thyroid, cricoid and tracheal cartilages; carry the incision through the septum of nose, nasopharynx, tongue, and both the palates.

Cut through the centre of the remaining occipital bone and cervical vertebrae. This will complete the sagittal section of head and neck.

Identify the structures in the interior of three parts of pharynx, i.e. nasopharynx, oropharynx and laryngopharynx. Clean the surfaces of buccinator muscle and adjoining superior constrictor muscles by removing connective tissue and buccopharyngeal fascia over these muscles. Detach the medial pterygoid muscle from its origin and reflect it downwards. This will expose the superior constrictor muscle completely.

Dimensions of pharynx

Length: About 12 cm.

Width: (a) Upper part is widest (3.5 cm) and noncollapsible; (b) middle part is narrow; and (c) the lower end is the narrowest part of the gastrointestinal tract (except for the appendix).

Boundaries

Superiorly: Base of the skull, including the posterior part of the body of the sphenoid and the basilar part of the occipital bone, in front of the pharyngeal tubercle.

Inferiorly: The pharynx is continuous with the oesophagus at the level of the sixth cervical vertebra, corresponding to the lower border of the cricoid cartilage.

Posteriorly: The pharynx glides freely on the prevertebral fascia which separates it from the cervical spine.

Anteriorly: It communicates with the nasal cavity, the oral cavity and the larynx. Thus the anterior wall of the pharynx is incomplete.

On each side: (A) The pharynx is attached to: (a) The medial pterygoid plate; (b) the pterygo-mandibular raphe; (c) the mandible; (d) the tongue; (e) the hyoid bone; and (f) the thyroid and cricoid cartilages.

(B) It communicates on each side with the middle ear cavity through the auditory tube.

(C) The pharynx is related on either side to: (a) The styloid process and the muscles attached to it; and (b) the common carotid, internal carotid, and external carotid arteries, and the cranial nerves related to them.

Parts of the Pharynx

The cavity of the pharynx is divided into: (a) The nasal part, nasopharynx; (b) the oral part, oropharynx; and (c) the laryngeal part, laryngopharynx (Fig 14.7).

Nasal Part of Pharynx/Nasopharynx

This is the upper part of the pharynx situated behind the nose, and above the lower border of the soft palate.

It resembles the nose structurally as well as functionally, (a) It is respiratory in function, and no food normally enters it. (b) Its walls are rigid and non-collapsible, so that the air passage is kept patent. (c) It is lined by ciliated columnar epithelium. (d) Its mucous membrane is supplied by the pharyngeal branch of pterygopalatine ganglion suspended by maxillary branch of trigeminal nerve. (Note: The other parts of the pharynx are supplied by cranial nerves IX and X.

The following facts may be noted.

1. The wall of the nasopharynx is formed by the *pharyngobasilar fascia* and the *posterior median pharyngeal ligament* or raphe.

2. *Anteriorly*, the nasopharynx communicates with the nasal cavities through the posterior nasal apertures.

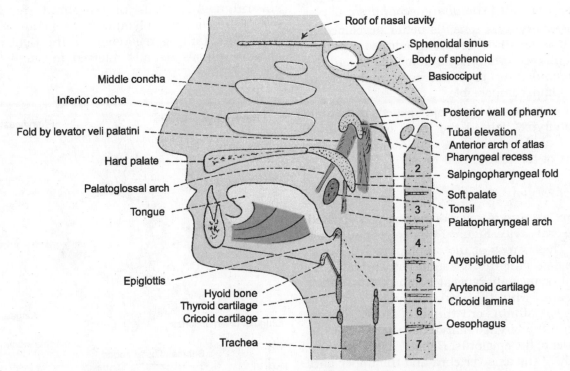

Fig. 14.7: *Sagittal section through the pharynx, the nose, the mouth and the larynx.*

3. *Inferiorly,* it communicates with the oropharynx at the pharyngeal isthmus or nasopharyngeal isthmus. The isthmus is an opening bounded by the lower border of the soft palate and the posterior wall of the pharynx formed by Passavant's ridge (Fig. 14.4B).

4. The *lateral wall* presents the following: (a) The pharyngeal *opening of the auditory* tube, at the level of the inferior nasal concha and 1.2 cm behind it. (b) The *tubal elevation* bounds the tubal opening. (c) The *salpingopharyngeal* fold is a vertical fold of mucous membrane running downwards from the posterior margin of the tubal elevation and gradually fading on the side wall of the pharynx. The fold is raised by a slip of muscle, the salpingo-pharyngeus. (d) The levator veli palatini, as it enters the soft palate, raises a fold of mucous membrane just below the tubal opening (e) Behind the tubal elevation there is a narrow vertical slit that leads into a flat pocket of mucous membrane called the *pharyngeal recess or lateral recess, or fossa of Rosenmuller.* The recess extends sideways for 1.2 cm or more between the auditory tube and prevertebral muscles, above the upper edge of the superior constrictor.

5. The *roof and posterior* wall form a continuous slope, opposite the posterior part of the body of the sphenoid, the basiocciput, and the anterior arch of the atlas. Under the mucous membrane, opposite the basiocciput, there is a collection of lymphoid tissue called the *pharyngeal or nasopharyngeal* tonsil. There is a small median recess in the mucosa covering this tonsil. It is called the *pharyngeal bursa.*

The nasopharyngeal tonsil is better developed in children. It is small or absent in adults. A pathologically enlarged pharyngeal tonsil is given the name *adenoids.* Its presence may make nasal breathing almost impossible.

Another collection of lymphoid tissue is present in the nasopharynx, behind the tubal opening. It is called the tubal tonsil. It is continuous with the lateral part of the pharyngeal tonsil.

Oral Part of Pharynx (Oropharynx)

Oropharynx is the middle part of the pharynx situated behind the oral cavity. Figure 14.8 depicts path of air and food. These cross at the oropharynx. Above, it communicates with the nasopharynx through the pharyngeal or nasopharyngeal isthmus. *In front,* it communicates with the oral cavity through the oropharyngeal isthmus or isthmus of fauces. *Below,* it opens into the laryngopharynx at the level of the upper border of the epiglottis. *Behind,* it is supported by the body of the axis vertebra and the upper part of the body of the third cervical vertebra. Its *lateral*

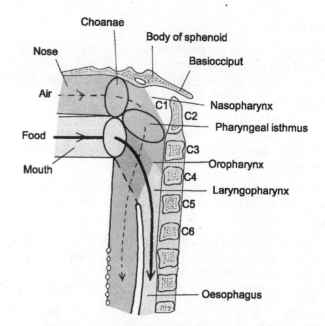

Fig. 14.8: *Path of air and food through the pharynx.*

wall presents the palatine tonsil which lies in the tonsillar fossa. This fossa is bounded anteriorly by the palatoglossal arch, and posteriorly by the palatopharyngeal arch. The wall of the oropharynx is formed posteriorly by the superior, middle and inferior constrictors of the pharynx.

Waldeyer's Lymphatic Ring

In relation to the oropharyngeal isthmus, there are several aggregations of lymphoid tissue that constitute Waldeyer's lymphatic ring (Fig. 14.9). The most important aggregations are the right and left palatine tonsils usually referred to simply as the

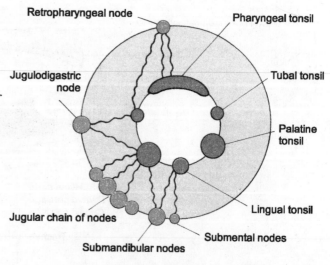

Fig. 14.9: *Waldeyer's lymphatic ring.*

tonsils. Posteriorly and above there is the pharyngeal tonsil; laterally and above there are the tubal tonsils, and inferiorly there is the lingual tonsil over the posterior part of the dorsum of the tongue.

Palatine Tonsil (The Tonsil)

Surface Marking

It is marked by an oval (almond-shaped) area over the masseter just anterosuperior to the angle of the mandible.

Features

The palatine tonsil occupies the tonsillar sinus or fossa between the palatoglossal and palatopharyngeal arches (Figs 14.2, 14.3). It can be seen through the mouth.

The tonsil is almond-shaped. It has two surfaces medial and lateral; two borders, anterior and posterior and two poles, upper and lower.

The *medial surface* is covered by stratified squamous epithelium continuous with that of the mouth. This surface has 12 to 15 crypts. The largest of these is called the *intratonsillar cleft*.

The *lateral surface* is covered by a sheet of fascia which forms the capsule of the tonsil. The capsule is an extension of the pharyngobasilar fascia. It is only loosely attached to the muscular wall of the pharynx, formed here by the superior constrictor and by the styloglossus, but anteroinferiorly the capsule is firmly adherent to the side of the tongue just in front of the insertion of the palatoglossus and the palatopharyngeus muscles. This firm attachment keeps the tonsil in place during swallowing. The tonsillar artery enters the tonsil by piercing the superior constrictor just behind the firm attachment.

The palatine vein or external palatine or paratonsillar vein descends from the palate in the loose areolar tissue on the lateral surface of the capsule, and crosses the tonsil before piercing the wall of the pharynx. The vein may be injured during removal of the tonsil or tonsillectomy.

The bed of the tonsil is formed from within outwards by: (a) The pharyngobasilar fascia; (b) the superior constrictor and palatopharyngeus muscles; (c) the buccopharyngeal fascia; and (d) in the lower part the styloglossus and the (e) glossopharyngeal nerve (Fig. 14.10).

Still more laterally there are the facial artery with its tonsillar and ascending palatine branches. The internal carotid artery is 2.5 cm posterolateral to the tonsil.

The *anterior border* is related to the palatoglossal arch with its muscle (Fig. 14.3).

The *posterior border* is related to the palatopharyngeal arch with its muscle.

The *upper pole* is related to the soft palate, and the lower pole, to the tongue.

The *plica triangularis* is a triangular vestigial fold of mucous membrane covering the anteroinferior part of the tonsil. The plica semilunaris, is a similar semilunar fold that may cross the upper part of the tonsillar sinus.

The *intratonsillar cleft* is the largest crypt of the tonsil. It is present in its upper part (Fig. 14.11). It is sometimes wrongly named the supratonsillar fossa. The mouth of the cleft is semilunar in shape and parallel to the dorsum of the tongue. It represents the internal opening of the second pharyngeal pouch.

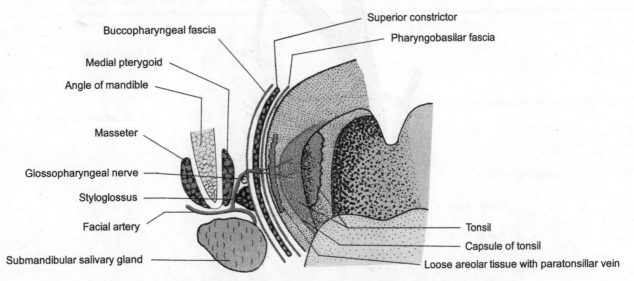

Fig. 14.10: Horizontal section through the right palatine tonsil showing its deep relations.

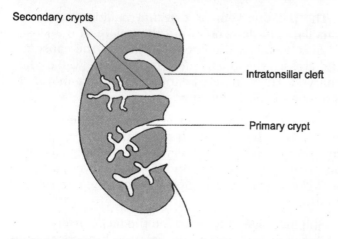

Fig. 14.11: Medial surface of the palatine tonsil to show its crypts.

A peritonsillar abscess or quinsy often begins in this cleft.

Arterial Supply of Tonsil

1. Main source: Tonsillar branch of facial artery.
2. Additional sources: (a) Ascending palatine branch of facial artery; (b) dorsal lingual branches of the lingual artery; (c) ascending pharyngeal branch of the external carotid artery; and (d) the greater palatine branch of the maxillary artery (Fig. 14.12).

Venous Drainage

One or more veins leave the lower part of the deep surface of the tonsil, pierce the superior constrictor, and join the palatine, pharyngeal, or facial veins.

Lymphatic Drainage

Lymphatics pass to the jugulodigastric node (Fig. 12.29).

Nerve Supply

Glossopharyngeal and lesser palatine nerves.

Histology

The palatine tonsil is situated at the oropharyngeal isthmus. Its oral aspect is covered with stratified squamous nonkeratinised epithelium, which dips into the underlying tissue to form the crypts. The lymphocytes lie on the sides of the crypts in the form of nodules. The structure of tonsil is not differentiated into cortex and medulla.

Development

The epithelium over the tonsil develops from ventral part of second pharyngeal pouch. The lymphocytes are mesodermal in origin.

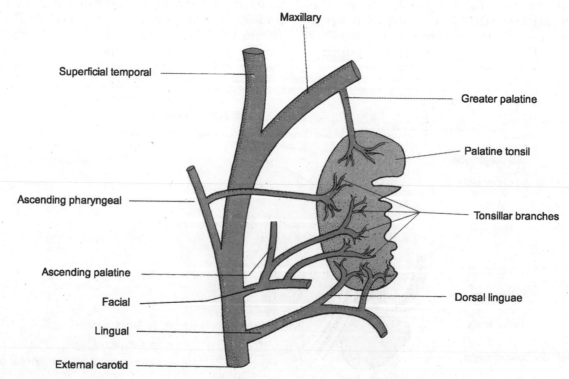

Fig. 14.12: Arterial supply of the palatine tonsil.

CLINICAL ANATOMY

1. The tonsils are large in children. They retrogress after puberty.

2. The tonsils are frequently sites of infection, specially in children. Infection may spread to surrounding tissue forming a peritonsillar abscess.

3. Enlarged and infected tonsils often require surgical removal. The operation is called tonsillectomy. A knowledge of the relationship of the tonsil is of importance to the surgeon.

4. Tonsillectomy is usually done by the guillotine method. Haemorrhage after tonsillectomy is checked by removal of clot from the raw tonsillar bed. This is to be compared with the method for checking postpartum haemorrhage from the uterus. These are the only two organs in the body where bleeding is checked by removal of clots. In other parts of the body, clot formation is encouraged.

5. Tonsillitis may cause referred pain in the ear as glossopharyngeal nerve supplies both these areas.

6. Suppuration in the peritonsillar area is called quinsy. A peritonsillar abscess is drained by making an incision in the most prominent point of the abscess.

7. Tonsils are often sites of a septic focus. Such a focus can lead to serious disease like pulmonary tuberculosis, meningitis, etc. and is often the cause of general ill health.

Laryngeal Part of Pharynx (Laryngopharynx)

This is the lower part of the pharynx situated behind the larynx. It extends from the upper border of the epiglottis to the lower border of the cricoid cartilage.

The *anterior wall* presents: (a) The inlet of the larynx; and (b) the posterior surfaces of the cricoid and arytenoid cartilages (Fig. 14.13).

The *posterior wall* is supported mainly by the fourth and fifth cervical vertebrae, and partly by the third and sixth vertebrae. In this region, the posterior wall of the pharynx is formed by the superior, middle and inferior constrictors of the pharynx.

The *lateral wall* presents a depression called the piriform fossa, one on each side of the inlet of the larynx. The fossa is bounded medially by the aryepiglottic fold, and laterally by the thyroid cartilage and the thyrohyoid membrane. Beneath the mucosa of fossa there lies the internal laryngeal nerve. Removal of foreign bodies from the piriform fossa may damage the internal laryngeal nerve, leading to anaesthesia in the supraglottic part of the larynx.

Structure of Pharynx

The wall of the pharynx is composed of the following five layers from within outwards.

(1) *Mucosa*

(2) *Submucosa*

(3) *Pharyngobasilar fascia* or pharyngeal aponeurosis. This is a fibrous sheet internal to the

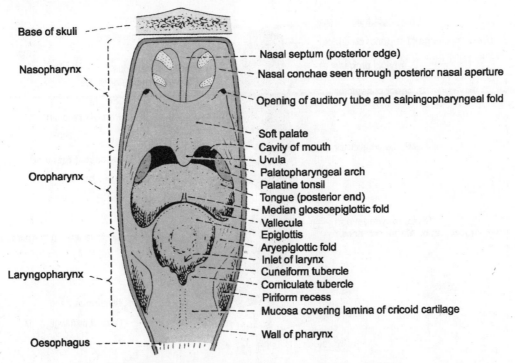

Base of skull

Nasopharynx

Oropharynx

Laryngopharynx

Oesophagus

Nasal septum (posterior edge)

Nasal conchae seen through posterior nasal aperture

Opening of auditory tube and salpingopharyngeal fold

Soft palate
Cavity of mouth
Uvula
Palatopharyngeal arch
Palatine tonsil
Tongue (posterior end)
Median glossoepiglottic fold
Vallecula
Epiglottis
Aryepiglottic fold
Inlet of larynx
Cuneiform tubercle
Corniculate tubercle
Piriform recess
Mucosa covering lamina of cricoid cartilage

Wall of pharynx

Fig. 14.13: *Anterior wall of the pharynx seen from behind.*

pharyngeal muscles. It is thickest in the upper part where it fills the gap between the upper border of the superior constrictor and the base of the skull, and also posteriorly where it forms the pharyngeal raphe. Superiorly, the fascia is attached to the basiocciput, the petrous temporal bone, the auditory tube, the posterior border of the medial pterygoid plate, and the pterygomandibular raphe. Inferiorly, it is gradually lost deep to muscles, and hardly extend beyond the superior constrictor (Figs 14.14, 14.15).

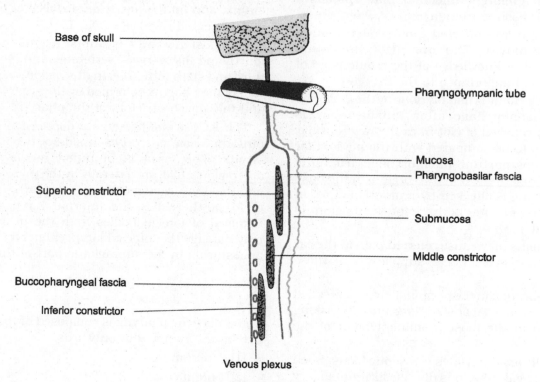

Fig. 14.14: Structure of the pharynx.

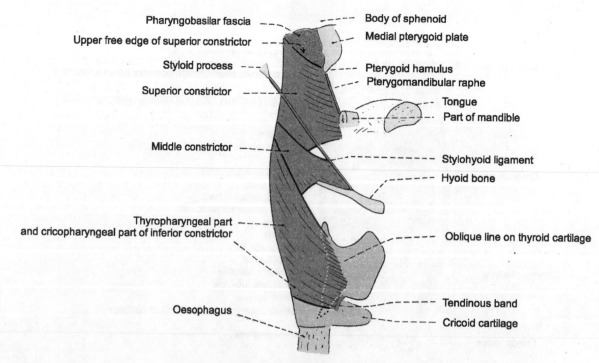

Fig. 14.15: Origin of the constrictors of the pharynx.

(4) The *muscular coat* consists of an outer circular layer made up of the three constrictors, and an inner longitudinal layer made up of the stylopharyngeus, the salpingopharyngeus and the palatopharyngeus muscles. These muscles are described later.

(5) The *buccopharyngeal fascia* covers the outer surface of the constrictors of the pharynx and extends forwards across the pterygomandibular raphe to cover the buccinator. Like the pharyngobasilar fascia, the buccopharyngeal fascia is best developed in the upper part of the pharynx.

Between the buccopharyngeal fascia, and the muscular coat there are the pharyngeal plexuses of veins and nerves (Fig. 14.14).

Muscles of the Pharynx

Preliminary Remarks about the Constrictors of the Pharynx

The muscular basis of the wall of the pharynx is formed mainly by the three pairs of constrictors—superior, middle and inferior. The origins of the constrictors are situated anteriorly in relation to the posterior openings of the nose, the mouth and the larynx. From here their fibres pass into the lateral and posterior walls of the pharynx, the fibres of the two sides meeting in the middle line in a fibrous raphe. The three constrictors are so arranged that the inferior overlaps middle which in turn overlaps the superior. The fibres of the superior constrictor reach the base of the skull posteriorly, in the middle line. On the sides, however, there is a gap between the base of the skull and the upper edge of the superior constrictor. This gap is closed by the pharyngobasilar fascia which is thickened in this situation (Fig. 14.15). The lower edge of the inferior constrictor becomes continuous with the circular muscle of the oesophagus.

DISSECTION

Define the attachments of middle and inferior constrictors of pharynx, and the structures situated/traversing through the gaps between the three constrictor muscles. Identify structures above the superior constrictor muscle and below the inferior constrictor muscle.

Cut through the tensor veli palatini and reflect it downwards. Remove the fascia and identify the mandibular nerve again with otic ganglion medial to it. Identify the branches of the mandibular nerve. Locate the middle meningeal artery at the foramen spinosum, as it lies just posterior to mandibular nerve.

Details of Origin of Constrictors

1. The *superior constrictor* takes origin from the following (from above downwards):
   a. Pterygoid hamulus (Fig. 14.15).
   b. Pterygomandibular raphe.
   c. Medial surface of the mandible at the posterior end of the mylohyoid line, i.e. near the lower attachment of the pterygomandibular raphe (Fig. 1.27).
   d. Side of posterior part of tongue.
2. The *middle constrictor* takes origin from:
   a. The lower part of the stylohyoid ligament
   b. Lesser cornua of hyoid bone
   c. Upper border of the greater cornu of the hyoid bone (Figs 14.16, 1.32).
3. The *inferior constrictor* consists of two parts. One part the *thyropharyngeus* arises from the thyroid cartilage. The other part the *cricopharyngeus* arises from the cricoid cartilage. Details of their origin are as follows.

The thyropharyngeus arises from:
   a. The oblique line on the lamina of the thyroid cartilage, including the inferior tubercle (Fig. 14.16).
   b. A tendinous band that crosses the cricothyroid muscle and is attached above to the inferior tubercle of the thyroid cartilage.
   c. The inferior cornua of the thyroid cartilage.

The cricopharyngeus arises from the cricoid cartilage behind the origin of the cricothyroid muscle.

Insertion of Constrictors of Pharynx

All the constrictors of the pharynx are inserted into a median raphe on the posterior wall of the pharynx. The upper end of the raphe reaches the base of the skull where it is attached to the pharyngeal tubercle on the basilar part of the occipital bone (Fig. 14.17).

Longitudinal Muscle Coat of the Pharynx

The pharynx has three muscles that run longitudinally. The *stylopharyngeus* arises from the styloid process. It passes through the gap between the superior and middle constrictors to run downwards on the inner surface of the middle and inferior constrictors. The fibres of the *palatopharyngeus* descend from the sides of the palate and run longitudinally on the inner aspect of the constrictors (Fig. 14.5). The *salpingopharyngeus* descends from the auditory tube to merge with the palatopharyngeus (Fig. 14.16).

Gaps Between Pharyngeal Muscles and Structures Related to them

1. The *large gap between the upper concave border of the superior constrictor and the base of the skull* is

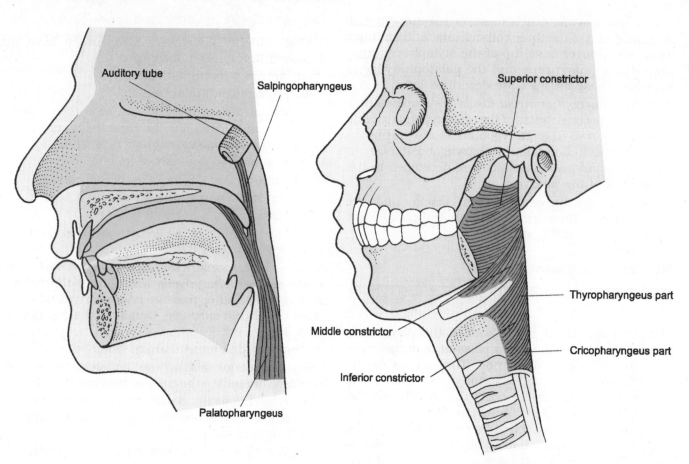

Fig. 14.16: *Muscles of the pharynx.*

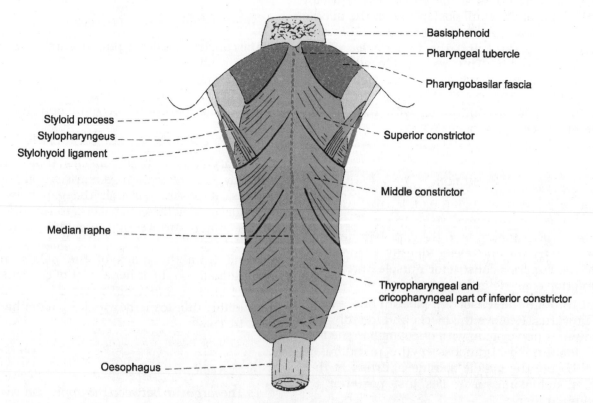

Fig. 14.17: *Wall of the pharynx, seen from behind.*

semilunar and is known as the *sinus of Morgagni*. It is closed by the upper strong part of the pharyngo-basilar fascia (Fig. 14.17). The structures passing through this gap are: (a) The auditory tube; (b) the levator veli palatini muscle; and (c) the ascending palatine artery (Fig. 14.18).

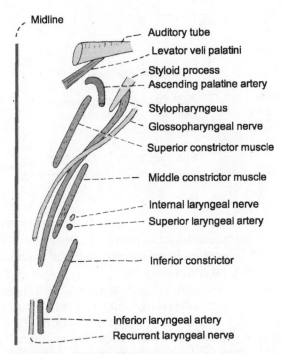

Fig. 14.18: *Schematic coronal section through the pharynx, showing the gaps between pharyngeal muscles and the structures related to them.*

2. The structures passing through the *gap between the superior and middle constrictors* are the stylopharyngeus and the glossopharyngeal nerve.

3. The internal laryngeal nerve and the superior laryngeal vessels pierce the thyrohyoid membrane in the *gap between the middle and inferior constrictors*.

4. The recurrent laryngeal nerve and the inferior laryngeal vessels pass through the *gap between the lower border of the inferior constrictor and the oesophagus*.

Killian's Dehiscence

In the posterior wall of the pharynx, the lower part of the thyropharyngeus is a single sheet of muscle, not overlapped internally by the upper and middle constrictors. This weak part lies below the level of the vocal folds or upper border of the cricoid lamina and is limited inferiorly by the thick cricopharyngeal sphincter. This area is known as *Killian's dehiscence*. Pharyngeal diverticula are formed by outpouching of the dehiscence. Such diverticula are normal in the pig. Pharyngeal diverticula are often attributed to

neuromuscular incoordination in this region which may be due to the fact that different nerves supply the two parts of the inferior constrictor. The propulsive thyropharyngeus is supplied by the pharyngeal plexus, and the sphincteric cricopharyngeus, by the recurrent laryngeal nerve. If the cricopharyngeus fails to relax when the thyropharyngeus contracts, the bolus of food is pushed backwards, and tends to produce a diverticulum.

Nerve Supply and Actions

The nerve supply of the muscles of the pharynx is considered below (also see Table 14.2). For actions see section on deglutition.

Nerve Supply

The pharynx is supplied by the pharyngeal plexus of nerves which lies chiefly on the middle constrictor. The plexus is formed by: (1) The pharyngeal branch of the vagus carrying fibres of the cranial accessory nerve; (2) the pharyngeal branches of the glosso-pharyngeal nerve; and (3) the pharyngeal branches of the superior cervical sympathetic ganglion.

Motor fibres are derived from the cranial accessory nerve through the branches of the vagus. They supply all muscles of the pharynx, except the stylopharyngeus which is supplied by the glossopharyngeal nerve. The inferior constrictor receives an additional supply from the external and recurrent laryngeal nerves. The plexus also supplies all muscles of the soft palate except the tensor veli palatini which is supplied by the mandibular nerve.

Sensory fibres or general visceral afferent from the pharynx travel mostly through the glosso-pharyngeal nerve, and partly through the vagus. However, the nasopharynx is supplied by the maxillary nerve through the pterygopalatine ganglion; and the soft palate and tonsil, by the lesser palatine and glossopharyngeal nerves.

Taste sensations from the vallecula and epiglottic area pass through the internal laryngeal branch of the vagus.

The parasympathetic *secretomotor* fibres to the pharynx are derived from the greater petrosal nerve, branch of facial nerve and through the lesser palatine branches of the pterygopalatine ganglion (Table 1.3).

Blood Supply

The arteries supplying the pharynx are as follows.

(1) Ascending pharyngeal branch of the external carotid artery; (2) ascending palatine and tonsillar branches of the facial artery; (3) dorsal lingual branches of the lingual artery; and (4) the greater

Table 14.2: Mesodermal derivatives of pharyngeal arches

Arch	Muscles of Arch	Nerve of Arch
I	Muscles of mastication (masseter, temporalis, medial and lateral pterygoids, tensor veli palatini, tensor tympani mylohyoid and anterior belly of digastric	Mandibular division of trigeminal
II	Muscles of facial expression, occipitofrontalis, auricular muscles, platysma, stapedius, stylohyoid and posterior belly of digastric	Facial nerve
III	Stylopharyngeus	Glossopharyngeal nerve
IV	Cricothyroid Constrictors of pharynx (3) Levator veli palatini	External laryngeal, pharyngeal branch of vagus through vagoaccessory complex
VI	All other intrinsic muscles of larynx	Recurrent laryngeal branch of vagus

palatine, pharyngeal and pterygoid branches of the maxillary artery (Fig. 14.12).

The veins form a plexus on the posterolateral aspect of the pharynx. The plexus receives blood from the pharynx, the soft palate and the prevertebral region. It drains into the internal jugular and facial veins.

Lymphatic Drainage

Lymph from the pharynx drains into the retropharyngeal and deep cervical lymph nodes.

Deglutition (Swallowing)

Swallowing of food occurs in three stages described below.

First Stage

1. This stage is voluntary in character.

2. The anterior part of the tongue is raised and pressed against the hard palate by the intrinsic muscles of the tongue, especially the superior longitudinal and transverse muscles. The movement takes place from anterior to the posterior side. This pushes the food bolus into the posterior part of the oral cavity.

3. The soft palate closes down on to the back of the tongue, and helps to form the bolus.

4. Next, the hyoid bone is moved upwards and forwards by the suprahyoid muscles. The posterior part of the tongue is elevated upwards and backwards by the styloglossi; and the palatoglossal arches are approximated by the palatoglossi. This pushes the bolus through the oropharyngeal isthmus to the oropharynx, and the second stage begins.

Second Stage

1. It is involuntary in character. During this stage the food is pushed from the oropharynx to the lower part of the laryngopharynx.

2. The nasopharyngeal isthmus is closed by elevation of the soft palate by levator veli palatini and tenser veli palatini and by approximation to it of the posterior pharyngeal wall (ridge of Passavant). This prevents the food bolus from entering the nose.

3. The inlet of larynx is closed by approximation of the aryepiglottis folds by aryepiglottic and oblique arytenoid. This prevents the food bolus from entering the larynx (Fig. 16.8).

4. Next, the larynx and pharynx are elevated behind the hyoid bone by the longitudinal muscles of the pharynx, and the bolus is pushed down over the posterior surface of the epiglottis, the closed inlet of the larynx and the posterior surface of the arytenoid cartilages, by gravity, and by contraction of the superior and middle constrictors and of the palatopharyngeus.

Third Stage

1. This is also involuntary in character. In this stage, food passes from the lower part of the pharynx to the oesophagus.

2. This is brought about by the inferior constrictors of the pharynx.

Development

The primitive gut extends from the buccopharyngeal membrane cranially, to the cloacal membrane caudally. It is divided into four parts — the pharynx, the foregut, the midgut and the hindgut. The pharynx extends from buccopharyngeal membrane to the tracheobronchial diverticulum. It is divided into upper part, the nasopharynx; middle part, the oropharynx; and the lower part, the laryngopharynx.

Auditory Tube

It is also known as the pharyngotympanic tube or the Eustachian tube.

The auditory tube is a trumpet-shaped channel which connects the middle ear cavity with the nasopharynx. It is about 4 cm long, and is directed downwards, forwards and medially. It forms an angle of 45 degrees with the sagittal plane and 30 degrees with the horizontal plane. The tube is divided into bony and cartilaginous parts (Figs 14.14, 14.19).

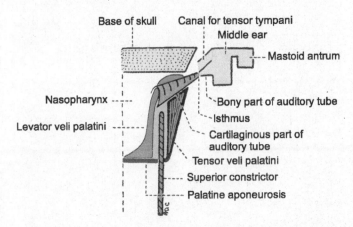

Fig. 14.19: Scheme showing anatomy of left auditory tube.

Bony Part

The bony part forms the posterior and lateral one-third of the tube. It is 12 mm long, and lies in the petrous temporal bone near the tympanic plate. Its lateral end is wide and opens on the anterior wall of the middle ear cavity. The medial end is narrow (isthmus) and is jagged for attachment of the cartilaginous part. The lumen of the tube is oblong being widest from side to side.

Relations. (a) *Superior:* Canal for the tensor tympani (Fig. 18.10). (b) *Medial:* Carotid canal. (c) *Lateral:* Chorda tympani, spine of the sphenoid, auriculotemporal nerve and the temporomandibular joint.

Cartilaginous Part

The cartilaginous part forms the anterior and medial two-thirds of the tube. It is 25 mm long, and lies in the sulcus tubae, a groove between the greater wing of the sphenoid and the apex of the petrous temporal (Fig. 14.16).

It is made up of a triangular plate of cartilage which is curled to form the superior and medial walls of the tube. The lateral wall and floor are completed by a fibrous membrane. The apex of the plate is attached to the medial end of the bony part. The base is free and forms the tubal elevation in the nasopharynx.

Relations. (a) *Anterolaterally:* Tensor veli palatini, mandibular nerve and its branches, otic ganglion, chorda tympani, middle meningeal artery and medial pterygoid plate. (b) *Posteromedially:* Petrous temporal and levator veli palatini. (c) The levator veli palatini is attached to its inferior surface, and the salpingopharyngeus to lower part near the pharyngeal opening (Fig. 10.14).

Vascular Supply

The arterial supply of the tube is derived from the ascending pharyngeal and middle meningeal arteries and the artery of the pterygoid canal.

The veins drain into the pharyngeal and pterygoid plexuses of veins. Lymphatics pass to the retropharyngeal nodes.

Nerve Supply

(1) At the ostium, by the pharyngeal branch of the pterygopalatine ganglion suspended by the maxillary nerve; (2) cartilaginous part, by the nervus spinosus branch of mandibular nerve; and (3) bony part, by the tympanic plexus formed by glossopharyngeal nerve (Fig. 10.14).

Function

The tube provides a communication of the middle ear cavity with the exterior, thus ensuring equal air pressure on both sides of the tympanic membrane.

The tube is usually closed. It opens during swallowing, yawning and sneezing, by the actions of the tensor and levator veli palatini muscles.

CLINICAL ANATOMY

1. Infections may pass from the throat to the middle ear through the auditory tube. This is more common in children because the tube is shorter and straighter in them.

2. Inflammation of the auditory tube (Eustachian catarrh) is often secondary to an attack of common cold, or of sore throat. This causes pain into the ear which is aggravated by swallowing, due to blockage of the tube. Pain is relieved by instillation of decongestant drops in the nose, which help to open the ostium. The ostium is commonly blocked in children by enlargement of the tubal tonsil.

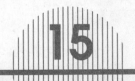

The Nose and Paranasal Sinuses

Sense of smell perceived in the upper part of nasal cavity by olfactory nerve rootlets ends in olfactory bulb, which is connected to uncus and also to the dorsal nucleus of vagus in medulla oblongata. Good smell of food, thus stimulates secretion of gastric juice through vagus nerve.

Most of the mucous membrane of the nasal cavity is respiratory and is continuous with various paranasal sinuses. Since nose is the most projecting part of the face, its integrity must be maintained and efforts should be made to see that nose is "not cut". Great mythological war has been fought for "cutting the nose".

Environmental pollution causes inhalation of unwanted gases and particles, leading to frequent attacks of sinusitis, respiratory diseases including asthma.

Nasal mucous membrane is quite vascular. Sometimes picking of the nose may cause bleeding from "Little's area", called the epistaxis.

THE NOSE

The nose performs two functions. It is a respiratory passage. It is also the organ of smell. The receptors for smell are placed in the upper one-third of the nasal cavity. This part is lined by olfactory mucosa. The rest of the nasal cavity is lined by respiratory mucosa. The respiratory mucosa is highly vascular and warms the inspired air. The secretions of numerous serous glands make the air moist; while the secretions of mucous glands trap dust and other particles. Thus the nose acts as an air conditioner where the inspired air is warmed, moistened and cleansed before it is passed on to the delicate lungs.

The *olfactory mucosa* lines the upper one-third of the nasal cavity including the roof formed by cribriform plate and the medial and lateral walls up to the level of the superior concha. It is thin and less vascular than the respiratory mucosa. It contains receptors called olfactory cells.

For descriptive purposes the nose is divided into two main parts, the external nose and the nasal cavity.

External Nose

Some features of the external nose have been described in Chapter 2. The external nose has a skeletal framework that is partly bony and partly cartilaginous. The bones are the nasal bones, which form the bridge of the nose, and the frontal processes of the maxillae. The cartilages are the superior and inferior nasal cartilages, the septal cartilage, and some small cartilages (Fig. 15.1A, B). The skin over the external nose is supplied by the external nasal, infratrochlear and infraorbital nerves (Fig. 2.19).

Nasal Cavity

The nasal cavity extends from the external nares or nostrils to the posterior nasal apertures, and is subdivided into right and left halves by the nasal septum. Each half has a roof, a floor, and medial and lateral walls. Each half measures about 5 cm in height, 5–7 cm in length, and 1.5 cm in width near the floor. The width near the roof is only 1–2 mm.

DISSECTION

Dissect and remove mucous membrane of the septum of nose in small pieces. The mucous membrane is covering both surfaces of the septum of the nose.

Dissect and preserve the nerves lying in the mucous membrane. Remove the entire mucous membrane to see the details in the interior of the nasal cavity.

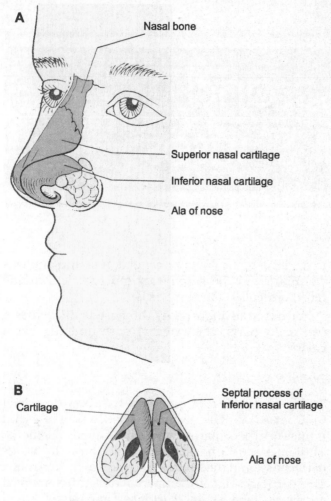

Fig. 15.1: *Skeleton of the external nose.*

The *roof* is about 7 cm long and 2 mm wide. It slopes downwards, both in front and behind. The <u>middle horizontal</u> part is formed by the <u>cribriform plate</u> of the ethmoid. The <u>anterior slope</u> is formed by the <u>nasal part</u> of the <u>frontal bone</u>, nasal bone, and the <u>nasal</u>

cartilages. The posterior slope is formed by the inferior surface of the body of the sphenoid bone.

The *floor* is about 5 cm long and 1.5 cm wide. It is formed by the <u>palatine process</u> of the <u>maxilla</u> and the <u>horizontal plate</u> of the <u>palatine</u> bone. It is concave from side to side and is slightly higher anteriorly than posteriorly (Fig. 15.2).

Nasal Septum

The *nasal septum* is median osseocartilaginous <u>partition</u> between the <u>two halves</u> of the <u>nasal cavity</u>. On each side, it is covered by <u>mucous membrane</u> and forms the medial wall of both nasal cavities.

The *bony part* is formed almost entirely by (1) the vomer, and (2) the perpendicular plate of the ethmoid. However, its margins receive contributions from the <u>nasal spine of the frontal bone</u>, the rostrum of the sphenoid, and the <u>nasal crests of the nasal</u>, <u>palatine</u> and <u>maxillary bones</u>. (Fig. 15.3).

The *cartilaginous part* is formed by (1) the <u>septal cartilage</u>, and (2) the <u>septal processes</u> of the <u>inferior nasal cartilages</u> (Fig. 15.1B).

The *cuticular part* or <u>lower end</u> is formed by <u>fibro-fatty tissue</u> covered by skin. The lower margin of the septum is called the columella.

The nasal septum is rarely strictly median. Its central part is usually *deflected* to one or the other side. The deflection is produced by overgrowth of one or more of the constituent parts.

The septum has (a) four borders, superior, inferior, anterior and posterior; and (b) two surfaces, right and left.

Arterial Supply

Anterosuperior part is supplied by the <u>anterior ethmoidal artery</u> (Fig. 15.4).

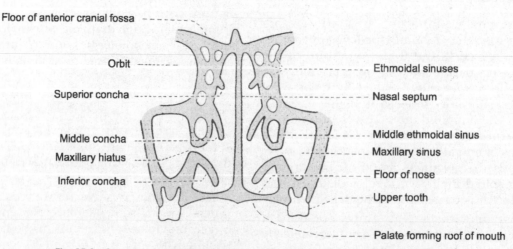

Fig. 15.2: *Coronal section through the nasal cavity and the maxillary air sinuses.*

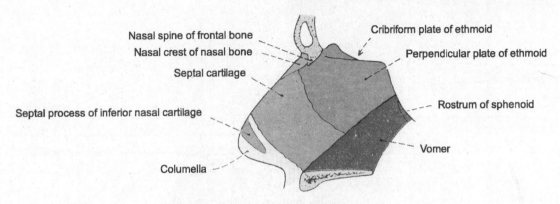

Fig. 15.3: *Formation of the nasal septum.*

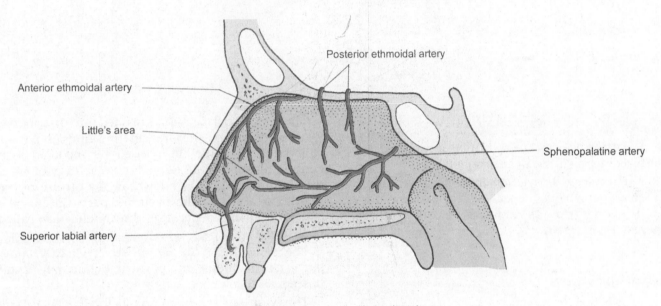

Fig. 15.4: *Arterial supply of nasal septum.*

Posteroinferior part: is supplied by the sphenopalatine artery.

Anteroinferior part: by the superior labial branch of facial artery.

Posterosuperior part: by the posterior ethmoidal artery.

The anteroinferior part or vestibule of the septum contains anastomoses between the septal ramus of the superior labial branch of the facial artery, branch of sphenopalatine artery, and of anterior ethmoidal artery. These form a large capillary network called the Kiesselbach's plexus. This is a common site of bleeding from the nose or epistaxis, and is known a *Little's area.*

Venous Drainage

The veins form a plexus which is more marked in the lower part of the septum or Little's area. The plexus drains anteriorly into the facial vein, posteriorly through the sphenopalatine vein to pterygoid venous plexus.

Nerve Supply

I. *General sensory nerves,* arising from trigeminal nerve, are distributed to whole of the septum (Fig. 15.5).

1. The anterosuperior part of the septum is supplied by the internal nasal branch of the anterior ethmoidal nerve.

2. The posteroinferior part is supplied by the nasopalatine branch of the pterygopalatine ganglion.

3. The posterosuperior part is supplied by the medial posterior superior nasal branches of the pterygopalatine ganglion

II. *Special sensory nerves* or *olfactory* nerves are confined to the upper part or olfactory area.

Lymphatic Drainage

Anterior half to the submandibular nodes.

Posterior half to the retropharyngeal and deep cervical nodes.

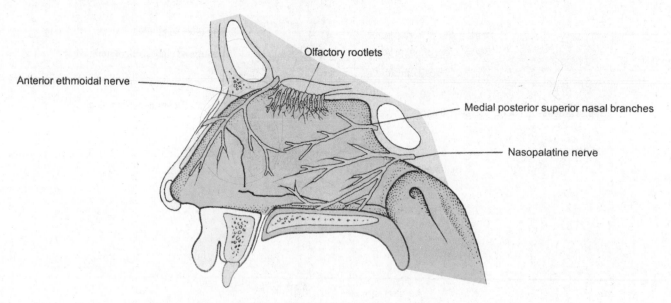

Anterior ethmoidal nerve

Olfactory rootlets

Medial posterior superior nasal branches

Nasopalatine nerve

Fig. 15.5: *Nerve supply of nasal septum.*

Lateral Wall of Nose

The lateral wall of the nose is irregular owing to the presence of three shelf-like bony projections called *conchae*. The conchae increase the surface area of the nose for effective air-conditioning of the inspired air (Fig. 15.2).

The lateral wall separates the nose: (a) From the orbit above, with the ethmoidal air sinuses intervening; (b) from the maxillary sinus below; and (c) from the lacrimal groove and nasolacrimal canal in front.

The lateral wall can be subdivided into three parts. (a) A small depressed area in the anterior part is called the vestibule. It is lined by modified skin containing short, stiff, curved hairs called vibrissae. (b) The middle part is known as the atrium of the middle meatus. (c) The posterior part contains the conchae. Spaces separating the conchae are called meatuses (Fig. 15.6).

The *skeleton of the lateral wall* is partly bony, partly cartilaginous, and partly made up only of soft tissues as follows.

The *bony part* is formed from before backwards by the following bones: (1) Nasal; (2) frontal process of maxilla; (3) lacrimal; (4) labyrinth of ethmoid with superior and middle conchae; (5) inferior nasal concha; (6) perpendicular plate of the palatine bone together with its orbital and sphenoidal processes; and (7) medial pterygoid plate (Fig. 15.6).

The *cartilaginous part* is formed by: (a) The superior nasal cartilage; (b) the inferior nasal cartilage; and (c) 3 or 4 small cartilages of the ala.

The *cuticular lower part* is formed by fibrofatty tissue covered with skin.

Chonchae and Meatuses

The *nasal conchae* are curved bony projections directed downwards and medially. The following three conchae are usually found:

1. The *inferior concha* is an independent bone.

2. The *middle concha* is a projection from the medial surface of the ethmoidal labyrinth (Fig. 15.6).

3. The *superior concha* is also a projection from the medial surface of the ethmoidal labyrinth. This is

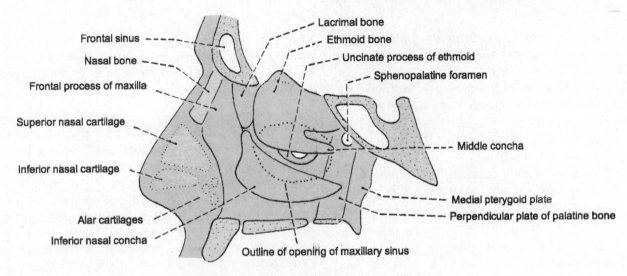

Fig. 15.6: Formation of the lateral wall of the nose.

Labels in figure 15.6:
Frontal sinus
Nasal bone
Frontal process of maxilla
Superior nasal cartilage
Inferior nasal cartilage
Alar cartilages
Inferior nasal concha
Outline of opening of maxillary sinus
Lacrimal bone
Ethmoid bone
Uncinate process of ethmoid
Sphenopalatine foramen
Middle concha
Medial pterygoid plate
Perpendicular plate of palatine bone

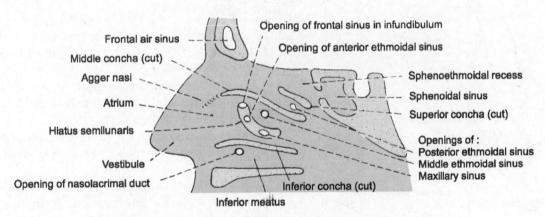

Fig. 15.7: Lateral wall of the nose seen after removing the conchae.

Labels in figure 15.7:
Frontal air sinus
Middle concha (cut)
Agger nasi
Atrium
Hiatus semilunaris
Vestibule
Opening of nasolacrimal duct
Inferior meatus
Opening of frontal sinus in infundibulum
Opening of anterior ethmoidal sinus
Sphenoethmoidal recess
Sphenoidal sinus
Superior concha (cut)
Openings of :
Posterior ethmoidal sinus
Middle ethmoidal sinus
Maxillary sinus
Inferior concha (cut)

the smallest concha situated just above the posterior part of the middle concha.

The *meatuses of the nose* are passages beneath the overhanging conchae. Each meatus communicates freely with the nasal cavity proper (Fig. 15.7).

1. The *inferior meatus* lies underneath the inferior concha, and is the largest of the three meatuses. The nasolacrimal duct opens into it at the junction of its anterior one-third and posterior two-thirds. The opening is guarded by the lacrimal fold, or Hasner's valve.

2. The *middle meatus* lies underneath the middle concha. It presents the following features: (a) The *ethmoidal bulla,* is a rounded elevation produced by the underlying middle ethmoidal sinuses. (b) The *hiatus semilunaris,* is a deep semicircular sulcus below the bulla. (c) The *infundibulum* is a short passage at the anterior end of the hiatus. (d) The *opening of the frontal air sinus* is seen in the anterior

part of the hiatus semilunaris. (f) The *opening of the maxillary air sinus* is located in the posterior part of the hiatus semilunaris. It is often represented by two openings. (g) The *opening of the middle ethmoidal air sinus* is present at the upper margin of the bulla (Fig. 15.7).

3. The *superior meatus* lies below the superior concha. This is the shortest and shallowest of the three meatuses. It receives the *openings of the posterior ethmoidal air sinuses.*

The *sphenoethmoidal recess* is a triangular fossa just above the superior concha. It receives the *opening of the sphenoidal air sinus* (Fig. 15.7).

The *atrium of the middle meatus* is a shallow depression just in front of the middle meatus and above the vestibule of the nose. It is limited above by a faint ridge of mucous membrane, the *agger nasi,* which runs forwards and downwards from the upper end of the anterior border of the middle concha (Fig. 15.7).

Arterial Supply of Lateral Wall

1. The *anterosuperior quadrant* is supplied by the anterior ethmoidal artery assisted by the posterior ethmoidal and facial arteries.

2. The *anteroinferior quadrant*, is supplied by branches from the facial and greater palatine arteries (Fig. 15.8).

3. The *posterosuperior quadrant*, is supplied by the sphenopalatine artery.

4. The *posteroinferior quadrant* is supplied by branches from the greater palatine artery which pierce the perpendicular plate of the palatine bone.

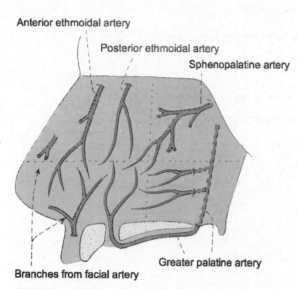

Fig. 15.8: *Arteries supplying the lateral wall of the nose.*

Venous Drainage

The veins form a plexus which drains anteriorly into the facial vein; posteriorly, into the pharyngeal plexus of veins; and from the middle part, to the pterygoid plexus of veins.

DISSECTION

Trace the nasopalatine nerve till the sphenopalatine foramen. Try to find few nasal branches of the greater palatine nerve.

Gently break the perpendicular plate of palatine bone to expose the greater palatine nerve, branch of the pterygopalatine ganglion. Follow the nerve and its accompanying vessels to the hard palate. Identify the lesser palatine nerves and trace them till the soft palate.

Nerve Supply

I. *General sensory nerves* derived from the branches of trigeminal nerve are distributed to whole of the lateral wall:

1. The *anterosuperior quadrant* is supplied by the anterior ethmoidal nerve branch of ophthalmic nerve (Fig. 15.9).

2. The *anteroinferior quadrant* is supplied by the anterior superior alveolar nerve, branch of maxillary nerve.

3. The *posterosuperior quadrant* is supplied by the posterior superior lateral nasal branches from the pterygopalatine ganglion suspended by the maxillary nerve.

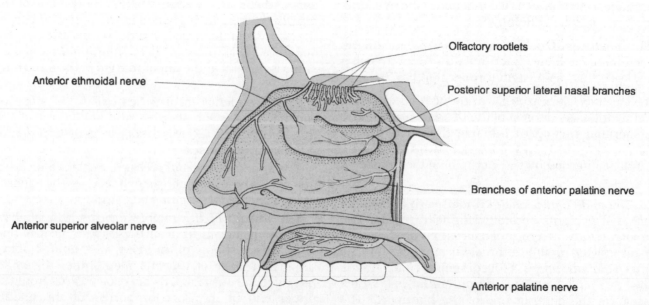

Fig. 15.9: *Nerve supply of lateral wall of nasal cavity.*

4. The *posteroinferior quadrant* is supplied by the anterior or greater palatine branch from the pterygopalatine ganglion suspended by the maxillary nerve.

II. *Special sensory nerves* or *olfactory* are distributed to the upper part of the lateral wall just below the cribriform plate of the ethmoid up to the superior concha.

Note that the olfactory mucosa lies partly on the lateral wall and partly on the nasal septum.

Lymphatic Drainage

Lymphatics from the anterior half of the lateral wall pass to the submandibular nodes, and from the posterior half, to the retropharyngeal and upper deep cervical nodes.

PARANASAL SINUSES

Paranasal sinuses are air filled spaces present within some bones around the nasal cavities. The sinuses, are *frontal, maxillary, sphenoidal and ethmoidal*. All of them open into the nasal cavity through its lateral wall (Fig. 15.10). The *function* of the sinuses is to make the skull lighter and add resonance to the voice. In infections of the sinuses or *sinusitis*, the voice is altered.

The sinuses are rudimentary, or even absent at birth. They enlarge rapidly during the ages of six to seven years, i.e. time of eruption of permanent teeth and then after puberty. From birth to adult life the growth of the sinuses is due to enlargement of the bones; in old age it is due to resorption of the surrounding cancellous bone.

The anatomy of individual sinuses is important as they are frequently infected.

CLINICAL ANATOMY

1. Common cold or rhinitis is the commonest infection of the nose.

2. The paranasal air sinuses may get infected from the nose. Maxillary sinusitis is the commonest of such infections.

3. The relations of the nose to the anterior cranial fossa through the cribriform plate, and to the lacrimal apparatus through the nasolacrimal duct are important in the spread of infection.

4. Hypertrophy of the mucosa over the inferior nasal concha is a common feature of allergic rhinitis, which is characterized by sneezing, nasal blockage and excessive watery discharge from the nose.

DISSECTION

Remove the thin medial walls of the ethmoidal air cells, and look for the continuity with the mucous membrane of the nose. Remove the medial wall of maxillary air sinus extending anteriorly from opening of nasolacrimal duct till the greater palatine canal posteriorly. Now maxillary air sinus can be seen. Remove part of the roof of the maxillary air sinus so that the maxillary nerve and pterygopalatine ganglion are identifiable in the pterygopalatine fossa.

Trace the infraorbital nerve in the infraorbital canal in the floor of the orbit. Try to locate the sinuous course of anterior superior alveolar nerve into the upper incisor teeth.

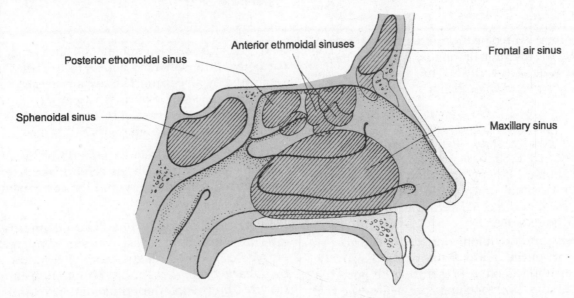

Fig. 15.10: *Lateral wall of nasal cavity with location of paranasal sinuses.*

Frontal Sinus

Surface Marking

It is marked by a triangular area formed by joining the following three points.

 a. The first point at the nasion.

 b. The second point 2.5 cm above the nasion.

 c. The third point at the junction of medial one-third and lateral two-thirds of the supraorbital margin, i.e. at the supraorbital notch.

Features

1. The frontal sinus lies in the frontal bone deep to the superciliary arch. It extends upwards above the medial end of the eyebrow, and backwards into the medial part of the roof of the orbit (Fig. 15.10).

2. It *opens* into the middle meatus of nose at the anterior end of the hiatus semilunaris either through the infundibulum or through the frontonasal duct (Fig. 15.6).

3. The right and left sinuses are usually unequal in size; and rarely one or both may be absent. Their *average* height, width and anteroposterior depth are each about 2.5 cm. The sinuses are better developed in males than in females.

4. They are rudimentary or absent at birth. They are well developed between seven and eight years of age, but reach full size only after puberty.

5. *Arterial supply:* Supraorbital artery. *Venous drainage:* Into the anastomotic vein between the supraorbital and superior ophthalmic veins, in the supraorbital notch. *Lymphatic drainage:* To the submandibular nodes. *Nerve supply:* Supraorbital nerve.

Maxillary Sinus

Surface Marking

The *roof* is represented by the inferior orbital margin; the *floor*, by the alveolus of the maxilla, the *base*, by the lateral wall of the nose. The *apex* lies in the zygomatic process of the maxilla.

Features

1. The maxillary sinus lies in the body of the maxilla (Fig. 15.2), and is the largest of all the paranasal sinuses. It is pyramidal in shape, with its base directed medially towards the lateral wall of the nose, and the apex directed laterally in the zygomatic process of the maxilla.

2. It *opens* into the middle meatus of the nose in the lower part of the hiatus semilunaris (Fig. 15.6). A second opening is often present at the posterior end of the hiatus. Both openings are nearer the roof than the floor of the sinus.

3. In an isolated maxilla, the opening or hiatus of the maxillary sinus is large. However, in the intact skull the size of the opening is reduced to 3 or 4 mm as it is overlapped by the following: (a) From above, by the uncinate process of the ethmoid, and the descending part of the lacrimal bone; (b) from below, by the inferior nasal concha; and (c) from behind, by the perpendicular plate of the palatine bone (Fig. 15.7). It is further reduced in size by the thick mucosa of the nose.

4. The size of the sinus is variable Average measurements are: height, 3.5 cm; width, 2.5 cm; and anteroposterior depth, 3.5 cm (Fig. 15.10).

5. Its *roof* is formed by the floor of orbit, and is traversed by the infraorbital nerve. The *floor* is formed by the alveolar process of the maxilla, and lies about 1 cm below the level of the floor of the nose. The level corresponds to the level of the lower border of the ala of the nose. The floor is marked by several conical elevations produced by the roots of the upper molar and premolar teeth. The roots may even penetrate the bony floor to lie beneath the mucous lining. The canine tooth may project into the anterolateral wall.

6. The maxillary sinus is the first paranasal sinus to *develop*.

7. *Arterial supply:* Facial, infraorbital and greater palatine arteries. *Venous drainage:* Into the facial vein and the pterygoid plexus of veins. *Lymphatic drainage:* Into the submandibular nodes. *Nerve supply:* Infraorbital, and anterior, middle and posterior superior alveolar nerves.

Sphenoidal Sinus

Features

1. The right and left sphenoidal sinuses lie within the body of the sphenoid bone (Fig. 15.10). They are separated by a septum. The two sinuses are usually unequal in size. Each sinus opens into the sphenoethmoidal recess of the corresponding half of the nasal cavity (Figs 15.6, 15.7).

2. Each sinus is related superiorly to the optic chiasma and the hypophysis cerebri; and laterally to the internal carotid artery and the cavernous sinus (Fig. 6.6).

3. *Arterial supply:* Posterior ethmoidal and internal carotid arteries. *Venous drainage:* Into pterygoid venous plexus and cavernous sinus. *Lymphatic drainage:* To the retropharyngeal nodes. *Nerve Supply:* Posterior ethmoidal nerve and orbital branches of the pterygopalatine ganglion.

Ethmoidal Sinuses

Features

Ethmoidal sinuses are numerous small inter-communicating spaces which lie within the labyrinth of the ethmoid bone (Fig. 15.2). They are completed from above by the orbital plate of the frontal bone, from behind by the sphenoidal conchae and the orbital process of the palatine bone, and anteriorly by the lacrimal bone. The sinuses are divided into anterior, middle and posterior groups (Fig. 15.10).

The *anterior ethmoidal sinus* is made up of 1 to 11 air cells. It opens into the anterior part of the hiatus semilunaris of the nose. It is supplied by the anterior ethmoidal nerve and vessels. Its lymphatics drain into the submandibular nodes.

The *middle ethmoidal sinus* consisting of one to seven air cells open into the middle meatus of the nose. It is supplied by the posterior ethmoidal nerve and vessels and the orbital branches of the pterygopalatine ganglion. Lymphatics drain into the submandibular nodes (Fig. 15.6).

The *posterior ethmoidal sinus* consisting of one to seven air cells opens into the superior meatus of the nose. It is supplied by the posterior ethmoidal nerve and vessels and the orbital branches of the pterygopalatine ganglion. Lymphatics drain into the retropharyngeal nodes.

CLINICAL ANATOMY

1. Infection of a sinus is known as *sinusitis*. It causes headache and persistent, thick, purulent discharge from the nose. Diagnosis is assisted by transillumination and radiography. A diseased sinus is opaque.

The maxillary sinus is most commonly involved. It may be infected from the nose or from a caries tooth. *Drainage of the sinus is difficult because its ostium lies at a higher level than its floor.* Another factor is that cilia in the lining mucosa are destroyed by chronic infection. Hence, the sinus is drained surgically by making an artificial opening near the floor in one of the following two ways. (a) Antrum puncture can be done by breaking the lateral wall of the inferior meatus. (b) An opening can be made at the canine fossa through the vestibule of the mouth, deep to the upper lip (Caldwell-Luc operation).

2. Carcinoma of the maxillary sinus arises from the mucosal lining. Symptoms depend on the direction of growth.

(a) Invasion of the orbit causes proptosis and diplopia. If the infraorbital nerve is involved there is facial pain and anaesthesia of the skin over the maxilla.

(b) Invasion of the floor may produce a bulging and even ulceration of the palate.

(c) Forward growth obliterates the canine fossa and produces a swelling of the face.

(d) Backward growth may involve the palatine nerves and produce severe pain referred to the upper teeth.

(e) Growth in a medial direction produces nasal obstruction, epistaxis and epiphora.

(f) Growth in a lateral direction produces a swelling on the face and a palpable mass in the labiogingival groove.

3. Frontal sinusitis can produce a brain abscess in the frontal lobe. A similar abscess may result from ethmoiditis.

PTERYGOPALATINE FOSSA

Definition

This is small pyramidal space situated deeply, below the apex of the orbit (Fig. 15.11).

Boundaries

Anterior: Superomedial part of the posterior surface of the maxilla.

Posterior: Root of the pterygoid process and adjoining part of the anterior surface of the greater wing of the sphenoid.

Medial: Upper part of the perpendicular plate of the palatine bone. The orbital and sphenoidal processes of the bone also take part.

Lateral: The fossa opens into the infratemporal fossa through the pterygomaxillary fissure.

Superior: Undersurface of the body of the sphenoid.

Inferior: Closed by the pyramidal process of the palatine bone in the angle between the maxilla and the pterygoid process.

Communications

Anteriorly: With the orbit through the medial end of the inferior orbital fissure.

Posteriorly: (a) With the middle cranial fossa through the foramen rotundum; (b) with the foramen lacerum through the pterygoid canal; and (c) with the pharynx through the palatinovaginal canal.

Medially: With the nose through the sphenopalatine foramen.

Laterally: With the infratemporal fossa through the pterygomaxillary fissure.

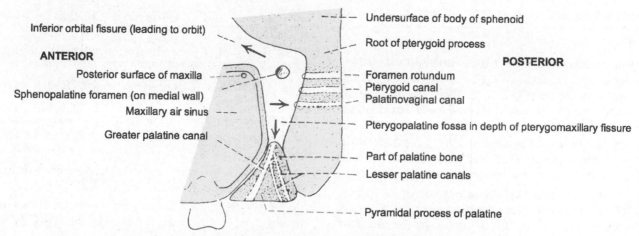

Inferior orbital fissure (leading to orbit)

ANTERIOR

Posterior surface of maxilla

Sphenopalatine foramen (on medial wall)

Maxillary air sinus

Greater palatine canal

Undersurface of body of sphenoid

Root of pterygoid process

POSTERIOR

Foramen rotundum
Pterygoid canal
Palatinovaginal canal

Pterygopalatine fossa in depth of pterygomaxillary fissure

Part of palatine bone

Lesser palatine canals

Pyramidal process of palatine

Fig. 15.11: *Scheme to show the pterygopalatine fossa and its communications.*

Inferiorly: With the oral cavity through the greater and lesser palatine canals.

Contents

1. Third part of the maxillary artery and its branches which bear the same names as the branches of the pterygopalatine ganglia and accompany all of them.

2. Maxillary nerve and its two branches, zygomatic and posterior superior alveolar.

3. Pterygopalatine ganglion and its numerous branches containing fibres of the maxillary nerve mixed with autonomic nerves.

MAXILLARY NERVE

It arises from the trigeminal ganglion, runs forwards in the lateral wall of the cavernous sinus below the ophthalmic nerve, and leaves the middle cranial fossa by passing through the foramen rotundum (Figs 6.6, 6.14). Next, the nerve crosses the upper part of the pterygopalatine fossa, beyond which it is continued as the infraorbital nerve (Figs 2.19, 2.20).

In the pterygopalatine fossa, the nerve is intimately related to the pterygopalatine ganglion, and gives off the zygomatic and posterior superior alveolar nerves.

The posterior superior alveolar nerve enters the posterior surface of the body of the maxilla, and supplies the three upper molar teeth and the adjoining part of the gum.

Pterygopalatine Ganglion (Sphenopalatine Ganglion)

Pterygopalatine is the largest parasympathetic peripheral ganglion. It serves as a relay station for secretomotor fibres to the lacrimal gland and to the mucous glands of the nose, the paranasal sinuses,

the palate and pharynx. Topographically, it is related to the maxillary nerve, but functionally it is connected to the facial nerve through its greater petrosal branch.

The flattened ganglion lies in the pterygopalatine fossa just below the maxillary nerve, in front of the pterygoid canal and lateral to the sphenopalatine foramen (Figs 15.11, 15.12).

DISSECTION

Trace the connections, and branches of pterygopalatine ganglion. It is responsible for supplying secretomotor fibres to the glands of nasal cavity, palate, pharynx and the lacrimal gland. It is also called *Hay fever ganglion* (allergic sinusitis).

Connections

1. The *motor or parasympathetic root* of the ganglion is formed by the nerve of the pterygoid canal. It carries preganglionic fibres that arise from neurons present near the superior salivatory and lacrimatory nuclei, and pass through the nervus intermedius, the facial nerve, the geniculate ganglion, the greater petrosal nerve and the nerve of the pterygoid canal to reach the ganglion. The fibres relay in the ganglion. Postganglionic fibres arise in the ganglion to supply secretomotor nerves to the lacrimal gland and to the mucous glands of the nose, the paranasal sinuses, the palate and the nasopharynx (Fig. 15.12).

2. The *sympathetic root* is also derived from the nerve of the pterygoid canal. It contains postganglionic fibres arising in the superior cervical sympathetic ganglion which pass through the internal carotid plexus, the deep petrosal nerve and the nerve of the pterygoid canal to reach the ganglion. The fibres

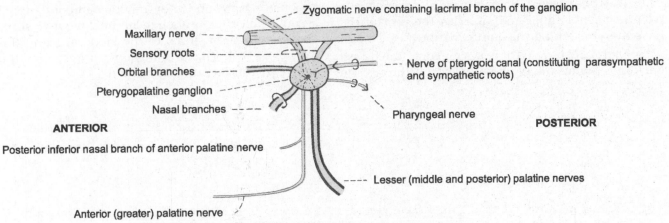

Fig. 15.12: Connections of the pterygopalatine ganglion.

pass through the ganglion without relay, and supply vasomotor nerves to the mucous membrane of the nose, the paranasal sinuses, the palate and the nasopharynx (Table 1.3).

The *sensory root* comes from the maxillary nerve. Its fibres pass through the ganglion without relay. They emerge in the branches described below (Fig. 15.12).

Branches

The branches of the ganglion are actually branches of the maxillary nerve. They also carry parasympathetic and sympathetic fibres which pass through the ganglion. The branches are as:

1. *Orbital branches* pass through the inferior orbital fissure, and supply the periosteum of the orbit, and the orbitalis muscle (Fig. 15.12).

2. *Palatine branches. The greater or anterior palatine nerve* descends through the greater palatine canal, and supplies the hard palate and the lateral wall of the nose, i.e. inferior concha and adjoining meatuses. The *lesser or middle and posterior palatine nerves* supply the soft palate and the tonsil (Fig. 15.13).

3. *Nasal branches* enter the nasal cavity through the sphenopalatine foramen (Fig. 15.11). The *lateral posterior superior nasal nerves*, about six in number supply the posterior parts of the superior and middle conchae (Fig. 15.9). The *medial posterior superior nasal nerves*, two or three in number supply the posterior part of the roof of the nose and of the nasal septum: the largest of these nerves is known as the *nasopalatine nerve* which descends up to the anterior part of the hard palate through the incisive foramen (Fig. 15.5).

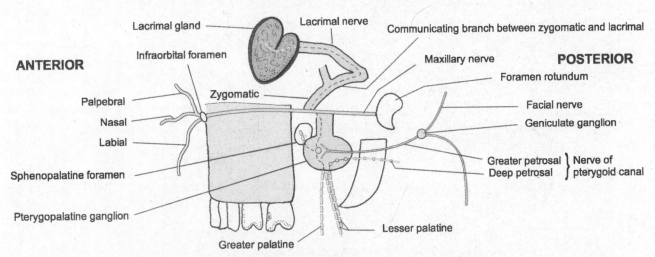

Fig. 15.13.: Maxillary nerve with pterygopalatine ganglion.

4. The *pharyngeal branch* passes through the palatinovaginal canal and supplies the part of the nasopharynx behind the auditory tube (Fig. 15.12).

5. *Lacrimal branch*. The postganglionic fibres pass back into the maxillary nerve to leave it through its zygomatic nerve and its zygomaticotemporal branch, a communicating branch to lacrimal nerve to supply the secretomotor fibres to the lacrimal gland (Figs 15.12, 15.13). The preganglionic fibres have their origin in the lacrimatory nucleus.

The Larynx

Larynx or voice box is well developed in humans. Its capabilities are greatly enhanced by the large "vocalisation area" in the lower part of motor cortex. Our speech is guided and controlled by the cerebral cortex. God has given us two ears and one mouth; to hear more, contemplate and speak less according to time and need.

A man's language is an "index of intellect". One speaks during the expiratory phase of respiration. Larynx is a part of the respiratory system allowing two-way flow of gases. It is kept patent because one adult is breathing about 15 times per minute, unlike the oesophagus which opens at the time of eating or drinking only. Abuse of the vocal cords by excessive talking may cause singer's nodules, or teacher's nodules, and even cancer of the vocal cords.

Introduction

The larynx is the organ for production of voice or phonation. It is also an air passage, and acts as a sphincter at the inlet of the lower respiratory passages. The upper respiratory passages include the nose, the nasopharynx and the oropharynx.

Situation and Extent

The larynx lies in the anterior midline of the neck, extending from the root of the tongue to the trachea. In the adult male, it lies in front of the third to sixth cervical vertebrae, but in children and in the adult female it lies at a little higher level (Fig. 14.7).

Size

The length of the larynx is 44 mm in males and 36 mm in females. At puberty the male larynx grows rapidly and becomes larger than the female larynx. The pubertal growth of the female larynx is negligible.

Constitution of Larynx

The larynx is made up of a skeletal framework of cartilages. The cartilages are connected by joints, ligaments and membranes; and are moved by a number of muscles. The cavity of the larynx is lined by mucous membrane.

The Skeleton or Cartilages of Larynx

The larynx contains nine cartilages, of which three are unpaired and three, paired.

Unpaired cartilages
1. Thyroid
2. Cricoid
3. Epiglottic

Paired cartilages
1. Arytenoid
2. Corniculate
3. Cuneiform

Thyroid Cartilage

This cartilage is V-shaped in cross-section. It consists of right and left laminae (Fig. 16.1). Each lamina is roughly quadrilateral. The laminae are placed obliquely relative to the midline: their posterior borders are far apart, but the anterior borders approach each other at an angle that is about 90 degrees in the male and about 120 degrees in the female. The lower parts of the anterior borders of the right and left laminae fuse and form a median projection called the *laryngeal prominence.* The upper parts of the anterior borders do not meet. They are separated by the *thyroid notch.* The posterior borders are free. They are prolonged upwards and downwards as the superior and inferior cornua or horns. The superior cornua is connected with the greater cornua of the hyoid bone by the lateral thyrohyoid ligament in which a small cartilago triticia may develop. The inferior cornua articulates with the cricoid cartilage to form the cricothyroid joint (Fig. 16.2). The inferior border of the thyroid cartilage is convex in front and concave behind. In the median plane, it is connected to the cricoid cartilage by the conus elasticus. The *outer surface* of each lamina is marked by an oblique line which extends from the superior thyroid tubercle in front of the root of the superior cornua to the inferior thyroid tubercle behind the middle of the inferior border. The thyrohyoid and the inferior constrictor of the pharynx are attached to the oblique line.

Cricoid Cartilage

This cartilage is shaped like a ring. It encircles the larynx below the thyroid cartilage. It is thicker and stronger than the thyroid cartilage. The ring has a narrow anterior part called the *arch*, and a broad posterior part, called the *lamina* (Fig. 16.2). The lamina projects upwards behind the thyroid cartilage, and articulates superiorly with the arytenoid cartilages. The inferior cornua of the thyroid cartilage articulates with the side of the cricoid cartilage at the junction of the arch and lamina.

Epiglottic Cartilage/Epiglottis

This is a *leaf-shaped* cartilage placed in the anterior wall of the upper part of the larynx. Its *upper end* is broad and free, and projects upwards behind the hyoid bone and the tongue. The *lower end* or *stalk* is pointed and is attached to the upper part of the angle between the two laminae of the thyroid cartilage (Figs 16.2, 16.3). The right and left margins of the cartilage provide attachment to the aryepiglottic folds. Its *anterior surface* is connected: (a) To the tongue by a median glossoepiglottic fold (Fig. 17.1); and (b) to the hyoid bone by the hyoepiglottic ligament (Fig. 16.4). The *posterior surface* is covered with mucous membrane, and presents a tubercle in the lower part.

Arytenoid Cartilage

These are two small *pyramid-shaped* cartilages lying on the upper border of the lamina of the cricoid cartilage. The *apex* of the arytenoid cartilage is curved posteromedially and articulates with the corniculate cartilage. Its *base* is concave and

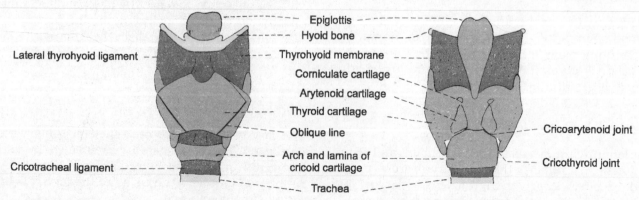

Fig. 16.1: *Skeleton of the larynx : anterior view.*

Fig. 16.2: *Skeleton of the larynx : posterior view.*

Labels (Fig. 16.1): Lateral thyrohyoid ligament; Cricotracheal ligament; Epiglottis; Hyoid bone; Thyrohyoid membrane; Corniculate cartilage; Arytenoid cartilage; Thyroid cartilage; Oblique line; Arch and lamina of cricoid cartilage; Trachea

Labels (Fig. 16.2): Cricoarytenoid joint; Cricothyroid joint articulates with the lateral part of the upper border of the cricoid lamina. It is prolonged anteriorly to form the vocal process, and laterally to form the muscular process (see Fig. 16.10). The *surfaces* of the cartilage are anterolateral, medial and posterior (Figs 16.2, 16.3, 16.4).

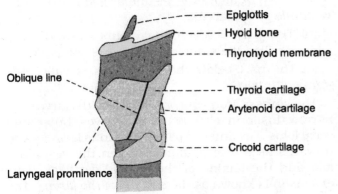

Fig. 16.3: *Cartilages of the larynx: lateral view.*

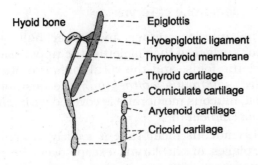

Fig. 16.4: *Cartilages of the larynx as seen in sagittal section.*

Corniculate Cartilages

These are two small conical nodules which articulate with the apex of the arytenoid cartilages, and are directed posteromedially. They lie in the posterior parts of the aryepiglottic folds (Fig. 16.5).

Cuneiform Cartilages

These are two small rod-shaped pieces of cartilage placed in the aryepiglottic folds just ventral to the corniculate cartilages.

Histology of Laryngeal Cartilages

The thyroid and cricoid cartilages, and the basal parts of the arytenoid cartilages are made up of hyaline cartilage. They may ossify after the age of 25 years. The other cartilages of the larynx, e.g. epiglottis corniculate, cuneiform and processes of the arytenoid are made of elastic cartilage and do not ossify.

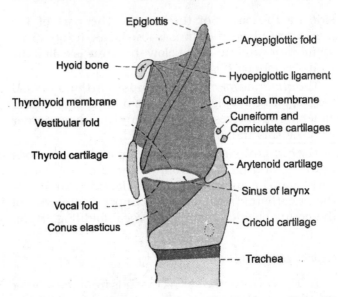

Fig. 16.5: *Ligaments and membranes of the larynx. Note the quadrate membrane and the conus elasticus.*

Laryngeal Joints

The *cricothyroid joint* is a *synovial* joint between the inferior cornua of the thyroid cartilage and the side of the cricoid cartilage. It permits rotatory movements around a transverse axis, and also gliding movements in different directions.

The *cricoarytenoid joint* is also a *synovial* joint between the base of the arytenoid cartilage and the upper border of the lamina of the cricoid cartilage. It permits rotatory movements around a vertical axis, and also gliding movements in all directions (Fig. 16.2).

Laryngeal Ligaments and Membranes

Extrinsic

(1) The *thyrohyoid membrane* connects the thyroid cartilage to the hyoid bone. Its median and lateral parts are thickened to form the median and lateral thyrohyoid ligaments. The membrane is pierced by the internal laryngeal nerves, and by the superior laryngeal vessels (Fig. 16.5).

(2) The *hyoepiglottic ligament* connects the upper end of the epiglottic cartilage to the hyoid bone.

(3) The *cricotracheal ligament* connects the cricoid cartilage to the upper end of the trachea (Fig. 16.1).

Intrinsic

The intrinsic ligaments are part of a broad sheet of fibroelastic tissue, known as the *fibroelastic membrane of the larynx*. This membrane is placed just outside the mucous membrane. It is interrupted on each side by the sinus of the larynx. The part of the membrane above the sinus is known as the quadrate membrane, and the part below the sinus is called the conus elasticus (Fig. 16.5).

The *quadrate membrane* extends from the arytenoid cartilage to the epiglottis. It has a lower free border which forms the vestibular fold; and an upper border which forms the aryepiglottic fold.

The *conus elasticus* or *cricovocal membrane* extends upwards and medially from the arch of the cricoid cartilage. The anterior part is thick and is known as the cricothyroid ligament. The upper free border of the conus elasticus forms the vocal fold (Fig. 16.5).

Cavity of Larynx

1. The cavity of the larynx extends from the inlet of the larynx to the lower border of the cricoid cartilage. The *inlet of the larynx* is placed obliquely. It looks backwards and upwards, and opens into the laryngopharynx. The inlet is *bounded anteriorly*, by the epiglottis; *posteriorly*, by the interarytenoid fold of mucous membrane; and *on each side*, by the aryepiglottic fold (Fig. 16.6).

2. Within the cavity of larynx, there are two folds of mucous membrane on each side. The upper fold is the *vestibular fold*, and the lower fold is the *vocal fold*. The space between the right and left vestibular folds is the *rima vestibuli*; and the space between the vocal folds is the *rima glottidis*. The vocal fold is attached anteriorly to the middle of the angle of the thyroid cartilage on its posterior aspect; and posteriorly to the vocal process of the arytenoid cartilage. The rima glottidis is limited posteriorly by an interarytenoid

fold of mucous membrane. The rima, therefore, has an anterior intermembranous part (three-fifth) and a posterior intercartilaginous part (see Fig. 16.11A). The rima is the narrowest part of the larynx. It is longer (23 mm) in males than in females (17 mm).

3. The vestibular and vocal folds divide the cavity of the larynx into three parts.

(a) The part above the vestibular fold is called the *vestibule* of the larynx.

(b) The part between the vestibular and vocal folds is called the sinus or *ventricle* of the larynx.

(c) The part below the vocal folds is called the *infraglottic part.*

The *sinus of Morgagni* or *ventricle of the larynx* is a narrow fusiform cleft between the vestibular and vocal folds. The anterior part of the sinus is prolonged upwards as a diverticulum between the vestibular fold and the lamina of the thyroid cartilage. This extension is known as the *saccule of the larynx*. The saccule contains mucous glands which help to lubricate the vocal folds (Fig. 16.6).

Mucous Membrane of Larynx

1. The anterior surface and upper half of the posterior surface of the epiglottis, the upper parts of aryepiglottic folds, and the vocal folds are lined by *stratified squamous epithelium*. The rest of the laryngeal mucous membrane is covered with *ciliated columnar epithelium.*

2. The mucous membrane is loosely attached to the cartilages of the larynx except over the vocal ligaments and over the posterior surface of the epiglottis where it is thin and firmly adherent.

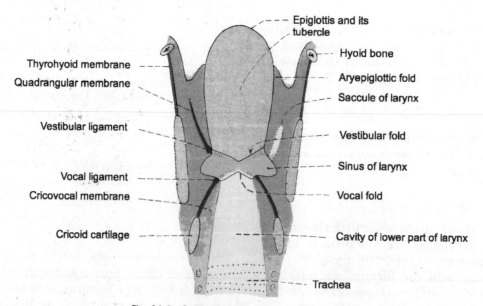

Fig. 16.6: *Coronal section through the larynx.*

3. *Mucous glands* are absent over the vocal cords, but are plentiful over the anterior surface of the epiglottis, around the cuneiform cartilages and in the vestibular folds. The glands are scattered over the rest of the larynx.

Intrinsic Muscles of Larynx

The attachments of intrinsic muscles of larynx are described these are also presented in Table 16.1 and their main action in Table 16.2.

Cricothyroid

This is the only intrinsic muscle lying on the external aspect of the larynx (Fig. 16.7).

Origin

Lower border and lateral surface of the cricoid cartilage.

Insertion

Its fibres pass backwards and upwards to be inserted into the inferior cornua and lower border of the thyroid cartilage.

Table 16.2: Muscles acting on the larynx

Movement	Muscles
1. Elevation of larynx	Thyrohyoid, mylohyoid
2. Depression of larynx	Sternothyroid, sternohyoid
3. Opening inlet of larynx	Thyroepiglotticus
4. Closing inlet of larynx	Aryepiglotticus
5. Abductor of vocal cords	Posterior cricoarytenoid only
6. Adductor of vocal cords	Lateral cricoarytenoid transverse, oblique arytenoids
7. Tensor of vocal cords	Cricothyroid
8. Relaxor of vocal cords	Thyroarytenoid

Posterior Cricoarytenoid

This is a triangular muscle (Fig. 16.8).

Origin

Posterior surface of the lamina of the cricoid cartilage. Origin is medial to insertion.

Table 16.1: Intrinsic muscles of the larynx (Fig. 15.4)

Muscle	Origin	Fibres	Insertion
1. *Cricothyroid* The only muscle outside the larynx (Fig. 16.7)	Lower border and lateral surface of cricoid	Fibres pass backwards and upwards	Inferior cornua and lower border of thyroid cartilage
2. *Posterior cricoarytenoid* Triangular muscle (Fig. 16.8)	Posterior surface of the lamina of cricoid	Upwards and laterally	Muscular process of arytenoid
3. *Lateral cricoarytenoid* (Figs 16.9, 16.10)	Lateral part of upper border of arch of cricoid	Upwards and backwards	Muscular process of arytenoid
4. *Transverse arytenoid* Unpaired muscle (Fig. 16.8)	Posterior surface of one arytenoid	Transverse	Posterior surface of another arytenoid
5. *Oblique arytenoid* and *aryepiglotticus* (Fig. 16.8)	Muscular process of one arytenoid	Oblique	Apex of the other arytenoid. Some fibres are continued as *aryepiglottic* muscle to the edge of the epiglottis
6. *Thyroarytenoid* and *Thyroepiglottic* (Fig. 16.9)	Thyroid angle and adjacent cricothyroid ligament	Backwards and upwards	Anterolateral surface of arytenoid cartilage. Some fibres project into the vocal fold and are known as *vocails*. Some of the upper fibres of thyroarytenoid curve upwards into the aryepiglottic fold to reach the edge of epiglottis. This is known as *thyroepiglottic*

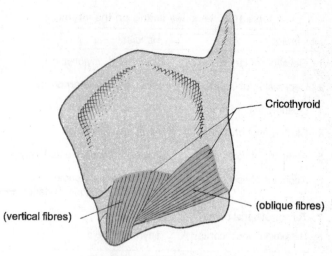

Fig. 16.7: Cricothyroid muscle.

Insertion

Its fibres pass upwards and laterally and are inserted into posterior aspect of muscular process of the arytenoid cartilage.

Lateral Cricoarytenoid

Origin

Lateral part of the upper border of the arch of the cricoid cartilage, origin is lateral to insertion.

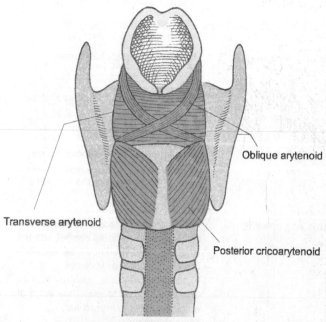

Fig. 16.8: Muscles of larynx: posterior view.

Insertion

Its fibres pass upwards and backwards to the inserted into, the anterior aspect of muscular process of the arytenoid cartilage.

Transverse Arytenoid

This is the only unpaired intrinsic muscle of the larynx. Its fibres run transversely from the posterior surface of one arytenoid cartilage to that of the opposite arytenoid cartilage.

Oblique Arytenoid

These are slips of muscle that run obliquely across the midline crossing each other. Each slip arises from the muscular process of one arytenoid cartilage and is inserted into the apex of the opposite arytenoid cartilage (Fig. 16.8).

Aryepiglotticus

This is made up of some fibres of the oblique arytenoid which are continued into the aryepiglottic fold to reach the edge of the epiglottic cartilage.

Thyroarytenoid

Origin

From the posterior aspect of the angle of the thyroid cartilage and the adjacent part of the cricothyroid ligament (Fig. 16.9).

Insertion

The fibres run backwards and upwards to reach the anterolateral surface of the arytenoid cartilage.

Vocalis

The vocalis is made up of some fibres of the thyroarytenoid that gain attachment to the vocal ligament.

Thyroepiglotticus

Some of the upper fibres of the thyroarytenoid curve upwards into the aryepiglottic fold to reach the edge of the epiglottis. These constitute the thyroepiglotticus (Fig. 16.9).

Nerve Supply of Muscles

All intrinsic muscles of the larynx are supplied by the recurrent laryngeal nerve except for the cricothyroid which is supplied by the external laryngeal nerve.

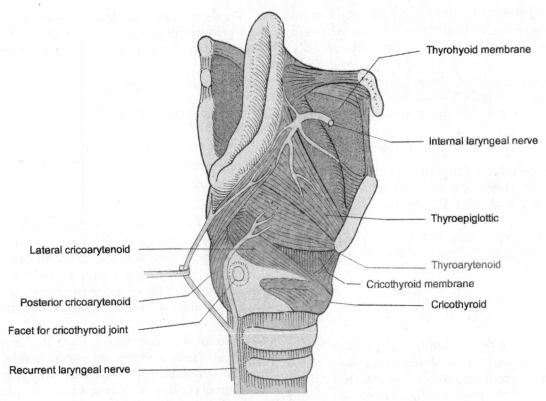

Fig. 16.9: Muscles of the larynx: Lateral view.

Actions

The vocal process and muscular processes move in opposite directions. Any muscle which pulls the muscular process medially, pushes the vocal process laterally, resulting in abduction of vocal cords. This is done by only one pair of muscle, the posterior cricoarytenoid. Muscles which pull the muscular process forward and laterally will push the vocal process medially causing adduction of vocal cords. This is done by lateral cricoarytenoid, transverse arytenoid. The cricothyroid causes rocking movement of thyroid forwards, increasing the distance between two attachments of vocal cords, thus tensing the vocal cords. The thyroarytenoid pulls the arytenoid forward, relaxing the vocal cords (Table 16.2).

1. Muscles which abduct the vocal cords: Only posterior cricoarytenoids.

2. Muscles which adduct the vocal cords: (1) Lateral cricoarytenoids; (2) transverse arytenoid; (3) cricothyroids; and (4) thyroarytenoids (Fig. 16.10).

3. Muscles which tense the vocal cords: Cricothyroids.

4. Muscles which relax the vocal cords: (1) Thyroarytenoids; and (2) vocalis (Fig. 16.9).

5. Muscles which close the inlet of the larynx: (1) Oblique arytenoids; and (2) aryepiglotticus.

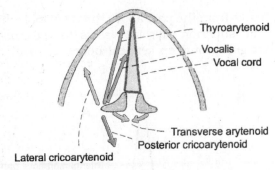

Fig. 16.10: Scheme to show the direction of pull of some intrinsic muscles of the larynx.

6. Muscles which open the inlet of larynx: Thyroepiglotticus (Fig. 16.9).

Movements of Vocal Folds

Movements of the vocal folds affect the shape and size of the rima glottidis.

1. During quiet breathing or condition of rest, the intermembranous part of the rima is triangular, and the intercartilaginous part is quadrangular (Fig. 16.11A).

2. During phonation or speech, the glottis is reduced to a chink by the adduction of the vocal folds (Fig. 16.11 B).

3. During forced inspiration, both parts of the rima are triangular, so that the entire rima is lozenge-shaped; the vocal folds are fully abducted (Fig. 16.11 C).

4. During whispering, the intermembranous part of the rima glottidis is closed, but the intercartilaginous part is widely open (Fig. 16.11 D).

Arterial Supply and Venous Drainage of Larynx

Up to the vocal folds: by the superior laryngeal artery, a branch of the superior thyroid artery. The superior laryngeal vein drains into the superior thyroid vein.

Below the vocal folds: by the inferior laryngeal artery, a branch of the inferior thyroid artery. The inferior laryngeal vein drains into the inferior thyroid vein.

Nerve Supply of Larynx

Motor nerves. See nerve supply of the muscles.

Sensory nerves: The internal laryngeal nerve supplies the mucous membrane upto the level of the vocal folds. The recurrent laryngeal nerve supplies it below the level of the vocal folds.

Lymphatic Drainage

Lymphatics from the part above the vocal folds drain along the superior thyroid vessels to the antero-superior group of deep cervical nodes.

Those from the part below the vocal folds drain to the posteroinferior group of deep cervical nodes. A few of them drain through the prelaryngeal nodes.

Mechanism of Speech

The mechanism of speech involves the following four processes.

1. Expired air from lungs
2. Vibrators
3. Resonators
4. Articulators

Expired air: As the air is forced out of lungs and larynx, it produces voice. Loudness or intensity of voice depends on the force of expiration of air.

Vibrators: The expired air causes vibrations of the vocal cords. Pitch of voice depends on the rate of vibration of vocal cords. Vowels are produced in the larynx.

Resonators: The column of air between vocal cords and nose and lips act as resonators. Quality of sound depends on resonators. One can make out change of quality of voice even on the telephone.

Articulators: These are formed by palate, tongue, teeth and lips. These narrow or stop the exhaled air. Many of the consonants are produced by the intrinsic muscles of tongue. Consonants produced by lips are –B, P, M, Pa, Pha, Ba, Bha, Ma; by labiodental–T,D,N, Ta, Tha, Da, Dha, Na; Lingual – C, E, J, Cha, Ja, Jha; Palatal – K, A, Ka, Kha, Ga, Gha.

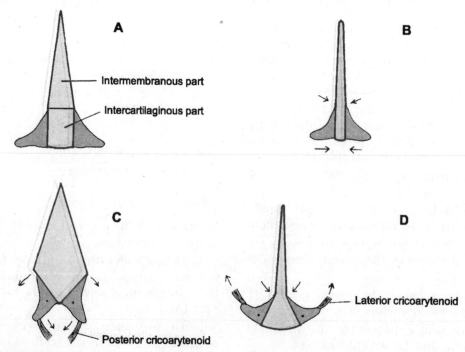

Fig. 16.11: *Rima glottidis (a) in quiet breathing, (b) in phonation or speech, (c) during forced inspiration, (d) during whispering.*

CLINICAL ANATOMY

1. When any foreign object enters the larynx severe protective coughing is excited to expel the object. However, damage to the internal laryngeal nerve produces anaesthesia of the mucous membrane in the supraglottic part of the larynx breaking the reflex arc so that foreign bodies can readily enter it.

2. Damage to the external laryngeal nerve causes some weakness of phonation due to loss of the tightening effect of the cricothyroid on the vocal cord.

3. When both recurrent laryngeal nerves are interrupted, the vocal cords lie in the cadaveric position in between abduction and adduction and phonation is completely lost. Breathing also becomes difficult through the partially opened glottis.

When only one recurrent laryngeal nerve is paralysed, the opposite vocal cord compensates for it and phonation is possible but there is hoarseness of voice. There is failure of forceful explosive part of voluntary and reflex coughing.

In progressive lesions of the recurrent laryngeal nerve, the only abductors of the vocal cords, the posterior cricoarytenoids are the first to be paralysed and the last to recover, as compared to the adductors. This is called as Semon's Law.

On the other hand, in functional paralysis of larynx, the adductors are the first to be paralysed.

4. The larynx can be examined either directly through a laryngoscope (*direct laryngoscopy*); or indirectly through a laryngeal mirror (*indirect laryngoscopy*). By these procedures one can inspect the base of the tongue, the valleculae, the epiglottis, the aryepiglottic folds, the piriform fossae, the vestibular folds, and the vocal folds (Fig. 16.12).

5. Since the larynx or glottis is the narrowest part of the respiratory passages, *foreign bodies* are usually lodged here.

6. Infection of the larynx is called *laryngitis*. It is characterized by hoarseness of voice.

7. *Laryngeal oedema* may occur due to a variety of causes. This can cause obstruction to breathing.

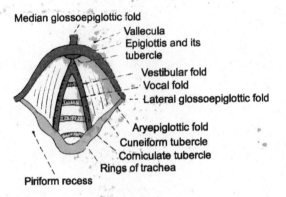

Median glossoepiglottic fold
Vallecula
Epiglottis and its tubercle
Vestibular fold
Vocal fold
Lateral glossoepiglottic fold
Aryepiglottic fold
Cuneiform tubercle
Corniculate tubercle
Rings of trachea
Piriform recess

Fig. 16.12: *Larynx as seen through a laryngoscope.*

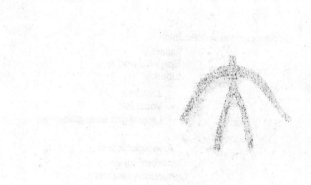

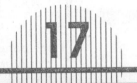

The Tongue

Tongue comprises skeletal muscle which is voluntary. These voluntary muscles start behaving as involuntary in any classroom – funny?

Thanks to the taste buds that the multiple hotels, restaurants, fast food outlets, *chat–pakori* shops, etc. are flourishing. One need not be too fussy about the taste of the food. Nutritionally, it should be balanced and hygienic.

"Tongue is barely three inches long, but it can kill a person six feet tall." Tongue appears very mobile, still it cannot be swallowed like food, because tongue is anchored to hyoid bone, mandible and soft palate. Four intrinsic and three extrinsic muscles of tongue are supplied by hypoglossal nerve. Only palatoglossus is supplied by vagoaccessory complex. In paralysis of hypoglossal nerve, the tip of tongue if protruded gets deviated to the paralysed side.

Introduction

The tongue is a muscular organ situated in the floor of the mouth. It is associated with the functions of taste, speech, mastication and deglutition. It has an oral part that lies in the mouth, and a pharyngeal part that lies in the pharynx. The oral and pharyngeal parts are separated by a V-shaped sulcus, the sulcus terminalis (Fig. 17.1).

DISSECTION

In the sagittal section, identify fan-shaped genioglossus muscle. Cut the attachments of buccinator, superior constrictor muscles and the intervening pterygomandibular raphe and reflect these downwards exposing the lateral surface of the tongue. Look at the superior, inferior surfaces of your own tongue with the help of hand lens.

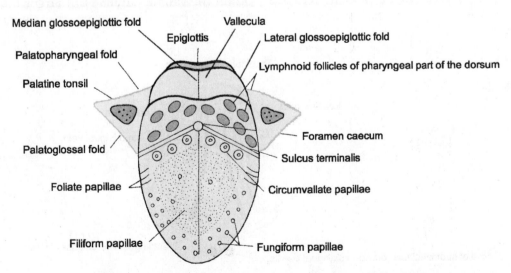

Fig. 17.1: The dorsum of the tongue, epiglottis and palatine tonsil.

External Features

The tongue has:

1. A root,

2. A tip, and

3. A body, which has (a) a curved upper surface or dorsum, and (b) an inferior surface. The dorsum is divided into oral and pharyngeal parts. The inferior surface is confined to the oral part only.

The *root* is attached to the mandible and soft palate above, and to the hyoid bone below (Figs 11.2, 14.2). Because of these attachments we are not able to swallow the tongue itself. In between the two bones, it is related to the geniohyoid and mylohyoid muscles.

The *tip* of the tongue forms the anterior free end which, at rest, lies behind the upper incisor teeth.

The *dorsum* of the tongue (Fig. 17.1) is convex in all directions. It is divided into: (a) An *oral part* or anterior two-thirds, and (b) a *pharyngeal part* or posterior one-third, by a faint V-shaped groove, the *sulcus terminalis*. The two limbs of the 'V' meet at a median pit, named the *foramen caecum*. They run laterally and forwards up to the palatoglossal arches. The foramen caecum represents the site from which the thyroid diverticulum grows down in the embryo. The oral and pharyngeal parts of the tongue differ in their development, topography, structure, and function.

The *oral or papillary part of the tongue* is placed on the floor of the mouth. Its *margins* are free and in contact with the gums and teeth. Just in front of the palatoglossal arch each margin shows 4 to 5 vertical folds, named the *foliate papillae*. The *superior surface* of the oral part shows a median furrow and is covered with papillae which make it rough. The *inferior surface* is covered with a smooth mucous membrane, which shows a median fold called the *frenulum linguae*. On either side of the frenulum there is a prominence produced by the deep lingual veins. More laterally there is a fold called the *plica fimbriata* that is directed forwards and medially towards the tip of the tongue (Fig. 17.2).

The *pharyngeal or lymphoid part of the tongue* lies behind the palatoglossal arches and the sulcus terminalis. Its posterior surface, sometimes called the base of the tongue, forms the anterior wall of the oropharynx. The mucous membrane has no papillae, but has many *lymphoid follicles* that collectively constitute the *lingual tonsil.* Mucous glands are also present.

The posteriormost part of the tongue is connected to the epiglottis by three folds of mucous membrane. These are the median glossoepiglottic fold and the right and left lateral glossoepiglottic folds. On either side of the median fold there is a depression called the vallecula (Fig. 17.1). The lateral folds separate the vallecula from the piriform fossa.

Papillae of the Tongue

These are projections of mucous membrane or corium which give the anterior two-thirds of the tongue its characteristic roughness. These are of the following three types.

1. *Vallate* or *circumvallate papillae.* They are large in size 1–2 mm in diameter and are 8–12 in number. They are situated immediately in front of the sulcus terminalis. Each papilla is a cylindrical projection surrounded by a circular sulcus. The walls of the papilla are raised above the surface (Fig. 17.1).

2. The *fungiform papillae* are numerous near the tip and margins of the tongue, but some of them are also scattered over the dorsum. These are smaller than the vallate papillae but larger than the filiform

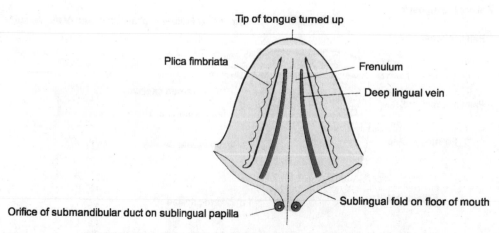

Fig. 17.2: *The inferior surface of the tongue and the floor of mouth.*

papillae. Each papilla consists of a narrow pedicle and a large rounded head. They are distinguished by their bright red colour.

3. The *filiform papillae* or *conical papillae* cover the presulcal area of the dorsum of the tongue, and give it a characteristic velvety appearance. They are the smallest and most numerous of the lingual papillae. Each is pointed and covered with keratin; the apex is often split into filamentous processes.

Muscles of the Tongue

A middle fibrous septum divides the tongue into right and left halves. Each half contains four intrinsic and four extrinsic muscles.

Intrinsic muscles
1. Superior longitudinal
2. Inferior longitudinal
3. Transverse
4. Vertical (Fig. 17.3)

Extrinsic muscles
1. Genioglossus (Fig. 17.4)
2. Hyoglossus, (Fig. 17.5)
3. Styloglossus (Fig. 17.5)
4. Palatoglossus (Fig. 14.5)

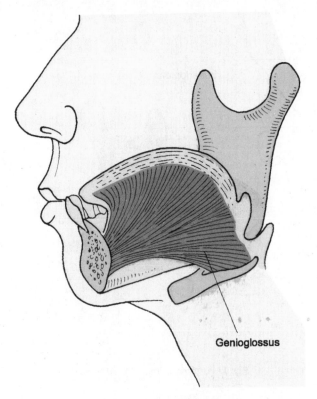

Fig. 17.4: Genioglossus.

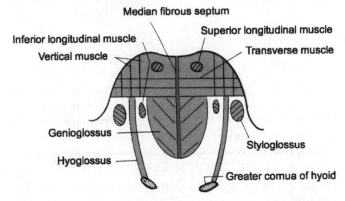

Fig. 17.3: Coronal section of the tongue showing arrangement of the intrinsic muscles and extrinsic muscles.

The *intrinsic muscles* (Fig. 17.6) occupy the upper part of the tongue, and are attached to the submucous fibrous layer and to the median fibrous septum. They alter the shape of the tongue. The *superior longitudinal muscle* lies beneath the mucous membrane. It shortens the tongue and makes its dorsum concave. The *inferior longitudinal muscle* is a narrow band lying close to the inferior surface of the tongue between the genioglossus and the hyoglossus. It shortens the tongue and makes its dorsum convex. The *transverse muscle* extends from the median

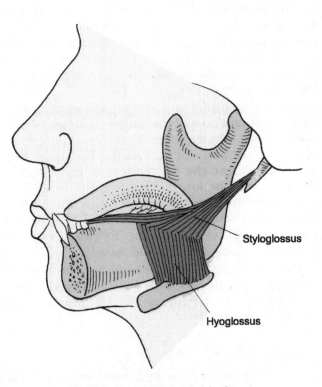

Fig. 17.5: Hyoglossus and styloglossus.

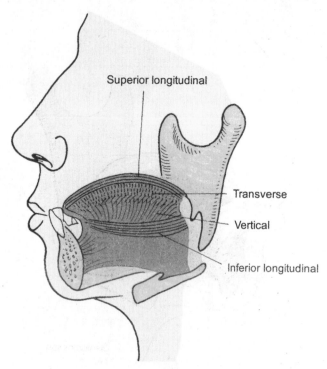

Fig. 17.6: *Intrinsic muscles of tongue.*

septum to the margins. It makes the tongue narrow and elongated. The *vertical muscle* is found at the borders of the anterior part of the tongue. It make the tongue broad and flattened (Fig. 17.3).

The *extrinsic muscles* connect the tongue to the mandible via genioglossus; to the hyoid bone through hyoglossus; to the styloid process via styloglossus, and the palate via palatoglossus. The genioglossus is described here. The hyoglossus has been described in Chapter 11; the styloglossus in Chapter 12 and the palatoglossus in Chapter 14.

The *genioglossus* is a fan-shaped muscle which forms the main bulk of the tongue. It arises from the upper genial tubercle of the mandible. From here the fibres fan out and run backwards. The upper fibres are inserted into the tip, the middle fibres into the dorsum, and the lower fibres into the hyoid bone. The upper fibres retract the tip, the middle fibres depress the tongue, and the lower fibres pull the posterior part of the tongue forwards and thus protrude the tongue from the mouth.

This muscle if paralysed will fall back on the oropharynx and block the air passage. During anaesthesia, the tongue is pulled forwards to clear the air passage.

Arterial Supply of Tongue

It is chiefly derived from the *lingual artery*, a branch of the external carotid artery. The root of the tongue

is also supplied by the tonsillar and ascending pharyngeal arteries (Figs 11.2, 14.12).

Venous Drainage

The arrangement of the vena comitantes/veins of the tongue is variable. Two venae comitantes accompany the lingual artery, and one vena comitantes accompanies the hypoglossal nerve. The deep lingual vein is the largest and principal vein of the tongue. It is visible on the inferior surface of the tongue. It runs backwards and crosses the genioglossus and the hyoglossus below the hypoglossal nerve.

These veins unite at the posterior border of the hyoglossus to form the lingual vein which ends either in the common facial vein or in the internal jugular vein.

Lymphatic Drainage

1. The tip of the tongue drains bilaterally to the submental nodes (Fig. 17.7).

2. The right and left halves of the remaining part of the anterior two-thirds of the tongue drain unilaterally to the submandibular nodes. A few central lymphatics drain bilaterally to the same nodes.

3. The posterior one-third of the tongue drains bilaterally to the jugulo-omohyoid nodes, these are known as the lymph nodes of the tongue.

Nerve Supply

Motor nerves. All the intrinsic and extrinsic muscles, except the palatoglossus, are supplied by the hypoglossal nerve. The palatoglossus is supplied by the cranial root of the accessory nerve through the pharyngeal plexus.

Sensory nerves. The lingual nerve is the nerve of general sensation and the chorda tympani is the nerve of taste for the anterior two-thirds of the tongue except vallate papillae.

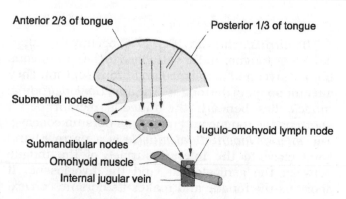

Fig. 17.7: *Lymphatic drainage of tongue.*

The glossopharyngeal nerve is the nerve for both general sensation and taste for the posterior one-third of the tongue including the circumvallate papillae. The posteriormost part of the tongue is supplied by the vagus nerve through the internal laryngeal branch (Table 17.1).

Histology

1. The bulk of the tongue is made up of striated muscles.

2. The *mucous membrane* consists of a layer of connective tissue (corium), lined by stratified squamous epithelium. On the oral part of the dorsum, it is thin, forms papillae, and is adherent to the muscles. On the pharyngeal part of the dorsum, it is very rich in lymphoid follicles. On the inferior surface, it is thin and smooth. Numerous glands, both mucous and serous lie deep to the mucous membrane.

3. *Taste buds* are most numerous on the sides of the vallate papillae, and on the walls of the surrounding sulci. Taste buds are numerous over the foliate papillae and over the posterior one-third of the tongue; and sparsely distributed on the fungiform papillae, the soft palate, the epiglottis and the pharynx. There are no taste buds on the mid-dorsal region of the oral part of the tongue.

Development of Tongue

I. Epithelium

(a) *Anterior two-thirds:* from two lingual swellings and one tuberculum impar, which arise from the first branchial arch. The tuberculum impar soon disappears. Therefore, it is supplied by lingual nerve (post-trematic) and chorda tympani (pretrematic).

(b) *Posterior one-third:* from cranial large part of the hypobranchial eminence, i.e. from the third arch. Therefore, it is supplied by the glossopharyngeal nerve (Table 17.1).

(c) Posteriormost part from the fourth arch. This is therefore supplied by the vagus nerve.

II. Muscles

The muscles develop from the occipital myotomes which are supplied by the hypoglossal nerve.

III. Connective Tissue

The connective tissue develops from the local mesenchyme.

CLINICAL ANATOMY

1. Injury to the hypoglossal nerve produces paralysis of the muscles of the tongue on the side of lesion. If the lesion is infranuclear, there is gradual atrophy of the affected half of the tongue or hemiatrophy. Muscular twitchings are also observed. Infranuclear lesions of the hypoglossal nerve are seen typically in motor neuron disease and in syringomyelia. Supranuclear lesions of the hypoglossal nerve produce paralysis without wasting. This is best seen in pseudobulbar palsy where the tongue is stiff, small and moves very sluggishly resulting in defective articulation.

2. Glossitis is usually a part of generalized ulceration of the mouth cavity or stomatitis. In certain anaemias, the tongue becomes smooth due to atrophy of the filiform papillae.

3. The presence of a rich network of lymphatics and of loose areolar tissue in the substance of the tongue is responsible for enormous swelling of the tongue in acute glossitis. The tongue fills up the mouth cavity and then protrudes out of it.

4. The undersurface of the tongue is a good site along with the bulbar conjunctiva for observation of jaundice.

Table 17.1: Parts of the tongue

Nerve supply	Anterior two-thirds	Posterior one-third	Posterior most part or vallecula
Sensory	Lingual	Glossopharyngeal	Internal laryngeal branch of vagus
Taste	Chorda tympani except vallate papillae	Glossopharyngeal including the vallate papillae	Internal laryngeal branch of vagus
Development of epithelium	Lingual swellings of I arch. Tuberculum impar which soon disappears	Third arch which forms large ventral part of hypobranchial eminence	Fourth arch which forms small dorsal part of hypobranchial eminence

Muscles develop from occipital myotomes, so the cranial nerve XII (hypoglossal nerve) supplies all intrinsic and three extrinsic muscles. Only palatoglossus is supplied by cranial root of accessory through pharyngeal plexus and is developed from mesoderm of sixth arch.

5. In unconscious patients, the tongue may fall back and obstruct the air passages. This can be prevented either by lying the patient on one side with head down (the 'tonsil position') or by keeping the tongue out mechanically.

6. In patients with grand mal epilepsy, the tongue is commonly bitten between the teeth during the attack. This can be prevented by hurriedly putting in a mouth gag at the onset of the seizure.

7. Carcinoma of the tongue is quite common. The affected side of the tongue is removed surgically. All the deep cervical lymph nodes are also removed, i.e. block dissection of neck because recurrence of malignant disease occurs in lymph nodes. Carcinoma of the posterior one-third of the tongue is more dangerous due to bilateral lymphatic spread.

The Ear and Vestibulocochlear Nerve

Tympanic membrane comprises all the three embryonic layers — outer layer is ectodermal, inner layer is endodermal while middle one is mesodermal in origin. The ossicles of the ear are the only bones fully formed at birth. Middle ear is a box-like cavity with six walls modified accordingly.

One hears with the ears. The centre for hearing is in the temporal lobe of brain above the ear. Reading aloud is a quicker way of memorising, as the ear, temporal lobes and motor speech area are also activated. The labyrinth is also supplied by an "end artery" like the retina.

Noise pollution within the four walls of the homes from the music albums and advertisements emitted from the television sets cause a lot of damage to the cochlear nerves and temporal lobes, besides causing irritation, hypertension and obesity. Addiction to TV works out to be extremely expensive in terms of both health and time. Time management is important for success on all fronts.

The ear is an organ of hearing. It is also concerned in maintaining the equilibrium of the body. It consists of three parts: The external ear, the middle ear and the internal ear.

EXTERNAL EAR

The external ear consists of: (a) The auricle or pinna; and (b) the external acoustic meatus.

Auricle/Pinna

The auricle is the part seen on the surface, the part the layman calls the ear. The greater part of it is made up of a single crumpled plate of elastic cartilage which is lined on both sides by skin. However, the lowest part of the auricle is soft and consists only of connective tissue covered by skin: This part is called

the *lobule* for wearing the ear rings. The rest of the auricle is divided into a number of parts that are shown in Fig. 18.1. In particular, note the large depression called the *concha*; it leads into the external acoustic meatus.

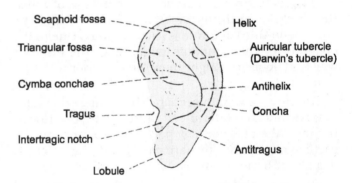

Scaphoid fossa
Triangular fossa
Cymba conchae
Tragus
Intertragic notch
Lobule
Helix
Auricular tubercle (Darwin's tubercle)
Antihelix
Concha
Antitragus

Fig. 18.1: *Named featured to be seen on the auricle.*

In relation to the auricle there are a number of muscles. These are vestigeal in man. In lower animals, the *intrinsic* muscles alter the shape of the auricle, while the *extrinsic* muscles move the auricle as a whole.

The *blood supply* of the auricle is derived from the posterior auricular and superficial temporal arteries. The *lymphatics* drain into the preauricular, postauricular and superficial cervical lymph nodes.

Nerve Supply: The upper two-thirds of the lateral surface of the auricle are supplied by the auriculotemporal nerve; and the lower one-third by the great auricular nerve. The upper two-thirds of the medial surface are supplied by the lesser occipital nerve; and the lower one-third by the great auricular nerve. The root of the auricle is supplied by the auricular branch of the vagus. The auricular muscles are supplied through branches of the facial nerve.

External Acoustic Meatus

The external auditory meatus conducts sound waves from the concha to the tympanic membrane. The canal is S-shaped. Its outer part is directed medially, forwards and upwards. The middle part is directed medially, backwards and upwards. The inner part is directed medially, forwards and downwards. The meatus can be straightened for examination by pulling the auricle upwards, backwards and slightly laterally.

DISSECTION

Expose the external auditory meatus by cutting the tragus of the auricle. Put a probe into the external auditory meatus and remove the anterior wall of cartilaginous and bony parts of the external auditory meatus with the scissors. Be slow and careful not to damage the tympanic membrane.

The meatus or canal is about 24 mm long, of which the medial two-thirds or 16 mm is bony, and the lateral one-third or 8 mm is cartilaginous. Due to the obliquity of the tympanic membrane, the anterior wall and floor are longer than the posterior wall and roof.

The canal is oval in section. The greatest diameter is vertical at the lateral end, and anteroposterior at the medial end. The bony part is narrower than the cartilaginous part. The narrowest point, the *isthmus*, lies about 5 mm from the tympanic membrane.

The *bony part* is formed by the tympanic plate of the temporal bone which is C-shaped in cross-section. The posterosuperior part of the plate is deficient. Here the wall of the meatus is formed by a part of the squamous temporal bone. The meatus is lined by thin skin, firmly adherent to the periosteum.

The *cartilaginous part* is also C-shaped in section; and the gap of the 'C' is filled with fibrous tissue. The lining skin is adherent to the perichondrium, and contains hairs, sebaceous glands, and ceruminous or wax glands. *Ceruminous glands* are modified sweat glands.

Blood supply: The outer part of the canal is supplied by the superficial temporal and posterior auricular arteries, and the inner part, by the deep auricular branch of the maxillary artery.

Lymphatics: The lymphatics pass to preauricular, postauricular and superficial cervical lymph nodes.

Nerve supply: The skin lining the anterior half of the meatus is supplied by the auriculotemporal nerve, and that lining the posterior half, by the auricular branch of the vagus.

CLINICAL ANATOMY

1. As already stated, for examination of the meatus and tympanic membrane the auricle should be drawn upwards, backwards and slightly laterally. However, in infants, the auricle is drawn downwards and backwards because the canal is only cartilaginous and the outer surface of the tympanic membrane is directed mainly downwards.

2. Boils and other infections of the external meatus cause little swelling but are extremely painful, due to the fixing of the skin to the underlying bone and cartilage.

3. Irritation of the auricular branch of the vagus in the external ear by ear wax or syringing may reflexly produce persistent cough called ear cough, vomiting or even death due to sudden cardiac inhibition. On the other hand, mild stimulation of this nerve may reflexly produce increased appetite.

4. Accumulation of wax in the external acoustic meatus is often a source of excessive itching, although fungal infection and foreign bodies should be excluded. Troublesome impaction of large foreign bodies like seeds, grains, insects is common.

5. Involvement of the ear in herpes zoster of the geniculate ganglion depends on the connection between the auricular branch of the vagus and the facial nerve within the petrous temporal bone.

6. Small pieces of skin from the lobule of the pinna are commonly used for demonstration of lepra bacilli to confirm the diagnosis of leprosy.

7. A good number of ear traits follow Mendelian inheritance.

Tympanic Membrane

This is a thin, translucent partition between the external acoustic meatus and the middle ear.

It is oval in shape, measuring 9 × 10 mm. It is placed obliquely at an angle of 55 degrees with the floor of the meatus. It faces downwards, forwards and laterally (Fig. 18.2).

The membrane has outer and inner surfaces.

The outer surface of the membrane is lined by thin skin. It is concave.

The inner surface provides attachment to the handle of the malleus which extends up to its centre. The inner surface is convex. The point of maximum convexity lies at the tip of the handle of the malleus and is called the *umbo*.

The membrane is thickened at its circumference which is fixed to the tympanic sulcus of the temporal

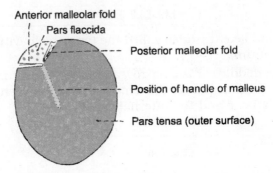

Anterior malleolar fold
Pars flaccida
Posterior malleolar fold
Position of handle of malleus
Pars tensa (outer surface)

Fig. 18.2: Left tympanic membrane : outer surface.

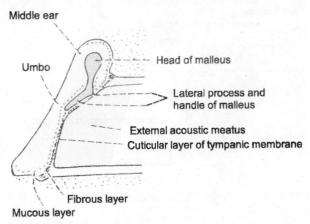

Middle ear
Umbo
Head of malleus
Lateral process and handle of malleus
External acoustic meatus
Cuticular layer of tympanic membrane
Fibrous layer
Mucous layer

Fig. 18.4: Tympanic membrane as seen in section.

bone on the tympanic plate. Superiorly, the sulcus is deficient. Here the membrane is attached to the tympanic notch. From the ends of the notch two bands, the anterior and posterior malleolar folds are prolonged to the lateral process of the malleus.

While the greater part of the tympanic membrane is tightly stretched and is, therefore, called the *pars tensa*, the part between the two malleolar folds is loose and is called the pars flaccida. The pars flaccida is crossed internally by the chorda tympani (Fig. 18.3). This part is more liable to rupture than the pars tensa.

The membrane is held tense by the inward pull of the tensor tympani muscle which is inserted into the upper end of the handle of the malleus.

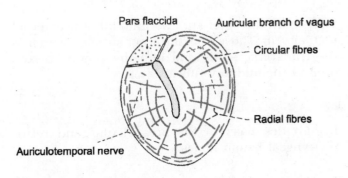

Pars flaccida
Auricular branch of vagus
Circular fibres
Radial fibres
Auriculotemporal nerve

Fig. 18.5: Arrangement of fibres in the tympanic membrane and its nerve supply.

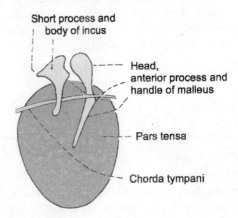

Short process and body of incus
Head, anterior process and handle of malleus
Pars tensa
Chorda tympani

Fig. 18.3: Left tympanic membrane : Inner surface.

Structure

The tympanic membrane is composed of the following three layers:

1. The *outer cuticular layer* of skin (Fig. 18.4).

2. The *middle fibrous layer* made up of superficial radiating fibres and deep circular fibres. The circular fibres are minimal at the centre and maximal at the periphery. The fibrous layer is replaced by loose areolar tissue in the pars flaccida (Fig. 18.5).

3. The *inner mucous layer* (Fig. 18.6) is lined by a low ciliated columnar epithelium.

Blood Supply

1. The outer surface is supplied by the deep auricular branch of the maxillary artery.

2. The inner surface is supplied by the anterior tympanic branch of the maxillary artery and by the posterior tympanic branch of the stylomastoid branch of the posterior auricular artery (Fig. 10.7).

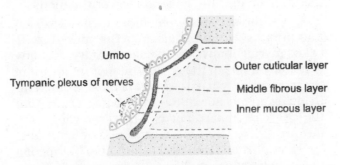

Umbo
Tympanic plexus of nerves
Outer cuticular layer
Middle fibrous layer
Inner mucous layer

Fig. 18.6: Curvatures of the tympanic membrane.

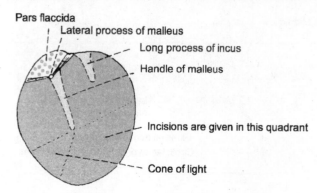

Fig. 18.7: The left tympanic membrane seen through the external acoustic meatus.

Venous Drainage

Veins from the outer surface drain into the external jugular vein. Those from the inner surface drain into the transverse sinus and into the venous plexus around the auditory tube.

Lymphatic Drainage

Lymphatics pass to the preauricular and retropharyngeal lymph nodes.

Nerve Supply

1. *Outer surface:* The anteroinferior part is supplied by the auriculotemporal nerve, and the posterosuperior part by the auricular branch of the vagus nerve.

2. *Inner surface:* This is supplied by the tympanic branch of the glossopharyngeal nerve through the tympanic plexus.

CLINICAL ANATOMY

1. When the tympanic membrane is illuminated for examination, the concavity of the membrane produces a 'cone of light' over the anteroinferior quadrant which is the farthest or deepest quadrant with its apex at the umbo (Fig. 18.7). Through the membrane one can see the underlying handle of the malleus and the long process of the incus.

2. The membrane is sometimes incised to drain pus present in the middle ear. The procedure is called myringotomy. The incision for myringotomy is usually made in the posteroinferior quadrant of the membrane where the bulge is most prominent. In giving an incision, it has to be remembered that the chorda tympani nerve runs downwards and forwards across the inner surface of the membrane, lateral to the long process of the incus, but medial to the neck of the malleus.

MIDDLE EAR

The middle ear is also called the tympanic cavity, or tympanum.

The middle ear is a narrow air filled space situated in the petrous part of the temporal bone between the external ear and the internal ear (Fig. 18.8).

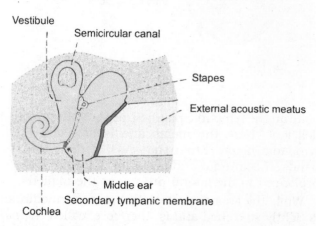

Fig. 18.8: Scheme to show the three parts of the ear.

Shape and Size

The middle ear is shaped like a cube. Its lateral and medial walls are large, but the other walls are narrow, because the cube is compressed from side to side. Its vertical and anteroposterior diameters are both about 15 mm. When seen in coronal section the cavity of the middle ear is biconcave, as the medial and lateral walls are closest to each other in the centre. The distances separating them are 6 mm near the roof, 2 mm in the centre, and 4 mm near the floor.

DISSECTION

Remove the dura mater and endosteum from the floor of the middle cranial fossa. Identify greater petrosal nerve emerging from a canaliculus on the anterior surface of petrous temporal bone. Trace it as it passes inferior to trigeminal ganglion to reach the carotid canal.

Carefully break the roof of the middle ear formed by tegmen tympani which is a thin plate of bone situated parallel and just lateral to the greater petrosal nerve. Cavity of the middle ear can be visualised. Try to put a probe in the anteromedial part of the cavity of middle ear till it appears at the opening in the lateral wall of nasopharynx. Identify the posterior wall of the middle ear which has an opening in its upper part. This is the aditus to mastoid antrum which in turn connects the cavity to the mastoid air cells.

Ear ossicles

Identify the bony ossicles. Locate the tendon of tensor tympani muscle passing from the malleus towards the medial wall of the cavity where it gets continuous with the muscle. Trace the tensor tympani muscle traversing in a semicanal above the auditory tube. Break one wall of the pyramid to visualise the stapedius muscle. Just superior to the attachment of tendon of tensor tympani, look for chorda tympani traversing the tympanic membrane.

Parts

The cavity of the middle ear can be subdivided into the tympanic cavity proper which is opposite the tympanic membrane; and the epitympanic recess which lies above the level of the tympanic membrane.

Communications

The middle ear communicates anteriorly with the nasopharynx through the auditory tube, and posteriorly with the mastoid antrum and mastoid air cells through the aditus to the mastoid antrum.

The middle ear is likened to a sump pit or trap in the sloping course of the aditus to the epitympanic recess and the auditory tube (Fig. 18.9)

Contents

The middle ear contains the following:

1. Three small bones or ossicles namely the malleus, the incus and the stapes. The upper half of the malleus, and the greater part of the incus lie in the epitympanic recess.

2. Ligaments of the ear ossicles.

3. Two muscles, the tensor tympani and the stapedius.

4. Vessels supplying and draining the middle ear.

5. Nerves: Chorda tympani and tympanic plexus.

The mucous membrane lining the middle ear cavity invests all the contents and forms several vascular folds which project into the cavity. This gives the cavity a honeycombed appearance.

Boundaries

The Roof or Tegmental Wall

1. The roof separates the middle ear from the middle cranial fossa. It is formed by a thin plate of bone called the tegmen tympani. This plate is prolonged backwards as the roof of the canal for the tensor tympani (Fig. 18.10).

2. In young children, the roof presents a gap at the unossified petrosquamous suture where the middle ear is in direct contact with the meninges. In adults, the suture is ossified and transmits a vein from the middle ear to the superior petrosal sinus.

The Floor or Jugular Wall

The floor is formed by a thin plate of bone which separates the middle ear from the superior bulb of the internal jugular vein. This plate is a part of the temporal bone (Fig. 18.10).

Near the medial wall the floor presents the tympanic canaliculus which transmits the tympanic branch of the glossopharyngeal nerve to the medial wall of the middle ear.

The Anterior or Carotid Wall

The anterior wall is narrow due to the approximation of the medial and lateral walls, and because of descent of the roof.

The uppermost part of the anterior wall bears the opening of the canal for the tensor tympani. The middle part has the opening of the auditory tube. The inferior part of the wall is formed by a thin plate of bone which forms the posterior wall of the carotid canal. The plate separates the middle ear from the internal carotid artery. This plate of bone is perforated by the superior and inferior sympathetic caroticotympanic nerves and the tympanic branch of the internal carotid artery (Fig. 18.11).

The bony septum between the canals for the tensor tympani and for the auditory tube is continued

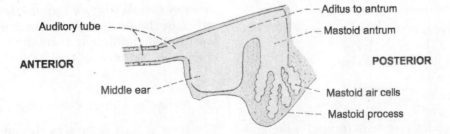

Fig. 18.9: *Scheme to show some relationships of the middle ear cavity. Note that the cavity resembles a sump-pit or trap.*

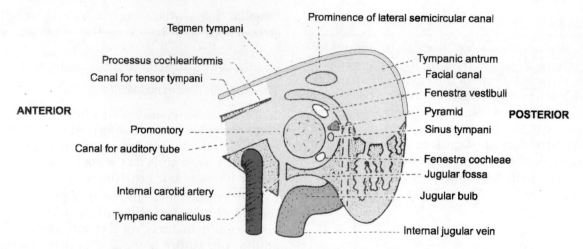

Fig. 18.10: *Scheme to show the landmarks on the medial wall of the middle ear. Some related structures are also shown.*

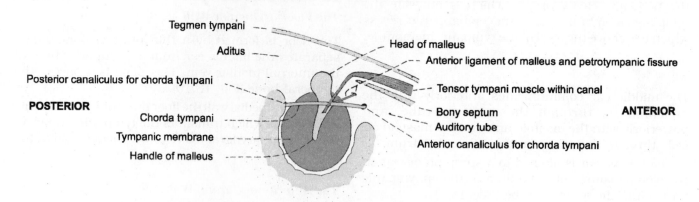

Fig. 18.11: *Lateral wall of the middle ear viewed from the medial side.*

posteriorly on the medial wall as a curved lamina called the *processus cochleariformis*. Its posterior end forms a pulley around which the tendon of the tensor tympani turns laterally to reach the upper part of the handle of the malleus.

The Posterior or Mastoid Wall

The posterior wall presents these features from above downwards.

1. Superiorly, there is an opening or *aditus* through which the epitympanic recess communicates with the mastoid or tympanic antrum (Figs 18.10, 18.11).

2. The *fossa incudis* is a depression which lodges the short process of the incus.

3. A conical projection, called the *pyramid*, lies near the junction of the posterior and medial walls. It has an opening at its apex for passage of the tendon of the stapedius muscle.

4. Lateral to pyramid and near the posterior edge of the tympanic membrane, there is the *posterior canaliculus for the chorda tympani* through which the nerve enters the middle ear cavity.

The Lateral or Membranous Wall

1. The lateral wall separates the middle ear from the external acoustic meatus. It is formed: (a) Mainly by the tympanic membrane along with the tympanic ring and sulcus and (b) partly by the squamous temporal bone, in the region of the epitympanic recess.

2. Near the tympanic notch there are two small apertures. (a) The *petrotympanic fissure* lies in front of the upper end of the bony rim. It lodges the anterior process of the malleus and transmits the tympanic branch of the maxillary artery. (b) The *anterior canaliculus for the chorda tympani* nerve lies either in the fissure or just in front of it. The nerve leaves the middle ear through this canaliculus to emerge at the base of the skull.

The *Medial or Labyrinthine Wall*

The medial wall separates the middle ear from the internal ear. It presents the following features.

(a) The *promontory* is a rounded bulging produced by the first turn of the cochlea. It is grooved by the tympanic plexus (Fig. 18.12).

(b) The *fenestra vestibuli* is an oval opening posterosuperior to the promontory. It leads into the vestibule of the internal ear and is closed by the footplate of the stapes.

(c) The *prominence of the facial canal* runs backwards just above the fenestra vestibuli, to reach the lower margin of the aditus. The canal then descends behind the posterior wall to end at the stylomastoid foramen.

(d) The *fenestra cochleae* is a round opening at the bottom of a depression posteroinferior to the promontory. It opens into the scala tympani of the cochlea, and is closed by the *secondary tympanic membrane.*

(e) The *sinus tympani* is a depression behind the promontory, opposite the ampulla of the posterior semicircular canal.

(f) The *processus cochleariformis* (see the anterior wall).

Arterial Supply

The main arteries of the middle ear are as follows.

1. The anterior tympanic branch of the maxillary artery which enters the middle ear through the petrotympanic fissure.

2. The posterior tympanic branch of the stylomastoid branch of the posterior auricular artery which enters through the stylomastoid foramen.

Small arteries supplying the middle ear are as follows.

1. The superior tympanic branch of the middle meningeal artery which enters through the canal for the tensor tympani.

2. The inferior tympanic branch of the ascending pharyngeal artery entering through the tympanic canaliculus.

3. The tympanic branch of the artery of the pterygoid canal by passing through the canal for the auditory tube.

4. The caroticotympanic branch of the internal carotid artery entering through the anterior wall.

5. The petrosal branch of the middle meningeal artery entering through the hiatus for the greater petrosal nerve.

Venous Drainage

Veins from the middle ear drain into the superior petrosal sinus and the pterygoid plexus of the veins.

Lymphatic Drainage

Lymphatics pass to the preauricular and retropharyngeal lymph nodes.

Nerve Supply

The nerve supply is derived from the tympanic plexus which lies over the promontory. The plexus is formed by the following.

1. The tympanic branch of the glossopharyngeal nerve. Its fibres are distributed to the mucous membrane of the middle ear, the auditory tube, the mastoid antrum and air cells. It also gives off the lesser petrosal nerve.

2. The superior and inferior caroticotympanic nerves arise from the sympathetic plexus around the internal carotid artery. These fibres are vasomotor to the mucous membrane.

Functions of the Middle Ear

1. It transmits sound waves from the external ear to the internal ear through the chain of ear ossicles, and thus transforms the airborne vibrations from the tympanic membrane to liquid borne vibrations in the internal ear.

2. The intensity of the sound waves is increased ten times by the ossicles. It may be noted that the frequency of sound does not change.

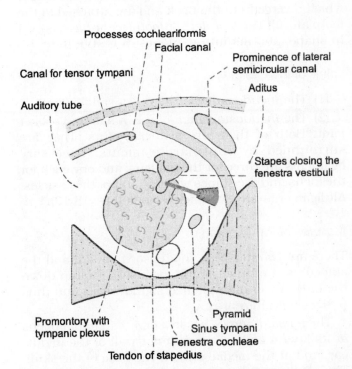

Fig. 18.12: *Features on the medial wall of the middle ear. The stapes and the tendon of the stapedius are also shown.*

Processes cochleariformis
Facial canal
Canal for tensor tympani
Prominence of lateral semicircular canal
Aditus
Auditory tube
Stapes closing the fenestra vestibuli
Promontory with tympanic plexus
Pyramid
Sinus tympani
Fenestra cochleae
Tendon of stapedius

CLINICAL ANATOMY

1. Throat infections commonly spread to the middle ear through the auditory tube and cause otitis media. The pus from the middle ear may take one of the following courses: (a) It may be discharged into the external ear following rupture of the tympanic membrane. (b) It may erode the roof and spread upwards, causing meningitis and brain abscess. (c) It may erode the floor and spread downwards, causing thrombosis of the sigmoid sinus and the internal jugular vein. (d) It may spread backwards, causing mastoid abscess and even thrombosis in the sigmoid sinus.

Chronic otitis media and mastoid abscess are responsible for persistent discharge of pus through the ear. Otitis media is more common in children than in adults.

2. Fracture of the middle cranial fossa breaks the roof of the middle ear, rupture the tympanic membrane, and thus cause bleeding through the ear along with discharge of CSF.

3. The inferior pouch of the outer attic or Prussak's pouch does not drain easily, the pouch is bounded laterally by the pars flaccida of the tympanic membrane; medially by the neck of the malleus; anteriorly and posteriorly by the malleolar folds; and superiorly by the lateral ligament of the malleus. Inflammatory exudates in the pouch often lead to perforation of the pars flaccida.

THE EAR OSSICLES

Malleus

The malleus is so called because it resembles a hammer. It is the largest, and the most laterally placed ossicle. It has the following parts. (a) The rounded *head* lies in the epitympanic recess. It articulates posteriorly with the body of the incus. It provides attachment to the superior and lateral ligaments. (b) The *neck* lies against the pars flaccida and is related medially to the chorda tympani nerve. (c) The *anterior process* is connected to the petrotympanic fissure by the anterior ligament. (d) The *lateral process* projects from the upper end of the handle and provides attachment to the malleolar folds. (e) The *handle* extends downwards, backwards and medially, and is attached to the upper half of the tympanic membrane (Fig. 18.13).

Incus or Anvil

It is so called because it resembles an anvil, used by blacksmiths. It resembles a molar tooth and has the following parts. (a) The *body* is large and bears an

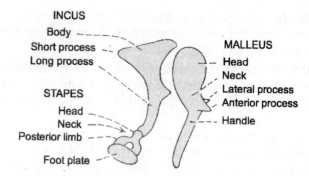

Fig. 18.13: *Ossicles of the left ear, seen from the medial side.*

articular surface that is directed forwards. It articulates with the head of the malleus. (b) The *long process* projects downwards just behind and parallel with the handle of the malleus. Its tip bears a lentiform nodule directed medially which articulates with the head of the stapes.

Stapes

This bone is so called because it is shaped like a stirrup. It is the smallest, and the most medially placed ossicle of the ear.

It has the following parts. (a) The small *head* has a concave facet which articulates with the lentiform nodule of the incus. (b) The narrow *neck* provides insertion, posteriorly, to the thin tendon of the stapedius. (c) *Two limbs* or crura; anterior, the shorter and less curved; and posterior, the longer which diverge from the neck and are attached to the footplate. (d) The *footplate*, a *footpiece* or *base*, is oval in shape, and fits into the fenestra vestibuli.

Joints of the Ossicles

(1) The *incudomalleolar joint* is a saddle joint.

(2) The *incudostapedial joint* is a ball and socket joint. Both of them are synovial joints. They are surrounded by capsular ligaments. Accessory ligaments are three for the malleus, and one each for the incus and the stapes which stabilize the ossicles. All ligaments are extremely elastic (Fig. 18.13).

Muscles of the Middle Ear

There are two muscles, the tensor tympani and the stapedius. Both act simultaneously to damp down the intensity of high-pitched sound waves and thus protect the internal ear.

The *tensor tympani* lies in a bony canal that opens at its lateral end on the anterior wall of the middle ear, and at the medial end on the base of the skull. The auditory tube lies just below this canal. The muscle arises from the walls of the canal in which it lies. Some fibres arise from the cartilaginous part of the auditory tube, and some from the base of the skull. The muscle ends in a tendon which reaches the medial wall of the middle ear and bends sharply around the processus cochleariformis. It then passes laterally across the tympanic cavity to be inserted into the handle of the malleus. The tensor tympani is supplied by the mandibular nerve. The fibres pass through the nerve to the medial pterygoid, and through the otic ganglion, without any relay. It develops from the mesoderm of first branchial arch.

The *stapedius* lies in a bony canal that is related to the posterior wall of the middle ear. Posteriorly, and below, this canal is continuous with the vertical part of the canal for the facial nerve. Anteriorly, the canal opens on the summit of the pyramid. The muscle arises from the walls of this canal. Its tendon emerges through the pyramid and passes forwards to be inserted into the posterior surface of the neck of the stapes. The stapedius is supplied by the facial nerve. It develops from the mesoderm of the second branchial arch.

CLINICAL ANATOMY

Otosclerosis
Sometimes bony fusion takes place between the foot plate of the stapes and the margins of the fenestra vestibuli. This leads to deafness. The condition can be surgically corrected.

TYMPANIC OR MASTOID ANTRUM

Mastoid antrum is a small, circular, air filled space situated in the posterior part of the petrous temporal bone. It is of adult size at birth, size of a small pea, or 1 cm in diameter and has a capacity of about one millilitre.

Boundaries

1. *Superiorly:* Tegmen tympani, and beyond it the temporal lobe of the cerebrum.
2. *Inferiorly:* Mastoid process containing the mastoid air cells.
3. *Anteriorly:* It communicates with the epitympanic recess through the aditus. The aditus is related medially to the ampullae of the superior and lateral semicircular canals, and posterosuperiorly to the facial canal.
4. *Posteriorly:* It is separated by a thin plate of bone from the sigmoid sinus. Beyond the sinus there is the cerebellum.
5. *Medially:* Petrous temporal bone.

6. *Laterally:* It is bounded by part of the squamous temporal bone. This part corresponds to the suprameatal triangle seen on the surface of the bone. This wall is 2 mm thick at birth, but increases in thickness at the rate of about 1 mm per year up to a maximum of about twelve to 15 mm.

DISSECTION

Clean the mastoid temporal bone off all the muscles and identify suprameatal triangle and supra-mastoid crest. Use a fine chisel to remove the bone of the triangle till the mastoid antrum is reached. Examine the extent of mastoid air cells.

Remove the posterior and superior walls of external auditory meatus till the level of the roof of mastoid antrum. Identify the chorda tympani nerve at the posterosuperior margin of tympanic membrane.

Look for arcuate eminence on the anterior face of petrous temporal bone. Identify internal acoustic meatus on the posterior face of petrous temporal bone, with the nerves in it. Try to break off the superior part of petrous temporal bone above the internal acoustic meatus. Identify the facial nerve as it passes towards the aditus. Identify the sharp bend of the facial nerve with the geniculate ganglion.

Identify the facial nerve turning posteriorly into the medial wall. Trace it above the fenestra vestibuli till it turns inferiorly in the medial wall of aditus.

Identify facial nerve at the stylomastoid foramen. Try to break the bone vertically along the lateral edge of the foramen to expose the whole of facial nerve canal. Facial nerve is described in detail in Chapter 9. Revise it from there.

Break off more of the superior surface of the petrous temporal bone. Remove the bone gently. Examine the holes in the bone produced by semicircular canals and look for the semicircular ducts lying within these canals. Note the branches of vestibulocochlear nerve entering the bone at the lateral end of the meatus. Study the internal ear from the models of the museum.

Mastoid Air Cells

Mastoid air cells are a series of intercommunicating spaces of variable size present within the mastoid process. Their number varies considerably. Sometimes there are just a few, and are confined to the upper part of the mastoid process. Occasionally, they may extend beyond the mastoid process into the squamous or petrous parts of the temporal bone.

Vessels, Lymphatics and Nerves

The mastoid antrum and air cells are supplied by the *posterior tympanic artery* derived from the stylomastoid branch of the posterior auricular artery. The *veins* drain into the mastoid emissary vein, the posterior auricular vein and the sigmoid sinus. *Lymphatics* pass to the postauricular and upper deep cervical lymph nodes. *Nerves* are derived from the tympanic plexus formed by the glossopharyngeal nerve and from the meningeal branch of the mandibular nerve.

CLINICAL ANATOMY

Mastoid infection is secondary to otitis media. It is difficult to treat. A proper drainage of pus from the mastoid requires on operation through the suprameatal triangle. The facial nerve can be injured during this operation.

Infection from the mastoid antrum and air cells can spread to any of the structures related to them including the temporal lobe of the cerebrum, the cerebellum, and the sigmoid sinus.

INTERNAL EAR

The internal ear, or labyrinth, lies in the petrous part of the temporal bone. It consists of the bony labyrinth within which there is a membranous labyrinth. The membranous labyrinth is filled with a fluid called endolymph. It is separated from the bony labyrinth by another fluid called the perilymph.

Bony Labyrinth

The bony labyrinth consists of three parts: (a) The cochlea anteriorly; (b) the vestibule, in the middle; and (c) the semicircular canals posteriorly (Fig. 18.14).

Cochlea

The bony cochlea resembles the shell of a common snail. It forms the anterior part of the labyrinth. It has a conical central axis known as the *modiolus* around which the cochlear canal makes two and three quarter turns. The modiolus is directed forwards and laterally. Its apex points towards the anterosuperior part of the medial wall of the middle ear and the base towards the fundus of the internal acoustic meatus. A spiral ridge of the bone, the *spiral lamina*, projects from the modiolus and partially divides the cochlear canal into the scala vestibuli above, and the scala tympani below. These relationships apply to the lowest part or basal turn of the cochlea. The division between the two passages is completed by the basilar membrane. The scala vestibuli communicates with the scala tympani at the apex of the cochlea by a small opening, called the *helicotrema*.

Vestibule

This is the central part of the bony labyrinth. It lies medial to the middle ear cavity. Its lateral wall opens into the middle ear at the fenestra vestibuli which is closed by the footplate of the stapes. Three semicircular canals open into its posterior wall. The medial wall is related to the internal acoustic meatus, and presents the *spherical recess* in front, and the

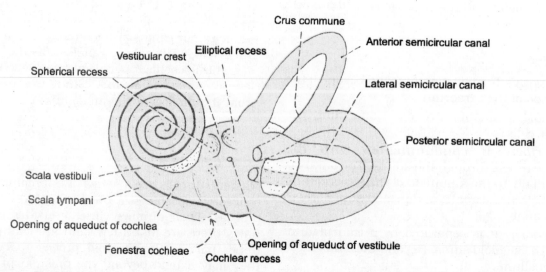

Fig. 18.14: *Scheme to the show some features of the bony labyrinth (seen from the lateral side).*

elliptical recess behind. The two recesses are separated by a *vestibular crest* which splits inferiorly to enclose the *cochlear recess* (Fig. 18.14). Just below the elliptical recess there is the opening of a diverticulum, the aqueduct of the vestibule which opens at a narrow fissure on the posterior aspect of the petrous temporal bone, posterolateral to the internal acoustic meatus. It is plugged in life by the ductus endolymphaticus and a vein; no perilymph escapes through it.

Semicircular Canals

There are three bony semicircular canals: An anterior or superior, posterior and lateral. They lie posterosuperior to the vestibule, and are set at right angles to each other. Each canal describes two-thirds of a circle, and is dilated at one end to form the *ampulla*. Three canals open into the vestibule by five openings.

The *anterior* or *superior semicircular canal* lies in a vertical plane at right angles to the long axis of the petrous temporal bone. It is convex upwards. Its position is indicated by the arcuate eminence seen on the anterior surface of the petrous temporal bone. Its ampulla is situated anterolaterally. Its posterior end unites with the upper end of the posterior canal to form the crus commune which opens into the medial wall of the vestibule.

The *posterior semicircular canal* also lies in a vertical plane parallel to the long axis of the petrous temporal bone. It is convex backwards. Its ampulla lies at its lower end. The upper end joins the anterior canal to form the crus commune.

The *lateral semicircular canal* lies in the horizontal plane with its convexity directed posterolaterally. The ampulla lies anteriorly, close to the ampulla of the anterior canal.

Note that the lateral semicircular canals of the two sides lie in the same plane, and that the anterior canal of one side lies in the plane of the posterior canal of the other side (Fig. 18.15).

Membranous Labyrinth

It is in the form of a complicated, but continuous closed cavity filled with endolymph. Parts of the epithelium of the membranous labyrinth are specialized to form receptors for sound organ of Corti, for static balance the maculae, and for kinetic balance the cristae.

Like the bony labyrinth, the membranous labyrinth also consists of three main parts: (a) The spiral duct of the cochlea or organ of hearing, anteriorly; (b) the utricle and saccule the organs of static balance, within the vestibule; and (c) the semicircular ducts the organs of kinetic balance, posteriorly (Fig. 18.16).

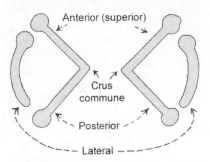

Fig. 18.15: *The semicircular canals. The lateral canals of the two sides lie in the same plane. The anterior canal of one side lies in the plane of the posterior canal of the other side.*

The Duct of the Cochlea or the Scala Media

The spiral duct occupies the middle part of the cochlear canal between the scala vestibuli and the scala tympani. It is triangular in cross-section. The floor is formed by the *basilar membrane;* the roof by the *vestibular* or *Reissner's membrane;* and the outer wall by the bony wall of the cochlea. The basilar membrane supports the spiral *organ of Corti* which is the end organ for hearing (Fig. 18.17). The organ of Corti is innervated by peripheral processes of bipolar cells located in the spiral ganglion. This ganglion is located in the spiral canal present within the modiolus at the base of the spiral lamina. The central processes of the ganglion cells form the cochlear nerve.

Posteriorly the duct of the cochlea is connected to the saccule by a narrow ductus reuniens.

The sound waves reaching the endolymph through the vestibular membrane make appropriate parts of the basilar membrane vibrate, so that different parts of the organ of Corti are stimulated by different frequencies of sound. The loudness of the sound depends on the amplitude of vibration.

Saccule and Utricle

The *saccule* lies in the anteroinferior part of the vestibule, and is connected to the basal turn of the cochlear duct by the ductus reuniens.

The *utricle* is larger than the saccule and lies in the posterosuperior part of the vestibule. It receives three semicircular ducts through five openings. The duct of the saccule unites with the duct of the utricle to form the ductus endolymphaticus. The ductus endolymphaticus ends in a dilatation, the saccus endolymphaticus. The ductus and saccus occupy the aqueduct of the vestibule.

The medial walls of the saccule and utricle are thickened to form a *macula* in each chamber. The maculae are end organs that give information about

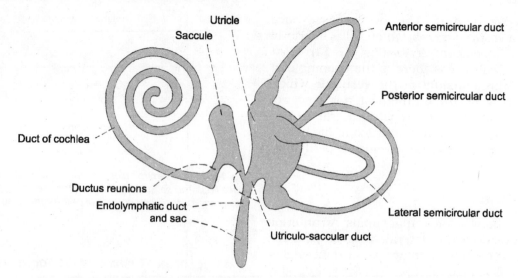

Fig. 18.16: Parts of the membranous labyrinth (as seen from the lateral side).

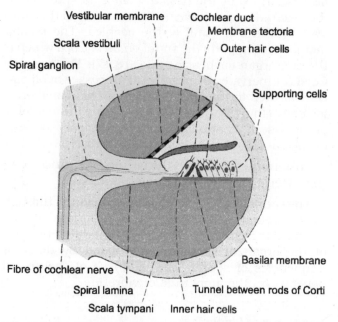

Fig. 18.17: Schematic section through one turn of the cochlea.

the position of the head. They are static balance receptors. They are supplied by peripheral processes of neurons in the vestibular ganglion.

Semicircular Ducts

The three semicircular ducts lie within the corresponding bony canals. Each duct has an ampulla corresponding to that of the bony canal. In each ampulla, there is an end organ called the ampullary crest or crista. Cristae respond to pressure changes in the endolymph caused by movements of the head.

Blood Supply of Labyrinth

The arterial supply is derived mainly from the labyrinthine branch of the basilar artery which accompanies the vestibulocochlear nerve; and partly from the stylomastoid branch of the posterior auricular artery.

The labyrinthine vein drains into the superior petrosal sinus or the transverse sinus. Other inconstant veins emerge at different points and open separately into the superior and inferior petrosal sinuses and the internal jugular vein.

Development

• External auditory meatus: *Dorsal part of 1st ectodermal cleft.*

• Auricle: *Tubercles appearing on 1st and 2nd branchial arches around the opening of external auditory meatus.*

• Middle ear cavity and auditory tube: *Tubotympanic recess* (Table 1.5).

Ossicles

• Malleus and incus: From *1st arch cartilage;*

• Stapes: From *2nd arch cartilage.*

Muscles:

• Tensor tympani: From *1st pharyngeal arch mesoderm*

• Stapedius: From *2nd pharyngeal arch mesoderm*

Internal Ear

Membranous labyrinth from ectodermal vesicle on each side of hind brain vesicle. Organ of Corti - ectodermal.

VESTIBULOCOCHLEAR NERVE
(Stato-acoustic or Auditory Nerve)

Vestibulocochlear is the eighth cranial nerve which has two distinct parts, a cochlear part concerned with hearing (Fig. 18.17), and a vestibular part concerned with equilibrium. Both parts contain special somatic afferent nerve fibres.

Nuclei

Of the cochlear nerve: The dorsal and ventral cochlear nuclei are situated in relation to the inferior cerebellar peduncle.

Of the vestibular nerve: The four vestibular nuclei, superior, inferior, medial and lateral, are situated partly in the medulla and partly in the pons in relation to the floor of the fourth ventricle.

Cochlear Nerve

1. The auditory receptors are the hair cells of the organ of Corti, situated in the cochlear duct of the internal ear.

2. They are innervated by peripheral processes of bipolar neurons of the spiral ganglion which are situated in a canal within the modiolus near the base of the spiral lamina. The central processes of these neurons form the cochlear nerve which ends in the dorsal and ventral cochlear nuclei.

The auditory pathway is described in Chapter 30.

Vestibular Nerve

The vestibular receptors are the maculae of the saccule and utricle, for static balance and the cristae of the ampullae of semicircular ducts, for kinetic balance. They are innervated by peripheral processes of bipolar neurons of the vestibular ganglion. This ganglion is situated in the internal acoustic meatus. The central processes of these neurons form the vestibular nerve which ends in the vestibular nuclei.

The related pathways are described in Chapter 30.

CLINICAL ANATOMY

Lesions of cochlear nerve cause hearing defects. Hearing power can be tested by means of a watch in one ear at a time. If there is any impairment of hearing one must determine whether it is really due to disease of the nerve, i.e. nerve deafness, or merely due to disease of the middle ear, i.e. conductive deafness. This is done by Rinne's test and Weber's test. The tests are based on the principle that normally aerial conduction of sound is better than bony conduction. In conductive deafness, bony conduction becomes better than aerial conduction. In nerve deafness, both types of conduction are lost.

In *Rinne's test*, a vibrating tuning fork is held opposite the ear and then placed on the mastoid process. The patient is asked to compare the relative loudness of the fork in the two instances.

In *Weber's test*, the vibrating tuning fork is placed on the centre of the forehead. The fork is heard better on the side of middle ear disease than on the normal side.

The Eyeball

Sense of sight appreciated through retina of the eyeball is one of the five special senses. Its importance is obvious in the varied ways of natural protection. Bony orbit, projecting nose and various coats protect the precious retina. Each and every component of its three coats is assisting the retina to focus the light properly. Lots of advances have been made in correcting the defects of the eye. Eyes can be donated at the time of death, and "will" can be prepared accordingly.

Eye sees the outside world. The inside of the eyeball can be seen through the ophthalmoscope whereby health of small vessels can be visualised in normal subjects, in diabetics and in hypertensive individuals. About 75% of afferents reach the brain through the eyes. Adequate rest to eye muscles is important. Could a good place for rest be the "classroom" where palpebral part of orbicularis oculi closes the eyes gently?

Introduction

The eyeball is the organ of sight. The camera closely resembles the eyeball in its structure. It is almost spherical in shape and has a diameter of about 2.5 cm. It is made up of three concentric coats. The outer or *fibrous coat* comprises the sclera and the cornea. The middle or *vascular coat* also called the uveal tract consists of the choroid, the ciliary body and the iris. The inner or *nervous coat* is the retina (Fig. 19.1).

Light entering the eyeball passes through several *refracting media*. From before backwards these are the cornea, the aqueous humour, the lens and the vitreous body.

THE OUTER COAT

Sclera

The sclera (*skleros*=hard) is opaque and forms the posterior five-sixths of the eyeball. It is composed of

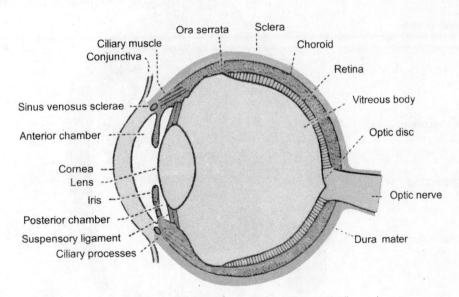

Fig. 19.1: *Sagittal section through the eyeball.*

dense fibrous tissue which is firm and maintains the shape of the eyeball. It is thickest behind, near the entrance of the optic nerve, and thinnest about 6 mm behind the sclerocorneal junction where the recti muscles are inserted. However, it is weakest at the entrance of the optic nerve. Here the sclera shows numerous perforations for passage of fibres of the optic nerve. Because of its sieve-like appearance this region is called the *lamina cribrosa* (*crib*=sieve).

DISSECTION

Use the fresh eyeball of the goats for this dissection. Clean the eyeball by removing all the tissues from its surface. Cut through the fascial sheath around the margin of the cornea. Clean and identify the nerve with posterior ciliary arteries and ciliary nerves close to the posterior pole of the eyeball. Identify venae vorticosae piercing the sclera just behind the equator.

Incise only the sclera at the equator and then cut through it all around and carefully strip it off from the choroid. Anteriorly, the ciliary muscles are attached to the sclera, offering some resistance. As the sclera is steadily separated the aqueous humour will escape from the anterior chamber of the eye. On dividing the optic nerve fibres the posterior part of sclera can be removed.

The *outer surface* of the sclera is white and smooth, it is covered by Tenon's capsule (Fig. 7.3). Its anterior part is covered by conjunctiva through which it can be seen as the white of the eye. The *inner surface* is brown and grooved for the ciliary nerves and vessels. It is separated from the choroid by the *perichoroidal space* which contains a delicate cellular tissue, termed the *suprachoroidal lamina* or *lamina fusca of the sclera*.

The sclera is continuous anteriorly with the cornea at the *sclerocorneal junction or limbus* (Fig. 19.1). The deep part of the limbus contains a circular canal, known as the *sinus venosus sclerae or the canal of Schlemm*. The aqueous humour drains into the anterior scleral or ciliary veins through this sinus.

The sclera is fused posteriorly with the *dural sheath of the optic nerve*. It provides insertion to the extrinsic muscles of the eyeball: The recti in front of the equator, and the oblique muscles behind the equator.

The sclera is pierced by a number of structures: (a) The *optic nerve* pierces it a little inferomedial to the posterior pole of the eyeball. (b) The *ciliary nerves and arteries* pierce it around the entrance of the optic nerve. (c) The *anterior ciliary arteries* derived from muscular arteries to the recti pierce it near the limbus. (d) Four *venae vorticosae* or the choroid veins pass out through the sclera just behind the equator (Figs 19.2, 19.3).

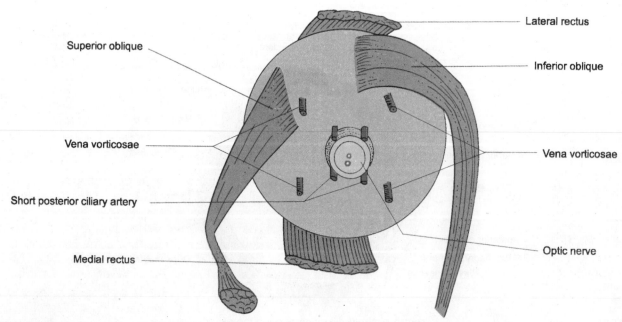

Fig. 19.2: *Structures piercing the posterior aspect of the eyeball.*

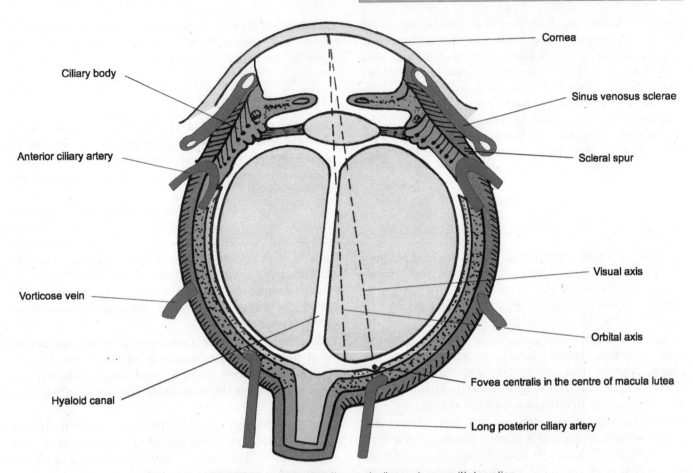

Fig. 19.3: *Structures piercing the eyeball seen in a sagittal section.*

The sclera is almost avascular. However, the loose connective tissue between the conjunctiva and sclera called as the *episclera* is vascular.

Cornea

The cornea is transparent. It replaces the sclera over the anterior one sixth of the eyeball. Its junction with the sclera is called the *sclerocorneal junction or limbus.*

DISSECTION

Identify the cornea. Make an incision around the corneoscleral junction and remove the cornea so that the iris is exposed for examination. Identify the choroid, ciliary body and iris deep to the sclera. Lateral to iris is the ciliary body with ciliary muscles and ciliary processes.

Strip off the iris, ciliary processes, anterior part of choroid. Remove the lens and put it in water. As the lens is removed the vitreous body also escapes. Only the posterior part of choroid and subjacent retina is left.

The cornea is more convex than the sclera, but the curvature diminishes with age. It is separated from the iris by a space called the anterior chamber of the eye.

The cornea is avascular and is nourished by lymph which circulates in the numerous corneal spaces.

It is supplied by branches of the ophthalmic nerve (through the ciliary ganglion) and the short ciliary nerves. Pain is the only sensation aroused from the cornea (Fig. 7.15).

Histology

Structurally, the cornea consists of these layers, from before backwards: (a) *Corneal epithelium* (stratified squamous nonkeratinized type) is continuous with that of the conjunctiva. (b) *Bowman's membrane* (anterior elastic lamina) is a structureless homogenous layer. It contains no elastic fibres. (c) The *substantia propria* consists of bundles of dense collagen fibres separated by corneal spaces. Each bundle contains parallel fibres, and alternate bundles cross at right angles. Corneal corpuscles which are modified fibroblasts lie between the bundles. (d) *Descemet's membrane* or posterior elastic lamina is also structureless and homogenous, but contains elastic fibres. At the peripheral margin its fibres divide into 3 groups. The inner fibres turn medially on to the iris and constitute the ligamentum pectinatum. The middle fibres give origin to the ciliary muscle. The outer fibres are continuous with the sclera. (e) Simple squamous *mesothelium* lines the posterior surface of the cornea (Fig. 19.4).

THE MIDDLE COAT

Choroid

Choroid is a thin pigmented layer which separates the posterior part of the sclera from the retina. Anteriorly, it ends at the ora serrata by merging with the ciliary body. Posteriorly, it is perforated by the optic nerve to which it is firmly attached.

Its *outer surface* is separated from the sclera by the suprachoroidal lamina which is traversed by the ciliary vessels and nerves. Its attachment to the sclera is loose, so that it can be easily stripped. The *inner surface* is firmly united to the retina.

Structurally, it consists of: (a) Suprachoroidal lamina made of collagen fibres, elastic fibres and pigment cells. *(b) Vascular lamina* composed of arteries and short posterior ciliary veins, the latter being arranged in the form of whorls which converge to form 4 to 5 venae vorticosae, loose areolar tissue, and pigment cells. (c) The *choriocapillary lamina* forms the most prominent feature of the choroid. It nourishes the rods and cones of the retina by diffusion. (d) The inner *basal lamina* or lamina vitrea or membrane of

Bruch is a thin structureless transparent membrane which is firmly adherent to the outer, pigmented layer of the retina (Fig. 19.5).

Ciliary Body

Ciliary body is a thickened part of the uveal tract lying just posterior to the corneal limbus. It is continuous anteriorly with the iris and posteriorly with the choroid. It suspends the lens and helps it in accommodation for near vision.

1. The ciliary body is triangular in cross-section. It is thick in front and thin behind (Fig. 19.6). The scleral surface of this body contains the ciliary muscle. The posterior part of the vitreous surface is smooth and black (pars plana). The anterior part is ridged anteriorly (pars plicata) to form about 70 ciliary processes. The central ends of the processes are free and rounded.

2. Ciliary zonule is thickened vitreous membrane fitted to the posterior surfaces of ciliary processes. The posterior layer lines hyaloid fossa and anterior thick layer forms the suspensory ligament of the lens (Fig. 19.7).

3. The *ciliary muscle* (Fig. 19.8) is a ring of unstriped muscle which are longitudinal or meridional, radial and circular. The longitudinal or meridional fibres arise from a projection of sclera or scleral spur near the limbus. They radiate backwards to the suprachoroidal lamina. The radial fibres are obliquely placed and get continuous with the circular fibres. The circular fibres lie within the anterior part of the ciliary body and are nearest to the lens. The contraction of all the parts relaxes the suspensory

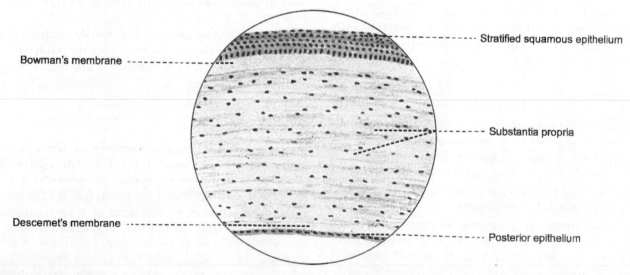

Bowman's membrane

Stratified squamous epithelium

Substantia propria

Descemet's membrane

Posterior epithelium

Fig. 19.4: *Histological structure of the cornea (Courtesy: Garg, Bahl and Kaul: A Text Book of Histology, 3rd edition, CBS Publishers and Distributors, New Delhi).*

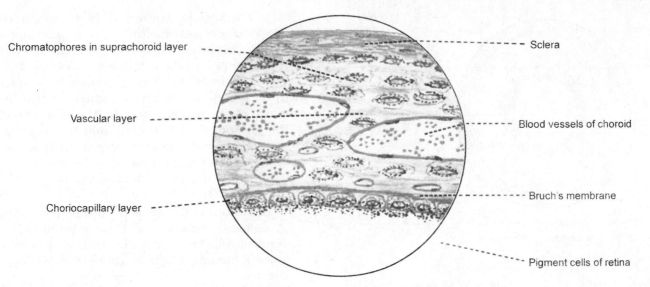

Fig. 19.5: *Histological structure of the choroid (Courtesy: Garg, Bahl and Kaul: A Text Book of Histology, 3rd edition, CBS Publishers and Distributors, New Delhi).*

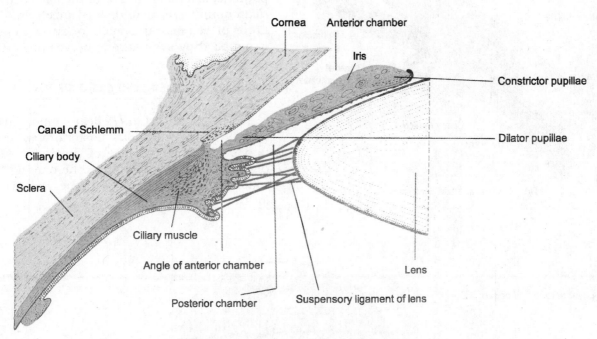

Fig. 19.6: *Components of ciliary body and iris.*

ligament so that the lens becomes more convex. All parts of the muscle are supplied by parasympathetic nerves. The pathway involves the Edinger-Westphal nucleus, oculomotor nerve and the **ciliary ganglion** (Fig. 7.12).

Iris

1. This is the anterior part of the uveal tract. It forms a circular curtain with an opening in the centre, called the *pupil*. By adjusting the size of the pupil it controls the amount of light entering the eye, and thus behaves like an adjustable diaphragm (Fig. 19.6).

2. It is placed vertically between the cornea and the lens, thus divides the anterior segment of the eye into anterior and posterior chambers, both containing aqueous humour. Its *peripheral margin* is attached to the middle of the anterior surface of the ciliary body and is separated from the cornea by the iridocorneal angle or angle of the anterior chamber. The *central free margin* forming the boundary of the pupil rests against the lens.

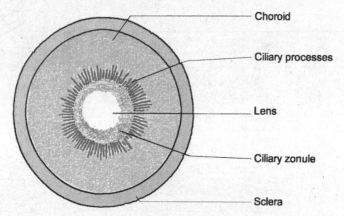

Fig. 19.7: *Anterior part of the inner aspect of the eyeball seen after vitreous has been removed.*

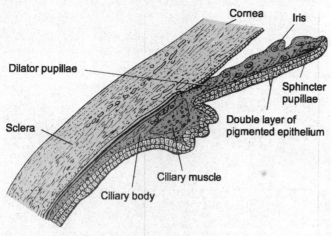

Fig. 19.8: *Epithelium lining the iris.*

3. The anterior surface of the iris is covered by a single layer of mesothelium, and the posterior surface by a double layer of deeply pigmented cells which are continuous with those of the ciliary body (Fig. 19.8). The main bulk of the iris is formed by stroma made up of blood vessels and loose connective tissue in which there are pigment cells. The long posterior and the anterior ciliary arteries join to form the *major arterial circle* at the periphery of the iris. From this circle vessels converge towards the free margin of the iris and join together to form the *minor arterial circle* of the iris (Fig. 7.9).

The colour of the iris is determined by the number of pigment cells in its connective tissue. If the pigment cells are absent, the iris is blue in colour due to the diffusion of light in front of the black posterior surface.

4. The iris contains a well-developed ring of muscle called the *sphincter pupillae* which lies near the margin of the pupil. Its nerve supply (parasympathetic) is similar to that of the ciliary muscle. The *dilator pupillae* is an ill-defined sheet of radial muscle fibres placed near the posterior surface of the iris. It is supplied by sympathetic nerves (Fig. 19.6).

THE INNER COAT/RETINA

1. This is the thin, delicate inner layer of the eyeball. It is continuous posteriorly with the optic nerve. The outer surface of the retina (formed by pigment cells) is attached to the choroid, while the inner surface is in contact with the hyaloid membrane (of the vitreous).

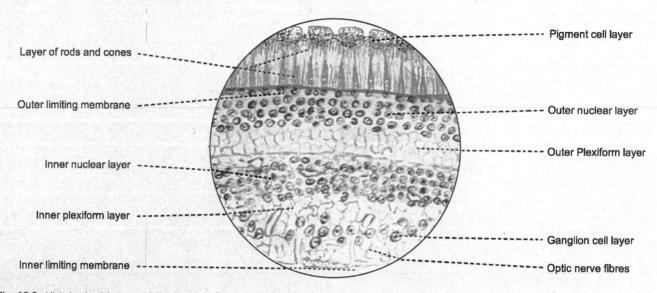

Fig. 19.9: *Histological layers of the retina (Courtesy: Garg, Bahl and Kaul: A Text Book of Histology, 3rd edition, CBS Publishers and Distributors, New Delhi).*

Opposite the entrance of the optic nerve (inferomedial to the posterior pole) there is a circular area known as the *optic disc.* It is 1.5 mm in diameter.

2. The retina diminishes in thickness from behind forwards and is divided into optic, ciliary and iridial parts. The *optic part of the retina* contains nervous tissue and is sensitive to light. It extends from the optic disc to the posterior end of the ciliary body. The anterior margin of the optic part of the retina forms a wavy line called the ora serrata (Fig. 19.1).

Beyond the ora serrata the retina is continued forwards as a thin, non-nervous insensitive layer that covers the ciliary body and iris, forming the *ciliary and iridial parts of the retina.* These parts are made up of two layers of epithelial cells (Fig. 19.8).

3. The depressed area of the optic disc is called the *physiological cup.* It contains no rods or cones and is therefore insensitive to light, i.e. it is the *physio-logical blind spot.* At the posterior pole of the eye 3 mm lateral to the optic disc there is another depression of similar size, called the *macula lutea.* It is avascular and yellow in colour. The centre of the macula is further depressed to form the *fovea centralis.* This is the thinnest part of the retina. It contains cones only, and is the site of maximum acuity of vision (Fig. 19.3).

4. The rods and cones are the light receptors of the eye. The *rods* contain a pigment called *visual purple.* They can respond to dim light (*scotopic vision*). The periphery of the retina contains only rods, but the fovea has none at all. The *cones* respond only to bright light (*photopic vision*) and are sensitive to colour. The fovea centralis has only cones. Their number diminishes towards the periphery of the retina.

5. The retina is composed of ten layers: (a) The outer pigmented layer; (b) layer of rods and cones; (c) external limiting membrane; (d) outer nuclear layer; (e) outer plexiform layer; (f) inner nuclear layer (bipolar cells); (g) inner plexiform layer; (h) ganglion cell layer; (i) nerve fibre layer; and (j) the internal limiting membrane (Fig. 19.9).

In detachment of the retina, the outer pigmented layer remains attached to the choroid, but the remaining layers of the retina separate from the pigmented layer and are displaced inwards.

6. The retina is supplied by the *central artery.* This is an end artery. In the optic disc it divides into an upper and a lower branch, each giving off nasal and temporal branches. The artery supplies the deeper layers of the retina up to the bipolar cells. The rods and cones are supplied by diffusion from the capillaries of the choroid. The retinal veins run with the arteries (Figs 19.10, 7.9).

AQUEOUS HUMOUR

This is a clear fluid which fills the space between the cornea in front and the lens behind the anterior segment. This space is divided by the iris into anterior and posterior chambers which freely communicate with each other through the pupil.

The aqueous humour is secreted into the posterior chamber from the capillaries in the ciliary processes. It passes into the anterior chamber through the pupil. From the anterior chamber it is drained into the anterior ciliary veins through the spaces of the

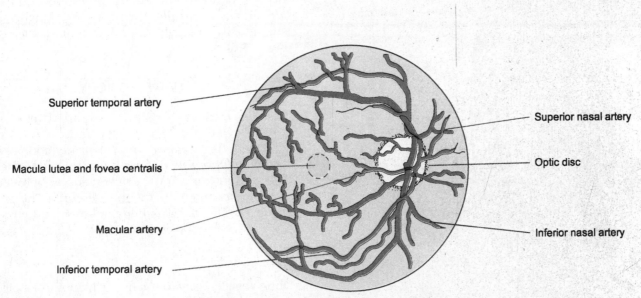

Superior temporal artery

Macula lutea and fovea centralis

Macular artery

Inferior temporal artery

Superior nasal artery

Optic disc

Inferior nasal artery

Fig. 19.10: *Distribution of central artery of the retina.*

iridocorneal angle or angle of anterior chamber (located between the fibres of the ligamentum pectinatum) and the canal of Schlemm (Fig. 19.6).

Interference with the drainage of the aqueous humour into the canal of Schlemm results in an increase of intraocular pressure (glaucoma). This produces cupping of the optic disc and pressure atrophy of the retina causing blindness.

The intraocular pressure is due chiefly to the aqueous humour which maintains the constancy of the optical dimensions of the eyeball. The aqueous is rich in ascorbic acid, glucose and amino acids, and nourishes the avascular tissues of the cornea and lens.

THE LENS

The lens is a transparent biconvex structure which is placed between the anterior and posterior segments of the eye. It is circular in outline and has a diameter of 1 cm. The central points of the anterior and posterior surfaces are called the anterior and posterior *poles* (Fig. 19.11). The line connecting the poles constitutes the *axis* of the lens, while the marginal circumference is termed the *equator*. The chief

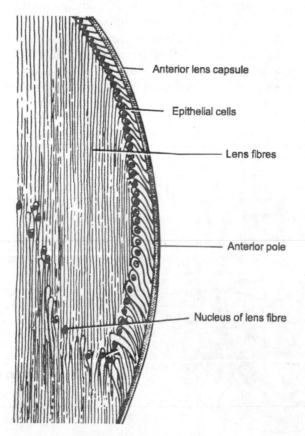

Fig. 19.11: The lens.

advantage of the lens is that it can vary its dioptric power. It contributes about 15 dioptres to the total of 58 dioptric power of the eye (A dioptre is the inverse of the focal length in meters. A lens having a focal length of half meter has a power of two dioptres).

The posterior surface of the lens is more convex than the anterior. The anterior surface is kept flattened by the tension of the suspensory ligament. When the ligament is relaxed by contraction of the ciliary muscle, the anterior surface becomes more convex due to elasticity of the lens substance.

The lens is enclosed in a transparent, structureless elastic *capsule* which is thickest anteriorly near the circumference. Deep to capsule, the anterior surface of the lens is covered by a *capsular epithelium*. At the centre of the anterior surface, the epithelium is made up of a single layer of cubical cells, but at the periphery, the cells elongate to produce the *fibres* of the lens. The fibres are concentrically arranged to form the lens substance. The centre (nucleus) of the lens is firm (and consists of the oldest fibres), whereas the periphery (cortex) is soft and is made up of more recently formed fibres (Fig. 19.11).

The *suspensory ligament of the lens* (or the zonule of Zinn) retains the lens in position and its tension keeps the anterior surface of the lens flattened. The ligament is made up of a series of fibres which are attached peripherally to the ciliary processes, to the furrows between the ciliary processes, and to the ora serrata. Centrally, the fibres are attached to the lens, mostly in front, and a few behind, the equator (Fig. 19.6).

VITREOUS BODY

It is a colourless, jellylike transparent mass which fills the posterior segment (posterior 4/5th) of the eyeball. It is enclosed in a delicate homogeneous *hyaloid membrane*. Behind it is attached to the optic disc, and in front to the ora serrata; in between it is free and lies in contact with the retina. The anterior surface of the vitreous body is indented by the lens and ciliary processes (Fig. 19.1).

Development

Optic vesicle forms optic cup. The optic vesicle is an out pouching from the *forebrain* vesicle.

Lens from *lens placode (ectodermal)*

Retina — pigment layer from the *outer layer of optic cup;* nervous layers from the *inner layer of optic cup.*

Choroid, sclera—*mesoderm*

Cornea—*surface ectoderm*

CLINICAL ANATOMY

Eye is a very sensitive organ and even a dust particle gives rise to pain.

Cornea can be grafted from one person to the other, as it is avascular.

Injury to cornea may cause opacities. These opacities may interfere with vision.

Overproduction of aqueous humour or lack of its drainage or combination of both raise the intraocular pressure. The condition is called glaucoma. It must be treated urgently.

The central artery of retina is an end-artery. Blockage of the artery leads to sudden blindness.

Bulbar conjunctiva is vascular. Inflammation of the conjunctiva leads to conjunctivitis. The look of palpebral conjunctiva is used to judge haemoglobin level.

The anteroposterior diameter of the eyeball and shape and curvature of the cornea determine the focal point. Changes in these result in myopia or short-sightedness, hypermetropia or long-sightedness, astigmation or presbyopia.

Retinal detachment occurs between outer single pigmented layer and inner nine nervous layers. Actually, it is an inter-retinal detachment.

Eye sees everyone. One can see the interior of the eye by ophthalmoscope. Through the ophthalmoscope one can see the small vessels in the retina and judge the changes in diabetes and hypertension. In addition, one can also examine the optic disc for evidence of papilloedema, caused by raised intracranial pressure.

Lens becomes opaque with increasing age. Since the opacities cause difficulty in vision, lens has to be replaced.

20

Surface Marking, Radiology and Imaging Anatomy

The bony and soft tissue landmarks on the head, face and neck help in surface marking of various structures. These landmarks are of immense value to the clinician for locating the part to be examined or to be operated.

SURFACE LANDMARKS

Landmarks on the Face

Some important named features to be identified on the living face have been described on page 45. Other landmarks are as follows.

1. The *supraorbital margin* lies beneath the upper margin of the eyebrow. The *supraorbital notch* is palpable at the junction of the medial one-third with the lateral two-thirds of the supraorbital margin (except in those cases in which the notch is converted into a foramen). A vertical line drawn from the supraorbital notch to the base of the mandible, passing midway between the lower two premolar teeth, crosses the infraorbital foramen 5 mm below the infraorbital margin, and the mental foramen midway between the upper and lower borders of the mandible (Fig. 1.5).

2. The *superciliary arch* is a curved bony ridge situated immediately above the medial part of each supraorbital margin. The *glabella* is the median elevation connecting the two superciliary arches, and corresponds to the elevation between the two eyebrows.

3. The *nasion* is the point where the internasal and frontonasal sutures meet. It lies a little above the floor of the depression at the root of the nose, below the glabella (Fig. 1.5).

Landmarks on the Lateral Side of the Head

The external ear or pinna is a prominent feature on the lateral aspect of the head. The named features on the pinna are shown in Fig. 18.1. Other landmarks on the lateral side of the head are as follows.

1. The *zygomatic bone* forms the prominence of the cheek at the inferolateral corner of the orbit. The *zygomatic arch* bridges the gap between the eye and the ear. It is formed anteriorly by the temporal process of the zygomatic bone, and posteriorly by the zygomatic process (zygoma) of the temporal bone. The *preauricular point* lies on the posterior root of the zygoma immediately in front of the upper part of the tragus (Fig. 1.8).

2. The head of the mandible lies in front of the tragus. It is felt best during movements of the lower jaw. The *coronoid process* of the mandible can be felt below the lowest part of the zygomatic bone when the mouth is opened. The process can be traced downwards into the anterior border of the *ramus* of the mandible. The posterior border of the ramus, though masked by the parotid gland, can be felt through the skin. The outer surface of the ramus is covered by the masseter which can be felt when the teeth are clenched. The lower border of the mandible can be traced posteriorly into the *angle* of the mandible (Fig. 1.8).

3. The *parietal eminence* is the most prominent part of the parietal bone, situated far above and a little behind the auricle.

4. The *mastoid process* is a large bony prominence situated behind the lower part of the auricle. The *supramastoid crest*, about 2.5 cm long, begins immediately above the external acoustic meatus and soon curves upwards and backwards. The crest is continuous anteriorly with the posterior root of the zygoma, and posterosuperiorly with the temporal line (Fig. 1.8).

5. The *temporal line* forms the upper boundary of the temporal fossa which is filled up by the temporalis muscle. The upper margin of the contracting temporalis helps in defining this line

which begins at the zygomatic process of the frontal bone, arches posterosuperiorly across the coronal suture, passes a little below the parietal eminence, and turns downwards to become continuous with the supramastoid crest. The area of the temporal fossa on the side of the head, above the zygomatic arch, is called the *temple* or temporal region (Fig. 1.8).

6. The *pterion* is the area in the temporal fossa where four bones (frontal, parietal, temporal and sphenoid) adjoin each other across an H-shaped suture. The centre of the pterion is marked by a point 4 cm above the midpoint of the zygomatic arch, falling 3.5 cm behind the frontozygomatic suture. Deep to the pterion lie the anterior branch of the middle meningeal artery, the middle meningeal vein, and deeper still the stem of the lateral sulcus of the cerebral hemisphere (at the *Sylvian point*) dividing into three rami. The pterion is a common site for trephining (making a hole in) the skull during operation (Fig. 1.9).

7. The junction of the back of the head with the neck is indicated by the external occipital protuberance and the superior nuchal lines. The *external occipital protuberance* is a bony projection felt in the median plane on the back of the head at the upper end of the nuchal furrow. The *superior nuchal lines* are indistinct curved ridges which extend from the protuberance to the mastoid processes. The back of the head is called the *occiput*. The most prominent median point situated on the external occipital protuberance is known as the *inion*. However, the posteriormost point on the occiput lies a little above the protuberance (Fig. 1.3).

Landmarks on the Side of the Neck

1. The *sternocleidomastoid* muscle is seen prominently when the face is turned to the opposite side. The ridge raised by the muscle extends from the sternum to the mastoid process (Fig. 3.1).

2. The *external jugular vein* crosses the sternocleidomastoid obliquely, running downwards and backwards from near the auricle to the clavicle. It is better seen in old age (Fig. 3.6).

3. The *greater supraclavicular fossa* lies above and behind the middle one-third of the clavicle. It overlies the cervical part of the brachial plexus and the third part of the subclavian artery (Fig. 3.5).

4. The *lesser supraclavicular fossa* is a small depression between the sternal and clavicular parts of the sternocleidomastoid. It overlies the internal jugular vein.

5. The *mastoid process* is a large bony projection behind the auricle (concha) (Fig. 3.1).

6. The *transverse process of the atlas vertebra* can be felt on deep pressure midway between the angle of the mandible and the mastoid process, immediately anteroinferior to the tip of the mastoid process. The *fourth cervical transverse process* is just palpable at the level of the upper border of the thyroid cartilage; and the *sixth cervical transverse process* at the level of the cricoid cartilage. The anterior tubercle of the *transverse process of the sixth cervical vertebra* is the largest of all such processes and is called the *carotid tubercle* (of Chassaignac). The common carotid artery can be best pressed against this tubercle, deep to the anterior border of the sternocleidomastoid muscle.

7. The *anterior border of the trapezius muscle* becomes prominent on elevation of the shoulder against resistance (Fig. 3.5).

Landmarks on the Anterior Aspect of the Neck

1. The *mandible* forms the lower jaw. The lower border of its horseshoe-shaped body is known as the *base of the mandible* (Fig. 1.26). Anteriorly, this base forms the *chin*, and posteriorly it can be traced to the *angle of the mandible* (Fig. 1.26).

2. The body of the U-shaped *hyoid bone* can be felt in the median plane just below and behind the chin, at the junction of the neck with the floor of the mouth. On each side the body of hyoid bone is continuous posteriorly with the *greater cornua* which is overlapped in its posterior part by the sterno-cleidomastoid muscle (Fig. 8.6).

3. The *thyroid cartilage* of the larynx forms a sharp protuberance in the median plane just below the hyoid bone. This protuberance is called the *laryngeal prominence or Adam's apple*. It is more prominent in males than in females (Fig. 8.10).

4. The rounded arch of the *cricoid cartilage* lies below the thyroid cartilage at the upper end of the trachea (Fig. 8.6).

5. The trachea runs downwards and backwards from the cricoid cartilage. It is identified by its cartilagineous rings. However, it is partially masked by the *isthmus of the thyroid gland* which lies against the second to fourth tracheal rings. The trachea is commonly palpated in the *suprasternal notch* which lies between the tendinous heads of origin of the right and left sternocleidomastoid muscles. In certain diseases, the trachea may shift to one side from the median plane. This indicates a shift in the mediastinum (Fig. 8.6).

Other Important Landmarks

1. The *frontozygomatic suture* can be felt as a slight depression in the upper part of the lateral orbital margin.

2. The *marginal tubercle* lies a short distance below the frontozygomatic suture along the posterior border of the frontal process of the zygomatic bone.

3. The *Frankfurt plane* is represented by a horizontal line joining the infraorbital margin to the centre of the external acoustic meatus. Posteriorly, the line passes through a point just below the external occipital protuberance.

4. The *jugal point* is the anterior end of the upper border of the zygomatic arch where it meets the frontal process of the zygomatic bone.

5. The *mandibular notch* is represented by a curved line concave upwards, extending from the head of the mandible to the anterior end of the zygomatic arch. The notch is 1–2 cm deep.

SURFACE MARKING OF VARIOUS STRUCTURES

Arteries

1. Facial Artery

It is marked on the face by joining these three points.
  a. A point on the base of the mandible at the anterior border of the masseter muscle.
  b. A second point 1.2 cm lateral to the angle of the mouth.
  c. A point at the medial angle of the eye.

The artery is tortuous in its course and is more so between the first two points (Fig. 1.9).

2. Common Carotid Artery

It is marked by a broad line along the anterior border of the sternocleidomastoid muscle by joining the following two points.
  a. A point on the sternoclavicular joint.
  b. A second point on the anterior border of the sternocleidomastoid muscle at the level of the upper border of the thyroid cartilage.

The thoracic part of the left common carotid artery is marked by a broad line extending from a point a little to the left of the centre of the manubrium to the left sternoclavicular joint (Fig. 12.10).

3. Internal Carotid Artery

It is marked by a broad line joining these two points.
  a. A point on the anterior border of the sternocleidomastoid muscle at the level of the upper border of the thyroid cartilage.
  b. A second point on the posterior border of the condyle of the mandible.

4. External Carotid Artery

The artery is marked by joining these two points.
  a. A point on the anterior border of the sternocleidomastoid muscle at the level of the upper border of the thyroid cartilage.
  b. A second point on the posterior border of the neck of the mandible.

The artery is slightly convex forwards in its lower half and slightly concave forwards in its upper half (Fig. 12.10).

5. Subclavian Artery

It is marked by a broad curved line, convex upwards, by joining these two points.
  a. A point on the sternoclavicular joint.
  b. A second point at the middle of the lower border of the clavicle.

The artery rises about 2 cm above the clavicle.

The thoracic part of the left subclavian artery is marked by a broad vertical line along the left border of the manubrium a little to the left of the left common carotid artery (Fig. 12.10).

6. Middle Meningeal Artery

It is marked by joining these points.
  a. A point immediately above the middle of the zygoma. The artery enters the skull opposite this point.
  b. A second point 2 cm above the first point. The artery divides deep to this point.
  c. A third point (centre of pterion) 3.5 cm behind and 1.5 cm above the frontozygomatic suture.
  d. A fourth point midway between the nasion and inion.
  e. A fifth point (lambda) 6 cm above the external occipital protuberance.

The line joining points a and b represents the stem of the middle meningeal artery inside the skull.

The line joining points b, c and d represents the anterior (frontal) branch. It first runs upwards and forwards (b-c) and then upwards and backwards, towards the point 'd'.

The line joining points b and e represents the posterior (parietal) branch. It runs backwards and upwards, towards the point 'e' (Fig. 1.9).

Veins

1. Facial Vein

It is represented by a line drawn just behind the facial artery.

2. External Jugular Vein

The vein is usually visible through the skin and can be made more prominent by blowing with the mouth and nostrils closed.

It can be marked, if not visible, by joining these points.

a. The first point a little below and behind the angle of the mandible.
b. The second point on the clavicle just lateral to the posterior border of the sternocleido-mastoid (Fig. 3.6).

3. Internal Jugular Vein

Internal jugular vein is marked by a broad line by joining these two points.

a. The first point on the neck medial to the lobule of the ear.
b. The second point at the medial end of the clavicle.

The lower bulb of the vein lies beneath the lesser supraclavicular fossa between the sternal and clavicular heads of the sternocleidomastoid muscle.

4. Subclavian Vein

Subclavian vein is represented by a broad line along the clavicle extending from a little medial to its midpoint to the medial end of the bone.

5. Superior Sagittal Sinus

Superior sagittal sinus is marked by two lines (diverging posteriorly) joining these two points.

a. One point at the glabella.
b. Two points at the inion, situated side by side, 1.2 cm apart (Fig. 6.9).

6. Transverse Sinus

Transverse sinus is marked by two parallel lines, 1.2 cm apart extending between the following two points.

a. Two points at the inion, situated one above the other and 1.2 cm apart.
b. Two points at the base of the mastoid process, situated one in front of the other and 1.2 cm apart.

The sinus is convex upwards, reaching 2 cm above Reid's base line (Fig. 6.9).

7. Sigmoid Sinus

Sigmoid sinus is marked by two parallel lines situated 1.2 cm apart and extending between these two points.

a. Two points at the base of the mastoid process, situated one in front of the other and 1.2 cm apart.
b. Two similar points near the posterior border and 1.2 cm above the tip of the mastoid process.

Nerves

1. Facial Nerve

Facial nerve is marked by a short horizontal line joining these two points.

a. A point at the middle of the anterior border of the mastoid process. The stylomastoid foramen lies 2 cm deep to this point.
b. A second point behind the neck of the mandible. Here the nerve divides into its five branches to the facial muscles (Fig. 9.5C, 10.13).

2. Auriculotemporal Nerve

Auriculotemporal nerve is marked by a line drawn first backwards from the posterior part of the mandibular notch (site of mandibular nerve) across the neck of the mandible, and then upwards across the preauricular point (Fig. 10.13).

3. Mandibular Nerve

Mandibular nerve is marked by a short vertical line in the posterior part of the mandibular notch just in front of the head of the mandible.

4. Lingual and Inferior Alveolar Nerves

Lingual nerve is marked by a curved line running downwards and forwards by joining these points (Fig. 10.13).

a. The first point on the posterior part of the mandibular notch, in line with the mandibular nerve.
b. The second point a little below and behind the last lower molar tooth.
c. The third point opposite the first lower molar tooth.

The concavity in the course of the nerve is more marked between the points b and c and is directed upwards.

Inferior alveolar nerve lies a little below and parallel to the lingual nerve.

5. Glossopharyngeal Nerve

Glossopharyngeal nerve is marked by joining the following points.

a. The first point on the anteroinferior part of the tragus.

b. The second point anterosuperior to the angle of the mandible.

From point 'b' the nerve runs forwards for a short distance along the lower border of the mandible. The nerve describes a gentle curve in its course (Fig. 12.20).

6. Vagus Nerve

The nerve runs along the medial side of the internal jugular vagus vein. It is marked by joining these two points.

a. The first point at the anteroinferior part of the tragus.

b. The second point at the medial end of the clavicle (Fig. 12.20).

7. Accessory Nerve (Spinal Part)

Accessory nerve spinal part is marked by joining the following four points.

a. The first point at the anteroinferior part of the tragus.

b. The second point at the tip of the transverse process of the atlas.

c. The third point at the middle of the posterior border of the sternocleidomastoid muscle.

d. The fourth point on the anterior border of the trapezius 6 cm above the clavicle.

8. Hypoglossal Nerve

Hypoglossal nerve is marked by joining these points.

a. The first point at the anteroinferior part of the tragus.

b. The second point posterosuperior to the tip of the greater cornua of the hyoid bone.

c. The third point midway between the angle of the mandible and the symphysis menti.

The nerve describes a gentle curve in its course (Fig. 12.20).

9. Phrenic Nerve

Phrenic nerve is marked by a line joining the following points.

a. A point on the side of the neck at the level of the upper border of the thyroid cartilage and 3.5 cm from the median plane.

b. The second point at the medial end of the clavicle (Fig. 12.25).

10. Cervical Sympathetic Chain

Cervical sympathetic chain is marked by a line joining the following points.

a. A point at the sternoclavicular joint.

b. The second point at the posterior border of the condyle of the mandible.

The *superior cervical ganglion* extends from the transverse process of the atlas to the tip of the greater cornua of the hyoid bone. The *middle cervical ganglion* lies at the level of the cricoid cartilage, and the *inferior cervical ganglion*, at a point 3 cm above the sternoclavicular joint (Fig. 12.25).

11. Trigeminal Ganglion

Trigeminal ganglion lies a little in front of the preauricular point at a depth of about 4.5 cm.

Glands

1. Parotid Gland

Parotid gland is marked by joining these four points with each other.

a. The first point at the upper border of the head of the mandible.

b. The second point just above the centre of the masseter muscle.

c. The third point posteroinferior to the angle of the mandible.

d. The fourth point on the upper part of the anterior border of the mastoid process.

The anterior border of the gland is obtained by joining the points a-b-c; the posterior border, by joining the points c-d; and the superior curved border with its concavity directed upwards and backwards, by joining the points a-d across the lobule of the ear (Fig. 9.3).

2. Parotid Duct

To mark this duct first draw a line joining these two points.

a. One point at the lower border of the tragus.

b. A second point midway between the ala of the nose and the red margin of the upper lip.

The middle-third of this line represents the parotid duct.

3. Thyroid Gland

The isthmus of thyroid gland is marked by two transverse parallel lines (each 1.2 cm long) on the trachea, the upper 1.2 cm and the lower 2.5 cm below the arch of the cricoid cartilage.

Each lobe extends up to the middle of the thyroid cartilage, below to the clavicle, and laterally to be overlapped by the anterior border of the sterno-cleidomastoid muscle. The upper pole of the lobe is pointed, and the lower pole is broad and rounded (Fig. 12.1).

4. Submandibular Gland

The submandibular salivary gland is marked by an oval area over the posterior half of the base of the mandible, including the lower border of the ramus. The areas extends 1.5 cm above the base of the mandible, and below to the greater cornua of the hyoid bone.

Palatine Tonsil

Palatine tonsil is marked by an oval (almond-shaped) area over the masseter just anterosuperior to the angle of the mandible (Fig. 9.3).

Paranasal Sinuses

1. Frontal Sinus

Frontal sinus is marked by a triangular area formed by joining these three points.

a. The first point at the nasion
b. The second point 2.5 cm above the nasion.
c. The third point at the junction of the medial one-third and lateral two-thirds of the supraorbital margin, i.e. at the supraorbital notch.

2. Maxillary Sinus

The roof of maxillary sinus is represented by the inferior orbital margin; the floor, by the alveolus of the maxilla; the base, by the lateral wall of the nose. The apex lies on the zygomatic process of the maxilla.

RADIOLOGICAL ANATOMY

In routine clinical practice, the following X-ray pictures of the skull are commonly used.

1. Lateral view for general survey of the skull.
2. A special posteroanterior view (in Waters' position) to study the paranasal sinuses.
3. Anteroposterior and oblique views for the study of cervical vertebrae.

LATERAL VIEW SKULL (PLAIN SKIAGRAM)

The radiogram is studied systematically as described here.

Cranial Vault

1. *Shape and size:* It is important to be familiar with the normal shape and size of the skull so that abnormalities, like oxycephaly (a type of craniostenosis), hydrocephalus, microcephaly, etc. may be diagnosed.

2. *Structure of cranial bones:* The bones are unilamellar during the first three years of life. Two tables separated by diploe appear during the fourth year, and the differentiation reaches its maximum by about 35 years when diploic veins produce characteristic markings in radiograms. The sites of the external occipital protuberance and frontal bone are normally thicker than the rest of the skull. The squamous temporal and the upper part of the occipital bone are thin.

Generalized thickened bones are found in Paget's disease. Thalassaemia, a congenital haemolytic anaemia, is associated with thickening and a characteristic sun-ray appearance of the skull bones. A localized hyperostosis may be seen over a meningioma. In multiple myeloma and secondary carcinomatous deposits, the skull presents large punched out areas. Fractures are more extensive in the inner table than in the outer table.

3. *Sutures:* The coronal and lambdoid sutures are usually visible clearly. The coronal suture runs downwards and forwards in front of the central sulcus of the brain. The lambdoid suture traverses the posteriormost part of the skull.

Obliteration of sutures begins first on the inner surface (between 30 and 40 years) and then on the outer surface (between 40 and 50 years). Usually the lower part of the coronal suture is obliterated first, followed by the posterior part of the sagittal suture. Premature closure of sutures occurs in craniostenosis, a hereditary disease. Sutures are opened up in children by an increase in intracranial pressure.

4. *Vascular markings.*

(a) *Middle meningeal vessels:* The anterior branch runs about 1 cm behind the coronal suture. The posterior branch runs backwards and upwards at a lower level across the upper part of the shadow of the auricle.

(b) The *transverse sinus* may be seen as a curved dark shadow, convex upwards, extending from the internal occipital protuberance to the petrous temporal.

(c) The *diploic venous markings* are seen as irregularly anastomosing, worm like, shadows produced by the frontal, anterior temporal, posterior temporal and occipital diploic veins.

These markings become more prominent in raised intracranial pressure.

5. *Cerebral moulding*, indicating normal impressions of cerebral gyri, can be seen. In raised intracranial tension, the impressions become more pronounced and produce a characteristic *silver beaten (or copper beaten) appearance* of the skull.

6. *Arachnoid granulations* may indent the parasagittal area of the skull to such an extent as to simulate erosion by a meningioma.

7. *Normal intracranial calcifications:*

(a) Pineal concretions (brain sand) appear by the age of 17 years. The pineal body is located 2.5 cm above and 1.2 cm behind the external acoustic meatus. When visible it serves as an important radiological landmark.

(b) Other structures which may become calcified include the choroid plexuses, arachnoid granulations, falx cerebri, and other dural folds.

8. *The auricle:* The curved margin of the auricle is seen above the petrous temporal.

9. The *frontal sinus* produces a dark shadow in the anteroinferior part of the skull vault.

Base of Skull

1. The *floor of the anterior cranial fossa* slopes backwards and downwards. The shadows of the two sides are often seen situated one above the other. The surface is irregular due to gyral markings. It also forms the roof of the orbit (Fig. 20.1).

2. The *hypophyseal fossa* represents the middle cranial fossa in this view. It is overhung anteriorly by the anterior clinoid process (directed posteriorly), and posteriorly by the posterior clinoid process. It measures 8 mm vertically and 14 mm antero-posteriorly. The interclinoid distance is not more than 4 mm. The fossa is enlarged in cases of pituitary tumours, arising particularly from acidophil or chromophobe cells.

3. The *sphenoidal air sinus* lies anteroinferior to the hypophyseal fossa. The shadows of the orbit, the nasal cavities, and the ethmoidal and maxillary sinuses lie superimposed on one another, below the anterior cranial fossa.

4. The *petrous part of the temporal bone* produces a dense irregular shadow posteroinferior to the hypophyseal fossa. Within this shadow there are two dark areas representing the external acoustic meatuses of the two sides; each shadow lies immediately behind the head of the mandible of that side. Similar dark shadows of the internal acoustic meatuses may also be seen. The posterior part of the dense shadow merges with the mastoid air cells producing a honeycomb appearance.

5. In addition to the features mentioned above, the *mandible* lies anteriorly forming the lower part of the facial skeleton. The *upper cervical vertebrae*

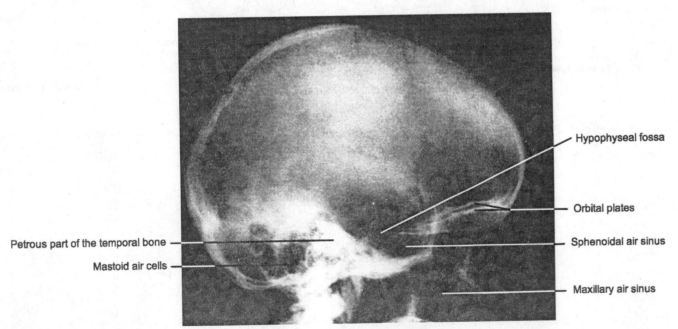

Petrous part of the temporal bone

Mastoid air cells

Hypophyseal fossa

Orbital plates

Sphenoidal air sinus

Maxillary air sinus

Fig. 20.1: Lateral view of the skull.

lie posteriorly and are seen as a pillar supporting the skull.

SPECIAL PA VIEW OF SKULL FOR PARANASAL SINUSES

This picture is taken with the head extended in such a way that the chin rests against the film and the nose is raised from it (Waters' position). This view shows the frontal and maxillary sinuses clearly.

The frontal sinuses are seen immediately above the nose and medial parts of the orbits. The nasal cavities are flanked on each side by the orbits above, and the maxillary sinuses below. The normal sinuses are clear and radiolucent, i.e. they appear dark. If a sinus is infected, the shadow is either hazy or radiopaque.

Cervical Vertebrae

The cervical vertebrae can be visualised in anteroposterior view of the neck and in oblique view of the neck. In the anteroposterior view, the body of cervical vertebrae, intervertebral discs, pedicles and spines are seen. In the oblique view, the adjacent inferior articular and superior articular processes and intervertebral foramen are visualised.

Ultrasound scans (Figs 20.2 and 20.3) through the thyroid gland reveal various relations of trachea.

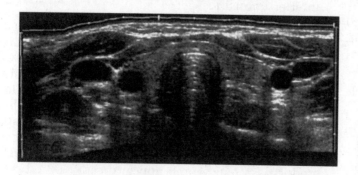
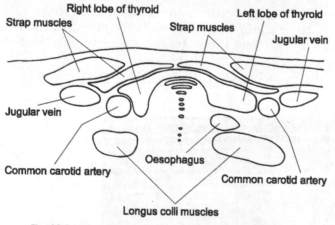

Fig. 20.2: Ultrasound scan showing relations of trachea.

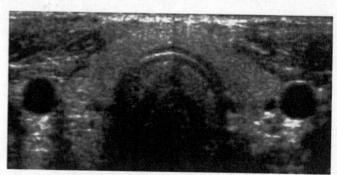
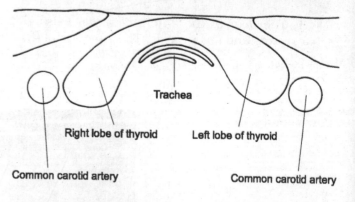

Fig. 20.3: Ultrasound scan showing thyroid gland and trachea.

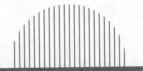

Appendix 1

CRANIAL NERVES

Olfactory/Cranial Nerve I: Olfactory Pathway

Olfactory epithelium of nose → olfactory rootlets → olfactory bulb → olfactory tract → lateral and medial olfactory striae (Fig. 29.8).

Lateral olfactory stria → pyriform lobe (comprises uncus and anterior part of parahippocampal gyrus).

Medial olfactory stria → septal nuclei.

Some impulses from uncus and septal nuclei travel via reticular formation to the dorsal nucleus of vagus where it may increase or decrease gastric secretion according to type of smell.

Optic/Cranial Nerve II: Visual Pathway

Retina → optic nerve → optic chiasma → optic tract → lateral geniculate body → optic radiation → visual area in occipital lobe (Fig. 30.4).

CLINICAL ANATOMY

Effect of lesions of different parts of visual pathways

1. Lesion in retina leads to scotoma, that is certain points may become blind spots.

2. Optic nerve damage results in complete blindness of that eye.

3. Optic chaisma lesion if central will lead to bitemporal hemianopia; but if peripheral on both sides will lead to binasal hemianopia.

4. Complete destruction of optic tract, lateral geniculate body, optic radiation or visual cortex of one side results in loss of the opposite half of field of vision.

5. A lesion on the right side leads to left homonymous hemianopia.

Oculomotor Nerve/Cranial Nerve III

Nuclear columns/functional components.

  i. General somatic efferent (GSE) column–nucleus of oculomotor
 ii. General visceral efferent (GVE) nucleus of Edinger-Westphal for the supply of intraocular muscles.
iii. General somatic afferent (GSA) – spinal nucleus of CN V. It receives proprioceptive impulses from extraocular muscles.

Nuclei (i) and (ii) are situated in midbrain at the level of superior colliculus. Fibres of Edinger-Westphal nucleus join those of the oculomotor nerve. The nerve is seen at the medial end of crus cerebri of midbrain (Fig. 7.10).

It enters the cavernous sinus and is placed in its lateral wall most anteriorly. As it traverses the sinus it divides into its two divisions in its anterior part. Both the divisions pass through the middle part of the superior orbital fissure (Fig. 7.11).

The superior division turns upwards lateral to optic nerve and supplies superior rectus and superficially placed levator palpebrae superioris.

The inferior division in orbit passes below the optic nerve and divides into three branches: for medial rectus, inferior rectus and inferior oblique muscles.

The nerve to inferior oblique gives a branch for the ciliary ganglion. This branch brings the fibres of Edinger-Westphal nucleus (GVE) to the ganglion for relay. The postganglionic fibres end up in supplying the ciliaris for enhancing the anterior curvature of the lens and the sphincter pupillae for narrowing the size of the pupil. Both these are intraocular muscles required for accommodation.

CLINICAL ANATOMY

Paralysis of oculomotor nerve results in partial ptosis, dilation of pupil, loss of accommodation, diplopia and lateral squint.

Trochlear Nerve/Cranial Nerve IV

Trochlear/cranial nerve IV nerve nucleus is situated at the level of inferior colliculus of mid brain. This nerve supplies only the superior oblique muscle of the eyeball. If the nerve is injured, patient cannot turn the centre of cornea downwards and laterally. On attempting to do this action, the eye rotates medially resulting in diplopia or double vision (Fig. 7.13).

Trigeminal Nerve/Cranial Nerve V

Cranial nerve V/trigeminal nerve comprises three branches, ophthalmic, maxillary and mandibular. Their branches are given:

Ophthalmic Nerve

Ophthalmic nerve is sensory. Its branches are as follows.

1. *Frontal*
   a. Supratrochlear: Upper eyelid, conjunctiva, lower part of forehead
   b. Supraorbital: Frontal air sinus, upper eyelid, forehead, scalp till vertex

2. *Nasociliary*
   a. Posterior ethmoidal: Sphenoidal air sinus, posterior ethmoidal air sinuses (Fig. 7.15).
   b. Long ciliary: Sensory to eyeball
   c. Nerve to ciliary ganglion
   d. Infratrochlear: Both eyelids, side of nose, lacrimal sac
   e. Anterior ethmoidal:
      1. Middle and anterior ethmoidal sinuses.
      2. Medial internal nasal
      3. Lateral internal nasal
      4. External nasal
   External nasal: Skin of ala of vestibule and tip of nose.

3. *Lacrimal*

Lateral part of upper eyelid; conveys secretomotor fibres from zygomatic nerve to lacrimal gland.

Maxillary Nerve

In Middle Cranial Fossa

1. Meningeal branch

In Pterygopalatine Fossa

2. Ganglionic branches (Fig. 15.13)
3. Zygomatic :
   a. Zygomaticotemporal
   b. Zygomaticofacial
4. Posterior superior alveolar

In Infraorbital Canal

5. Middle superior alveolar
6. Anterior superior alveolar

On Face

7. Infraorbital :
   a. Palpebral
   b. Labial
   c. Nasal

Mandibular Nerve

Trunk

1. Meningeal (Fig. 10.14)
2. Nerve to medial pterygoid:
   Tensor veli palatini
   Tensor tympani
   Medial pterygoid

Anterior Division

3. Deep temporal
4. Lateral pterygoid
5. Masseteric
6. Buccal—Skin of cheek

Posterior Division

7. Auriculotemporal
   a. Auricular
   b. Superficial temporal
   c. Articular to temporomandibular joint
   d. Secretomotor to parotid gland.
8. Lingual—General sensation from anterior two-thirds of tongue
9. Inferior alveolar—Lower teeth and
   a. Nerve to mylohyoid :
      1. Mylohoid
      2. Anterior belly of digastric

CLINICAL ANATOMY

In case of injury to ophthalmic nerve, there is loss of "corneal blink reflex"

Injury to maxillary nerve causes loss of "sneeze reflex"

Injury to mandibular nerve results in loss of "jaw jerk reflex".

Abducent/Cranial Nerve VI

Abducent nerve only supplies the lateral rectus of the eyeball. Paralysis of the nerve results in medial squint and diplopia (Fig. 7.14).

Facial Nerve/Cranial Nerve VII

It is called facial nerve as this nerve supplies all the muscles of facial expression developed from 2nd pharyngeal/branchial arch. Its various nuclear components are:

1. Special visceral efferent for the supply of muscles of facial expression. Nucleus is at lower pons.
2. General visceral efferent for the supply of lacrimal, nasal, palatal, pharyngeal glands through greater petrosal nerve (which forms nerve to pterygoid canal by joining with deep petrosal nerve (sympathetic fibres) and for submandibular and sublingual salivary glands through chorda tympani nerve. Nuclei are lacrimatory and superior salivatory nuclei.
3. Special visceral afferent for receiving taste fibres from anterior two-thirds of tongue except the circumvallate papillae and general visceral afferent from various glands. Nucleus is tractus solitarius.
4. General somatic afferent column for receiving proprioceptive fibres from muscles of facial expression. Nucleus is spinal nucleus of V CN.

The main nerve emerges at the lower border of pons above the olive.

The nervus intermedius composed of 2nd and 3rd nuclear components join the main nerve. These two enter the internal acoustic meatus. The two nerves run laterally in the petrous temporal bone where these fuse to form a single trunk. Then the nerve forms a bend, which is enlarged to form geniculate ganglion. It runs posteriorly in the medial wall of middle ear. Finally, it curves downwards traversing the facial canal. Lastly, the nerve exits through the cranial cavity by passing through the stylomastoid foramen as purely motor nerve (see Chapter 9).

Intracranial Branches

1. Through geniculate ganglion-greater petrosal nerve (from nervus intermedius) joins with deep petrosal (sympathetic fibres) to form nerve of pterygoid canal.
2. Branch to stapedius given off from facial nerve as it traverses the facial canal.
3. Chorda tympani nerve → also arises from nervus intermedius 6 mm above the stylomastoid foramen. This nerve passes through posterior wall → lateral wall → anterior wall → petrotympanic fissure → joins lingual nerve, lies on medial side of spine of sphenoid (Fig. 9.10).

Extracranial course : The nerve gives two branches numbered 4 and 5 and then enters posteromedial surface of parotid gland. It divides rejoins and finally emerge as 5 main branches.

4. Posterior auricular branch for the supply of auricular muscles and occipital belly of occipitofrontalis muscles.
5. Muscular branch which supplies posterior belly of digastric and stylohyoid muscles.

Then it passes through parotid gland and divides into various branches:

6. Temporal branches emerge from the upper border or base of the gland cross zygomatic arch to supply frontalis part of occipitofrontalis muscle.
7. Zygomatic branches supply orbicularis oculi. Paralysis of this muscle causes epiphora and prevents blinking.
8. Buccal branches usually pass above and below the parotid duct. These supply buccinator, muscles of nose and upper lip. Their paralysis causes dribbling from the mouth.
9. Marginal mandibular usually runs along the lower border of mandible. Injury of this nerve causes paralysis of depressors of lower lip.
10. Cervical lies in the neck and supplies platysma.

CLINICAL ANATOMY

1. Bells's palsy: Sudden paralysis of facial nerve at the stylomastoid foramen. Result is asymmetry of corner of mouth, inability to close the eye, disappearance of nasolabial fold and loss of wrinkling of skin of forehead on the same side.

2. Lesion above the origin of chorda tympani nerve will show symptoms of Bell's palsy plus loss of taste from anterior two-thirds of tongue except vallate papillae.

3. Lesion above the origin of nerve to stapedius will cause symptoms 1 and 2 and further causes hyperacusis.

Lesions 1, 2 and 3 are lower motor neuron type. Upper motor neuron paralysis will not affect the upper part of face, i.e. orbicularis oculi, only lower half of opposite side of face is affected. The upper half of face has bilateral representation, whereas lower half has only ipsilateral representation.

Vestibulocochlear/Cranial Nerve VIII

Auditory pathway

The auditory receptors are the hair cells of the organ of Corti, situated in the cochlear duct of the internal ear.

   i. The first sensory neuron lies in the spiral ganglion of bipolar cell, situated around modiolus at the base of spiral lamina. The peripheral processes are distributed to the organ of Corti, and the central processes form cochlear nerve which ends in the dorsal and ventral cochlear nuclei lying in relation to inferior cerebellar peduncle.

ii. The second neuron fibres start from the dorsal and ventral cochlear nuclei: their axons form trapezoid body and end in dorsal nucleus of trapezoid body of the same as well as the opposite side.

iii. The third neuron fibres from dorsal nuclei of trapezoid body ascend as lateral lemniscus on both sides. Some of the fibres of lateral lemniscus end in the inferior colliculus for auditory reflex activities, mediated through tectobulbar and tectospinal tracts. The rest of the lateral lemniscus relays in medial geniculate body.

iv. The fourth neuron fibres from medial geniculate body give rise to auditory radiations which pass through sublentiform part of internal capsule and are projected to auditory cortex of temporal lobe.

Damage to cochlear nerve produces tinnitis and sensorineuronal deafness.

Vestibular Pathway

The vestibular nerve innervates the maculae of the utricle and saccule. These are sensitive to static changes in equilibrium. The ampullae of the semicircular canals are sensitive to dynamic changes in equilibrium. Impulses pass along the vestibular nerve to vestibular nuclei situated at pontomedullary junction. Fibres from vestibular nuclei pass via inferior cerebellar peduncle to the cerebellum.

Damage to vestibular nerve results in vertigo or dizziness and nystagmus i.e., pendular movements of the eyes.

Glossopharyngeal Nerve/Cranial Nerve IX

It is named so, as it supplies one muscle of the pharynx—the stylopharyngeus and carries general sensation and taste from posterior one-third of the tongue and vallate papillae. It is the nerve of 3rd brachial arch.

Nuclear columns/functional components:

1. Special visceral efferent (nucleus ambiguus) for the supply only one muscle—the stylopharyngeus.

2. General visceral efferent—the inferior salivatory nucleus for the supply of parotid salivary gland after relay in the otic ganglion.

3. General visceral afferent and special visceral afferent. Nucleus of tractus solitarius as it receives general sensations from posterior one-

third of tongue, tonsil, pharynx, carotid body, carotid sinus, it also receives taste from posterior one third of tongue and vallate papillae. All these sensations reach the inferior ganglion of the nerve via the peripheral process of the ganglion cells. Their central process reach the nucleus of tractus solitarius.

4. General somatic afferent—carries proprioceptive impulses from pharyngeal muscle to spinal tract of V.

Intracranial Course

The fibres of the nerve arise from the respective nuclear columns at the level of medulla oblongata. The nerve fibres pass between olive and inferior cerebellar peduncle.

It is attached at the base of the brain in the posterolateral sulcus between olive and inferior cerebellar peduncle by 3–4 rootlets.

The rootlets join to form the nerve which enters the middle part of the jugular foramen in a separate sheath of dura mater.

Extracranial Course

The superior ganglion is small and is a detached part of the inferior ganglion.

The inferior ganglion is larger and its central processes carry all the sensory fibres (general and special sensation) of the nerve.

It curves medially across the stylopharyngeus muscle and supplies it.

It enters the pharynx through the interval between superior and middle constrictor muscles and ends by dividing into its terminal branches (Fig. 14.18).

Branches

1. Communicating to V, X and superior cervical ganglion of sympathetic chain.

2. Distribution to:

   a. Tympanic branch enters middle ear cavity → tympanic plexus on promontory → supplies middle ear, auditory tube and gives → lesser petrosal nerve relay in otic ganglion join auriculotemporal nerve → parotid salivary gland (Fig. 12.19).

   b. Sinocarotid nerve for carrying baroreceptor and chemoreceptor sensations from carotid sinus and carotid body respectively.

   c. Tonsillary and palatal branches for the supply of sensory fibres to the palatine tonsil and soft palate.

d. Lingual branches for the supply of general sensations and taste fibres from posterior one-third of tongue including the circumvallate papillae present anterior to the sulcus terminalis of the tongue.

e. Pharyngeal branch is sensory to the mucous membrane of pharynx.

f. Stylopharyngeus muscle.

CLINICAL ANATOMY

On tickling the posterior wall of pharynx, there is reflex contraction of muscles of pharynx. If cranial nerve IX is paralysed, no such contraction occurs. Further taste from posterior one-third of tongue and circumvallate papillae is not appreciated in cranial nerve IX paralysis. The cranial nerve IX is mostly paralysed along with cranial nerve X.

Vagus/Cranial Nerve X

Vagus leaves the cranial cavity through jugular foramen. It courses through neck, thorax and abdomen and supplies organs developed from foregut and midgut. Since it has too much to supply it borrows the cranial root of accessory to supply muscles of soft palate except tensor veli palatini, (supplied by mandibular); all muscles of pharynx except stylopharyngeus (supplied by CN IX) and all intrinsic muscles of larynx (Fig. 12.21). If vagus is damaged the effects are :

(a) Paralysis of muscles of soft palate resulting in nasal regurgitation of fluids

(b) Nasal tone of the voice

(c) Hoarseness of voice

Voice becomes monotonous because of paralysis of external laryngeal nerve.

It both recurrent laryngeal nerves are injured, there is inability to speak, and dyspnoea.

Accessory/Cranial Nerve XI

The accessory nerve comprises two roots, the cranial and spinal. The cranial root joins vagus to form vagoaccessory complex and gets distributed through branches of vagus to soft palate, pharynx and larynx. The spinal root supplies two big muscles of neck, the sternocleidomastoid and the trapezius (Fig. 12.22).

Injury to spinal root causes paralysis of both the above mentioned muscles. Paralysis of sterno-cleidomastoid turns the chin towards the side of injury. Paralysis of trapezius causes limitation in overhead abduction and inability to shrug the shoulder on the affected side.

Hypoglossal Nerve/Cranial Nerve XII

As the name implies it is the nerve supplying muscles of tongue (glossal means tongue) and is purely motor nerve. Functional components or nuclear columns:

It belongs to general somatic efferent column. Its nucleus is situated in the medulla in the floor of IV ventricle deep to hypoglossal triangle.

The rootlets are attached in the groove between the pyramid and olive. The rootlets join to form two bundles which pierce the dura mater separately near the anterior condylar canal or hypoglossal canal.

• It enters the neck through anterior condylar canal and is placed deeper than cranial nerves IX, X and XI.

• It descends between internal jugular vein and internal carotid artery.

• It curves around the vagus nerve as it passes deep to posterior belly of digastric muscle.

• The hypoglossal nerve makes a wide curve, crossing the internal carotid, external carotid and the loop of the lingual artery.

• The nerve passes above the hyoid bone in submandibular region, superficial to hyoglossus where it ends by dividing into its muscular branches.

Branches

1. Of communication with vagus, ventral ramus of first cervical nerve, lingual nerve and superior cervical ganglion of sympathetic chain.

2. Of distribution:

a. To the three extrinsic muscles of tongue namely styloglossus, genioglossus and hyoglossus and to four intrinsic muscles namely superior longitudinal, inferior longitudinal, transverse and vertical muscles. The fourth extrinsic muscle namely the palatoglossus is supplied by vagoaccessory complex (Fig. 12.24).

b. It carries fibres of ventral rumus of first cervical which gets distributed as meningeal branch, superior limb of ansa cervicalis, branch to thyrohyoid and geniohyoid muscles.

CLINICAL ANATOMY

If this nerves is injured the intrinsic and most of the extrinsic muscles of the same side to tongue are paralysed. If paralysed tongue is protruded, its tip gets deviated to the affected side.

HORNER'S SYNDROME

Preganglionic fibres from lateral horn of T1 segment of spinal cord enter sympathetic trunk via white ramus communicans of T1, pass upto superior cervical ganglion where these relay. The post-ganglionic fibres accompany internal carotid artery leave the artery to join ophthalmic nerve, nasociliary nerve-long ciliary nerve to supply cornea, choroid of eyeball, dilator pupillae and smooth part of levator palpebrae superioris muscle. If these fibres get interrupted the losses lead to Horner's syndrome:

1. Constriction of pupil due to loss of dilator pupillae.

2. Ptosis (partial drooping due to loss of sympathetic nerve supplying part of levator palpebrae superioris).

3. Anhydrosis—loss of sweating on the head and neck of the same side.

4. Enophthalamos—due to loss of paralysis of muscle fibres in the orbital cavity supplied by sympathetic nerves.

PHRENIC NERVE

Phrenic nerve arises primarily from ventral rami of C4 with small contributions from C3 and C5 nerve roots or through nerve to subclavius. It is the only motor supply to its own half of diaphragm and sensory to mediastinal pleura, peritoneum and fibrous pericardium. Inflammation of peritoneum under diaphragm causes referred pain in the area of supraclavicular nerves supply, especially tip of the shoulders as their root value is also ventral rami of C3 and C4 (Fig. 12.28).

CERVICAL PLEXUS

Ventral rami of C1, C2, C3, C4 form the cervical plexus. C1 runs along hypoglossal and supplies geniohyoid and thyrohyoid. It also gives superior limb of ansa cervicalis, which supplies superior belly of omohyoid and joins with inferior limb to form ansa. Inferier limb of ansa cervicalis is formed by ventral rami of C2, C3. Branches from ansa supply sternohyoid, sternothyroid, inferior belly of omohyoid. Cervical plexus also gives four cutaneous branches lesser occipital (C2), great auricular (C2, C3), supraclavicular (C3, C4) and transverse or anterior nerve of neck (C2, C3) (Figs 3.7, 8.13 and 12.28).

PARASYMPATHETIC GANGLIA

Submandibular Ganglion

Situation: The submandibular ganglion lies superficial to hyoglossus muscle in the sub-mandibular region. Functionally, it is connected to facial nerve, while topographically it is connected to lingual branch of mandibular nerve (Fig. 11.11).

Roots: The ganglion has sensory, sympathetic and secretomotor roots.

• Sensory root is from the lingual nerve. It is suspended by two roots of lingual nerve

• Sympathetic root is from the sympathetic plexus around the facial artery. This plexus contains pastganglionic fibres from the superior cervical ganglion of sympathetic trunk. These fibres pass express through the ganglion and are vasomotor to the gland

• Secretomotor root is from superior salivatory nucleus through nervus intermedius via chorda tympani which is a branch of cranial nerve VII. Chorda tympani joins lingual nerve. The parasympathetic fibres get relayed in the submandibular ganglion

Branches: The ganglion gives direct branches to the submandibular salivary gland.

Some postganglionic fibres reach the lingual nerve to be distributed to sublingual salivary gland.

Pterygopalatine Ganglion

Situation: Pterygopalatine or sphenopalatine is the largest parasympathetic ganglion, suspended by two roots of maxillary nerve. Functionally it is related to cranial nerve VII. It is called the ganglion of "Hay fever."

Roots: The ganglion has sensory, sympathetic and secretomotor roots (Figs 15.12, 15.13).

• Sensory root is from maxillary nerve. The ganglion is suspended by 2 roots of maxillary nerve.

• Sympathetic root is from postganglionic plexus around internal carotid artery. The nerve is called deep petrosal. It unites with greater petrosal to form nerve of pterygoid canal. The fibres of deep petrosal do not relay in the ganglion.

• Secretomotor root is from greater petrosal nerve which arises from geniculate ganglion of cranial nerve VII. These fibres relay in the ganglion.

Branches: The ganglion gives number of branches. These are

   i. *For lacrimal gland:* The postganglionic fibres pass → zygomatic branch of maxillary nerve. These fibres hitch hike through zygomatico-temporal nerve into the communicating branch between zygomatico-temporal and lacrimal nerve, then to the lacrimal nerve for supplying the lacrimal gland.

ii. *Nasopalatine nerve:* This nerve runs on the nasal septum and ends in the anterior part of hard palate. It supplies secretomotor fibres to both nasal and palatal glands.

iii. *Palatine branches:* These are one greater palatine and 2–3 lesser palatine branches. These pass through the respective foramina to supply sensory and secretomotor fibres to mucous membrane and glands of soft palate and hard palate.

iv. *Nasal branches:* These are posterior superior medial for the supply of glands and mucous membrance of nasal septum; the largest is named nasopalatine; and posterior superior lateral for the supply of glands and mucous membrane of lateral wall of nasal cavity.

v. *Orbital branches* for the orbital periosteum.

vi. Pharyngeal branches for the glands of pharynx.

Otic Ganglion

Situation: The otic ganglion lies deep to the trunk of mandibular nerve, between the nerve and the tensor veli palatini muscle in the infratemporal fossa, just distal to the foramen ovale. Topographically, it is connected to mandibular nerve, while functionally it is related to cranial nerve IX.

Roots: This ganglion has sensory, sympathetic, secretomotor and motor roots (Figs 10.15, 10.16).

• Sensory root is by the auriculotemporal nerve.

• Sympathetic root is by the sympathetic plexus around middle meningeal artery.

• Secretomotor root is by the lesser petrosal nerve from the tympanic plexus formed by tympanic branch of cranial nerve IX. Fibres of lesser petrosal nerve relay in the otic ganglion. Postganglionic fibres reach the parotid gland through auriculo-temporal nerve.

• Motor root is by a branch from nerve to medial pterygoid. This branch passes unrelayed through the ganglion and divides into two branches to supply tensor veli palatini and tensor tympani.

Branches: The postganglionic branches of the ganglion pass through auriculotemparal nerve to supply the parotid gland.

The motor branches supply the two muscles mentioned above.

Ciliary Ganglion

Situation: The ciliary ganglion is very small ganglion present in the orbit. Topographically the ganglion is related to nasociliary nerve, branch of ophthalmic division of trigeminal nerve, but functionally it is related to oculomotor nerve. This ganglion has no secretomotor fibres.

Roots: It has three roots, the sensory, sympathetic and motor. Only the motor root fibres relay to supply the intraocular muscles.

• Sensory root is from the long ciliary nerve.

• Sympathetic root is by the long ciliary nerve from plexus around ophthalmic artery.

• Motor root is from a branch to inferior oblique muscle. These fibres arise from Edinger-Westphal nucleus, join oculomotor nerve and leave it via the nerve to inferior oblique, to be relayed in the ciliary ganglion (Fig. 7.12).

Branches: The ganglion gives 10–12 short ciliary nerves containing postganglionic fibres for the supply of constrictor or sphincter pupillae for narrowing the size of pupil and ciliaris muscle for increasing the curvature of anterior surface of lens required during accommodation of the eye.

CLINICOANATOMICAL PROBLEMS

1. A 12-year-boy complained of sore throat and ear ache. He had 102° F temperature and difficulty in swallowing. He was also a mouth breather.

   Clinicoanatomical problem:
   ❑ What is Waldeyer's lymphatic ring ?
   ❑ Explain the basis of boy's earache ?
   ❑ What lymph node would likely be swollen and tender ?

   Ans. Major collections of lymphoid tissue at the oropharyngeal junction are called the tonsils. These lie in a ring form called the Waldeyer's lymphatic ring. The components of this ring are lingual tonsil anteriorly, palatine tonsil laterally, tubal tonsil posterolaterally and pharyngeal tonsil posteriorly.

   The earache is due to infection of the throat reaching the middle ear. The pharyngotympanic tube from the region of nasopharynx communicates with the anterior wall of the middle ear cavity carrying the infection from pharynx to the ear causing the earache.

   The jugulodigastric lymph node belonging to upper group of deep cervical group is most likely to be tender and swollen, as the lymphatics from the tonsil penetrate the wall of the pharynx to reach these lymph nodes.

2. A middle-aged women had a deep cut in the middle of her right posterior triangle of neck. The bleeding was arrested and wound was sutured. The patient later felt difficulty in combing her hair.

Clinicoanatomical problem:
☐ What blood vessel is severed ?
☐ Why did the patient have difficulty in combing her hair ?

Ans. The external jungular vein was severed. It passes across the sternocleidomastoid muscle to join the subclavian vein above the clavicle. Her accessory nerve is also injured as it crosses the posterior triangle close to its roof, causing paralysis of trapezius muscle. The trapezius with serratus anterior causes overhead abduction required for combing the hair. Due to paralysis of trapezius, she felt difficulty in combing her hair.

3. A 40-year-woman complained of a swelling in front of her neck, nervousness and loss of weight. Her diagnosis was hyperthyroidism. Partial thyroidectomy was performed, and she complained of hoarseness after the operation.

Clinicoanatomical problem:
☐ Why does thyroid swelling move up and down during deglutition ?
☐ Why does she complain of hoarseness after the operation ?
☐ Which other gland can be removed with thyroid ?

Ans. The thyroid gland is suspended from cricoid cartilage by the pretracheal fascia and ligament of Berry. So all the swellings of thyroid gland move with deglutition.

She complains of hoarsensess due to injury to the recurrent laryngeal nerve as it lies close to the inferior thyroid artery near the lower pole of the gland. Hoarseness can also result from postoperative oedema.

The parathyoid gland lying on the back of thyroid gland can be removed. Parathyroid controls calcium level in the blood.

4. A young man complained of fever and sore throat, noted a swelling and felt pain on both sides of his face in front the ear. Within a few days he noted swellings below his jaw and below his chin. He suddenly started looking very healthy by facial appearance The pain increased while chewing or drinking lemon juice. The physician noted enlargement of all three salivary glands on both sides of the face.

Clinicoanatomical problem:
☐ Where do the ducts of the salivary glands open ?
☐ Why did the pain increase while chewing ?
☐ Why did the pain increase while drinking lemon juice ?

Ans. The duct of the parotid gland opens at a papilla in the vestibule of mouth opposite the 2nd upper molar tooth. The duct of submandibular gland opens at the papilla on the sublingual fold. The sublingual gland opens by 10–12 ducts on the sublingual fold. The investing layer of cervical fascia encloses both the parotid and the submandibular glands and is attached to the lower border of the mandible. As mandible moves during chewing, the fascia gets stretched which results in pain. The fascia and skin are supplied by the great auricular nerve. While drinking lemon juice, there is lot of pain, as the salivary secretion is stimulated by the acid of the lemon juice. The investing layer of cervical fascia encloses : Two muscles, the trapezius and the sternocleidomastoid; two spaces, the suprasternal space and the supraclavicular space; two glands, the parotid and the submandibular glands; and forms two pulleys, one for the intermediate tendon of digastric and one for the intermediate tendon of omohyoid muscle.

5. A man aged 55 years complained of dysphagia in eating solid and even soft food and liquids. There was a large lymph node felt at the anterior border of sternocleidomastoid muscle. The diagnosis on biopsy was cancer of cervical part of oesophagus.

Clinicoanatomical problem:
☐ How was the large lymph node formed ?
☐ Why did the patient have dysphagia ?
☐ Where can the cancer spread around oesophagus ?

Ans. The pain during eating or drinking is due to cancer of the oesophagus. The cancer obliterates increasing part of the lumen, giving rise to pain. The lymphatic drainage from cervical part of oesophagus goes to inferior group of deep cervical lymph nodes. The cancer had metastasized to the lymph node at the anterior border of sternocleidomastoid muscle. Since trachea lies just anterior to oesophagus, the cancer can spread to trachea or any of the principal bronchi.

MULTIPLE CHOICE QUESTIONS

(A) Select the best response:

1. All of the following are the branches of external carotid except:
   a. Facial
   b. Ophthalmic
   c. Occipital
   d. Posterior auricular

2. Which of the laryngeal nerves accompanies the inferior thyroid artery:
   a. Internal
   b. External
   c. Recurrent
   d. Superior

3. Which of the following subdivision of anterior triangle is unpaired:
   a. Muscular
   b. Submental
   c. Digastric
   d. Carotid

4. Which part of internal carotid artery has no branch:
   a. Cerebral
   b. Petrous
   c. Cervical
   d. Cavernous

5. Only one muscle depresses the mandible. Which one is it?
   a. Medial pterygoid
   b. Temporalis
   c. Lateral pterygoid
   d. Masseter

6. Which muscles may elevate the larynx:
   a. Thyrohyoid
   b. Sternothyroid
   c. Sternohyoid
   d. Omohyoid — inferior belly

7. One of the following nerves does not traverse the superior orbital fissure. Which one is it?
   a. Nasociliary
   b. Maxillary
   c. Abducent
   d. Trochlear

8. Which of the following nerve supplies the cornea:
   a. Supraorbital
   b. Nasociliary
   c. Lacrimal
   d. Infraorbital

9. Tegmen tympani forms the roof of all of the following except:
   a. Mastoid antrum
   b. Tympanic cavity
   c. Canal for tensor tympani
   d. Internal acoustic meatus

10. By how many openings do the semicircular canals open into the vestibule:
    a. 3
    b. 5
    c. 4
    d. 2

11. The maxillary artery is a branch of:
    a. External carotid artery
    b. Internal carotid artery
    c. Facial artery
    d. Superficial temporal artery

12. The vocal folds are abducted by:
    a. Cricothyroid muscle
    b. Lateral cricoarytenoid muscle
    c. Posterior cricoarytenoid muscle
    d. Aryepiglottic

13. Greater cornua of hyoid bone is developed from— pharyngeal arch:
    a. I
    b. II
    c. III
    d. IV

14. Stylopharyngeus muscle is supplied by nerve:
    a. VII
    b. IX
    c. X
    d. XII

15. Temporomandibular joint is a:
    a. Plane joint
    b. Condyloid joint
    c. Ball and socket joint
    d. Saddle-shaped joint

B. Each question contains four suggested answers, out of which one or more are correct. Choose the answer:
    A. If 1, 2, 3 are correct
    B. If 1 and 3 are correct
    C. If 2 and 4 are correct
    D. If only 4 is correct
    E. If all are correct

16. The lesion of oculomotor nerve leads to:
    1. Diplopia
    2. Ptosis
    3. Dilatation of pupil
    4. Lateral squint

17. A fracture of cranial cavity passing through jugular foramen will cause paralysis of:
    1. Accessory nerve
    2. Vagus nerve
    3. Glossopharyngeal nerve
    4. Facial nerve

18. The superior colliculus of midbrain is:
    1. Visual reflex center
    2. Higher center for vision
    3. Situated in midbrain
    4. Visual relay center

19. The optic nerve is considered a tract because:
    1. The sheaths covering the optic nerve are derived from the three meninges.
    2. Its fibres have no neurilemma sheath
    3. It is attached to forebrain
    4. It cannot regenerate

20. The lateral geniculate body receives:
    1. Contralateral temporal retinal fibres
    2. Ipsilateral temporal retinal fibres
    3. Ipsilateral nasal retinal fibres
    4. Contralateral nasal retinal fibres

Answers to Multiple Choice Questions

1. b
2. c
3. b
4. c
5. c
6. a
7. b
8. b
9. d
10. b
11. a
12. c
13. c
14. b
15. b
16. E
17. A
18. A
19. E
20. C

Section 2

BRAIN

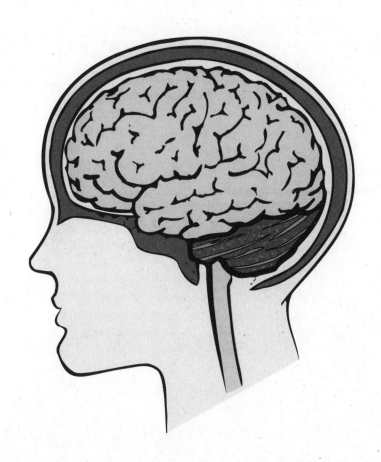

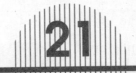

Introduction to the Brain

Human nervous system is responsible for judgement, intelligence and memory. Nervous system is highly evolved at the cost of regeneration. The activities of nervous system are linked with every aspect of our lives, that is physical, psychological and intellectual. It is the most complex system of the body.

Introduction

Nervous system is the chief controlling and coordinating system of the body. It adjusts the body to the surroundings and regulates all bodily activities both voluntary and involuntary. The sensory part of the nervous system collects information from the surroundings and helps in gaining knowledge and experience, whereas the motor part is responsible for responses of the body.

CELLULAR ARCHITECTURE

The nervous tissue is made up of: (a) Nerve cells or neurons; (b) neuroglial cells (neuroglia), forming the supporting (connective) tissue of the CNS. In peripheral nervous system, these are replaced by Schwann cells and the loose connective tissue;

(c) both types of cells are supplied with blood by abundant blood vessels.

Neuron

Each neuron is made up of the following.

a. A cell body. Collectively they form grey matter and the nuclei in the CNS, and ganglia in the peripheral nervous system (Fig. 21.1).

b. *Numerous cell processes of two varieties:* (i) Dendrites are many, short, richly branched and often varicose; (ii) the axon is a single elongated process. Collectively the axons form tracts (white matter) in the CNS, and nerves in the peripheral nervous system. The branches of axons often arise at right angles and are called the collaterals.

Functionally, each neuron is specialized for sensitivity and conductivity. The impulses can flow in them with great rapidity, in some cases about 125 metres per second. A neuron shows *dynamic polarity* in its processes. The impulse flows towards the cell body in the dendrites, and away from the cell body in the axon.

The neurons are connected to one another by their processes, forming long chains along which the

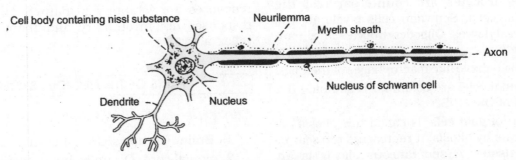

Fig. 21.1: *A nerve cell.*

impulses are conducted. The site of contact (contiguity without continuity) between the nerve cells in known as 'synapse'. One cell may establish such contacts through its dendrites with as many as 1000 axonal terminals. However, it must be remembered that each neuron is an independent unit and the contact between neurons is by contiguity and not by continuity ('neuron theory' of Waldeyer, 1891). The impulse is transmitted across a synapse through biochemical neurotransmitters (acetylcholine).

Classification of Neurons

A. According to the number of their processes, into four types.

    a. *Multipolar neurons.* Most of the neurons in man are multipolar. For example, all motor and internuncial neurons.

    b. *Bipolar neurons* are confined to the first neuron of the retina, ganglia of eighth cranial nerve, and the olfactory mucosa.

    c. *Pseudounipolar neurons* are actually unipolar to begin with but become bipolar functionally and are found in dorsal nerve root ganglia and sensory ganglia of the cranial nerves.

    d. *Unipolar neurons* are present in the mesencephalic nucleus of trigeminal nerve and also occur during foetal life. These cells are more common in lower vertebrates.

B. According to the length of axon, into two types.

    a. Golgi type I, with long axon.

    b. Golgi type II, with short axon.

Mature nerve cells are incapable of dividing and, therefore, cannot form tumours. Brain tumours arise from the neuroglial cells and the immature nerve cells.

Neuroglial Cells

Various types of neuroglial cells are as follows:

    a. Astrocytes are concerned with nutrition of the nervous tissue.

    b. Oligodendrocytes are counterparts of the Schwann cells. Schwann cells myelinate the peripheral nerves. Oligodendrocytes myelinate the tracts.

    c. Microglia behave like macrophages of the CNS.

    d. Ependymal cells are columnar cells lining the cavities of the CNS.

Proliferation of glial cells is called the 'gliosis'. A CNS lesion heals by gliosis. It represents the scar of the nervous tissue. A spontaneous gliosis is an indication of a degenerative change in the nervous

CLINICAL ANATOMY

If a nerve (axons) is injured or cut a series of degenerative and then regenerative changes follow. The degenerative changes occur in : (a) Cell body: It undergoes chromatolysis. Nissl granules disappear; cell becomes swollen and rounded; and the nucleus is pushed to the periphery. (b) The proximal part of the cut fibre: So long the mother cell is intact, it survives, and only a part near the cut end degenerates in a way similar to the distal part. (c) The distal part of the cut fibre: It degenerates completely. Axis cylinder becomes fragmented; myelin sheath breaks up into fat droplets; and the nuclei of Schwann cells multiply and fill up the neurilemmal tube. During regeneration, the tip of the axon still connected with the cell body begins to grow through the neurilemmal tube. The rate of growth is about 1–2 mm per day in man. Myelin sheath is reformed. Restoration of function may be considerable but rarely complete. The role of neurilemmal tube as a guiding factor to the regenerating proximal axon is considered to be of paramount importance. Thus a nerve can regenerate because it has a neurilemmal sheath. A tract cannot regenerate because it has no such sheath. However, a tract after demyelination can remyelinate, as is seen in demyelinating diseases.

tissue. Since the glial cells are capable of dividing, they can form the CNS tumours.

Reflex Arc

A reflex arc is the functional unit of the nervous system. In its simplest form, (monosynaptic reflex arc) it consists of : (a) a receptor, e.g. the skin; (b) the sensory neuron; (c) the motor neuron; and (d) the effector, e.g. the muscle. In complex forms of the reflex arc, the internuncial neurons (interneurons) are interposed between the sensory and motor neurons. An involuntary motor response to a sensory stimulus is known as the reflex action. Only cortical responses are voluntary in nature. All subcortical responses are involuntary and therefore are the reflex activities.

PARTS OF THE NERVOUS SYSTEM

Central Nervous System (CNS)

1. Brain. Occupies cranial cavity.
2. Spinal cord. Occupies upper two-thirds of the vertebral canal

Peripheral Nervous System

1. Somatic (cerebrospinal) nervous system. It is made up of 12 pairs of cranial nerves and 31 pairs of spinal nerves. Its efferent fibres reach the effectors without interruption.
2. Autonomic (splanchnic) nervous system. It consists of sympathetic and parasympathetic systems. Its efferent fibres first relay in a ganglion, and then the postganglionic fibres pass to the effectors.

Parts of Brain

The main parts and their subdivisions are shown in Table 21.1 (Fig. 21.2).

The brainstem includes the midbrain, pons and medulla. Hindbrain includes pons, medulla and cerebellum. The dilated part of the central canal of spinal cord within the conus medullaris is known as the terminal ventricle. Similarly, the cavity of septum pellucidum is sometimes called as the fifth ventricle.

Table 21.1: Parts of brain

	Parts		Subdivisions	Cavity
1.	Forebrain (prosencephalon)	A.	Telencephalon (cerebrum), made up of two cerebral hemispheres and the median part in front of the interventricular foramen	Lateral ventricle
		B.	Diencephalon (thalamencephalon), hidden by the cerebrum, consists of : a. Thalamus b. Hypothalamus c. Metathalamus, including the medial and lateral geniculate bodies, and d. Epithalamus, including the pineal body, habenular trigone and posterior commissure e. Subthalamus	Third ventricle
2.	Midbrain (mesencephalon)		Crus cerebri, substantia nigra, tegmentum, and tectum, from before backwards	Cerebral aqueduct
3.	Hindbrain (rhombencephalon)	A.	Metencephalon, made up of pons and cerebellum	Fourth ventricle
		B.	Myelencephalon or medulla oblongata	

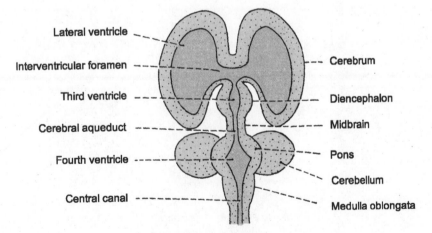

Fig. 21.2: Parts of brain.

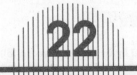

Meninges of the Brain and Cerebrospinal Fluid

The central nervous system is highly protected and safely secured in the cranial cavity. Its security is enhanced by the three meninges and fluid layers between them. So the brain almost floats in the cerebrospinal fluid without putting "its weight" on the neck. The outermost meninx, the dura mater not only separates the right and left cerebral hemisphere, but also partitions the cerebrum from cerebellum and hypophysis cerebri. In addition, it encloses various venous sinuses. The CSF forms watery cushions around the blood vessels to give them shock-free environment.

Introduction

The brain is a very important but delicate organ. It is protected by the following coverings.

1. Bony covering of the cranium.

2. Three membranous coverings (meninges): (a) The outer dura mater (pachymeninx); (b) the middle arachnoid mater; and (c) the inner pia mater. The arachnoid and pia are together known as the leptomeninges.

3. The cerebrospinal fluid fills the space between the arachnoid and the pia (subarachnoid space) and acts as a water cushion.

DURA MATER

The cerebral dura mater has been studied in detail with the head and neck in Chapter 6. However, it may be recapitulated that it is made up of two layers, an outer endosteal layer and an inner meningeal layer, enclosing the cranial venous sinuses between the two. The meningeal layer forms four folds which divide the cranial cavity into intercommunicating compartments for different parts of the brain (Table 22.1).

ARACHNOID MATER

The arachnoid mater is a thin transparent membrane that loosely surrounds the brain without dipping into its sulci. It bridges all irregularities of the brain, with the exception of the stem of the lateral sulcus. It cannot be identified in the hypophyseal fossa.

Relations

It is separated from the dura by the subdural space, and from the pia by the subarachnoid space containing cerebrospinal fluid (CSF).

Prolongations

1. It provides sheaths for the cranial nerves as far as their exit from the skull.

2. Arachnoid villi are small, fingerlike processes of arachnoid tissue, projecting into the cranial venous sinuses. They absorb CSF. With advancing age the arachnoid villi enlarge in size to form pedunculated tufts, called arachnoid granulations. These granulations may produce depressions in bone.

PIA MATER

The pia mater is a thin vascular membrane which closely invests the brain, dipping into various sulci and other irregularities of its surface. It is better defined around the brainstem.

Prolongations

1. It provides sheaths for the cranial nerves merging with the epineurium around them.

2. It also provides perivascular sheaths for the minute vessels entering and leaving the brain substance.

Table 22.1: The meningeal layer sends inwards following folds of dura mater

Folds	Shape	Attachments	Venous sinuses enclosed
Falx cerebri	Sickle-shaped, separates the right from left cerebral hemisphere	Superior, convex margins are attached to sides of the groove lodging the superior sagittal sinus	Superior sagittal sinus
		Inferior concave margin is free. Anterior attachment to crista galli, posterior to upper surface of tentorium cerebelli	Inferior sagittal sinus / Straight sinus
Tentorium cerebelli	Tent-shaped separates the cerebral hemispheres from hindbrain and lower part of mid-brain. Lifts off the weight of occipital lobes from the cerebellum	Has a free anterior margin. Its ends are attached to anterior clinoid processes. Rest is free and concave. Posterior margin is attached to the to the lips of groove containing transverse sinuses, superior petrosal sinuses and to posterior clinoid processes	Transverse sinuses, superior petrosal sinuses
Falx cerebelli	Small sickle shaped fold partly separating two cerebellar hemispheres	Base is attached to posterior part of inferior surface of tentorium cerebelli. Apex reaches till foramen magnum	Occipital sinus
Diaphragma sellae	Small horizontal fold	Anterior attachment is to tuberculum sellae, Posterior attachment is to dorsum sellae; laterally continuous with dura mater of middle cranial fossa	Anterior and posterior intercavernous sinuses

3. Folds of pia mater enclosing tufts of capillaries form the *telachoroidea*. Such pia mater lined by secretory ependyma form the choroid plexus.

EXTRADURAL (EPIDURAL) AND SUBDURAL SPACES

The extradural or epidural space is a potential space between the inner aspect of skull bone and the endosteal layer of dura mater. The subdural space is also a potential space between the dura and arachnoid maters. These become actual spaces in pathological conditions.

SUBARACHNOID SPACE

This is the space between the arachnoid and the pia mater. It is traversed by a network of arachnoid trabeculae which give it a sponge-like appearance.

It surrounds the brain and spinal cord, and ends below at the lower border of the second sacral vertebra.

The subarachnoid space contains CSF, and large vessels of the brain. Cranial nerves pass through the space.

Dilatations

At the base of the brain and around the brainstem the subarachnoid space forms intercommunicating pools, called *cisterns*, which reinforce the protective effect of CSF on the vital centres situated in the medulla. The subarachnoid cisterns are as follows.

1. The *cerebellomedullary cistern (cisterna magna)* lies between the medulla and the undersurface of the cerebellum. It is utilized for cisternal puncture. The CSF passes from the fourth ventricle to this cistern through the median and lateral apertures of the fourth ventricle.

2. The *pontine cistern (cisterna pontis)* contains the vertebral and basilar arteries.

3. The *interpeduncular cistern (basal cistern)* contains the circulus arteriosus (circle of Willis).

4. The *cistern of the lateral sulcus* contains the middle cerebral artery.

5. The *cistern of the great cerebral vein (cisterna ambiens)* contains the same vein.

6. The *cisterna chiasmatis* lies below and in front of the optic chiasma.

The arterial pulsations within the cisterns help to force the CSF from the cisterns on to the surface of the hemispheres. The cisterns themselves form cushions around the medulla.

Communications

The subarachnoid space communicates with the ventricular system of the brain at: (a) A median foramen (of Magendie); and (b) two lateral foramina (of Luschka), situated in the roof of the fourth ventricle. The CSF passes through these foramina from the fourth ventricle to the subarachnoid space (Fig. 27.2).

Prolongations

1. The space is prolonged into the arachnoid sheaths around nerves where it communicates with the neural lymphatics, particularly around the first, second and eighth cranial nerves.

DISSECTION

Cut through the fused endosteum and dura mater on the ventral aspect of brain from the inferolateral borders extending along the superolateral margin. Pull upwards the endosteum along with the fold of dura mater present between the adjacent medial surfaces of cerebral hemispheres, extending from the frontal lobe till the occipital lobe. This is falx cerebri. Pull backwards a similar but much smaller fold between two adjacent lobes of cerebellum—the falx cerebelli.

Separating the cerebrum and the cerebellum is another fold of dura mater called the tentorium cerebelli. Pull it on a horizontal plane. Thus the fused endosteum and dura mater get separated from the underlying subarachnoid mater, pia mater and the brain.

Identify various venous sinuses between the endosteum and folds of dura mater. Underneath the dura mater and separated by a flimsy subdural space is the cobweb like arachnoid mater. It is separated from the underlying pia mater by the subarachnoid space, containing cerebrospinal fluid and blood vessels of the brain. Cranial nerves also pass through this space. Near the superior sagittal sinus, arachnoid mater forms arachnoid villi. The subarachnoid space is dilated around the brainstem and at the base of the brain forming the subarachnoid cisterns.

Cerebrospinal fluid formed and flows through the ventricles of the brain into the subarachnoid space to be absorbed via subarachnoid villi into the superior sagittal sinus.

---

2. The space also extends into the pial sheaths around the vessels entering the brain substance (perivascular space). Thus CSF comes into direct contact with nerve cells.

CEREBROSPINAL FLUID (CSF)

The cerebrospinal fluid is a modified tissue fluid. It is contained in the ventricular system of the brain and in the subarachnoid space around the brain and spinal cord. CSF replaces lymph in the CNS (Figs 22.1, 22.2).

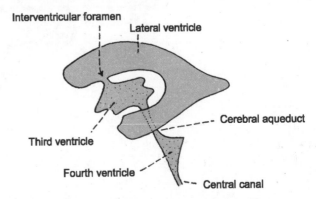

Fig. 22.1: Lateral view of the ventricular system.

Formation

1. The bulk of the CSF is formed by the choroid plexuses of the lateral ventricles, and lesser amounts by the choroid plexuses of the third and fourth ventricles.

2. Possibly, it is also formed by the capillaries on the surface of the brain and spinal cord.

The total quantity of CSF is about 150 ml. It is formed at the rate of about 200 ml per hour or 5000 ml per day. The normal pressure of CSF is 60 to 100 mm of CSF (or of water).

Circulation

CSF passes from each lateral ventricle to the third ventricle through the interventricular foramen (of Monro). From the third ventricle it passes to the fourth ventricle through the cerebral aqueduct. From the fourth ventricle the CSF passes to the subarachnoid space through the median and lateral apertures of the fourth ventricle (Table 22.2).

Absorption

1. CSF is absorbed chiefly through the arachnoid villi and granulations, and is thus drained into the cranial venous sinuses.

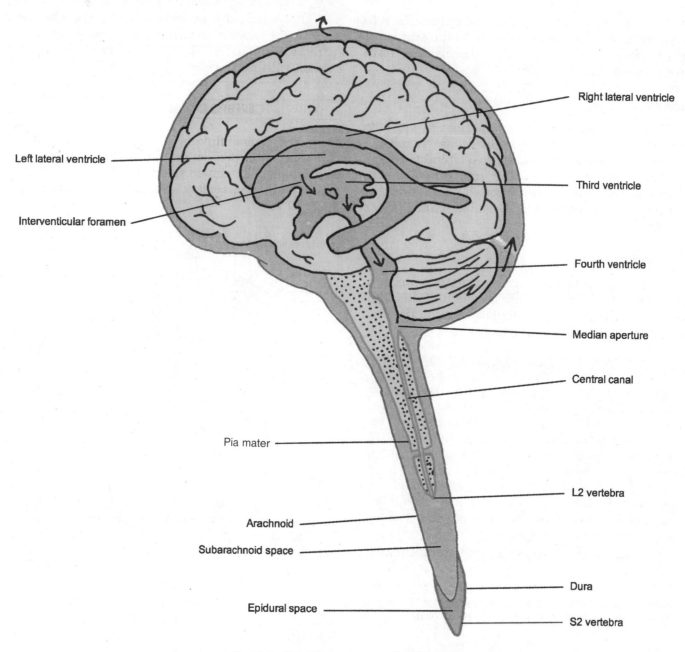

Fig. 22.2: *Circulation of cerebrospinal fluid.*

2. It is also absorbed partly by the perineural lymphatics around the first, second and eighth cranial nerves.

3. It is also absorbed by veins related to spinal nerves.

Functions

It is (a) protective, (b) nutritive, and (c) a pathway for metabolites from the CNS.

3. Obstruction to the flow of CSF in the ventricular system of the brain leads to *hydrocephalus* in children, and raised intracranial pressure in adults.

4. Drainage of CSF at regular intervals is of therapeutic value in meningitis. Certain intractable headaches of unknown aetiology are also known to have been cured by a mere lumbar puncture with drainage of CSF.

5. Obstruction in the vertebral canal produces *Froin's syndrome or loculation syndrome.* This is characterized by yellowish discolouration of CSF (xanthochromia) below the level of obstruction, and its spontaneous coagulation after withdrawal due to a high protein content. Biochemical examination of such fluid reveals that the protein content is raised, but the cell content is normal. This is known as *albumino-cytologic dissociation.*

Table 22.2: Cerebrospinal fluid (CSF)

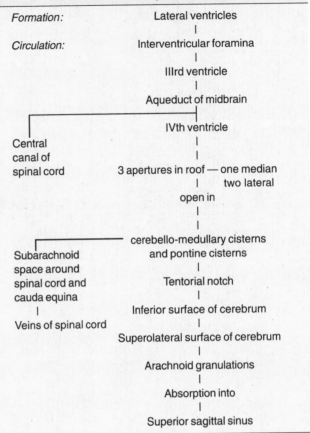

The Spinal Cord

Spinal cord is the lower part of central nervous system, responsible for establishing contacts between the brain in the cranial cavity and the peripheral end organs. The descending and ascending tracts course through the spinal cord. It is a centre for reflex activities.

Introduction

The spinal cord is the lower elongated, cylindrical part of the CNS. It occupies the upper two-thirds of the vertebral canal. It extends from the level of the upper border of the atlas to the lower border of vertebra L1, or the upper border of vertebra L2. It is about 45 cm long. The lower end is conical and is called the *conus medullaris.* The apex of the conus is continued down as the *filum terminale.* Along its length, the cord presents two thickenings, the *cervical and lumbar enlargements,* which give rise to large nerves for the limbs.

The spinal cord gives off 31 pairs of spinal nerves.

As the spinal cord is much shorter than the length of the vertebral column, the spinal segments *do not* lie opposite the corresponding vertebrae. In estimating the position of a spinal segment in relation to the surface of the body, it is important to remember that a vertebral spine is always *lower* than the corresponding spinal segment. As a rough guide it may be stated that in the cervical region there is a difference of one segment; in the upper thoracic region there is a difference of two segments; and in the lower thoracic region there is a difference of three segments (Fig. 23.1).

Internal Structure

When seen in transverse section the grey matter of the spinal cord forms an H-shaped mass. In each half of the cord, the grey matter is divisible into: (1) The *anterior grey column* (or horn), and (2) the *posterior grey column* (or horn). In some parts of the spinal cord, a small *lateral grey column* is also present. The grey matter of the right and left halves of the spinal cord is connected across the midline by the *grey commissure* which is traversed by the central canal.

The white matter of the spinal cord is divisible into right and left halves, in front by a deep *anterior median fissure;* and behind by the *posterior median septum.* In each half, the white matter is divided into: (i) The *posterior white column* or posterior funiculus; (ii) the *lateral white column* or lateral funiculus; and (iii) the *anterior white column* or anterior funiculus. The white matter of the right and left sides is continuous across the midline through the white commissure which lies anterior to the grey commissure (Fig. 23.2).

The spinal cord gives attachment, on either side, to a series of spinal nerves. Each spinal nerve arises by two roots: (i) Anterior (or ventral); and (ii) posterior (or dorsal). Each root is made up of a number of rootlets. The length of the spinal cord giving origin to the rootlets for one pair of spinal nerves constitutes one *spinal segment.*

Nuclei of Spinal Cord

The grey matter of spinal cord is arranged in three horns. Anterior is motor, lateral being visceral efferent and afferent in function, and posterior is sensory in function.

Nuclei in Anterior Grey Column or Horn

The anterior horn is divided into a ventral part, the head and a dorsal part, the base. The nuclei in anterior horn innervate the skeletal muscles. The cells in the anterior horn are arranged in the following three main groups.

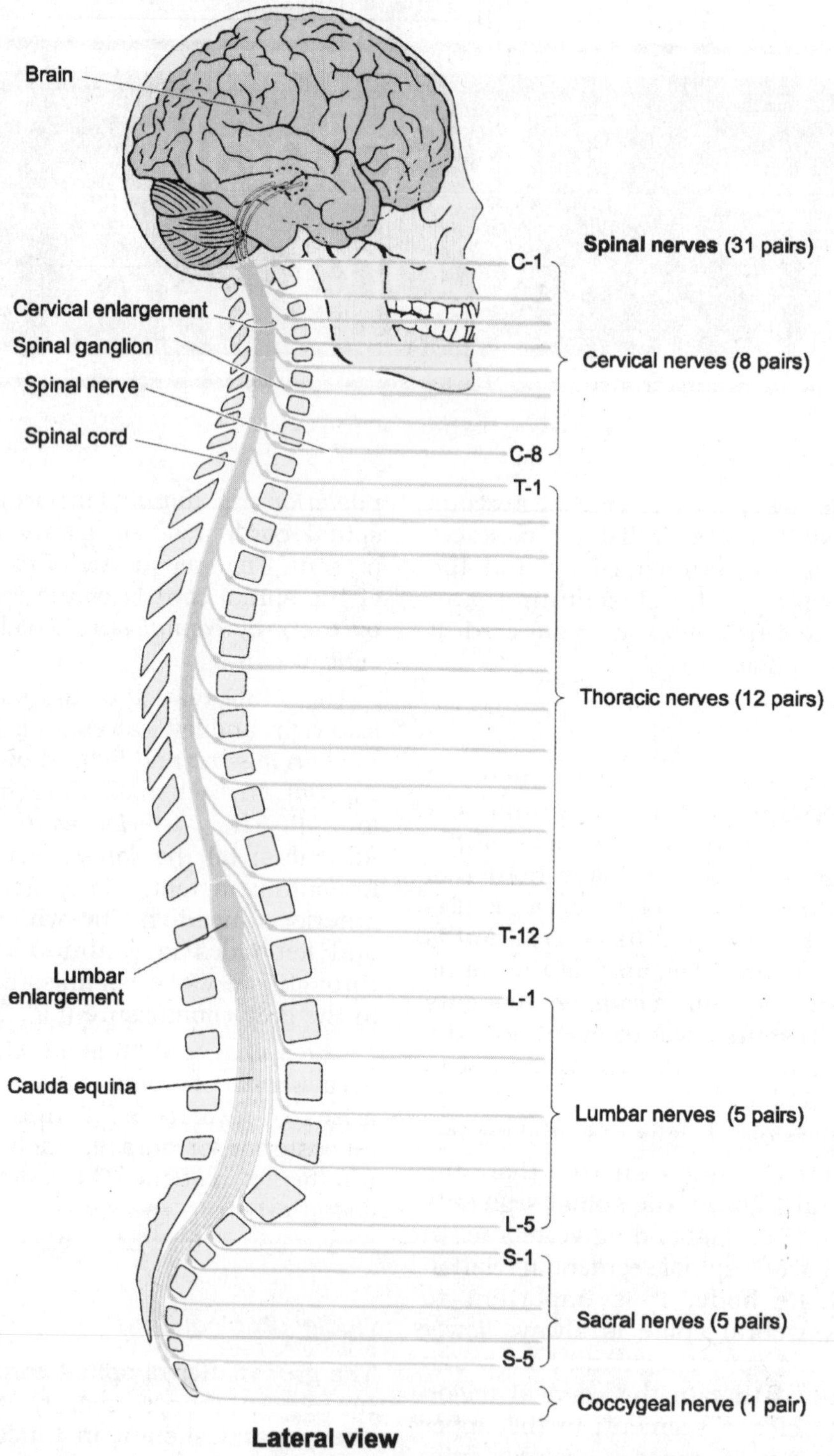

Lateral view

Fig. 23.1: Spinal cord with its 31 pairs of spinal nerves.

(a) Medial group: It is present throughout the entire extent of spinal cord and innervates the axial muscles of the body.

(b) Lateral group: Present only in the cervical and lumbar enlargements and supplies musculature of limbs. It is subdivided into three subgroups.

(i) Anterolateral supplying proximal muscles of limbs (shoulder and arm/gluteal region and thigh).

(ii) Posterolateral supplying intermediate muscles of limbs (forearm/leg) (Fig. 23.3).

(iii) Post posterolateral innervating the distal segment (hand/foot).

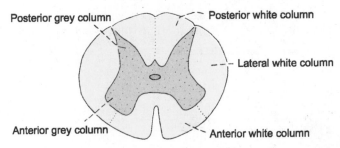

Fig. 23.2: Internal structure of spinal cord.

(c) *Central group:* Only in upper cervical segments as phrenic nerve nucleus and nucleus of spinal root of accessory nerve.

Nuclei in Lateral Horn

Nuclei in Lateral horn are as follows:

(a) *Intermediolateral nucleus:* This acts as both efferent and afferent nuclear columns. This nucleus is seen at two levels. .

(i) From T1 to L2 segments, giving rise to preganglionic sympathetic fibres (thoracolumbar outflow).

(ii) From S2 to S4 segments giving rise to preganglionic parasympathetic fibres chiefly for the pelvic viscera.

At these two levels, the intermediolateral cell column receives visceral afferent fibres.

(b) *Intermediomedial nucleus:* This is mostly internuncial neuronal column.

Nuclei in Posterior Grey Column

Afferent nuclear group column: The four main afferent nuclei are seen in this are:

(i) *Posteromarginal nucleus:* Thin layer of neurons caps the posterior horn. It receives some of incoming dorsal root fibres.

(ii) *Substantia gelatinosa:* This is found at the tip of posterior horn through the entire extent of spinal cord. It acts as a relay station for pain and temperature fibres and is concerned with sensory associative mechanism. Its axons give rise to the lateral spinothalamic tract.

(iii) *Nucleus proprius:* It lies subjacent to the substantia gelatinosa throughout the entire extent of cord.

It is concerned with sensory associative mechanism.

(iv) Nucleus dorsalis also known as thoracic nucleus at the medial part of base of posterior horn extending from C8 to L3 segments. It is a relay nuclear column for reflex or unconscious proprioceptive impulses to the cerebellum and its axons give rise to the posterior spinocerebellar tract.

Laminar Organisation in Spinal Cord

In thick sections, spinal cord neurons appear to have a laminar (layered) arrangement. Ten layers of neurons are recognised, known also as Laminae of Rexed. These are numbered consecutively by Roman numerals, starting at the tip of the dorsal horn and moving ventrally into ventral horn (Fig. 23.4).

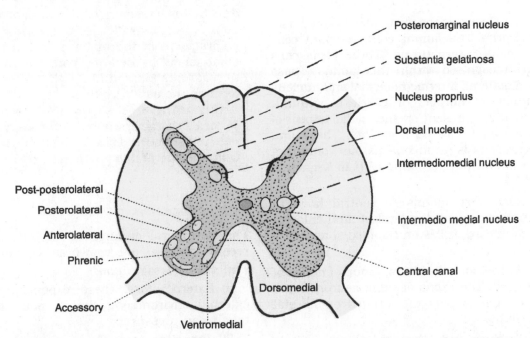

Fig. 23.3: Nuclei in the grey matter of spinal cord. (Courtesy: Garg, Kaul and Bahl: Text Book of Neuroanatomy, 2nd edition, CBS Publishers and Distributors, New Delhi).

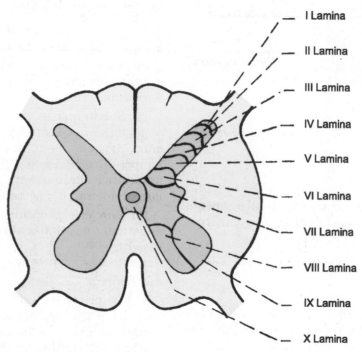

I Lamina
II Lamina
III Lamina
IV Lamina
V Lamina
VI Lamina
VII Lamina
VIII Lamina
IX Lamina
X Lamina

Fig. 23.4: *Laminar organisation in the spinal cord. (Courtesy: Garg, Kaul and Bahl: Text Book of Neuroanatomy, 2nd edition, CBS Publishers and Distributors, New Delhi).*

Lamina I: Corresponds to posteromarginal nucleus.

Lamina II: Corresponds to the substantia gelatinosa.

Laminae III and *IV:* Correspond to nucleus proprius.

Laminae V and VI: Correspond to base of dorsal column.

Lamina VII: Occupies the territory between dorsal and ventral horns. This lamina contains many cells that function as interneurons. Three clear cells columns are recognised within this lamina. These are intermediolateral, intermediomedial and nucleus dorsalis (nucleus thoracis or Clarke's column). Nucleus dorsalis is present on the medial aspect of dorsal horn from C8 to L3 segments. The sacral autonomic nucleus is an inconspicuous column of cells in the lateral part of lamina VII in segments S2, S3 and S4.

Lamina VIII: Corresponds to ventral horn in thoracic segments but at the level of limb enlargements of spinal cord, it lies on the medial aspect of ventral horn.

Lamina IX: Includes the lateral group of nuclei of the ventral horn. The axons of these neurons leave the spinal cord to supply the striated or skeletal muscles of limbs.

Lamina X: Surrounds the central canal. It is composed of decussating axons, neuroglia and some neurons in the grey matter surrounding central canal that have properties of interneurons.

DISSECTION

Study the spinal cord after it was removed from vertebral canal and separated from the dura mater and arachnoid mater. Identify the dorsal root due to the presence of dorsal root ganglion or spinal ganglion. Note the position of cervical enlargement in the upper part and lumbosacral enlargement in the lower part. See the numerous nerve roots surrounding the filum terminale forming the cauda equina.

Cut transverse sections of spinal cord at cervical, thoracic, lumbar, and sacral regions to note the shape and size of the horns in relation to white matter (Table 23.1).

Sensory Receptors

The peripheral endings of afferent fibres which receive impulses are known as receptors.

Functional classification:

(i) *Exteroceptors:* These respond to stimuli from external environment, that is pain, temperature, touch and pressure.

(ii) *Proprioceptors:* These respond to stimuli in deeper tissues that is contraction of muscles,

Table 23.1: Shape of horns in different segments of spinal cord

Segments of spinal cord	Posterior Horn	Lateral Horn	Anterior Horn
Cervical	Slender	Absent	Broad in C 5–8 segments for supply of upper limbs
Thoracic	Slender	Present for thoraco-lumbar outflow	Slender
Lumbar	Bulbous	Present only in lumbar 1–2 segments	Bulbous for supply of lower limbs
Sacral	Thick	Present in sacral 2–4 segments for sacral outflow	Bulbous for supply of lower limbs

movements, position and pressure related to joints. These are responsible for coordination of muscles, maintenance of body posture and equilibrium. These actions are perceived at unconscious level.

(iii) *Interoceptors/Enteroceptors:* These include receptor end-organs in the walls of viscera, gland, blood vessels and specialised structures in the carotid sinus, carotid bodies and osmoreceptors.

(iv) *Special sense receptors:* These are concerned with vision, hearing, smell and taste.

TRACTS OF THE SPINAL CORD

A collection of nerve fibres that connects two masses of grey matter within the central nervous system is called a tract. Tracts may be ascending or descending. They are usually named after the masses of grey matter connected by them. Some tracts are called fasciculi or lemnisci.

The following tracts are seen in a transverse section through the spinal cord. Their location should be identified in (Figs 23.5, 23.6).

Descending Tracts

A. The pyramidal or *corticospinal tract* descends from the cerebral cortex to the spinal cord. It consists of two parts:

1. The lateral corticospinal tract, which lies in the lateral funiculus; and

2. The anterior corticospinal tract which lies in the anterior funiculus (Fig. 30.1).

B. Extrapyramidal tracts. These are:

1. The *rubrospinal tract.*

2, 3. The *medial and lateral reticulospinal tracts.*

4. The *olivospinal tract.*

5. The *vestibulospinal tract.*

6. The *tectospinal tract.*

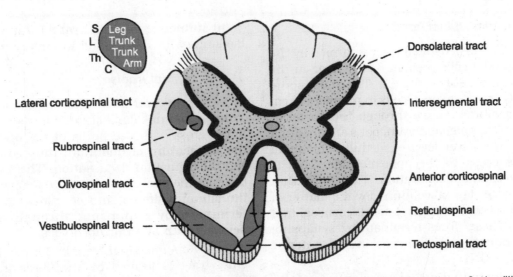

Fig. 23.5: *Descending tracts of spinal cord. (Courtesy: Garg, Kaul and Bahl: Text Book of Neuroanatomy, 2nd edition, CBS Publishers and Distributors, New Delhi).*

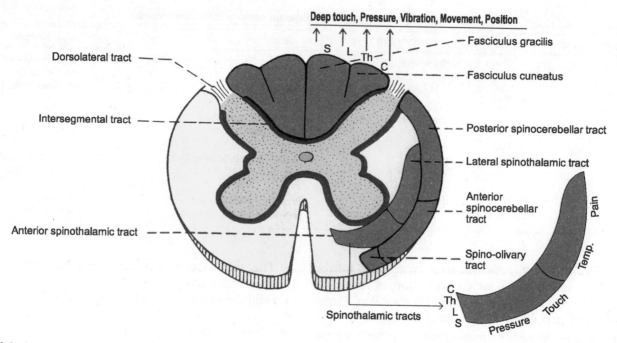

Fig. 23.6: Ascending tracts in spinal cord. (Courtesy: Garg, Kaul and Bahl: *Text Book of Neuroanatomy, 2nd edition, CBS Publishers and Distributors, New Delhi*).

Ascending Tracts

1. Lateral spinothalamic tract (Fig. 23.6).
2. Anterior spinothalamic tract (Fig. 23.7).
3. Fasciculus gracilis (medially)
4. Fasciculus cuneatus (laterally) (Fig. 23.6).
5. Dorsal or posterior spinocerebellar tracts.
6. Ventral or anterior spinocerebellar tract
7. Spino-olivary tract.
8. Spinotectal tract.

Descending Tracts

Pyramidal or Corticospinal Tract

The pyramidal or corticospinal tract is formed by the axons of pyramidal cells predominantly lying in the motor area of cerebral cortex. There is some contribution to it from axon of cells in premotor area. From here the fibres course through the posterior limb of internal capsule, midbrain, pons and medulla oblongata. At the lower level of medulla oblongata 80% of fibres cross to the opposite side. This is known as pyramidal decussation. The fibres that have crossed enter lateral column of white matter of spinal cord and descend as lateral corticospinal tract. Most of these fibres terminate by synapsing through the internuncial neurons at the anterior horn cells (Fig. 30.1).

The 20% of fibres that do not cross enter anterior white column of spinal cord to form anterior corticospinal tract. The fibres of this tract also cross at appropriate levels to reach grey matter of the opposite half of spinal cord and synapse with internuncial neurons similar to those of lateral corticospinal tract (Fig. 23.5).

Thus the cerebral cortex through lateral and anterior corticospinal tracts controls anterior horns cells of opposite half of spinal cord (Table 23.2).

Functional Significance

(i) The cerebral cortex controls voluntary movements of opposite half of body through anterior horn cells.

(ii) Influence of this tract is supposed to be facilitatory for flexors and inhibitory for extensors.

Extrapyramidal Tracts

1. *Rubrospinal tract:* This tract is formed by the axons of red nucleus, situated in the midbrain. The fibres cross with the fibres of the opposite side in the tegmentum of midbrain; thus constituting the ventral tegmental decussation. The tract descends through the pons and medulla oblongata and enters the lateral white column of spinal cord. The fibres terminate by synapsing through internuncial neurons with anterior horn cells.

2, 3. *Reticulospinal tracts:* The medial reticulospinal tract is formed by the fibres from reticular formation in pons and descends to the cervical segments only. It lies in the anterior white column

Table 23.2: The descending tracts

S. No.	Name	Function	Crossed uncrossed	Spinal segment	Beginning	1st termination
The Ascending Tracts						
A1.	Lateral corticospinal	Main motor tract	Crossed	C_1 to S_5	Motor area of cortex (upper neurons)	Anterior grey column cells alpha motor neurons
A2.	Anterior corticospinal	Main motor tract	Uncrossed	C_1 to S_5	Motor area of cortex (upper motor neurons)	Anterior grey column alpha motor neurons
B1.	Rubrospinal	Efferent pathway for cerebellum and corpus stratum	Crossed	C_1 to C_5	Red nucleus of midbrain	Anterior grey column cells
B2.	Medial reticulo-spinal	Extrapyramidal tract	Uncrossed mainly	C_1 to S_5	Reticular formation of grey matter of pons	Anterior grey column cells (interneurons)
B3.	Lateral reticulospinal	Extrapyramidal tract	Crossed	C_1 to S_5	Reticular formation of grey matter of medulla oblongota	Anterior grey column cells (interneurons)
B4.	Olivospinal	Extrapyramidal tract	Uncrossed	C_1 to C_5	Inferior olivary nucleus	Anterior grey column cells
B5.	Vestibulospinal	Efferent pathway for equilibratory control	Uncrossed	C_1 to S_5	Lateral vestibular nucleus	Anterior grey column cells
B6.	Tectospinal	Efferent pathway for visual reflexes	Crossed	C_1 to C_5	Superior colliculus	Anterior grey column

of spinal cord. It has uncrossed fibres. The lateral reticulospinal tract originate from reticular formation in medulla olongata, descend upto thoracic segments of spinal cord. It has both crossed and uncrossed fibres. It lies in the anterolateral white column of spinal cord. Both the tracts terminate by synapsing with the neurons in laminae VII of the spinal cord.

4. *Olivospinal tract:* Its fibres originate from the inferior olivary nucleus in medulla oblongata, descend to spinal cord, lie in the anterolateral column of white matter and synapse with the anterior horn cells.

5. *Vestibulospinal tract:* The fibres arise from lateral vestibular nucleus lying at pontomedullary junction. The fibres descend uncrossed to spinal cord. This tract is situated in the anterior white column of spinal cord. These fibres synapse with anterior horn cells.

6. *Tectospinal tract:* The tract is formed by the axons of neurons lying in the superior colliculus of the midbrain. The fibres cross to the opposite side thus forming dorsal tegmental decussation in midbrain. The tract descends through pons, medulla and anterior white column of spinal cord. The fibres terminate on the cells of anterior horn through internuncial neurons.

All these descendimg tracts control the voluntary movements of skeletal muscles of the body through anterior horn cells.

Ascending Tracts

For the sensory pathways the first neuron fibres always start in the dorsal root ganglia which has pseudounipolar cells. The peripheral process of these cells form the sensory fibres of peripheral nerves which carry various types of sensations from sensory end organs. The central process of the neurons in the dorsal root ganglia enter the spinal cord through dorsal nerve root and terminate either by synapsing with cells in posterior grey column of spinal cord or at higher level in the medulla oblongata with the cells of nucleus gracilis and nucleus cuneatus. After relay in the nuclei second neuron fibres start and ascend to either thalamus or cerebellum. The cerebellum finally recieves second neurons fibres, whereas from the thalamus relayed third neuron fibres are projected to the sensory areas in the cerebral cortex (Table 23.3).

1. *Lateral spinothalamic tract:* This tract carries the sensation of pain and temperature. The first neuron fibres start in the dorsal root ganglia. These relay by synapsing with neurons lying in the grey matter of lamina II and III. Pain fibres relay in Lamina II (substantia gelatinosa). The second neuron fibres cross immediately to opposite side close to the central canal and ascend as tract in the lateral white column of spinal cord.

2. *Anterior spinothalamic tract:* This tract carries the fibres for crude touch and pressure. First neuron fibres are in the dorsal root ganglia. These relay in the grey matter of posterior horn or nucleus proprius (Laminae III–IV). The second neuron fibres ascend for 1-2 segments and cross to opposite side in the white commissure and ascend as a tract in the anterior white column of spinal cord.

The anterior and lateral spinothalamic tracts carry sensations from the opposite half of body.

These lie in continuity with each other in the anterolateral white column of spinal cord showing somatotopic lamination. The sensations of pressure, touch, temperature and pain are lying medial to lateral. Pressure sensations are medial most near the anterior median fissure. Cervical segments are facing medially and sacral segments face laterally.

The sensations like deep touch, pressure, tactile localisation (the ability to locate exactly the proprioceptive part touched), tactile discrimination (the ability to localise two separate points on the skin that is touched), stereognosis (ability to recognise shape of object held in hand), sense of vibration are carried by fasciculus gracilis and fasciculus cuneatus.

3. *Fasciculus gracilis (tract of Goll):* It commences at the caudal limit of spinal cord and is composed mainly of the long ascending branches of the medial division of fibres of dorsal nerve roots. These are the first order neuron fibres from dorsal root ganglia. These run directly upwards (without relaying in the spinal grey matter) in the posterior column of white

Table 23.3: Neurons of sensory tracts

	1st	2nd	3rd	Clinical tests
Lateral spinothalamic	Dorsal root ganglion	Substantia gelatinosa	Posterolateral ventral nucleus of thalamus	1. Pain with pin prick 2. Temperature with hot and cold water in the test tubes
Anterior spinothalamic	,,	Nucleus proprius		1. Joint sense 2. Vibration sense 3. Tactile localization 4. Tactile discrimination 5. Rhomberg's test 6. Stereognosis 7. Crude touch 8. Crude pressure
Fasciculus gracilis	,,	Nucleus gracilis in medulla oblongata	,,	
Fasciculus cuneatus	,,	Nucleus cuneatus in medulla oblongata	,,	
Dorsal spinocerebellar	,,	Clark's column	Nil	All cerebellar tests, like the finger-nose and heel-knee tests for intention tremors
Ventral spinocerebellar	,,	Neurons of posterior horn	Nil	

matter of spinal cord. As the tract ascends, it recieves accession from each dorsal root. The fibres which enter in the coccygeal and lower sacral region are thrust medially by fibres which enter at higher levels. Fasciculus gracilis which contains fibres derived from lower thoracic, lumbar, sacral and coccygeal segments of spinal cord occupies the

medial part of posterior column of upper part of spinal cord is separated from fasciculus cuneatus by postero-intermediate septum (Fig. 23.7).

4. *Fasciculus cuneatus (tract of Burdach):* It commences in mid-thoracic region. It derives its fibres from upper thoracic and cervical segments.

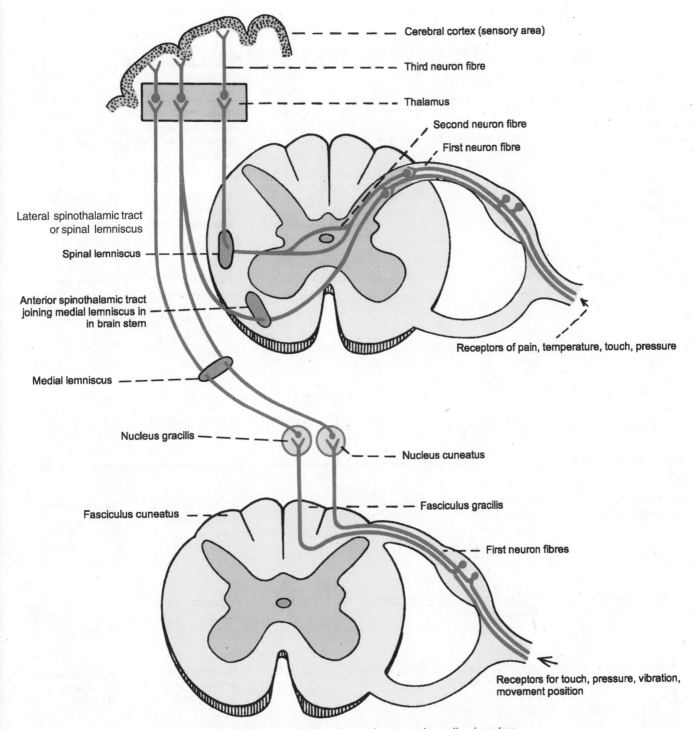

Fig. 23.7: Exteroceptive and conscious proprioceptive impulses.

Both fasciculi contain first neuron fibres from central process of dorsal root ganglia and end by synapsing with the neurons in nucleus gracilis and nucleus cuneatus, situated in the medulla oblogata from where second neuron fibres take origin.

The reflex proprioceptive sensations are carried by dorsal and ventral spinocerebellar tracts. They convey to the cerebellum both exteroceptive (touch) and unconscious proprioceptive impulses arising in

Golgi tendon organ and muscle spindle and are essential for the control of posture (Table 23.4).

5. *Dorsal or posterior spinocerebellar tract:* It begins about the level of 2nd or 3rd lumbar segment of spinal cord. The first neuron fibres are the central processes of dorsal root ganglia. These relay in the dorsal nucleus (thoracic or Clark's column) which lies on the medial side of the base of posterior grey column in segments. This relay gives rise to second

Table 23.4: The ascending tracts of the spinal cord

S. No.	Name	Function	Crossed uncrossed	Spinal segment	Beginning	1st termination
1.	Lateral spinothalamic	Pain and temperature from opposite half of body	Crossed	C_1 to S_5	Substantia gelatinosa of posterior grey column	Posterolateral ventral nucleus of thalamus
2.	Anterior spinothalamic	Touch (crude) and pressure from opposite half of body	Crossed	C_1 to S_5	Posterior grey column of opposite side	Posterolateral ventral nucleus of thalamus
3.	Fasciculus gracilis	Conscious proprioception, Discriminatory touch	Uncrossed	S_5 to T_7	Dorsal root ganglion cells	Nucleus gracilis
4.	Fasciculus cuneatus	Vibratory sense Stereognosis	Uncrossed	T_1 to T_5	Dorsal root ganglion cells	Nucleus cuneatus
5.	Posterior spino-cerebellar	Unconscious proprioception to cerebellum	Uncrossed	C_1 to L_2	Thoracic nucleus of posterior grey column	Vermis of cerebellum (via inferior cerebellar peduncle)
6.	Anterior spino-cerebellar	Cerebellum adjustments of muscle tone	Crossed	C_1 to L_2	Posterior grey column same side	Vermis of cerebellum (via superior cerebellar peduncle) via re-crossing
7.	Spino-olivary	Proprioceptive sense	Uncrossed	C_1 to S_5	Posterior grey column	Dorsal and medial accessory olivary nuclei
8.	Spinotectal	Afferent limb of reflex movements of eyes and head towards source of stimulation	Crossed	C_1 to C_6	Posterior grey column of opposite side	Tectum or superior colliculus of mid-brain

neuron fibres which form dorsal spinocerebellar tract. This uncrossed tract ascends in the lateral column of white matter of spinal cord. Here it is situated as a flattened band at the posterior region of lateral column, medially in contact with lateral corticospinal tract. It ascends to the level of medulla oblongata where its fibres pass through inferior cerebellar peduncle to reach the cerebellum (Fig. 23.8).

6. *Ventral or anterior spinocerebellar tract:* The first neuron fibres are the central processes of dorsal root ganglia. The second neuron fibres are derived from the large cells of posterior grey column (laminae V, VI) in the lumbar and sacral segments. The second neuron fibres are from opposite side mainly, very few from the ipsilateral side. These ascend in the lateral white column of spinal cord anterior to the fibres of dorsal spinocerebellar tract to pass through the medulla oblongata and pons. These fibres finally curve along lateral aspect of superior cerebellar peduncle, and recross in the inferior cerebellar commissure to regain their original site of origin.

Functionally, both spinocerebellar tracts control the coordination and movements of muscles controlling posture of the body. The ventral tract conveys muscle and joint information from both upper and lower limbs, while the dorsal tract receives information from trunk and lower limbs.

7, 8. The other ascending tracts the spino-olivary and spinotectal, are responsible for visual and proprioceptive reflexes. ,

Intersegmental tracts: These are formed of fibres connecting various segments of spinal cord. These are present in anterior, posterior and lateral columns of white matter of spinal cord adjacent to the spinal cord.

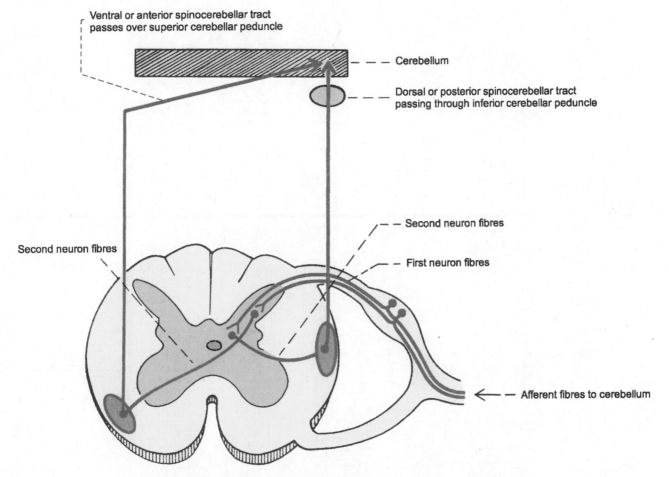

Fig. 23.8: *Path of dorsal and ventral spinocerebellar tracts.*

CLINICAL ANATOMY

Syringomyelia : It is the condition in which there is dilatation of central canal of spinal cord usually beginning in cervical region. Decussating fibres for pain and temperature in the grey commissure are interrupted. This leads to bilateral loss of pain and temperature in the affected region. But touch and proprioception is present. Thus patient has dissociation of sensory loss. Usually the patient gets severe infections in the fingers due to uncared cuts and bruises.

Poliomyelitis : It is a viral disease which involves anterior horn cells leading to flaccid paralysis of the affected segments. It is lower motor neuron paralysis.

Following is the comparison between upper motor neuron and lower motor neuron paralysis:

LMN Paralysis	UMN Paralysis
Muscle tone abolished	Muscle tone increased
Leads to flaccid paralysis	Leads to spastic paralysis
Muscles atropy later	No atrophy of muscles
Reaction of degeneration seen	Reaction of degeneration not seen
Tendon reflexes absent	Tendon reflexes exaggerated
Limited damage	Extensive damage

The Brainstem

The brainstem connects the spinal cord to cerebrum. The various ascending and descending tracts pass through the three components of the brainstem. Medulla contains the respiratory and vasomotor centers. In hanging or capital punishment, the dens of axis breaks and strikes on these centers causing immediate death. Midbrain contains nuclei of oculomotor and trochlear nerves. Pons has the nuclei of trigeminal, abducent, facial and stato-acoustic nerves while medulla houses the nuclei of last four cranial nerves, i.e. glossopharyngeal, vagus, accessory and hypoglossal nerves.

The brainstem consists of the medulla oblongata, the pons and the midbrain.

THE MEDULLA OBLONGATA

The medulla is the lowest part of the brainstem, extending from the lower border of the pons to a plane just above the first cervical nerve where it is continuous with the spinal cord. It lies in the anterior part of the posterior cranial fossa, extending down to the foramen magnum. Anteriorly, it is related to the clivus and meninges; and posteriorly, to the vallecula of the cerebellum. Along with other parts of the hindbrain, the medulla occupies the infratentorial space.

External Features

1. The medulla is divided into right and left halves by the anterior and posterior median fissures. Each half is further divided into anterior, lateral and posterior regions by the anterolateral and poste-rolateral sulci (Fig. 24.1).

2. The anterior region is in the form of a longitudinal elevation called the *pyramid*. The pyramid is made up of corticospinal fibres. In the lower part of the medulla, many fibres of the right and left pyramids cross in the midline forming the *pyramidal decussation*.

3. Some fibres run transversely across the upper part of the pyramid. These are the *anterior external arcuate fibres.*

4. The upper part of the lateral region shows an oval elevation, the *olive*. It is produced by an underlying mass of grey mater called the *inferior olivary nucleus*. A bundle of fibres curving around the lower edge of the olive is the *circumolivary bundle.*

5. The rootlets of the hypoglossal nerve emerge from the anterolateral sulcus between the pyramid and the olive.

6. The rootlets of the cranial nerves IX and X and of the cranial part of the accessory nerve emerge through the posterolateral fissure, behind the olive.

7. The posterolateral region lies between the posterolateral sulcus and the posterior median fissure. The upper part of this region is marked by a V-shaped depression which is the lower part of the floor of the fourth ventricle. Below the floor we see three longitudinal elevations. From medial to lateral side these are the fasciculus gracilis, the fasciculus cuneatus and the inferior cerebellar peduncle. The upper ends of the fasciculus gracilis and fasciculus cuneatus expand to form the *gracile and cuneate tubercles*. These tubercles are formed by underlying masses of grey matter called the *nucleus gracilis* and *nucleus cuneatus* (Fig. 24.2).

8. In the lower part of the medulla, there is another elevation the *tubercinerium* lateral to the fasciculus cuneatus. It is produced by a mass of grey matter called the *spinal nucleus of the trigeminal nerve.*

9. The medulla is divided in two parts: The lower *closed part* with a central canal; and the upper *open part* where the central canal opens out to form the fourth ventricle.

321

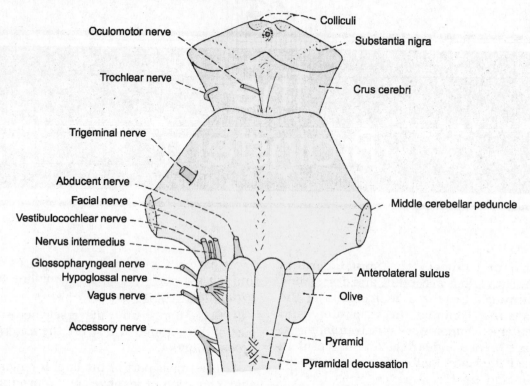

Oculomotor nerve

Trochlear nerve

Trigeminal nerve

Abducent nerve

Facial nerve

Vestibulocochlear nerve

Nervus intermedius

Glossopharyngeal nerve

Hypoglossal nerve

Vagus nerve

Accessory nerve

Colliculi

Substantia nigra

Crus cerebri

Middle cerebellar peduncle

Anterolateral sulcus

Olive

Pyramid

Pyramidal decussation

Fig. 24.1: *Surface features of the brainstem as seen from the front.*

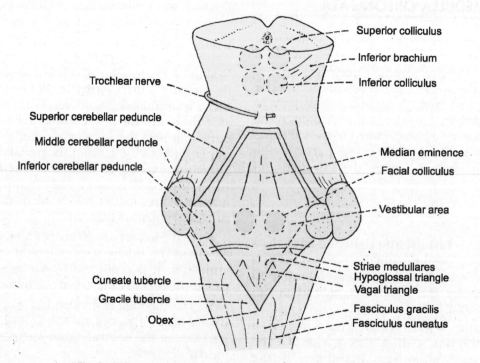

Trochlear nerve

Superior cerebellar peduncle

Middle cerebellar peduncle

Inferior cerebellar peduncle

Cuneate tubercle

Gracile tubercle

Obex

Superior colliculus

Inferior brachium

Inferior colliculus

Median eminence

Facial colliculus

Vestibular area

Striae medullares

Hypoglossal triangle

Vagal triangle

Fasciculus gracilis

Fasciculus cuneatus

Fig. 24.2: *Surface features of the brainstem as seen from behind.*

Remove the small blood vessels and pia mater from the medulla oblongata. Identify its dorsal and ventral surfaces including the attachments of cranial nerves IX-XII.

The internal structure of medulla oblongata is studied by making sections at the level of: (a) Pyramidal decussation; (b) sensory decussation; and (c) inferior cerebellar peduncles.

Identify the convex basilar or ventral surface of pons with the basilar sulcus lodging the basilar artery. Its dorsal surface is overlapped by the cerebellum. The structure of the basilar part of pons is similar in its whole extent. The structure of dorsal or tegmental part is different in the lower and upper part. Make sections through the pons in its upper and lower parts and identify its various nuclei and fibre components.

Midbrain is the highest part of the brainstem. Identify the four swellings on its dorsal surface. These are a pair of inferior and a pair of superior colliculi. Demarcate the subdivisions of the midbrain.

Make one transverse section through the midbrain at the level of inferior colliculus and another at the level of superior colliculus. Try to identify few parts of grey and white matters.

Internal Structure

The internal structure of the medulla can be studied conveniently by examining transverse sections through it at three levels.

Transverse Section through the Lower Part of the Medulla Passing through the Pyramidal Decussation

It resembles a transverse section of the spinal cord in having the same three funiculi and the same tracts. Identify the following in Fig. 24.3.

Grey Matter

1. The decussating pyramidal fibres separate the anterior horn from the central grey matter. The *separated anterior horn* forms the spinal nucleus of the accessory nerve laterally and the supraspinal nucleus for motor fibres of the first cervical nerve medially.

2. The central grey matter (with the central canal) is pushed backwards.

3. The nucleus gracilis and the nucleus cuneatus are continuous with the central grey matter.

4. Laterally, the central grey matter is continuous with the nucleus of the spinal tract of the trigeminal nerve. A bundle of fibres overlying this nucleus forms the spinal tract of the trigeminal nerve.

White Matter

1. The pyramids, anteriorly.

2. The decussation of the pyramidal tracts forms the most important features of the medulla at this level. The fibres of each pyramid run backwards and laterally to reach the lateral white column of the spinal cord where they form the lateral corticospinal tract.

3. The fasciculus gracilis and the fasciculus cuneatus occupy the broad posterior white column.

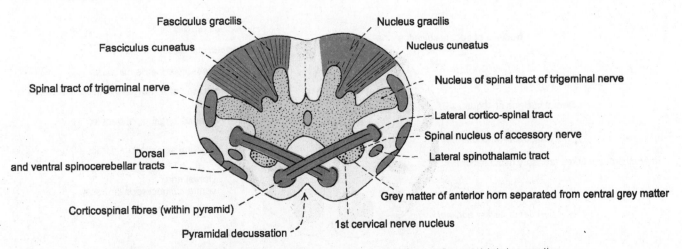

Fasciculus gracilis

Fasciculus cuneatus

Spinal tract of trigeminal nerve

Dorsal
and ventral spinocerebellar tracts

Corticospinal fibres (within pyramid)

Pyramidal decussation

Nucleus gracilis

Nucleus cuneatus

Nucleus of spinal tract of trigeminal nerve

Lateral cortico-spinal tract

Spinal nucleus of accessory nerve

Lateral spinothalamic tract

Grey matter of anterior horn separated from central grey matter

1st cervical nerve nucleus

Fig. 24.3: Transverse section of medulla oblongata at the level of pyramidal decussation.

4. The other features of the white matter are similar to those of the spinal cord.

Transverse Section through the Middle of Medulla (through the sensory decussation)

Identify the following features in Fig. 24.4.

Grey Matter

1. The nucleus gracilis and the nucleus cuneatus are much larger and are separate from the central grey matter. The fasciculus gracilis and the fasciculus cuneatus end in these nuclei.

2. Lateral to the cuneate nucleus we see the *accessory cuneate nucleus* which relays unconscious proprioceptive fibres from the upper limbs.

3. The *nucleus of the spinal tract of the trigeminal nerve* is also separate from the central grey matter.

4. The lower part of the *inferior olivary nucleus* is seen.

5. The central grey matter contains the following:
(a) Hypoglossal nucleus
(b) Dorsal nucleus of the vagus.
(c) Nucleus of tractus solitarius.

White Matter

1. The nucleus gracilis and cuneatus give rise to the *internal arcuate fibres*. These fibres cross to the opposite side where they form a paramedian band of fibres, called the *medial lemniscus*. In the lemniscus, the body is represented with the head posteriorly and the feet anteriorly.

2. The *pyramidal tracts* lie anteriorly.

3. The *medial longitudinal bundle* lies posterior to the medial lemniscus.

4. The *spinocerebellar* and *lateral spinothalamic tracts* (and other tracts) lie in the anterolateral area.

Transverse Section through the Upper Part of the Medulla Passing through the Floor of the Fourth Ventricle

Identify the following in Fig. 24.5.

Grey Matter

1. The nuclei of several cranial nerves are seen in the floor of the fourth ventricle: (a) The *hypoglossal nucleus*, in a paramedian position; (b) the *dorsal nucleus of the vagus*, lateral to the XII nerve nucleus; (c) the *nucleus of the tractus solitarius*, ventrolateral to the dorsal nucleus of the vagus; and (d) the *inferior and medial vestibular nuclei*, medial to the inferior cerebellar peduncle.

2. The *nucleus ambiguus* lies deep in the reticular formation of the medulla. It gives origin to motor fibres of the cranial nerves IX, X and XI.

3. The dorsal and ventral cochlear nuclei lie on the surface of the inferior cerebellar peduncle. These nuclei receive fibres of the cochlear nerve.

4. The *nucleus of the spinal tract* of the trigeminal nerve lies in the dorsolateral part.

5. The *inferior olivary nucleus* is the largest mass of grey matter seen at this level. It is responsible for producing the elevation of the olive. Its grey matter appears like a crumpled purse.

Close to the inferior olivary nucleus there are the medial and dorsal accessory olivary nuclei.

6. The *arcuate nucleus* lies anteromedial to the pyramidal tract.

Visceral centres are :

(i) Respiratory centre

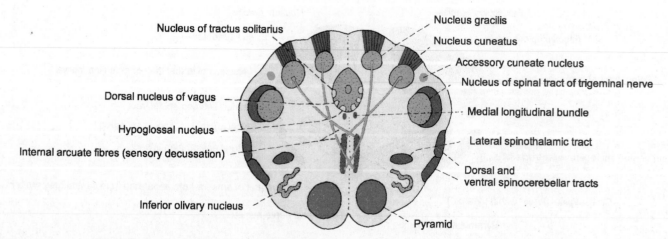

Fig. 24.4: *Transverse section through the medulla oblongata at the level of sensory decussation.*

Nucleus of tractus solitarius

Dorsal nucleus of vagus

Hypoglossal nucleus

Internal arcuate fibres (sensory decussation)

Inferior olivary nucleus

Nucleus gracilis

Nucleus cuneatus

Accessory cuneate nucleus

Nucleus of spinal tract of trigeminal nerve

Medial longitudinal bundle

Lateral spinothalamic tract

Dorsal and ventral spinocerebellar tracts

Pyramid

(ii) Cardiac centre for regulation of heart rate
(iii) Vasomotor centre for regulation of blood pressure

White Matter

It shows the following important features.

1. The inferior cerebellar peduncle occupies the posterolateral part, lateral to the fourth ventricle.

2. The *olivocerebellar fibres* are seen prominently in actual sections. The fibres emerge at the hilum of the inferior olivary nucleus and pass to the opposite inferior cerebellar peduncle, on their way to the opposite half of the cerebellum.

3. *Striae medullares* are seen in the floor of the fourth ventricle.

4. Identify the various tracts ascending from the spinal cord. They lie in the anterolateral part of the medulla.

cerebellar artery, and (b) thrombosis of the vertebral artery. The two lesions cause lateral and medial medullary syndromes, respectively.

THE PONS

The pons is the middle part of the brainstem, connecting the midbrain with the medulla. Literally, the word, pons, means 'bridge'.

External Features

The pons has *two surfaces*, ventral and dorsal. The *ventral or anterior surface* is convex in both directions and is transversely striated. In the median plane, it shows a vertical *basilar sulcus* which lodges the basilar artery (Fig. 24.1). Laterally, the surface is continuous with the middle cerebellar peduncle. The trigeminal nerve is attached to this surface at the junction of the pons with the peduncle. The nerve has two roots, a small motor root which lies medial to the much larger sensory root. The abducent, facial and vestibulocochlear nerves are attached at the lower border of the ventral surface.

The *dorsal or posterior surface* is hidden by the cerebellum, and forms the upper half of the floor of the fourth ventricle (Fig. 24.2).

Internal Structure of Pons

In transverse sections, the pons is seen to be divisible into ventral and dorsal parts. The ventral or *basilar part* is continuous inferiorly with the pyramids of the medulla, and on each side with the cerebellum through the middle cerebellar peduncle. The dorsal or tegmental part is a direct upward continuation of the medulla (excluding the pyramids).

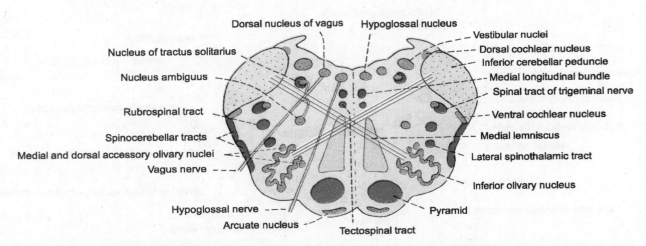

Fig. 24.5: *Transverse section through the olive of medulla oblongata.*

Basilar Part of Pons

The basilar part of the pons has a uniform structure throughout its length. However, the structure of the tegmental part differs in the upper and lower parts of the pons (Fig. 24.6).

Grey Matter

It is represented by the *pontine nuclei* which are scattered among longitudinal and transverse fibres. The pontine nuclei form an important part of the corticopontocerebellar pathway. Some of these nuclei get displaced during development, and form the arcuate nucleus (see medulla) and the pontobulbar body. Fibres from all these nuclei go to the opposite half of the cerebellum.

White Matter

It consists of longitudinal and transverse fibres.

1. The longitudinal fibres include: (a) The *corticospinal* and *corticonuclear* (pyramidal) tracts, and (b) the *corticopontine* fibres ending in the pontine nuclei.

2. The transverse fibres are *pontocerebellar* fibres beginning from the pontine nuclei and going to the opposite half of the cerebellum, through the middle cerebellar peduncle.

Tegmentum in the Lower Part of the Pons

Identify the following in Fig. 24.6.

Grey Matter

1. The *sixth nerve nucleus* lies beneath the facial colliculus.

2. The *seventh nerve nucleus* lies in the reticular formation of the pons.

3. The vestibular and cochlear nuclei lie in relation to the inferior cerebellar peduncle. The *vestibular nuclei* lie deep to the vestibular area in the floor of the fourth ventricle, partly in the medulla and partly in the pons. They are divisible into four parts, superior, inferior, medial and lateral (Fig. 25.3). They receive the fibres of the vestibular nerve, and give efferents to the cerebellum (vestibulocerebellar), the medial longitudinal bundle, the spinal cord (vestibulospinal tract arising in the lateral vestibular nucleus) and the lateral lemniscus. The dorsal and ventral *cochlear nuclei* are situated dorsal and ventral to the inferior cerebellar peduncle. They receive the fibres of the cochlear nerve, and give efferents mostly to the superior olivary nucleus and partly to nuclei of the corpus trapezoideum, and to nuclei of the lateral lemniscus. These fibres form the trapezoid body.

4. The spinal nucleus of the trigeminal nerve lies in the lateral part.

5. Other nuclei present include the salivatory and lacrimatory nuclei (not shown in figure).

White Matter

1. The *trapezoid body* is a transverse band of fibres lying just behind the ventral part of the pons. It consists of fibres that arise in the cochlear nuclei of both sides. It is a part of the auditory pathway (described in Chapter 30).

2. The medial lemniscus forms a transverse band on either side of the midline, just behind the trapezoid body.

3. The lateral spinothalamic tract (spinal lemniscus) lies lateral to the medial lemniscus.

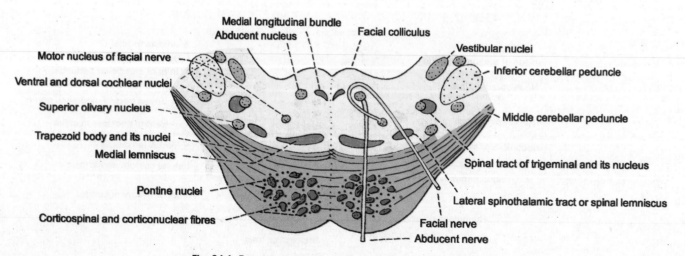

Fig. 24.6: *Transverse section through the lower part of pons.*

4. The inferior cerebellar peduncle lies lateral to the floor of the fourth ventricle.

5. The fibres of the facial nerve follow a peculiar course. They first pass backwards and medially to reach the medial side of the abducent nucleus. They then form a loop dorsal to the abducent nucleus. This loop is responsible for producing an elevation, the facial colliculus, in the floor of the fourth ventricle.

Tegmentum in the Upper Part of Pons

Identify the following in Fig. 24.7.

Grey Matter

The special features are the *motor and superior sensory nuclei of the trigeminal nerve*. The motor nucleus is medial to the superior sensory nucleus.

White Matter

1. Immediately behind the ventral part of the pons we see a transverse band of fibres that is made up (from medial to lateral side) of the medial lemniscus, the trigeminal lemniscus, the spinal leminscus, and the lateral leminscus (MTSL).

The trigeminal leminscus contains fibres arising in the spinal nucleus of the trigeminal nerve and travelling to the thalamus. The lateral leminscus is a part of the auditory pathway. It is formed by fibres arising in nuclei lying in close relation to the trapezoid body (superior olivary nucleus, nucleus of trapezoid body).

2. The superior cerebellar peduncles lie dorso-lateral to the fourth ventricle (replacing the inferior peduncle seen in the lower part of the pons).

3. The medial longitudinal bundle is made up of fibres that interconnect the nuclei of the cranial nerves III, IV, VI and VIII and the spinal part of the accessory nerve. It coordinates movements of the head and neck in response to stimulation of the cranial nerve VIII. However, the majority of fibres in the medial longitudinal bundle arise in the vestibular nuclei.

THE MIDBRAIN

The midbrain is also called the *mesencephalon*. It connects the hindbrain with the forebrain. Its cavity is known as the cerebral aqueduct: it connects the third ventricle with the fourth ventricle.

The midbrain passes through the tentorial notch, and is related on each side to the parahippocampal gyri, the optic tracts, the posterior cerebral artery, the basal vein, the trochlear nerve, and the geniculate bodies. Anteriorly, it is related to the interpeduncular structures, and posteriorly to the splenium of the corpus callosum, the great cerebral vein, the pineal body, and the posterior ends of the right and left thalami (Figs 28.5, 28.15).

Subdivisions

When we examine a transverse section through the midbrain we can make out the following major subdivisions.

A. The *tectum* is the part posterior to the aqueduct. It is made up of the right and left superior and inferior colliculi.

B. Each half of the midbrain anterior to the aqueduct is called the *cerebral peduncle*. Each cerebral peduncle is subdivided into: (a) The crus

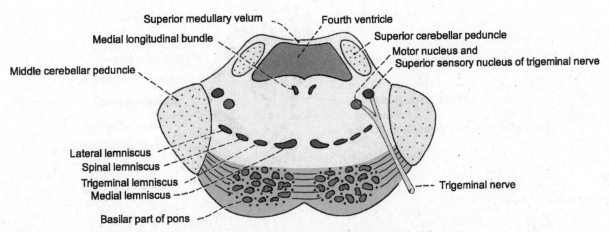

Fig. 24.7: *Transverse section through the upper part of the pons.*

cerebri, anteriorly; (b) the substantia nigra, in the middle; and (c) the tegmentum, posteriorly (Fig. 24.8).

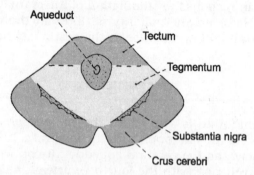

Fig. 24.8: *Transverse section of the midbrain to show its main subdivisions.*

The medial and lateral geniculate bodies (metathalamus) are situated on the posterolateral aspect of the midbrain. The superior colliculus is connected to the lateral geniculate body by the superior brachium. Likewise, the inferior colliculus is connected to the medial geniculate body by the inferior brachium (Fig. 28.11).

Internal Structure of Midbrain

It is studied conveniently by examining sections, at the level of the inferior colliculi and at the level of the superior colliculi.

Transverse Section of Midbrain at the Level of Inferior Colliculi

Grey Matter

1. The central (periaqueductal) grey matter contains: (a) The *nucleus of the trochlear nerve* in the ventromedial part; and (b) the *mesencephalic nucleus* of the trigeminal nerve in the lateral part. The mesencephalic nucleus is made up of unipolar cells (first neuron) and receives proprioceptive impulses from the muscles of mastication, the facial and ocular muscles, and the teeth (Fig. 24.9).

2. The *inferior colliculus* receives afferents from the lateral lemniscus, and gives efferents to the medial geniculate body. In the past it has been considered as the centre for auditory reflexes, but the available evidence indicates that it helps in localizing the source of sounds.

3. The *substantia nigra* is a lamina of grey matter made up of deeply pigmented nerve cells. It is concerned with muscle tone.

White Matter

1. The *crus cerebri* contains: (a) The corticospinal tract in the middle; (b) frontopontine fibres in the medial one-sixth; and (c) temporopontine, parietopontine and occipitopontine fibres in the lateral one-sixth.

2. The *tegmentum* contains ascending tracts as follows.

(a) The *lemnisci* (medial, trigeminal, spinal, and lateral) are arranged in the form of a band in which they lie in the order mentioned (from medial to lateral side).

(b) The *decussation of the superior cerebellar peduncles* is seen in the median plane.

(c) The *medial longitudinal bundle* lies in close relation to the trochlear nucleus (somatic efferent column).

(d) The tectospinal tract and the rubrospinal tract, are present.

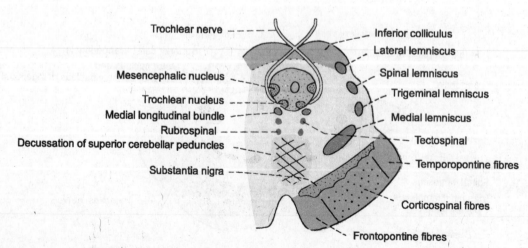

Fig. 24.9: *Transverse section of midbrain at the level of inferior colliculus.*

3. The trochlear nerve passes laterally and dorsally round the central grey matter. It decussates in the superior medullary velum, and emerges lateral to the frenulum veli.

Transverse Section of Midbrain at the Level of Superior Colliculi

Grey Matter

1. The central grey matter contains: (a) the nucleus of the *oculomotor nerve* including Edinger-Westphal nucleus in the ventromedial part, and (b) the *mesencephalic nucleus* of the trigeminal nerve in the lateral part. The oculomotor nuclei of the two sides are fused in the median plane (Fig. 24.10).

2. The *superior colliculus* receives afferents from the retina (visual), and various other centres. It gives efferents to the spinal cord (tectospinal tract). It controls reflex movements of the eyes, and of the head and neck in response to visual stimuli.

3. The *pretectal nucleus* lies deep to the superolateral part of the superior colliculus. It receives afferents from the lateral roots of the optic tract. It gives efferents to the Edinger-Westphal nuclei of both sides. The pretectal nucleus is an important part of the pathway for the light reflex and the consensual reflex. Its lesion causes Argyll-Robertson pupil in which the light reflex is lost but accommodation reflex remains intact (Chapter 30).

4. The *red nucleus* is about 0.5 cm in diameter. It receives afferents from the superior cerebellar peduncle, the globus pallidus, the subthalamic nucleus and the cerebral cortex. It gives efferents to the spinal cord (*rubrospinal tract*), the reticular formation, the thalamus, the olivary nucleus, the subthalamic nucleus, etc. It has an inhibitory influence on muscle tone.

5. The *substantia nigra* has already been described.

White Matter

1. The *crus cerebri* has the same tracts as described above.

2. The *tegmentum* contains the following.

(a) Lemnisci are arranged as medial, trigeminal and spinal. Lateral lemniscus is absent as it has terminated in the inferior colliculus.

(b) The decussation of the tectospinal and tectobulbar tracts forms the dorsal tegmental decussation.

(c) The decussation of the rubrospinal tracts forms the ventral tegmental decussation.

(d) Medial longitudinal bundle.

(e) Emerging fibres of oculomotor nerve.

3. The *tectum* shows the posterior commissure connecting the two superior colliculi.

DEVELOPMENT

Medulla oblongata: From caudal myelencephalic part of rhombencephalic vesicle. Olivary nucleus is formed by the migrated cells from alar lamina.

Pons: From cranial mesencephalic part of rhombencephalic vesicle. Cells of alar lamina migrate to form the pontine nuclei.

Midbrain: From middle vesicle, the mesencephalon. Alar lamina cells multiply and fuse to form 4 colliculi. Some cells also migrate ventrally to form red nucleus and substantia nigra. The basal lamina forms the crus cerebri.

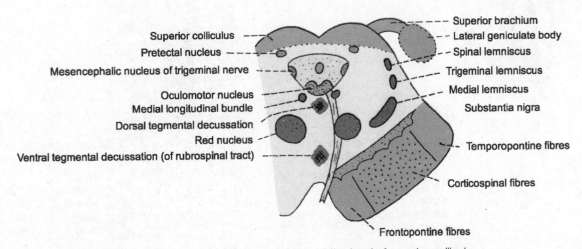

Superior colliculus
Pretectal nucleus
Mesencephalic nucleus of trigeminal nerve
Oculomotor nucleus
Medial longitudinal bundle
Dorsal tegmental decussation
Red nucleus
Ventral tegmental decussation (of rubrospinal tract)

Superior brachium
Lateral geniculate body
Spinal lemniscus
Trigeminal lemniscus
Medial lemniscus
Substantia nigra
Temporopontine fibres
Corticospinal fibres
Frontopontine fibres

Fig. 24.10: *Transverse section of midbrain at the level of superior colliculus.*

1. A unilateral lesion in the lower part of the pons results in paralysis of the facial nerve on the side of lesion, and paralysis of the limbs (hemiplegia) on the opposite side (crossed hemiplegia or Millard Gubler syndrome).

2. Argyll-Robertson pupil: This is the condition when light reflex is lost but the accommodation reflex remains intact. This is generally a result of lesion in the vicinity of pretectal nucleus. Causes include tertiary syphilis, diabetes, and encephalitis.

3. Lesions of tegmentum may involve the follwing.

(a) Third nerve leading to paralysis of extraocular muscles.

(b) Sensory tracts: resulting in loss of sensations.

(c) Substantia nigra and subthalamic nucleus, leading to involuntary movements.

4. Lesion in vicinity of cerebral peduncles leads to oculomotor paralysis of same side but hemiplegia of opposite side.

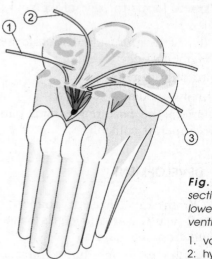

Fig. 24.11A: Brainstem sectioned at the level of the lower border of the fourth ventricle.

1. vagus nerve
2. hypoglossal nerve
3. olive

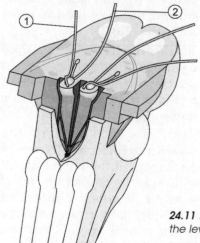

24.11 B: Brainstem sectioned at the level of lower pons.

1. facial nerve
2. abducent nerve

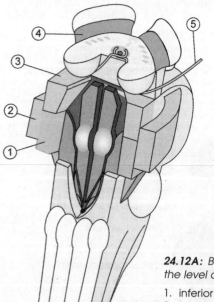

24.12A: Brainstem sectioned at the level of inferior colliculus.

1. inferior cerebellar peduncle
2. middle cerebellar peduncle
3. superior cerebellar peduncle
4. substantia nigra
5. trochlear nerve

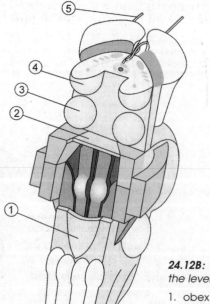

24.12B: Brainstem sectioned at the level of superior colliculus.

1. obex
2. superior medullary velum
3. inferior colliculi
4. superior colliculi
5. oculomotor nerve

(Courtesy, Dr. S. Sircar, Medical Physiology, CBS Publishers and Distributers, New Delhi).

Nuclei of Cranial Nerves and Reticular Formation

The twelve pairs of cranial nerves supply muscles of eyeball, face, palate, pharynx, larynx tongue and two large muscles of neck. Besides these are afferent to special senses like smell, sight, hearing, taste and touch. Some nerves form the afferent loop and others form the efferent loop of the reflex arc. Optic nerve is afferent from eye while III, IV and VI are efferent to the eye muscles. Statoacoustic nerve is afferent for hearing and balance while spinal root accessory acts as its efferent component for turning the face to the side from where sound is heard. VII, IX and X are carrying sensation of taste from tongue and efferent component is XII nerve for movements of tongue and nucleus ambiguus which gives fibres to IX, X, and cranial root of XI for the muscles of palate, pharynx and larynx.

Reticular formation is diffuse network. It forms "ascending reticular activating system". Many anaesthetic drugs act through this reticular formation. Olfactory takes the sense of smell and stimulates dorsal nucleus of vagus for enhanced secretion if the smell is good. CN V, the largest cranial nerve, is mainly sensory to the face. The motor nerve of face is VII nerve. To come close to V nerve nucleus, VII nucleus winds around VI nucleus so that a reflex arc can be mediated between the afferent and efferent loops of the arc.

NUCLEI OF CRANIAL NERVES

There are 12 pairs of cranial nerves. Each cranial nerve has a number and a name as follows.

    I = Olfactory
    II = Optic
    III = Oculomotor
    IV = Trochlear
    V = Trigeminal
    VI = Abducent
    VII = Facial
    VIII = Vestibulocochlear (or Statoacoustic)
    IX = Glossopharyngeal
    X = Vagus
    XI = Accessory
    XII = Hypoglossal

Out of these the I and II nerves are attached to the forebrain; the III and IV to the midbrain; the V, VI, VII and VIII to the pons; and the IX, X, XI, and XII to the medulla (Fig. 25.1).

The olfactory and optic nerves are connected to the cerebrum and will be considered with it. The nuclei connected to the remaining nerves are as follows. Note that several cranial nerves are connected to more than one nucleus; and that some nuclei contribute fibres to more than one nerve.

Embryology

During early stages of development, the wall of the neural tube is made up of three layers: (a) The inner ependymal layer; (b) the middle mantle layer; and (c) the outer marginal layer. The mantle layer represents grey matter and the marginal layer, the white matter. Soon the mantle layer differentiates into a dorsal alar lamina (sensory) and a ventral basal lamina (motor), the two are partially separated internally by the sulcus limitans.

In the spinal cord, though grey matter forms a compact fluted column in the centre, it shows differentiation into two somatic and two visceral functional columns. The somatic columns are the general somatic efferent (motor or anterior horn) and the general somatic afferent (sensory or posterior horn); they supply structures derived from somites. The visceral columns are the general visceral efferent (motor) and the general visceral afferent (sensory); these are autonomic columns and supply the viscera, vessels and glands.

331

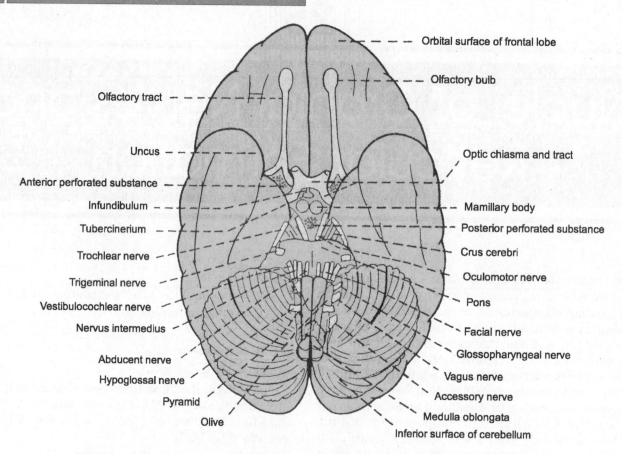

Fig. 25.1: *Inferior surface of brain with interpeduncular fossa and attachment of cranial nerves.*

In the brainstem, particularly hindbrain, the alar and basal laminae come to lie in the same ventral plane because of stretching of the roof plate (dorsal wall) of neural tube by pontine flexure. Further, the grey matter forms separate longitudinal functional columns, where the motor columns (from basal lamina) are medial and the sensory columns (from alar lamina) lateral in position. In addition to the four functional columns differentiated in the spinal cord, there appear two more columns (a motor and a sensory) for the branchial apparatus of the head region, namely the special visceral (branchial) efferent and the special visceral afferent; and one column more for the special senses, namely the special somatic afferent. Thus a total of seven columns (3 motor and 4 sensory) are formed. Each column, in its turn, breaks up into smaller fragments to form nuclei of the cranial nerves.

Nuclei

The details of the nuclei of cranial nerves are summarized in Table 25.1.

General Somatic Efferent Nuclei (GSE)

These nuclei supply skeletal muscle of somatic origin.

1. The *oculomotor nucleus* is situated in the midbrain at the level of the superior colliculus. Its fibres enter the oculomotor nerve and supply five extrinsic muscles of the eyeball except the lateral rectus and the superior oblique (Fig. 25.2).

2. The *trochlear nucleus* is situated in the midbrain at the level of the inferior colliculus. It supplies the superior oblique muscle through the trochlear nerve.

3. The *abducent nucleus* is situated in the lower part of the pons. It supplies the lateral rectus muscle through the abducent nerve.

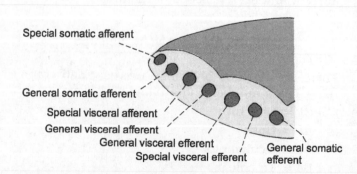

Fig. 25.2: *Transverse section of the hindbrain of an embryo showing the arrangement of functional columns of cranial nerve nuclei.*

4. The *hypoglossal nucleus* lies in the medulla. It is elongated and extends into both the open and closed parts of the medulla. It supplies most of the muscles of the tongue through the hypoglossal nerve.

Special Visceral Efferent/Branchial Efferent Nuclei

These nuclei supply striated muscle derived from the branchial arches.

1. The *motor nucleus of the trigeminal nerve* lies in the upper part of the pons. It supplies the muscles of mastication through the mandibular nerve.

2. The *nucleus of the facial nerve* lies in the lower part of the pons. It supplies the various muscles innervated by the facial nerve.

3. The *nucleus ambiguus* lies in the medulla. It forms an elongated column lying in both the open and closed parts of the medulla. It supplies:

(a) The stylopharyngeus muscle through the glossopharyngeal nerve; and

(b) the muscles of the pharynx, the soft palate and the larynx through the vagus and the cranial part of the accessory nerve (Fig. 25.3).

General Visceral Efferent Nuclei

These nuclei give origin to preganglionic neurons that relay in a peripheral autonomic ganglion.

Postganglionic fibres arising in the ganglion supply smooth muscle or glands.

1. The *Edinger-Westphal nucleus* lies in the midbrain in close relation to the oculomotor nucleus. Its fibres pass through the oculomotor nerve to the ciliary ganglion to supply the sphincter pupillae and the ciliaris muscle.

2. The *superior salivatory nucleus* lies in the lower part of the pons. It sends fibres through the facial nerve and its chorda tympani branch to the submandibular ganglion for supply of the submandibular and sublingual salivary glands.

3. The *inferior salivatory nucleus* lies in the lower part of the pons just below the superior nucleus. It sends fibres through the glossopharyngeal nerve to the otic ganglion for supply of the parotid gland.

4. The *lacrimatory nucleus* lies near the salivatory nuclei (in the lower pons). It gives off fibres that pass through the facial nerve and its branch greater petrosal nerve to relay in the pterygopalatine ganglion and supply the lacrimal, nasal, palatal gland.

5. The *dorsal nucleus of the vagus* is a long column extending into the open and closed parts of the medulla. It gives off fibres that pass through the vagus nerve to be distributed to thoracic and abdominal viscera. (The ganglia concerned are present in the walls of the viscera supplied.)

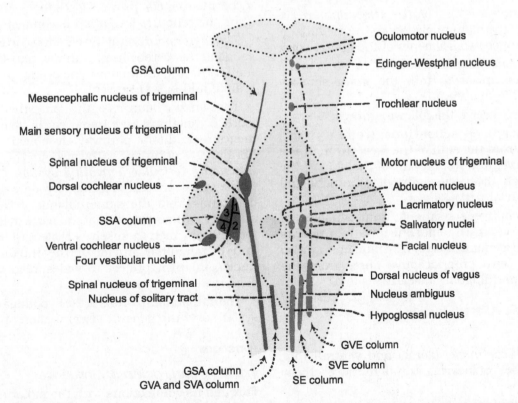

Fig. 25.3: *Scheme to show the cranial nerve nuclei as projected on to the posterior surface of the brainstem. Vestibular nuclei; 1. Superior; 2. medial; 3. lateral, 4. spinal.*

General Visceral Afferent Nucleus and Special Visceral Afferent Nucleus

The only nucleus in this category is the *nucleus of the solitary tract.* It lies in the medulla and extends into both its closed and open parts.

It receives *general visceral sensations* through:-

(i) The glossopharyngeal nerve, from the tonsil, pharynx and the posterior part of the tongue, carotid body and sinus.

(ii) Through the vagus nerve, from the pharynx, the larynx, the trachea, the oesophagus and other thoracic and abdominal viscera.

It also receives *sensations of taste* (special visceral afferent) as follows.

(a) From the anterior two-thirds of the tongue, and the palate except circumvallate papillae through the facial nerve.

(b) From the posterior one-third of the tongue through the glossopharyngeal nerve, including the circumvallate papillae.

(c) From the posterior most part of the tongue and from the epiglottis through the vagus nerve.

General Somatic Afferent Nuclei

These are all related to the trigeminal nerve.

1. The *main or superior sensory nucleus of the trigeminal nerve* lies in the upper part of the pons.

2. The *spinal nucleus of the trigeminal nerve* descends from the main nucleus into the medulla. It reaches the upper two segments of the spinal cord.

3. The *mesencephalic nucleus of the trigeminal nerve* extends upwards from the main sensory nucleus into the midbrain.

These nuclei receive the following fibres:

(a) Exteroceptive sensations (touch, pain, temperature) from the skin of the face, through the trigeminal nerve; and from a part of the skin of the auricle through the vagus (auricular branch) and through the facial nerve.

(b) Proprioceptive sensations from muscles of mastication reach the mesencephalic nucleus through the trigeminal nerve. The nucleus is also believed to receive proprioceptive fibres from the ocular, facial and lingual muscles.

Special Somatic Afferent Nuclei

These are:

1. The *cochlear nuclei* (dorsal and ventral) that receive impulses of hearing through the cochlear nerve.

2. The *vestibular nuclei* (superior, spinal, medial and lateral) that receive fibres from the semicircular canals, the utricle and the saccule through the vestibular nerves (Table 25.1).

RETICULAR FORMATION

Introduction

The reticular formation is a diffuse network of fine nerve fibres intermingled with numerous poorly defined nuclei. Phylogenetically, it is very old: in primitive vertebrates, it represents the largest part of the CNS. In man, it is best developed in the brainstem, although it can be traced to all levels of the CNS.

Location and Identity

1. The reticular formation, in general, is placed in the deep and dorsal parts of the neural axis.

2. It is very diffuse in its distribution, and has ill-defined boundaries.

3. It is better defined physiologically than anatomically.

Connections

The reticular formation is connected to all the principal parts of the nervous system, including the motor, sensory and autonomic pathways with their centres. The connections are reciprocal (to and from the areas to be mentioned) providing feedback mechanisms. Thus the reticular formation is connected to:

The *motor neurons* of the cerebral cortex, the basal ganglia, the cerebellum, various masses of grey matter in the brainstem including the nuclei of cranial and spinal nerves.

The *sensory neurons* of the somesthetic pathways (cortex, thalamus and spinal cord), visual pathway (tectum), auditory pathway, (cochlear), and equilibratory (vestibular) pathways. In this group the *ascending reticular activating system (ARAS)* is of prime importance. It is formed by a great number of collaterals from the spinothalamic, trigeminal and auditory pathways to the lateral parts of the reticular formation, which themselves project to the reticular and intralaminar nuclei of the thalamus. These nuclei, in turn, project to widespread area of the cerebral cortex.

The *autonomic neurons* of the hypothalamus, limbic system and the general visceral efferent columns.

Functions

Inhibitory and Facilitatory Influences

Through its connections with the motor areas of the nervous system, certain areas of the reticular formation inhibit voluntary and reflex activities of the

Table 25.1: Nuclei of the cranial nerves

Cranial nerve	Nuclei (n.)	Location	Functional components**	Function of the nerve component
I	—	—		Smell
II	—	—		Sight
III	Oculomotor nucleus	Midbrain, level of superior colliculus	GSE GVE GSA*	Movements of eyeball Contraction of pupil, accommodation Proprioceptive
IV	Trochlear nucleus	Midbrain, level of Inferior colliculus	GSE GSA*	Movement of eyeball (superior oblique m.) Proprioceptive
V	1. Motor nucleus 2. Mesencephalic nucleus 3. Superior sensory nucleus 4. Spinal nucleus	Upper pons Midbrain Upper pons From upper pons to C2 segment of spinal cord.	BE GSA GSA GSA	Movement of mandible Proprioceptive, muscles of mastication, face and eye. Touch and pressure from skin and mucous membrane of facial region Pain and temperature of face
VI	Abducent nucleus	Lower pons	GSE GSA*	Lateral movement of eyeball Proprioceptive
VII	1. Motor nucleus 2. Nucleus of tractus solitarius 3. Superior salivatory nucleus 4. Lacrimatory nucleus	Lower pons Lower pons Lower pons Lower pons	BE SVA GVE GVE GSA	Facial expressions, elevation of hyoid Taste, anterior two-thirds tongue Secretomotor, submandibular and sublingual salivary glands Secretomotor, lacrimal gland, nasal, etc. Proprioceptive
VIII Cochlear Vestibular	Two cochlear nuclei dorsal and ventral Four vestibular nuclei superior, spinal, medial and lateral	Junction of medulla and pons ,,	SSA SSA	Hearing Equilibrium of head
IX	1. Nucleus ambiguus 2. Inferior salivatory nucleus 3. Nucleus of tractus solitarius	Medulla ,, ,,	BE GVE SVA GVA* GSA*	Elevation of larynx Secretomotor to parotid gland Taste posterior one-third of tongue Sensations from mucous membrane of pharynx and posterior one-third of tongue go to dorsal nucleus of vagus (GVA) and spinal nucleus of 5th nerve (GSA)
X and cranial part of XI.	1. Nucleus ambiguus 2. Dorsal nucleus of vagus 3. Nucleus of tractus solitarius	Medulla ,, ,,	BE GVE GVA SVA GSA*	Movements of palate, pharynx and larynx Motor and secretomotor to bronchial tree and gut; inhibitory to heart Sensations from viscera Taste from post. most tongue and epiglottis Sensations from the skin of external ear go to the spinal nucleus of V nerve
Spinal part of XI	Spinal nucleus of accessory nerve	Spinal cord, Cl-5	BE	Sternocleidomastoid and trapezius
XII	Hypoglossal nucleus	Medulla	GSE GSA	Movements of tongue Proprioceptive

* These components do not have corresponding nuclei and terminate in the nuclei of different nerves.

** GSE = general somatic efferent; BE = branchial efferent; GVE = general visceral efferent; GVA = general visceral afferent; SVA = special visceral afferent; GSA = general somatic afferent; SVA = special somatic afferent.

body, whereas certain other areas can facilitate them.

State of Arousal, General Awareness and Alertness

The ascending reticular activating system (ARAS) is responsible for maintaining the state of wakefulness and alertness, by its connections with a great number of collaterals from sensory tracts. Thus sensory perception of any type is quickly and acutely appreciated, so that an appropriate motor response by the body may be synthesized and actuated.

Sleep is a normal, periodic inhibition of the reticular formation. Hypnotics and general anaesthetics produce their effects by acting on this system.

Autonomic Influences

Through its autonomic connections and certain specific centres, the reticular formation influences respiratory and vasomotor activities. They are stimulated or suppressed according to the needs.

Through its connections with the limbic system it participates in regulating emotional, behavioral and visceral activities. It also takes part in neuroendocrine regulation and the development of conditioned and learned reflexes.

Action of Drugs

(i) Narcotics act more on nonspecific sensory system and less on the specific sensory system. Their main action is depression of reticular activating system, precise effects of which depend upon the type of narcotics used and its dosage. Narcotics depress the diffuse thalamocortical system as well.

(ii) Barbiturates depress the afferent impulses reaching the reticular-activating pathways.

(iii) Analgesics act by suppression of reactions concerned with activation of reticular-activating pathways.

(iv) Morphine suppresses the cortico-reticular pathways, and stimulates the nonspecific thalamic system, rhinencephalon and its projections. It also depresses conduction along specific sensory pathways.

(v) Promedol increases the activity of reticular activating system.

CLINICAL ANATOMY

(a) In brain stem injuries, involvement of reticular activating system may result in loss of consciousness or interference in the arousal mechanism.

(b) Petit mal epilepsy is a disorder of reticular activating system. It is characterised by attacks of mental confusion, with patient staring ahead with open eyes, partial retention of consciousness during these attacks protects the patient from harm.

(c) Another manifestation of disorders of reticular activating system consists of two features:

(i) Necroplexy which is marked by recurrent attacks of somnolescence and compulsive demands for immediate sleep.

(ii) Cataplexy consists of paroxysmal attacks of general muscular weakness during heights of rage, mirth and laughter.

The Cerebellum

Cerebellum, though small in size, subserves important functions for maintaining tone, posture equilibrium and movements of the body. Cerebellum controls the same side of the body directly or indirectly. The grey matter is highly folded to accommodate millions of neurons in a small area and the arrangement is called "arbor vitae" (vital tree of life). The structure of cerebellum is uniform throughout, i.e. it is homotypical. Damage to cerebellum gives rise to very typical symptoms.

Introduction

The cerebellum (little brain) is the largest part of the hindbrain. It is situated in the posterior cranial fossa behind the pons and medulla. It is an infratentorial structure that coordinates voluntary movements of the body.

Relations

Anteriorly: Fourth ventricle, pons and medulla
Posteroinferiorly: Squamous occipital bone; and
Superiorly: Tentorium cerebelli (Fig. 26.1).

DISSECTION

Identify the cerebellum. Remove all the arachnoid and pia mater from its surface to be able to demarcate its developmental components– archicerebellum, paleocerebellum and neocerebellum; its lobes–flucculonodular lobe, anterior lobe and middle lobe; its fissures–fissura prima, horizontal fissure, posterolateral fissure; its vermis – superior vermis and inferior vermis; and superior medullary velum connecting the two superior cerebellar peduncles which connect cerebellum to the midbrain and inferior medullary velum forming the bed for the tonsils of cerebellum.

Put the edge of the knife behind the flocculus. Carry the edge of the knife medially along the line of fissura prima till the median plane. Carry the inferior part of the incision till behind the tonsil. This section will expose: (a) The complex folding of grey matter around the white matter, the arbor vitae pattern and (b) the crinkled biggest intracerebeller nucleus— the dentate nucleus.

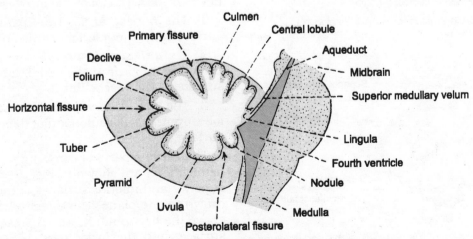

Fig. 26.1: *Sagittal section through the brainstem and cerebellum.*

Cut through the anterior lobe of the cerebellum and identify: (a) The middle cerebellar peduncle passing horizontally to the pons, (b) the superior cerebellar peduncle passing anterosuperiorly towards the midbrain. Identify the thin superior medullary velum between the adjacent superior cerebellar peduncles with a small part of cerebellar cortex—the lingula (a part of superior vermis) adherent to it.

External Features

The cerebellum consists of two cerebellar hemispheres that are united to each other through a median *vermis*. It has two surfaces *superior and inferior*. The superior surface is convex. The two hemispheres are continuous with each other on this surface (Fig. 26.2). The inferior surface shows a deep median notch called the *vallecula* which separates the right and left hemispheres (Fig. 26.3). The anterior aspect of the cerebellum is marked by a deep notch in which the pons and medulla are lodged. Posteriorly, there is a narrow and deep notch in which the falx cerebelli lies.

Each hemisphere is divided into three *lobes*. The *anterior lobe* lies on the anterior part of the superior

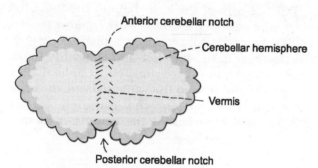

Fig. 26.2: Cerebellum as seen from above.

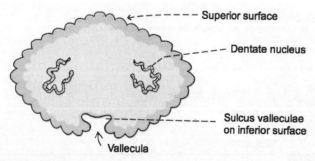

Fig. 26.3: Coronal section of the cerebellum showing its superior and inferior surfaces.

surface. It is separated from the middle lobe by the *fissura prima*. The *middle lobe* (sometimes known as the posterior lobe) is the largest of three lobes. It is limited in front by the fissura prima (on the superior surface), and by the posterolateral fissure (on the inferior surface). The *flocculonodular lobe* is the smallest lobe of the cerebellum. It lies on the inferior surface, in front of the posterolateral fissure (Fig. 26.4).

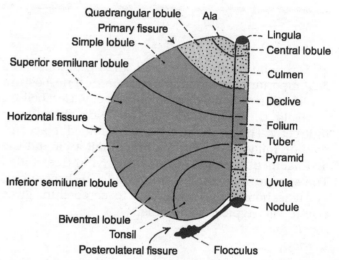

Fig. 26.4: Scheme to show the subdivision of the cerebellum. The parts above the horizontal fissure form the superior surface of the cerebellum; and those below the fissure are seen on the inferior surface.

Parts of Cerebellum

The cerebellum is subdivided into numerous small parts by fissures. Each fissure cuts the vermis and both hemispheres. Out of the numerous fissures, however, only the following are worth remembering.

1. The *horizontal fissure* separates the superior surface from the inferior surface (Fig. 26.1).

2. The *primary fissure (fissure prima)* separates the anterior lobe from the middle lobe on the superior surface of the cerebellum.

3. The *posterolateral fissure* separates the middle lobe from the flocculonodular lobe on the inferior surface.

The various parts of cerebellum (both vermis and hemisphere) are shown in Fig. 26.4 where both the superior and inferior surfaces of the cerebellum are drawn in one plane. The upper part of the diagram, above the horizontal fissure represents the superior surface; and the lower part, below the horizontal fissure represents the inferior surface.

The *parts of the vermis* are: (1) Lingula; (2) central lobule; (3) culmen; (4) declive; (5) folium; (6) tuber; (7) pyramid; (8) uvula; and (9) nodule.

The *subdivisions of the cerebellar hemisphere* are: (2) ala; (3) quadrangular lobule; (4) simple lobule; (5) superior semilunar lobule; (6) inferior semilunar lobule; (7) biventral lobule; (8) tonsil; and (9) flocculus.

In Fig. 26.4 note that each part of the vermis has a lateral extension. However, the lingula does not have any lateral extension.

Morphological and Functional Divisions of Cerebellum

1. The *archicerebellum* phylogenetically is the oldest part of the cerebellum. It is made up of the flocculonodular lobe and the lingula. It is chiefly vestibular in its connections. It controls the axial musculature and the bilateral movements used for locomotion and maintenance of equilibrium (Fig. 26.4).

2. The *paleocerebellum* is the next part of the cerebellum to appear. It is made up of the anterior lobe (minus lingula), and the pyramid and uvula of the inferior vermis. Its connections are chiefly spinocerebellar. It controls tone, posture and crude movements of the limbs.

3. The *neocerebellum* is the newest part of the cerebellum to develop. It is made up of the middle lobe (the largest part of the cerebellum) minus the pyramid and uvula of the inferior vermis. It is primarily concerned with the regulation of fine movements of the body.

Connections of Cerebellum

The fibres entering or leaving the cerebellum are grouped to form three peduncles which connect the cerebellum to the midbrain, the pons and the medulla. The constituent fibres in them are given in Table 26.1.

It is clear from Table 26.1 that the middle and inferior peduncles are chiefly afferent to the cerebellum and that the superior cerebellar peduncle is chiefly efferent in nature.

Grey Matter of Cerebellum

It consists of the cerebellar cortex and the cerebellar nuclei. There are four pairs of nuclei: (1) The *nucleus dentatus* is neocerebellar; (2) the *nucleus globosus* and (3) the *nucleus emboliformis* are paleocerebellar; and (4) the *nucleus fastigii* is archicerebellar (Fig. 26.5).

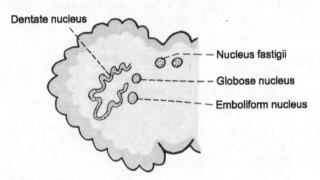

Fig. 26.5: *Horizontal section of the cerebellum showing the cerebellar nuclei.*

Table 26.1: Constituents of the cerebellar peduncles		
Peduncle	*Afferent tracts*	*Efferent tracts*
A. Superior cerebellar peduncle	1. Anterior spinocerebellar 2. Tectocerebellar 3. Dentatoolivary 4. Fastigioreticular	1. Cerebellorubral 2. Dentatothalamic
B. Middle cerebellar peduncle	Pontocerebellar (part of the corticopontocerebellar pathway)	——
C. Inferior cerebellar peduncle	1. Posterior spinocerebellar 2. Cuneocerebellar (posterior external arcuate fibres) 3. Olivocerebellar 4. Parolivocerebellar 5. Reticulocerebellar 6. Vestibulocerebellar 7. Anterior external arcuate fibres 8. Striae medullares 9. Trigeminocerebellar	1. Cerebellovestibular 2. Cerebelloolivary 3. Cerebelloreticular

Functions of Cerebellum

The cerebellum controls the same side of the body, i.e. its influence is ipsilateral. This is in marked contrast to other parts of the brain most of which control the opposite half (contralateral) of the body. The functions of the cerebellum are as follows:

1. The cerebellum coordinates voluntary movements so that they are smooth, balanced and accurate. This is chiefly done by the neocerebellum. Cerebellar dysfunction gives rise to incoordination of movements.

2. The cerebellum controls tone, posture and equilibrium. This is chiefly done by the archicerebellum and the paleocerebellum. Cerebellar lesions, therefore, give rise to hypotonia, and disturbances of equilibrium.

Development

Cerebellum develops from the neurons of alar lamina of metencephalic part of the rhombencephalic vesicle. These neurons migrate dorsally and form the rhombic lip which forms the cerebellum. The earliest part to develop is the archicerebellum. In its centre, the paleocerebellum develops, splitting the archicerebellar parts into two parts. Lastly, the paleocerebellar part is also split by the development of neocerebellum in its centre.

CLINICAL ANATOMY

1. *Cerebellar syndrome:* Cerebellar lesions give rise to symptoms and signs which together constitute the cerebellar syndrome. It is characterized by: (i) Muscular *hypotonia;* (ii) *intention tremors* (tremors only during movements) tested by finger-nose and heel-knee tests; (iii) *adiadochokinesia* which is the inability to perform rapid and regular alternating movements, like pronation and supination; (iv) *nystagmus* (to and fro oscillatory movements of the eyeballs while looking to either side); (v) *scanning speech* (jerky and explosive); and (vi) *ataxic gait (unsteady gait).*

The Fourth Ventricle

Fourth ventricle is the last and lowest ventricle of the cerebrum. Its tent-shaped roof makes it more spacious. Its roof contains three apertures for the release of closely guarded CSF into the subarachnoid space for absorption into the superior sagittal sinus.

The cavity of the hindbrain is called the fourth ventricle. It is a tent-shaped space situated between the pons and the medulla in front, and the cerebellum behind (Fig. 26.1).

Communications

1. Superiorly, it communicates with the third ventricle through the cerebral aqueduct.

2. Inferiorly, it is continuous with the central canal of the medulla, and of the spinal cord.

3. Dorsally, in lower part of the roof there is a median aperture (foramen of Magendi). Through this aperture the ventricle communicates with the subarachnoid space (cisterna magna) (Fig. 27.2).

4. On either side, again it communicates with the subarachnoid space through two lateral apertures (foramina of Luschka) (Fig. 27.1).

Recesses of the Fourth Ventricle

1. *A median dorsal recess*, extends into the white core of the cerebellum, above the nodule (Fig. 26.1).

2. Two lateral dorsal recesses, one on each side, extend backwards, lying above the inferior medullary velum and below the cerebellar nuclei.

3. Two lateral recesses, one on each side, extend laterally between the inferior cerebellar peduncle (in front) and the stem of the flocculus (behind). They reach up to the flocculus itself. Each recess opens at its lateral end through the foramen of Luschka.

Lateral Boundaries

On each side, the fourth ventricle is bounded: (a) *Inferolaterally*, by the gracile tubercle, the fasciulus cuneatus, the cuneate tubercle, and the inferior cerebellar peduncle; and (b) *superolaterally*, by the superior cerebellar peduncle (Fig. 27.1).

Roof of Fourth Ventricle

The roof is tent-shaped, projecting into the cerebellum. It is formed by: (1) The superior cerebellar peduncles;

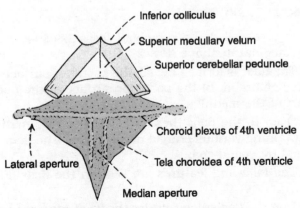

Fig. 27.1: *Boundaries of the fourth ventricle.*

Fig. 27.2: *Roof of the fourth ventricle.*

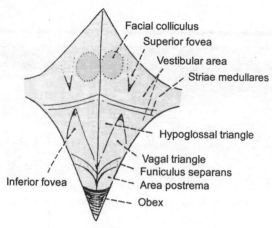

Fig. 27.3: *Floor of the fourth ventricle.*

(2) the superior medullary velum; (3) the inferior medullary velum; (4) the tela choroidea of the fourth ventricle, containing the choroid plexus; and (5) the taeniae with the obex. The taenia are white ependymal ridges covered with tela choroidea lying along the inferolateral margins of the roof. The two taeniae are continuous below with the obex which covers the inferior angle of the ventricle and is lined with ependyma both in front and behind (Fig. 27.2).

The *choroid plexus* of the fourth ventricle is supplied by a branch from the posterior inferior cerebellar artery. It lies within the tela choroidea of the fourth ventricle. The entire plexus is T-shaped, the vertical limb of the 'T' being double. The foramen of Magendie lies between the two limbs. The horizontal limbs extend into the lateral recesses and protrude through the foramina of Luschka into the subarachnoid space.

Floor of Fourth Ventricle

It is also called the rhomboid fossa because it is rhomboidal in shape (Fig. 27.3).

The floor is formed by: (a) The posterior surface of the pons; and (b) the posterior surface of the open part of the medulla.

Deep to the floor there is a layer of grey matter containing various cranial nerve nuclei. The floor is lined by ependyma.

The following features are seen in the floor (Fig. 27.3).

1. A *median sulcus* divides the floor into right and left halves.

2. On either side of the midline, there is an elevation called the *median eminence*. This eminences is bounded, laterally, by the *sulcus limitans*.

3. The following are seen in relation to the sulcus limitans.

(a) A bluish coloured area called the *locus coeruleus*, deep to which there is the *substantia ferruginea*.

(b) A depression, the *superior fovea*, which lies just lateral to the facial colliculus.

(c) Another depression, the *inferior fovea*, that lies just above the vagal triangle (see below).

4. The following features are seen in relation to the median eminence.

(a) The facial colliculus is an elevation over the upper part of the eminence. It lies opposite the superior fovea. It is produced by the underlying abducent nucleus, and the fibres of the facial nerve as they wind around the nucleus.

(b) The lower part of the eminence is occupied by the hypoglossal triangle. The hypoglossal nucleus lies deep to this triangle.

5. The *vestibular area* lies lateral to the fovea. Part of it extends into the lateral recess, and forms an elevation called the auditory tubercle. The tubercle overlies the dorsal cochlear nucleus and the cochlear nerve.

6. The *striae medullares* are transverse lines running across the floor. They represent fibres passing from the arcuate nucleus to the opposite half of the cerebellum.

7. The *vagal triangle* lies below the inferior fovea and between the hypoglossal triangle and the vestibular area. It overlies the dorsal nucleus of the vagus nerve.

Development

Fourth ventricle is the cavity of rhombencephalon. Roof plate here becomes thin and forms the roof of the fourth ventricle. The floor plate becomes thick due to migration of alar lamina lateral to basal lamina. It forms the floor of the fourth ventricle. Floor is formed by caudal part of pons and cranial part of medulla oblongata.

CLINICAL ANATOMY

1. Vital centres are situated in the vicinity of the vagal triangle. An injury to this area is therefore, fatal.

2. Infratentorial brain tumours block the median and lateral foramina situated in the roof of the ventricle. This results in a marked and early rise of intracranial pressure.

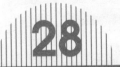

The Cerebrum

The appearance of sulci and gyri increases the surface area for the neurons many times, without increasing the size of the brain. There are specific areas on the brain for specific functions. Thalamus integrates sensory, motor and visceral activities. Hypothalamus controls various visceral and vaso-motor activities. It maintains a biological clock for our body. Parkinsonism occurs due to lesion of corpus striatum. There is reduction in speed or bradykinesia, i.e. slow movement or akinesia, i.e. no movement with muscle rigidity. There is free flow of information in the central nervous system, between two hemispheres through the commissural fibres; between various parts of one hemisphere through the association fibres and between upper and lower parts through the projection fibres.

Internal capsule contains lots of fibres packed in its "limbs". It is supplied by the "end artery". The rupture of "end artery" may cause the "end" of the human being concerned, if not treated properly.

Introduction

The cerebrum is made of two cerebral hemispheres which are incompletely separated from each other by the median *longitudinal fissure.* The two hemispheres are connected to each other across the median plane by the corpus callosum. Each hemisphere contains a cavity, called the lateral ventricle.

DISSECTION

Keep the cerebrum so that the longitudinal fissure faces superiorly. Identify the convex strong band of white matter, the corpus callosum binding parts of the medial surfaces of the two cerebral hemispheres. Define splenium as the thick rounded part of the corpus callosum.

Divide the corpus callosum in the median plane starting from the splenium towards the trunk, genu and rostrum. Inferior to the trunk of corpus callosum extend the incision into the tela choroidea of the lateral and third ventricles, and the interthalamic adhesion connecting the medial surfaces of two thalami.

Identify the thin septum pellucidum connecting the inferior surfaces of corpus callosum to a curved band of white matter - anterior column of the fornix. Look for the anterior commissure just at the anterior end of the anterior column of fornix.

Turn the brain upside down and identify optic chiasma. Divide the optic chiasma, anterior communicating artery, infundibulum and a thin groove between the adjacent mamillary bodies, posterior cerebral artery close to its origin. Carry the line of division around the midbrain to join the two ends of the median cut. Separate the right and the left cerebral hemispheres.

In the two hemisphere, identify the three surfaces, four borders three poles. Identify the central sulcus, posterior ramus of lateral sulcus, parieto-occipital sulcus and preoccipital notch and demarcate the four lobes of the superolateral surface of each cerebral hemisphere (Figs 28.1, 28.2).

Strip the meninges from the surfaces. Identify the vessels on the surfaces of hemisphere. Demarcate the main sulci and gyri on the supero-lateral surface, medial surface and inferior surface of hemisphere.

Make thin slice through the part of the calcarine sulcus, posterior to its junction with the parieto-occipital sulcus. Identify the stria running through it. On cutting series of thin slices try to trace the extent of visual stria.

345

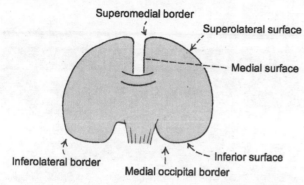

Fig. 28.1: *Borders and surfaces of the cerebrum at the coronal section.*

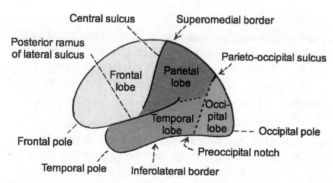

Fig. 28.2: *Some features of the superolateral surface of the cerebrum that are used to divide the hemisphere into lobes.*

CEREBRAL HEMISPHERE

External Features

Each hemisphere has the following features:

Three surfaces

1. The *superolateral surface* is convex and is related to the cranial vault.
2. The *medial surface* is flat and vertical. It is separated from the corresponding surface of the opposite hemisphere by the falx cerebri and the longitudinal fissure (Fig. 28.1).
3. The *inferior surface* is irregular. It is divided into an anterior part, the *orbital surface,* and a posterior part, the *tentorial surface.* The two parts are separated by a deep cleft called the stem of the lateral sulcus.

Four borders

1. The *superomedial border* separates the superolateral surface from the medial surface (Fig. 28.2).
2. The *inferolateral border* separates the superolateral surface from the inferior surface. The anterior part of this border is called the *superciliary border.* There is a depression on

the inferolateral border situated about 5 cm in front of the occipital pole: it is called the preoccipital notch.

3. The *medial orbital border* separates the medial surface from the orbital surface.
4. The *medial occipital border* separates the medial surface from the tentorial surface.

Three poles

1. *Frontal pole,* at the anterior end.
2. *Occipital pole,* at the posterior end.
3. *Temporal pole,* at the anterior end of the temporal lobe (Fig. 28.2).

Surface Marking of the Brain

Borders of Cerebral Hemisphere

Mark the following points.

1. First point just superolateral to the inion.
2. Second point just superolateral to the nasion.
3. Third point at the zygomatic process of the frontal bone just above the eyebrow.
4. Fourth point at the pterion (Fig. 1.8).
5. Fifth point at the middle of the upper border of the zygomatic arch.

The *superomedial border* is marked by joining points 1 and 2 by a paramedian line.

The *superciliary border* is marked by first joining points 2 and 3 by a line arching upwards just above the eyebrow, and then extending this line to point 4.

The *inferolateral border* is marked by first joining points 4 and 5 by a line convex forwards (temporal pole), and by then joining points 5 and 1 by a line convex upwards, passing just above the external acoustic meatus.

Central Sulcus

1. First point 1.2 cm behind the midpoint of a line joining the nasion with the inion.
2. Second point 5 cm above the preauricular point.

The sulcus is marked by joining these points by a sinuously curved line running downwards and forwards making an angle of 70 degrees with the median plane.

Lateral Sulcus

The following points are used to mark the lateral sulcus and its rami.

1. First point at the pterion.
2. Second point 2 cm below the parietal eminence.
3. Third point 2 cm above the pterion.

4. Fourth point 2 cm in front of the pterion.

Point 1 (pterion) is also called the Sylvian point. Here the stem of the lateral sulcus divides into its three rami.

The *posterior ramus* of the lateral sulcus is about 7 cm long and can be marked by joining points 1 and 2.

The *anterior ascending ramus* is marked by joining points 1 and 3.

The anterior horizontal ramus is marked by joining points 1 and 4.

Superior Temporal Sulcus

This is marked by a line parallel and 1 cm below the posterior ramus of the lateral sulcus.

Lobes of Cerebral Hemisphere

Each cerebral hemisphere is divided into four lobes—frontal, parietal, occipital and temporal. Their positions correspond, very roughly, to that of the corresponding bones. The lobes are best appreciated on the superolateral surface (Fig. 28.2). The sulci separating the lobes on this surface are as follows:

1. The *central sulcus* begins at the superomedial border of the hemisphere a little behind the midpoint between the frontal and occipital poles. It runs on the superolateral surface obliquely downwards and forwards and ends a little above the posterior ramus of the lateral sulcus.

2. We have seen that the *lateral sulcus* separates the orbital and tentorial parts of the inferior surface. Laterally, this sulcus reaches the superolateral surface where it divides into a number of branches. The largest of these, the *posterior ramus of the lateral sulcus* passes backwards and slightly upwards over the superolateral surface.

3. The *parieto-occipital* sulcus is a sulcus of the medial surface. Its upper end cuts off the supero-medial border about 5 cm in front of the occipital pole.

4. The *preoccipital notch* is an indentation on the inferolateral border, about 5 cm in front of the occipital pole.

The division is completed by drawing one line joining the parieto-occipital sulcus to the preoccipital notch; and another line continuing backwards from the posterior ramus of the lateral sulcus to meet the first line. The boundaries of each lobe will now be clear from Fig. 28.2.

Cerebral Sulci and Gyri

Cerebral cortex is folded into gyri which are separated from each other by sulci. This pattern increases the surface area of the cortex. In human brain, the total area of the cortex is estimated to be more than 2000 cm², and approximately two-thirds of this area is hidden from the surface within the sulci.

The pattern of folding of the cortex is not entirely haphazard. It is largely determined by the differential growth of specific functional areas of the cortex, because many of the sulci bear a definite topographical relation to these areas. A few types of sulci are given below.

1. Limiting sulcus separates at its floor two areas which are different functionally and structurally. An example is the central sulcus between the motor and sensory areas (Fig. 28.3A).

2. Axial sulcus develops in the long axis of a rapidly growing homogeneous area. An example is the postcalcarine sulcus in the long axis of the striate area (Fig. 28.3B).

3. Operculated sulcus separates by its lips two areas, and contains a third area in the walls of the sulcus. An example is the lunate sulcus (Fig. 28.3C).

4. Secondary sulcus is produced by factors other than the exuberant growth in the adjoining areas of the cortex. Examples are the lateral and parieto-occipital sulci.

5. Complete sulcus is very deep so as to cause elevation in the walls of the lateral ventricle. Examples are the collateral and calcarine sulci.

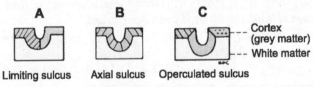

A   **B**   **C**

Cortex (grey matter)
White matter

Limiting sulcus   Axial sulcus   Operculated sulcus

Fig. 28.3: The types of sulci.

Sulci and Gyri of Superolateral Surface

These are shown in Fig. 28.4.

1. The *central sulcus* has been described above. The upper end of the sulcus extends for a short distance on to the medial surface (where it will be examined later).

2. We have seen that the *lateral sulcus* begins on the inferior surface. On reaching the lateral surface it divides into three rami. The largest of these is the *posterior ramus*. The posterior end of this ramus turns upwards into the temporal lobe. The other rami of the lateral sulcus are the *anterior horizontal and anterior ascending rami*. They extend into the lower part of the frontal lobe.

3. The frontal lobe is further divided by the following sulci.

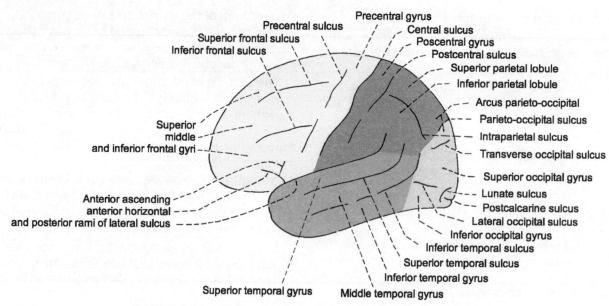

Fig. 28.4: *Sulci and gyri on the superolateral surface of the cerebrum.*

(a) The *precentral sulcus* runs parallel to the central sulcus, a little in front of it. The *precentral gyrus* lies between the two sulci (Table 28.1).

(b) The area in front of the precentral sulcus is divided into *superior, middle and inferior frontal gyri by the superior and inferior frontal sulci.*

(c) The anterior horizontal and anterior ascending rami of the lateral sulcus (see above) subdivide the inferior frontal gyrus into three parts, *(pars orbitalis, pars triangularis, and pars opercularis.*

4. The parietal lobe is further subdivided by the following sulci.

(a) The *postcentral sulcus* runs parallel to the central sulcus, a little behind it. The postcentral gyrus *lies between the two sulci.*

(b) *The area behind the postcentral gyrus is divided into the superior and inferior parietal lobules* by the *intraparietal sulcus.*

(c) The inferior parietal lobule is invaded by the upturned ends of the posterior ramus of the lateral sulcus, and of the superior and inferior temporal gyri (see below). They divide the inferior parietal lobule into anterior, middle and posterior parts. The anterior part is called the *supramarginal gyrus,* and the middle part is called the *angular gyrus.*

5. The *superior and inferior temporal sulci* divide the temporal lobe into *superior, middle and inferior temporal gyri.*

6. The occipital lobe is further subdivided by the following sulci.

(a) The *lateral occipital sulcus* divides this lobe into the *superior and inferior occipital gyri.*

(b) The *lunate sulcus* separates these gyri from the occipital pole.

(c) The area around the parieto-occipital sulcus is the *arcus parieto-occipitalis.* It is separated from the superior occipital gyrus by the *transverse occipital sulcus.*

Subdivisions of the Medial Surface

Confirm the following facts by examining Fig. 28.5.

The central part of the medial aspect of the hemisphere is occupied by the *corpus callosum.* The corpus callosum is divisible into the *genu* (anterior end), the *body,* and the *splenium* (posterior end). It is made up of nerve fibres connecting the two cerebral hemispheres. Below the corpus callosum there are the *septum pellucidum,* the *fornix* and the *thalamus.* In the remaining part of the medial surface, identify the following sulci.

1. The *cingulate sulcus* starts in front of the genu and runs backwards parallel to the upper margin of the corpus callosum. Its posterior end reaches the superomedial border a little behind the upper end of the central sulcus (Table 28.1).

2. The *suprasplenial sulcus* lies above and behind the splenium.

3. The *calcarine sulcus* begins a little below the splenium and runs towards the occipital pole. It gives off the *parieto-occipital sulcus* which reaches the superolateral surface.

4. A little below the genu there are two small anterior and posterior *parolfactory sulci.*

Table 28.1: Sulci and gyri of the cerebrum

Surface/Lobe	Sulci	Gyri
I. Superolateral surface		
1. Frontal lobe	A. Precentral B. Superior frontal C. Inferior frontal	a. Precentral b. Superior frontal c. Middle frontal d. Inferior frontal which also contains horizontal and anterior ascending rami of the lateral sulcus, and the pars orbitalis, pars triangularis and pars opercularis
2. Parietal lobe	A. Postcentral B. Intraparietal	a. Postcentral b. Superior parietal lobule c. Inferior parietal lobule, which is divided into 3 parts: (i) the anterior, supramarginal; (ii) the middle, angular; and (iii) the posterior, over the upturned end of inferior temporal sulcus.
3. Temporal lobe	A. Superior temporal B. Inferior temporal	a. Superior temporal, with 3 transverse temporal gyri b. Middle temporal c. Inferior temporal
4. Occipital lobe	A. Transverse occipital B. Lateral occipital C. Lunate D. Superior and inferior polar	a. Arcus parieto-occipitalis b. Superior occipital c. Inferior occipital d. Gyrus descendens
II. Medial surface	A. Anterior parolfactory B. Posterior parolfactory C. Cingulate D. Callosal E. Suprasplenial or subparietal F. Parieto-occipital G. Calcarine	a. Paraterminal b. Parolfactory (subcallosal area) c. Medial frontal d. Paracentral lobule e. Cingulate f. Cuneus g. Precuneus
III. Inferior surface	A. Olfactory B. H-shaped orbital sulci C. Collateral D. Rhinal E. Occipitotemporal	a. Gyrus rectus b. Anterior orbital c. Posterior orbital d. Medial orbital e. Lateral orbital f. Lingual g. Uncus h. Parahippocampal i. Medial occipitotemporal j. Lateral occipitotemporal

The following gyri can now be identified.

1. The *cingulate gyrus* lies between the corpus callosum and the cingulate sulcus. Its posterior part is bounded above by the *suprasplenial sulcus*.

2. The U–shaped gyrus around the end of the central sulcus is the *paracentral lobule*. It is usually limited posteriorly by the upturned end of the cingulate sulcus; and in front by a branch of the same sulcus.

3. The area between the gyrus cinguli and the superomedial border, in front of the paracentral lobule is called the *medial frontal gyrus*.

4. The quadrangular area between the suprasplenial gyrus and the superomedial border is called the *precuneus*.

5. The triangular area between the parieto-occipital sulcus (above) and the calcarine sulcus (below) is called the *cuneus*.

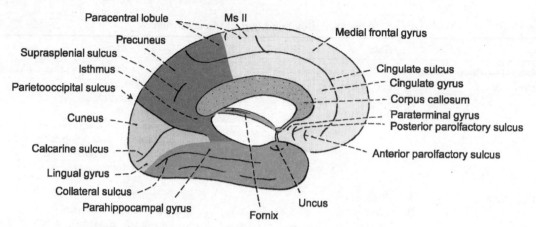

Fig. 28.5: Sulci and gyri on the medial surface of the cerebrum.

6. A narrow strip between the splenium and the stem of the calcarine sulcus is the *isthmus*.

7. The *paraterminal gyrus* lies just in front of the lamina terminalis.

8. The *parolfactory gyrus* lies between the anterior and posterior parolfactory sulci.

Sulci and Gyri on the Orbital Surface

1. Parallel to the medial orbital border there is the *olfactory sulcus:* between them there is the *gyrus rectus.* The rest of the orbital surface is subdivided by an H-shaped sulcus into *anterior, posterior, medial and lateral orbital gyri.*

2. The stem of the lateral sulcus lies deep between the temporal pole and the orbital surface (Fig. 28.6).

Sulci and Gyri on the Tentorial Surface

This area presents two sulci running antero-posteriorly. The medial one is the *collateral sulcus,* and the lateral is the *occipitotemporal sulcus.* On the medial side of the temporal pole there is the *rhinal sulcus.*

The gyri are as follows.

1. The part medial to the rhinal sulcus is the *uncus.*

2. The part medial to the collateral sulcus is the *parahippocampal gyrus.* Its posterior part is limited medially by the calcarine sulcus. It is joined to the cingulate gyrus through the isthmus.

3. The part lateral to the collateral sulcus is divided into *medial and lateral occipitotemporal gyri* by the *occipitotemporal sulcus.*

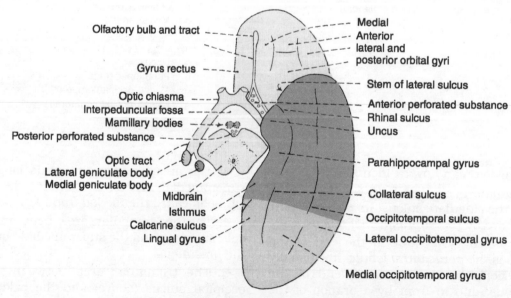

Fig. 28.6: Sulci and gyri on the inferior surface of the cerebrum.

Structural and Functional Type of the Cortex

A. *Allocortex (archipallium)*

It is the original olfactory cortex, and is represented by rhinencephalon (piriform area and hippocampal formation). Structurally, it is simple and is made up of only three layers.

B. *Isocortex (neopallium)*

It is the lately acquired cortex, containing various centres other than those for smell. Structurally, it is thick and six layered. It is subdivided into the following.

    a. Granular cortex (koniocortex or dust cortex). It is basically a sensory cortex.

    b. Agranular cortex. This is the motor cortex.

Main Functional Areas of Cerebral Cortex

The following areas are commonly referred to in clinical work (many others are described).

1. The *motor area* is located in the precentral gyrus on the superolateral surface of the hemisphere (Ms I), and in the anterior part of the paracentral lobule (Ms II) (Figs 28.5, 28.7). Stimulation of this area results in movements in the opposite half of the body. The body is represented upside down in this area (Table 28.2).

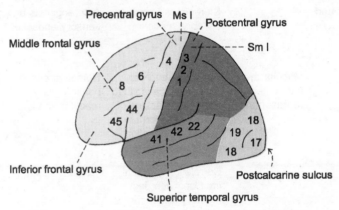

Fig. 28.7: *Diagram to show the numbers allotted by Brodmann to some areas of the cerebral cortex.*

2. The *premotor area* lies just anterior to the motor area. It occupies the posterior parts of the superior, middle and inferior frontal gyri. It is also called the psychomotor area. It is believed that patterns of movement are remembered in this area.

3. The *motor speech area* (of Broca) lies in the inferior frontal gyrus (in the left hemisphere in right handed persons). Injury to this area results in inability to speak (aphasia).

4. The *sensory area* is located in the postcentral gyrus (Sm I). It also extends into the posterior part of the paracentral lobule. As in the motor area, the body is represented upside down in the sensory area.

5. The *visual area* is located in the occipital lobe, mainly on the medial surface both above and below the calcarine sulcus.

6. The *acoustic area* (for hearing) is located in the temporal lobe. It lies partly on the surface of the temporal lobe, but mainly on that part of the superior temporal gyrus which forms the inferior wall of the posterior ramus of the lateral sulcus (on the anterior transverse temporal gyrus) (Table 28.2).

Mapping of the Cortex into Various Functional Areas

Investigations have shown the existence of areas in the cortex which differ from each other in structure, period of myelination of their associated fibres, and in function. Broadmann divided the cortex into 47 areas, each one of which is indicated by a number. Some of the important numbers frequently referred to are shown in Fig. 28.7.

Surface Marking of Functional Areas of Cerebral Cortex

1. The *motor area* is marked by a strip about 1 cm broad in front of the central sulcus.

2. The *sensory area* is marked by a strip about 1 cm broad, behind the central sulcus.

3. The *auditory area* is marked between the superior temporal sulcus and the posterior ramus of the lateral sulcus, immediately below the lower end of the central sulcus.

4. The *visual area* (the part extending on to the superolateral surface) is marked immediately in front of the occipital pole.

THE DIENCEPHALON

The diencephalon is a middle structure which is largely embedded in the cerebrum, and therefore hidden from surface view. Its cavity forms the greater part of the third ventricle. The hypothalamic sulcus, extending from the interventricular foramen to the cerebral aqueduct, divides each half of the diencephalon into dorsal and ventral parts. Further subdivisions are given below.

Dorsal part of diencephalon

1. Thalamus (dorsal thalamus).
2. Metathalamus, including the medial and lateral geniculate bodies, and (Fig. 28.6).

Table 28.2: Functional areas of the cerebral cortex

Lobe	Area	Area number	Location	Representation of body parts	Function	Effect of lesion
I. Frontal lobe	1. Motor area	4	Precentral gyrus and paracentral lobule	Upside down	Controls voluntary activities of the opposite half of body	Contralateral paralysis and Jacksonian fits
	2. Premotor area	6	Posterior parts of superior middle and inferior frontal gyri	—	Controls extra-pyramidal system	Often mixed with pyramidal effect
	3. Frontal eye field	6, 8	Posterior part of middle frontal gyrus	—	Controls horizontal conjugate move-ments of the eyes	Horizontal conjugate movements are lost
	4. Motor speech area (Broca's area)	44, 45	Pars triangularis and and pars opercularis	—	Controls the spoken speech	Aphasia (motor)
	5. Prefrontal area	—	The remaining large, anterior part of frontal lobe	—	Controls emotion, concentration, attention and judgement	Loss of orientation
II. Parietal lobe	1. Sensory (somesthetic) area	3, 1, 2	Postcentral gyrus and paracentral lobule	Upside down	Perception of extero-ceptive (touch, pain and temperature) and proprioceptive impulses	Loss of appreciation of the impulses received
	2. Parietal area	—	Between sensory and visual areas	—	Stereognosis and sensory speech	Astereognosis and sensory aphasias
III. Occipital lobe	1. Visuosensory area or striate area	17	In and around the postcalcarine sulcus	Macular area has largest representation	Reception and per-ception of the isolated visual impressions of colour, size, form, motion, illumination and transparency	Homonymous hemianopia with macular sparing
	2. Visuopsychic area parastriate and peristriate areas	18, 19	Surround the striate area	—	Correlation of visual impulses with past memory and recog-nition of objects seen, and also the depth	Visual agnosia
IV. Temporal lobe	1. Auditosensory area	41, 42	Posterior part of superior temporal gyrus and anterior transverse temporal gyrus	—	Reception and per-ception of isolated auditory impressions of loudness, quality and pitch	Impaired hearing
	2. Auditopsychic area	22	Rest of the superior temporal gyrus	—	Correlation of audi-tory impressions with past memory and identification (interpretation) of the sounds heard	Auditory agnosia

3. Epithalamus, including the pineal body and habenula.

Ventral part of diencephalon

1. Hypothalamus, and
2. Subthalamus (ventral thalamus).

THALAMUS

The thalamus is a large mass of grey matter situated in the lateral wall of the third ventricle and in the floor of the central part of the lateral ventricle. It has anterior and posterior ends; and superior, inferior, medial and lateral surfaces.

The *anterior end* with anterior nucleus is narrow and forms the posterior boundary of the interventricular foramen (Figs 28.8, 28.9).

The *posterior end* is expanded, and is known as the pulvinar. It overhangs the lateral and medial geniculate bodies, and the superior colliculus with its brachium.

The *superior surface* is divided into a lateral ventricular part which forms the floor of the central part of the lateral ventricle, and a medial extra-ventricular part which is covered by the tela choroidea of the third ventricle. It is limited laterally by the caudate nucleus, the stria terminalis and the thalamostriate vein, and medially by the habenular stria (stria medullaris thalami) (Fig. 28.10).

The *inferior surface* rests on the subthalamus and the hypothalamus.

The *medial surface* forms the posterosuperior part of the lateral wall of the third ventricle. The medial surfaces of two thalami are interconnected by an interthalamic adhesion (Fig. 28.11).

The *lateral surface* forms the medial boundary of the posterior limb of the internal capsule (Fig. 28.12).

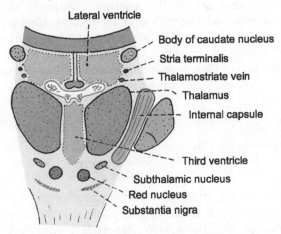

Fig. 28.8: *Coronal section through the thalami showing their relations.*

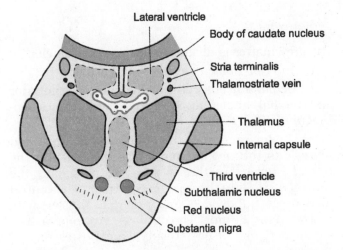

Fig. 28.10: *Relation of thalamus to the ventricles of brain.*

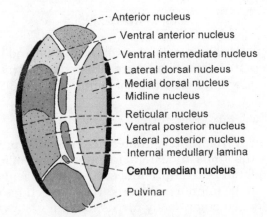

Fig. 28.9: *Subdivisions of the thalamus as seen in a horizontal section.*

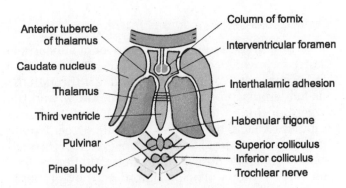

Fig. 28.11: *Superior view of the thalami.*

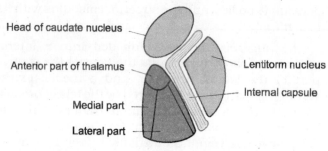

Fig. 28.12: Thalamus as seen in a horizontal section.

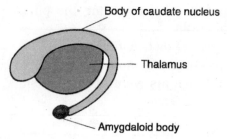

Fig. 28.13: Main connections of the amygdaloid body.

Structure and Nuclei of Thalamus

White Matter

The *external medullary lamina* covers the lateral surface.

The *internal medullary lamina* divides the thalamus into three parts, anterior, medial and lateral (Fig. 28.9).

Grey Matter

The grey matter is divided to form several nuclei.

1. *Anterior nucleus* in the anterior part.

2. *Medial nucleus* in the medial part. The anterior and medial nuclei together represent the *paleothalamus* (Fig. 28.9).

3. The lateral part of the thalamus is largest and represents the *neothalamus*. It is divided into the *lateral nucleus* in the dorsolateral part, and the *ventral nucleus* in the ventromedial part. The ventral nucleus is subdivided into anterior, intermediate and posterior groups. The posterior group is further subdivided into the posterolateral and posteromedial groups.

4. Intralaminar nuclei including centromedian nucleus (located in the internal medullary lamina), midline nuclei (periventricular grey on the medial surface) and reticular nuclei (on the lateral surface) are also present.

Connections and Functions of Thalamus

Afferent impulses from a large number of subcortical centres converge on the thalamus. Exteroceptive and proprioceptive impulses ascend to it through the medial lemniscus, the spinothalamic tracts and the trigeminothalamic tracts. Visual and auditory impulses reach the medial and lateral geniculate bodies. Sensations of taste are conveyed to it through solitariothalamic fibres. Although the thalamus does not receive direct olfactory impulses they probably reach it through the amygdaloid complex (Fig. 28.13). Visceral information is conveyed from the hypo-

thalamus and probably through the reticular formation. In addition to these afferents, the thalamus receives profuse connections from all parts of the cerebral cortex, the cerebellum, and the corpus striatum. The thalamus is, therefore, regarded as a great integrating centre where information from all these sources is brought together. This information is projected to almost the whole of the cerebral cortex through profuse thalamocortical projections. Efferent projections also reach the corpus striatum, the hypothalamus and the reticular formation. Besides its integrating function, the thalamus has some degree of ability to perceive exteroceptive sensations, especially pain. The connections and functions of nuclei of thalamus are presented in Table 28.3.

CLINICAL ANATOMY

1. Lesions of the thalamus cause impairment of all types of sensibilities; joint sense (posture and passive movements) being the most affected.

2. The *thalamic syndrome* is characterized by disturbances of sensations, hemiplegia, or hemiparesis together with hyperaesthesia and severe spontaneous pain. Pleasant as well as unpleasant sensations or feelings are exaggerated.

METATHALAMUS

The metathalamus consists of the medial and lateral geniculate bodies, which are situated on each side of the midbrain, below the thalamus (Fig. 28.6).

Medial Geniculate Body

It is an oval elevation situated just below the pulvinar of the thalamus and lateral to the superior colliculus. The inferior brachium connects the medial geniculate body to the inferior colliculus. The connections of the medial geniculate body are as follows.

Afferents: (1) lateral lemniscus; and (2) fibres from both inferior colliculi.

Table 28.3: Connection of thalamus

Nucleus	Afferents	Efferents	Function
1. Anterior nucleus	Mamillothalamic tract	To cingulate gyrus	Relay station for hippocampal impulses
2. Medial nucleus	From hypothalamus, frontal lobe in front of area 6, corpus striatum, and other thalamic nuclei	To same parts from which the afferents are received	Relay station for visceral impulses
3. Lateral nucleus	From precuneus and superior parietal lobule; also from ventral and medial nuclei	To precuneus and superior parietal lobule	Correlative in function
4. Anterior ventral nucleus	From globus pallidus (subthalamic fasciculus)	To area number 6 and 8 of cortex	Relay station for striatal impulses
5. Intermediate ventral nucleus	From cerebellum (dentatothalamic fibres) and red nucleus	To motor areas number 4 and 6	Relay station for cerebellar impulses
6. Posterolateral ventral nucleus	Spinal and medial lemnisci	To postcentral gyrus (area no. 3, 1, 2)	Relay station for exteroceptive (touch, pain and temperature) and proprioceptive impulses from body, except the face
7. Posteromedial ventral nucleus	Trigeminal and solitariothalamic lemnisci	To postcentral gyrus (areas no. 3, 1, 2)	Relay station for impulses from the face and taste impulses
8. Intralaminar, midline, and reticular nuclei	Reticular formation of brainstem	To all parts of cerebral cortex	Participate in arousal reactions
9. Centromedian nucleus	From parts of corpus striatum; collaterals from spinal, medial, trigeminal lemnisci, ascending reticulothalamic fibres. Impulses from area 4, 6 of cerebral cortex	Not connected to cerebral cortex, connected to other thalamic nuclei, corpus striatum	Receive pain fibres

Efferents: It gives rise to the acoustic (auditory) radiation going to the auditory area of the cortex (in the temporal lobe) through the sublentiform part of the internal capsule (Fig. 28.24).

Function

Medial geniculate body is the last relay station on the pathway of auditory impulses to the cerebral cortex.

Lateral Geniculate Body

It is a small oval elevation situated anterolateral to the medial geniculate body, below the thalamus. It is overlapped by the medial part of the temporal lobe, and is connected to the superior colliculus by the superior brachium (Fig. 28.6).

Structure

It is six-layered. Layers 1, 4 and 6 receive contralateral optic fibres, and layers 2, 3 and 5 ipsilateral optic fibres (Fig. 28.14).

Connections

Afferents: Optic tract (lateral root).

Efferents: It gives rise to optic radiations going to the visual area of cortex through retrolentiform part of internal capsule (Fig. 28.24).

Function

Lateral geniculate body is the last station on the visual pathway to the occipital cortex.

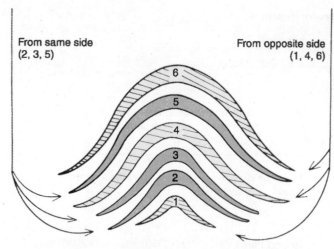

From same side (2, 3, 5)

From opposite side (1, 4, 6)

Fig. 28.14: Six layers of lateral geniculate body.

EPITHALAMUS

The epithalamus occupies the caudal part of the roof of the diencephalon and consists of: (1) The right and left habenular nuclei, each situated beneath the floor of the corresponding habenular trigone; (2) the pineal body or epiphysis cerebri; (3) the habenular commissure; and (4) the posterior commissure (Fig. 28.11).

Habenular Nucleus

The nucleus lies beneath the floor of the habenular trigone. The trigone is a small, depressed triangular area, situated above the superior colliculus and medial to the pulvinar of the thalamus. Medially, it is bounded by the stria medullaris thalami and the stalk of the pineal body.

The habenular nucleus forms a part of the limbic system.

Pineal Body

The pineal body is a small, conical organ, projecting backwards and downwards between the two superior colliculi. It is placed below the splenium of the corpus callosum, but is separated from it by the tela choroidea of the third ventricle and the contained cerebral veins (Fig. 28.11).

It consists of a conical *body* about 8 mm long, and a *stalk* or *peduncle* which divides anteriorly into two laminae separated by the pineal recess of the third ventricle. The superior lamina of the stalk contains the habenular commissure; and the inferior lamina contains the posterior commissure.

Morphological Significance

In many reptiles the epiphysis cerebri is represented by a double structure. The anterior part *(parapineal organ)* develops into the pineal or parietal eye. The posterior part is glandular in nature. The human pineal body represents the persistent posterior glandular part only. The parietal eye has disappeared.

Structure

The pineal gland is composed of two types of cells, pinealocytes and neuroglial cells, with a rich network of blood vessels and sympathetic fibres. The vessels and nerves enter the gland through the connective tissue septa which partly separate the lobules. Sympathetic ganglion cells may be present.

Calcareous concretions are constantly present in the pineal after the 17th year of life and may form aggregations *(brain sand)*. Spaces or cysts may also be present.

Functions

The pineal body has for long been regarded as a vestigial organ of no importance. Recent investigations have shown that it is an endocrine gland of great importance. It produces hormones that may have an important regulatory influence on many other endocrine organs (including the adenohypophysis, the neurohypophysis, the thyroid, the parathyroids, the adrenal cortex and medulla, and the gonads). The best known hormone is melatonin which causes changes in skin colour in some species. The synthesis and discharge of melatonin is remarkably influenced by exposure of the animal to light.

HYPOTHALAMUS

The hypothalamus is a part of the diencephalon. It lies in the floor and lateral wall of the third ventricle. It has been designated as the head ganglion of the autonomic nervous system because it takes part in the control of many visceral and metabolic activities of the body.

Anatomically, it includes: (1) The floor of the third ventricle, or structures in the interpeduncular fossa; and (2) the lateral wall of the third ventricle below the hypothalamic sulcus (Fig. 28.15).

Boundaries

As seen on the base of the brain, the hypothalamus is bounded *anteriorly* by the posterior perforated substance; and *on each side* by the optic tract and crus cerebri.

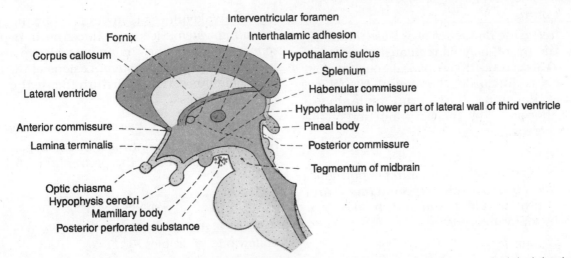

Fig. 28.15: *Sagittal section through the region of the third ventricle showing the hypothalamus and related structure.*

As seen in a sagittal section of the brain, it is bounded *anteriorly* by the lamina terminalis; *inferiorly* by the floor of the third ventricle (from the optic chiasma to the posterior perforated substance); and *posterosuperiorly* by the hypothalamic sulcus.

Parts of the Hypothalamus

The hypothalamus is subdivided into optic, tuberal and mamillary parts. The nuclei present in each part are as follows.

Optic part
1. Supraoptic nucleus, above the optic chiasma.
2. Paraventricular nucleus, just above the supraoptic nucleus (Fig. 28.16).

Tuberal part
3. Ventromedial nucleus.
4. Dorsomedial nucleus.
5. Tuberal nucleus, lateral to the ventromedial nucleus.

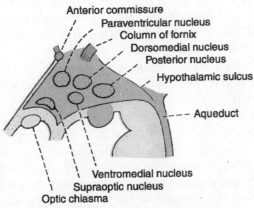

Fig. 28.16: *The hypothalamic nuclei.*

Mamillary part
6. Posterior nucleus, caudal to the ventromedial and dorsomedial nuclei.
7. Lateral nucleus, lateral to the posterior nucleus.

The nuclei 3, 4 and 6 (medial) are separated from nuclei 5 and 7 (lateral) by the column of the fornix, the mamillothalamic tract and the fasciculus retroflexus.

Important Connections

Afferents
The hypothalamus receives visceral sensations through the spinal cord and brainstem (reticular formation). It is also connected to several centres connected with olfactory pathways, including the piriform cortex; with the cerebellum; and with the retina.

Efferents
1. Supraopticohypophyseal tract from the optic nuclei to the pars posterior, the pars tuberalis and the pars intermedia of the hypophysis cerebri.
2. Mamillothalamic tract.
3. Mamillotegmental tract (periventricular system of fibres).

Functions of Hypothalamus

The hypothalamus is a complex neuroglandular mechanism concerned with regulation of visceral and vasomotor activities of the body. Its functions are as follows.

Endocrine Control

By forming *releasing hormones* or *release inhibiting hormones*, the hypothalamus regulates secretion of thyrotropin (TSH), corticotropin (ACTH), somatotropin (STH), prolactin, luteinizing hormone (LH), follicle stimulating hormone (FSH) and melanocyte stimulating hormone, by the pars anterior of the hypophysis cerebri.

Neurosecretion

Oxytocin and vasopressin (antidiuretic hormone, ADH) are secreted by the hypothalamus and transported to the infundibulum and the posterior lobe of the hypophysis cerebri.

General Autonomic Effect

The anterior parts of the hypothalamus chiefly mediate parasympathetic activity, and the posterior parts, chiefly mediate sympathetic activity, but the effects often overlap. Thus the hypothalamus controls cardiovascular, respiratory and alimentary functions.

Temperature Regulation

The hypothalamus maintains a balance between heat production and heat loss of the body. Raised body temperature is depressed through vasodilation, sweating, panting and reduced heat production. Lowered body temperature is elevated by shivering and in prolonged cases by hyperactivity of the thyroid.

Regulation of Food and Water Intake

The *hunger* or *feeding centre* is placed laterally, the *satiety centre*, medially. Stimulation of the feeding centre or damage of the satiety centre causes hyperphagia (overeating) leading to obesity. Stimulation of the satiety centre or damage of the feeding centre causes hypophagia or even aphagia and death from starvation.

The *thirst or drinking centre* is situated in the lateral part of the hypothalamus. Its stimulation causes copious drinking and overhydration.

Sexual Behaviour and Reproduction

Through its control of the anterior pituitary, the hypothalamus controls gametogenesis, various reproductive cycles (uterine, ovarian, etc.) and the maturation and maintenance of secondary sexual characteristics.

Through its connections with the limbic system, it participates in the elementary drives associated with food (hunger and thirst) and sex.

Biological Clocks

Many tissues and organ-systems of the body show a cyclic variation in their functional activity during the 24 hours of a day (circadian rhythm). Sleep and wakefulness is an outstanding example of a circadian rhythm. Wakefulness is maintained by the *reticular activating system*. Sleep is produced by the *hypnogenic zones*, mainly of the thalamus and hypothalamus and partly by the brainstem. Lesions of the anterior hypothalamus seriously disturb the rhythm of sleep and wakefulness.

Emotion, Fear, Rage, Aversion, Pleasure and Reward

These faculties are controlled by the hypothalamus, the limbic system and the prefrontal cortex.

CLINICAL ANATOMY

Lesions of the hypothalamus give rise to one of the following syndromes.

1. *Obesity.* Frolich's syndrome, or Laurence-Moon-Biedl syndrome.

2. *Diabetes insipidus.*

3. *Diencephalic autonomic epilepsy.*

This is characterized by flushing, sweating, salivation, lacrimation, tachycardia, retardation of respiratory rate, unconsciousness, etc.

4. *Sexual disturbance.* Either precocity or impotence.

5. *Disturbance of sleep.* Somnolence (persistent sleep), or narcolepsy (paroxysmal sleep).

6. *Hyperglycaemia and glycosurea.*

7. Acute ulcerations in the upper part of the gastrointestinal tract.

SUBTHALAMUS

The subthalamus lies between the midbrain and the thalamus, medial to the internal capsule and the globus pallidus. It consists of the following.

Grey matter: (1) The cranial ends of the red nucleus and substantia nigra extend into it; (2) subthalamic nucleus; and (3) zona incerta.

White matter. (1) Cranial ends of lemnisci, lateral to the red nucleus; (2) dentatothalamic tract along with the rubrothalamic fibres; (3) ansa lenticularis (ventral); (4) fasciculus lenticularis (dorsal); and (5) subthalamic fasciculus (intermediate fibres).

The *subthalamic nucleus* is biconvex (in coronal section) and is situated dorsolateral to the red nucleus and ventral to the zona incerta. From its connections it appears to be an important site for integration of a number of motor centres (Fig. 28.10).

The *zona incerta* is a thin lamina of grey matter situated between the thalamus and the subthalamic nucleus. Laterally, it is continuous with the reticular nucleus of the thalamus. Its functional significance is not known.

Discrete lesions of the subthalamic nucleus result in hemiballismus characterised by involuntary choreiform movements on the opposite side of the body. The condition is abolished by ablation of the globus pallidus or of its efferent tracts, the anterior ventral nucleus of the thalamus, area 4 of the cerebral cortex, or of the corticospinal tract. From these facts it appears that the subthalamic nucleus has an inhibitory control on the globus pallidus and on the cerebral cortex.

BASAL NUCLEI

The basal nuclei are subcortical, intracerebral masses of grey matter forming important parts of the extrapyramidal system. They include the following.

1. The *corpus striatum*, which is partially divided by the internal capsule into two nuclei: (a) The *caudate nucleus*; and (b) the *lentiform nucleus*. These two nuclei are interconnected by a few bands of grey matter below the anterior limb of the internal capsule. The bands give it a striped appearance, hence the name. The lentiform nucleus is divided into a lateral part, the putamen and a medial part, the globus pallidus. The caudate nucleus and putamen (neostriatum) are often grouped as the *striatum*, whereas the globus pallidus (paleostriatum) is the *pallidum*.

2. The *amygdaloid body* forms a part of the limbic system.

3. *Claustrum.*

The four nuclei (caudate, lentiform, amygdaloid and claustrum) are joined to the cortex at the anterior perforated substance.

CORPUS STRIATUM

Corpus striatum comprises the caudate nucleus and lentiform nucleus.

Caudate Nucleus

It is a C-shaped or comma-shaped nucleus which is surrounded by the lateral ventricle. The concavity of 'C' encloses the thalamus and the internal capsule (Figs 28.17, 28.18).

The nucleus has a head, a body, and a tail.

The *head* forms the floor of the anterior horn of the lateral ventricle, and the medial wall of the anterior limb of the internal capsule. Bands of grey matter connect it to the putamen across the anterior limb of

Raise the lower border of the insula, stripping a thin layer of grey matter situated deep to the white matter of insula. This grey matter is known as the claustrum. As the insula is gradually raised, the external capsule and on a deeper plane, a fan-shaped layer of white matter, the corona radiata, is identifiable. Its fibres pass on a deeper plane than that of superior longitudinal fasciculus.

To explore the lentiform nucleus, strip the external capsule and identify rounded lentiform nucleus. Dissect the striate branches of the middle cerebral artery on the lateral surface of the lentiform nucleus.

Remove the genu and rostrum of corpus callosum from the cerebral hemisphere, identify the head of the caudate nucleus and the anterior part of the corona radiata emerging from between the caudate and the lentiform nuclei. Identify the anterior commissure and trace its fibres reaching till the temporal lobe.

Internal capsule: To expose the internal capsule, remove the lentiform nucleus as it forms the lateral boundary of the internal capsule. It is difficult to separate as many fibres of internal capsule enter the lentiform nucleus. Some fibres form two medullary laminae and divide the lentiform nucleus into outer dark part—the putamen and two paler inner parts—the globus pallidus. Putamen is continuous with the caudate nucleus. Trace the continuity of the corona radiata with the internal capsule and of the internal capsule with the crus cerebri. The latter part is visible after stripping the optic tract from the lateral side of the internal capsule.

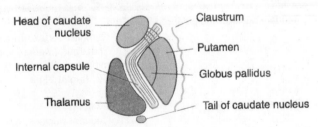

Fig. 28.17: *Horizontal section through the corpus striatum, the thalamus and the internal capsule.*

the internal capsule near the anterior perforated substance (Fig. 28.12).

The *body* forms the floor of the central part of the lateral ventricle, and lies medial to the posterior limb of the internal capsule. It is separated from the thalamus by the stria terminalis and the thala-

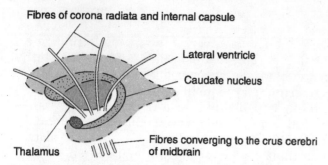

Fibres of corona radiata and internal capsule

Lateral ventricle

Caudate nucleus

Fibres converging to the crus cerebri of midbrain

Thalamus

Fig. 28.18: Relations of the caudate nucleus to the lateral ventricle, thalamus and internal capsule, seen in a lateral view.

mostriate vein. Superiorly, it is related to the fronto-occipital bundle and the corpus callosum (Fig. 28.13).

The tail forms the roof of the inferior horn of the lateral ventricle, and ends by joining the amygdaloid body at the temporal pole (Fig. 28.13). It is related medially to the stria terminalis, laterally to the tapetum, and superiorly to the sublentiform part of the internal capsule and to the globus pallidus.

Lentiform Nucleus

This is a large lens-shaped (biconvex) nucleus, forming the lateral boundary of the internal capsule. It lies beneath the insula and the claustrum (Fig. 28.12).

The lentiform nucleus has three surfaces.

1. The *lateral surface* is convex. It is related to the external capsule, the claustrum, the outermost capsule, insula, and is grooved by the lateral striate arteries.

2. The *medial surface* is more convex. It is related to the internal capsule, the caudate nucleus and the thalamus.

3. The *inferior surface* is related to the sublentiform part of the internal capsule which separates it from the optic tract, the tail of the caudate nucleus, and the inferior horn of the lateral ventricle. The surface is grooved by the anterior commissure just behind the anterior perforated substance.

The lentiform nucleus is divided into two parts by a thin lamina of white matter.

The larger lateral part is called the *putamen.* Structurally, it is similar to the caudate nucleus and contains small cells (Fig. 28.17).

The smaller medial part is called the *globus pallidus.* It is made up of large (motor) cells.

Morphological Divisions of Corpus Striatum

A. The *paleostriatum* is the older and primitive part. It is represented by the globus pallidus (pallidum).

B. The *neostriatum* is more recent in development. It is represented by the caudate nucleus and the putamen of the lentiform nucleus. The neostriatum is often called the striatum.

Connections of Corpus Striatum

The caudate nucleus and putamen are afferent nuclei, while the globus pallidus is the efferent nucleus, of the corpus striatum. The connections are shown in Table 28.4.

Table 28.4: Connections of the corpus striatum		
Nucleus	*Afferents*	*Efferents*
A. Caudate nucleus and putamen.	From: 1. Cerebral cortex (areas 4 and 6) 2. Thalamus (medial, intralaminar and midline nuclei) and 3. Substantia nigra	Chiefly to globus pallidus, but also to substantia nigra and thalamus.
B. Globus pallidus	Mainly from: 1. Caudate nucleus, and 2. Putamen Also from: 1. Thalamus 2. Subthalamic nucleus and 3. Substantia nigra	Efferents from three bundles, namely 1. Ansa lenticularis, ventrally 2. Fasciculus lenticularis, dorsally, and 3. Subthalamic fasciculus from the middle part of the globus pallidus These bundles terminate in the the following: a. Thalamus b. Hypothalamus c. Subthalamic nucleus d. Red nucleus e. Olivary nucleus f. Substantia nigra; and g. Reticular nuclei

Functions of Corpus Striatum

1. The corpus striatum regulates muscle tone and thus helps in smoothening voluntary movements.

2. It controls automatic associated movements, like the swinging of arms during walking. Similarly, it controls the coordinated movements of different parts of the body for emotional expression.

3. It influences the precentral motor cortex which is supposed to control the extrapyramidal activities of the body.

4. Lesions of the corpus striatum result in *Parkinsonism*. The rigidity and tremors associated with this condition can be controlled both medically and surgically.

Medically, L-dopa (a precursor of dopamine) is used as a replacement therapy in Parkinsonism because dopamine, the normal neurotransmitter in the striatum, is reduced in these cases. Nigro-striate fibres are considered to be important in the genesis of Parkinsonian tremor since their neurons utilize dopamine in neurotransmission.

Surgically, pallidotomy and thalamotomy have been used with success to control rigidity and tremors in different diseases of the corpus striatum. Such procedures are based on the belief that the disease is the result of overactivity of the pallidum which in turn leads to oscillating bursts of activity in the ventrolateral thalamic nuclei, the frequency of which corresponds to that of tremor.

| CLINICAL ANATOMY |

A. *Lesions of the corpus striatum* give rise to:

1. Hypertonicity, or lead–pipe type of muscular rigidity.

2. Loss of automatic associated movements and also of facial expressions. Reduction in speed known as bradykinesia, i.e. slow movement or akinesia, i.e. movement.

3. Involuntary movements, like tremors, and other types of abnormal movements like chorea, hemiballismus, athetosis.

| AMYGDALOID BODY |

This is a nuclear mass in the temporal lobe, lying anterosuperior to the inferior horn of the lateral ventricle. Topographically, it is continuous with the tail of the caudate nucleus, but functionally, it is related to the stria terminalis. It is a part of the limbic system (Fig. 28.19).

expose uncinate fasciculus. Also expose superior longitudinal fasciculus joining the frontal lobe to the occipital and temporal lobes. Lastly, scrape the grey matter between occipital and temporal lobes to expose the inferior longitudinal fasciculus.

Identify the various parts of the corpus callosum. Remove the fibres of the cingulum and identify the superficial fibres of the genu of corpus callosum passing into the medial aspect of hemisphere. Such fibres of the two sides form the forceps minor.

Expose the band of fibres passing from splenium of corpus callosum towards the superior part of occipital lobe. Trace the fibres of tapetum arising from the trunk and splenium of corpus callosum curving to reach the inferior parts of the occipital and temporal lobes.

Identify the anterior commissure lying just anterior to column of fornix and the interventricular foramen. Examine the posterior commissure situated dorsal to the upper part of aqueduct and inferior to the root of the pineal body. Look for habenular commissure present at the root of the pineal body. Lastly, identify the commissure of the fornix and the hypothalamic commissures.

Lift up a strip of superficial fibres of the genu of corpus callosum and tear these laterally. Identify the intersectioning fibres of corpus callosum and those of the vertically disposed fibres of the corona radiata.

Association (Arcuate) Fibres

These are the fibres which connect different cortical areas of the same hemisphere to one another. These are subdivided into the following two types.

A. *Short association fibres* connect adjacent gyri to one another (Fig. 28.20).

B. *Long association fibres* connect more widely separated gyri to one another. Some examples are: (1) The *uncinate fasciculus*, connecting the temporal pole to the motor speech area and to the orbital cortex; (2) the *cingulum*, connecting the cingulate gyrus to the parahippocampal gyrus; (3) the *superior longitudinal fasciculus*, connecting the frontal lobe to the occipital and temporal lobes; and (4) the *inferior longitudinal fasciculus*, connecting the occipital and temporal lobes.

Projection Fibres

These are fibres which connect the cerebral cortex to other parts of the CNS, e.g. the brainstem and spinal cord. Many important *tracts*, e.g. corticospinal and corticopontine are made up of projection fibres.

Commissural Fibres

These are the fibres which connect corresponding parts of the two hemispheres. They constitute the commissures of the cerebrum. They are: (1) The *corpus callosum* connecting the cerebral cortex of the two sides; (2) the *anterior commissure*, connecting the archipallia (olfactory bulbs, piriform area and anterior parts of temporal lobes) of the two sides; (3) the *posterior commissure*, connecting the superior colliculi, and also transmitting corticotectal fibres and fibres from the pretectal nucleus to the Edinger–Westphal nucleus of the opposite side; (4) the *commissure of the fornix (hippocampal commissure)*, connecting the crura of the fornix and thus the hippocampal formations of the two sides; (5) the *habenular commissure*, connecting the habenular nuclei; (6) and the *hypothalamic commissures*, including the anterior hypothalamic commissure (of Ganser), the ventral supraoptic commissure (of Gudden) and the dorsal supraoptic commissure (of Meynert).

Corpus Callosum

The corpus callosum is the largest commissure of the brain. It connects the two cerebral hemispheres. Since it is the neopallial commissure, it attains enormous size in man (10 cm long).

Parts of Brain Connected by it

The corpus callosum connects all parts of the cerebral cortex of the two sides, except the lower and anterior parts of the temporal lobes which are connected by the anterior commissure.

Parts of Corpus Callosum

1. The *genu* is the anterior end. It lies 4 cm behind the frontal pole. It is related anteriorly to the anterior cerebral arteries, and posteriorly to the anterior horn of the lateral ventricle (Fig. 28.21).

2. The *rostrum* is directed downwards and backwards from the genu, and ends by joining the

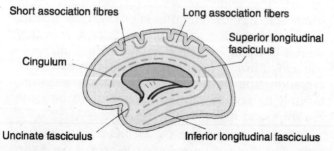

Fig. 28.20: *The short and long association fibres of the cerebrum.*

Short association fibres

Long association fibers

Superior longitudinal fasciculus

Cingulum

Uncinate fasciculus

Inferior longitudinal fasciculus

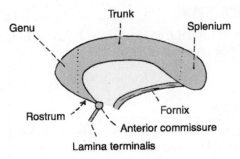

Fig. 28.21: *Parts of the corpus callosum as seen in a sagittal section.*

lamina terminalis, in front of the anterior commissure. It is related superiorly to the anterior horn of the lateral ventricle, and inferiorly to the indusium griseum and the longitudinal striae.

3. The *trunk* or body is the middle part, between the genu and the splenium. Its *superior surface* is convex from before backwards and concave from side to side. It is related to the anterior cerebral arteries and to the lower border of the falx cerebri. It is overlapped by the gyrus cinguli and is covered by the indusium griseum and the longitudinal striae. The *inferior surface* is concave from before backwards and convex from side to side. It provides attachment to the septum pellucidum and the fornix, and forms the roof of the central part of the lateral ventricle (Fig. 28.22).

4. The *splenium* is the posterior end forming the thickest part of the corpus callosum. It lies 6 cm in front of the occipital pole. Its *inferior surface* is related to the tela choroidea of the third ventricle, the pulvinar, the pineal body, and the tectum of the midbrain. The *superior surface* is related to the inferior sagittal sinus and the falx cerebri. *Posteriorly,* it is related to the great cerebral vein, the straight sinus and the free margin on the tentorium cerebelli (Fig. 28.15).

Fibres of Corpus Callosum

1. The rostrum connects the orbital surfaces of the two frontal lobes.

2. The *forceps minor* is made up of fibres of the genu that connect the two frontal lobes.

3. The *forceps major* is made up of fibres of the splenium connecting the two occipital lobes.

4. The *tapetum* is formed by some fibres from the trunk and splenium of the corpus callosum. The tapetum forms the roof and lateral wall of the posterior horn, and the lateral wall of the inferior horn of the lateral ventricle.

Functional Significance

The corpus callosum helps in coordinating activities of the two hemispheres.

INTERNAL CAPSULE

The internal capsule is a large band of fibres, situated in the inferomedial part of each cerebral hemisphere. In horizontal sections of the brain, it appears V-shaped with its concavity directed laterally. The concavity is occupied by the lentiform nucleus.

The internal capsule contains fibres going to and coming from the cerebral cortex. It can be compared to a narrow gate where the fibres are densely crowded. Small lesions of the capsule can give rise to widespread derangements of the body.

When traced *upwards*, the fibres of the capsule diverge and are continuous with the corona radiata. When traced *downwards* its fibres converge and many of them are continuous with the crus cerebri of the midbrain.

The internal capsule is divided into the following parts (Fig. 28.23).

1. The *anterior limb* lies between the head of the caudate nucleus and the lentiform nucleus.

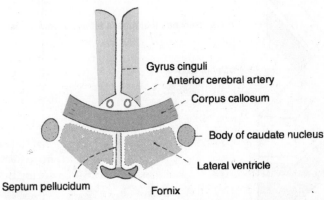

Fig. 28.22: *Coronal section of the trunk of the corpus callosum showing its relations.*

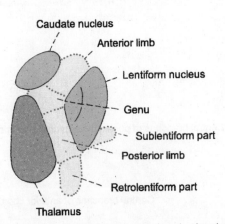

Fig. 28.23: *The internal capsule as seen in a horizontal section.*

2. The *posterior limb* lies between the thalamus and the lentiform nucleus.

3. The *genu* is the bend between the anterior and posterior limbs.

4. The *retrolentiform part* lies behind the lentiform nucleus.

5. The *sublentiform part* lies below the lentiform nucleus. It can be seen in a coronal section, whereas the rest of the parts are seen in a horizontal section.

Constituent Fibres

The fibres of internal capsule are shown in Fig. 28.24. These are presented in Table 28.5.

Blood Supply

The arteries supplying different parts of the internal capsule are depicted in Fig. 28.25.

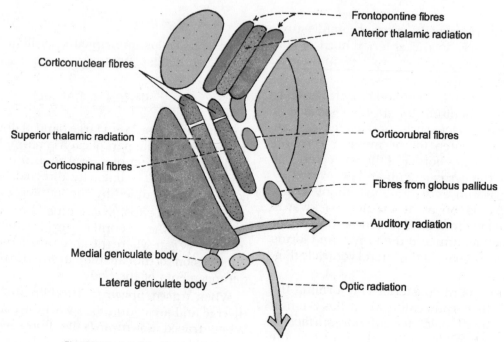

Fig. 28.24: *Scheme to show the fibres passing through the internal capsule.*

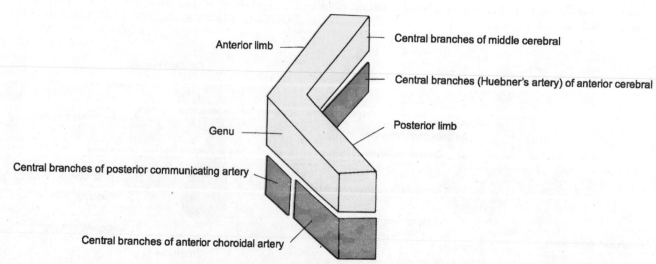

Fig. 28.25: *Arterial supply of the internal capsule.*

Table 28.5: Fibres in the internal capsule (Fig. 28.24)

Part	Descending tracts	Ascending tracts
1. Anterior limb	Frontopontine fibres (a part of the corticoponto-cerebellar pathway)	Anterior thalamic radiation (fibres from anterior and medial nuclei of thalamus)
2. Genu	Corticonuclear fibres (a part of the pyramidal tract going to motor nuclei of cranial nerves and forming their supranuclear pathway)	Anterior part of the superior thalamic radiation (fibres from posterior ventral nucleus of thalamus)
3. Posterior limb	1. Corticospinal tract (pyramidal tract for the upper limb, trunk and lower limb) 2. Corticopontine fibres 3. Corticorubral fibres	1. Superior thalamic radiation 2. Fibres from globus pallidus to subthalamic nucleus
4. Retrolentiform part	1. Parietopontine and occipitopontine fibres 2. Fibres from occipital cortex to superior colliculus and pretectal region	Posterior thalamic radiation made up of 1. Mainly by optic radiation 2. Partly by fibres connecting the parietal and occipital lobes to the thalamus (posterior part)
5. Sublentiform part	1. Parietopontine and temporopontine fibres 2. Interconnections between temporal lobe and thalamus	Auditory radiation

Development

Cerebral hemispheres arise as outgrowths from the lateral wall of prosencephalon during 5–6 weeks. These gradually enlarge to cover thalamus, midbrain and pons. Further growth results in formation of lobes and poles. Increased growth in a limited area result in formation of sulci and gyri. The basal part of the hemisphere increases in size to form two big nuclei connected together by fibres. These nuclei are the caudate and lentiform nuclei. Between these two nuclei pass fibres both ascending and descending. These form internal capsule (projection fibres). The commissural fibres develop in the lamina terminalis.

CLINICAL ANATOMY

Lesions of the internal capsule are usually vascular, due to involvement of the middle cerebral artery. They give rise to *hemiplegia* on the opposite half of the body (paralysis of one half of the body, including the face). It is an upper motor neuron type of paralysis.

Thrombosis of the recurrent branch of the anterior cerebral artery gives rise to an upper motor neuron type of paralysis of the opposite upper limb and of the face.

29

The Third and Lateral Ventricles and Limbic System

Third and lateral ventricles of brain secrete the cerebrospinal fluid with the help of their choroid plexuses (Figs 29.1A and B). Rhinencephalon and limbic system are related to smell and various visceral activities.

THE THIRD VENTRICLE

The third ventricle is a median cleft between the two thalami. Developmentally, it represents the cavity of the diencephalon, except for the area in front of the interventricular foramen which is derived from the median part of the telencephalon. The cavity is lined by ependyma.

DISSECTION

Identify the extent of the third ventricle from the lamina terminalis anteriorly to the upper end of the aqueduct and root of pineal body posteriorly. Examine its anterior wall, posterior wall, roof, floor and lateral walls.

Communications

Anterosuperiorly, on each side, it communicates with the lateral ventricle through the interventricular foramen (or foramen of Monro). This foramen is bounded anteriorly by the column of the fornix, and posteriorly by the tubercle of the thalamus.

Posteroinferiorly, in the median plane, it communicates with the fourth ventricle through the cerebral aqeduct (Fig. 29.2).

Recesses

Recesses are extensions of the cavity. These are: (a) Suprapineal; (b) pineal; (c) infundibular; and (d) optic (Fig. 29.2) Also see Fig. 29.7B.

Boundaries

Anterior wall: (1) Lamina terminalis; (2) anterior commissure; and (3) anterior columns of fornix. The two columns of the fornix diverge, pass downwards and backwards, and sink into the lateral wall of the third ventricle to reach the mamillary body (see Fig. 29.9).

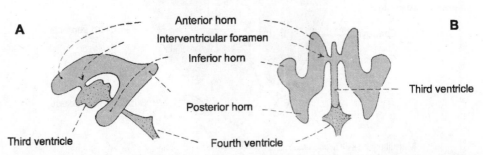

Fig. 29.1: *Anterior, posterior, inferior horns of lateral ventricle, third and fourth ventricles of the brain: (A) Lateral view, (B) superior view.*

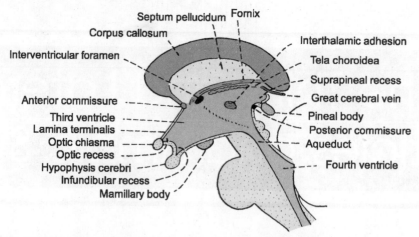

Fig. 29.2: *Sagittal section through the third ventricle and some related structures.*

Posterior wall: (1) Pineal body, (2) posterior commissure (in the lower lamina of the pineal stalk); and (3) cerebral aqueduct.

Roof: It is formed by the ependyma lining the under surface of the tela choroidea of the third ventricle. The choroid plexus of the third ventricle projects downwards from the roof (Fig. 29.3).

At the junction of the roof with the anterior and lateral walls, there are the interventricular foramina.

Floor: It is formed by hypothalamic structures: (1) Optic chiasma; (2) tubercinerium; (3) infundibulum (pituitary stalk); (4) mamillary bodies; (5) posterior perforated substance; and (6) tegmentum of the midbrain.

At the junction of the floor with the anterior wall, there is the optic recess.

Lateral wall: It is formed by the following: (1) Medial surface of thalamus (in its posterosuperior part); (2) hypothalamus, (in its anteroinferior part); and (3) the hypothalamic sulcus which separates the thalamus from the hypothalamus. The sulcus extends from the interventricular foramen to the cerebral aqueduct.

Note that: (a) The interthalamic adhesion connects the medial surfaces of the two thalami and crosses the ventricular cavity. (b) The habenular stria lies at the junction of the roof and the lateral wall. The two striae join posteriorly at the habenular commissure. (c) The columns of the fornix, as already indicated, run downwards and backwards to reach the mamillary bodies. The columns lie beneath the lateral wall of the ventricle.

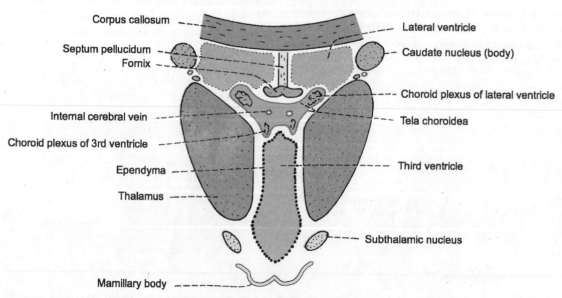

Fig. 29.3: *Coronal section through the third and lateral ventricles of the brain.*

1. The third ventricle is a narrow space which is easily obstructed by local brain tumours or by developmental defects. The obstruction leads to raised intracranial pressure in adults and hydrocephalus in infants.

2. Tumours in the lower part of the third ventricle give rise to hypothalamic symptoms, like diabetes insipidus, obesity, etc. (see hypothalamus).

3. The site of obstruction can be found out by CT scan/MRI (magnetic resonance imaging) scans, where, the third ventricle is seen, normally, as a narrow, vertical midline shadow. Dilatation of the third ventricle would indicate obstruction at a lower level, e.g. the cerebral aqueduct. If the obstruction is in the third ventricle, both the lateral ventricles are dilated symmetrically. Obstruction at an interventricular foramen causes unilateral dilatation of the lateral ventricle of that side.

THE LATERAL VENTRICLE

The lateral ventricles are two irregular cavities situated one in each cerebral hemisphere. Each lateral ventricle communicates with the third ventricle through an interventricular foramen (or foramen of Monroe).

Each lateral ventricle consists of: (1) A central part; and (2) three horns, anterior, posterior and inferior (Fig. 29.1).

DISSECTION

Take the right hemisphere and put the tip of the knife at the interventricular foramen. Give a vertical incision through the fornix, septum pellucidum, body of corpus callosum, the medial surface of the hemisphere till the superomedial border.

Turn the brain so that superolateral surface points towards you. Continue the previous incision on this surface for 2 cm. Carry the incision posteriorly and then curve it downwards till the end of the posterior ramus of the lateral sulcus.

Expose the insula by depressing the temporal lobe. Cut through the medial part of the gyri situated on the superior surface of the temporal lobe till the stem of the lateral sulcus.

Now try to separate the frontal lobe from the temporal lobe, and open up the stem of the lateral sulcus. Put the knife in the anterior part of stem of the lateral sulcus and extend the incision medially to the inferior part of stem of the lateral sulcus. Keep on opening the cut while making it and identify the choroid plexus entering the inferior horn of the lateral ventricle from its medial side.

Now brain is easily separable into an upper frontal part and a lower occipitotemporal part. Lift the fornix from the thalamus, separating the fornix from the choroid plexus. Identify the choroidal branches of the posterior cerebral artery. Identify structures in all horns of lateral ventricle with the help of the two parts, i.e. frontal part and occipitotemporal parts of the cerebral hemisphere.

Expose the anterior column of fornix by scraping the ependyma of anterior part of third ventricle. Trace the anterior column of fornix till the mamillary body. Trace another bundle the mamillothalamic tract till the anterior nucleus of the thalamus.

Central Part

This part of the lateral ventricle extends from the interventricular foramen in front to the splenium of the corpus callosum behind (see Fig. 29.7A).

Boundaries

Roof: It is formed by the undersurface of the corpus callosum (Fig. 29.3).

Floor: It is formed (from lateral to medial side by: (a) Body of caudate nucleus; (b) stria terminals; (c) thalamostriate vein; and (d) lateral portion of the upper surface of the thalamus.

Medial wall: It is formed by: (a) Septum pellucidum, and (b) body of fornix.

Choroid Fissure

The line along which the choroid plexus invaginates into the lateral ventricle is called the choroid fissure. It is a C-shaped slit in the medial wall of the cerebral hemisphere. It starts at the interventricular foramen (above and in front) and passes around the thalamus and cerebral peduncle to the uncus (in the temporal lobe). Thus it is present only in relation to the central part and inferior horn of the lateral ventricle. Its convex margin is bounded by the fornix (body and crus), the fimbria and the hippocampus and the concave margin is bounded by the thalamus (superior and posterior surfaces), the tail of the caudate nucleus and the stria terminalis. At the fissure, the pia mater and ependyma come into contact with each other and both are invaginated into the ventricle by the choroid plexus (see Fig. 29.6).

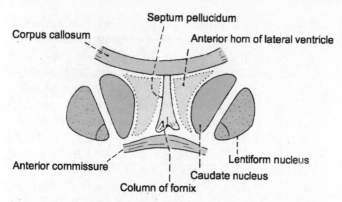

Fig. 29.4: Boundaries of the anterior horn of the lateral ventricle as seen in a coronal section.

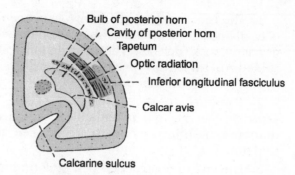

Fig. 29.5: Boundaries of the posterior horn of the lateral ventricle as seen in a coronal section.

In the central part of the lateral ventricle, the choroid fissure is a narrow gap between the edge of the fornix and the upper surface of the thalamus. The gap is invaginated by the choroid plexus.

Anterior Horn

This is the part of the lateral ventricle which lies in front of the interventricular foramen and extends into the frontal lobe. It is directed forwards, laterally and downwards, and is triangular on cross-section (Fig. 29.4).

Boundaries

Anterior: Posterior surface of genu and rostrum of the corpus callosum.

Roof: Anterior part of the trunk of the corpus callosum.

Floor: (a) Head of the caudate nucleus; and (b) upper surface of the rostrum of the corpus callosum.

Medial: (a) Septum pellucidum; and (b) column of fornix.

Posterior Horn

This is the part of the lateral ventricle which lies behind the splenium of the corpus callosum and extends into the occipital lobe. It is variable in size and may be absent. It is directed backwards and medially (Fig. 29.5).

Boundaries

Floor and medial wall: (a) Bulb of the posterior horn raised by the forceps major; and (b) calcar avis raised by the anterior part of the calcarine sulcus.

Roof and lateral wall: Tapetum.

Inferior Horn

This is the largest horn of the lateral ventricle. It begins at the junction of the central part with the

posterior horn of the lateral ventricle; and extends into the temporal lobe (Fig. 29.6, 29.7).

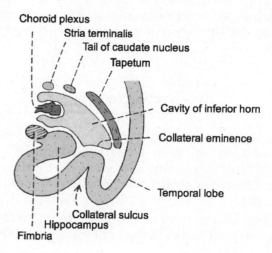

Fig. 29.6: Boundaries of the inferior horn of the lateral ventricle as seen in a coronal section.

Boundaries

Roof (and lateral wall): (a) Chiefly the tapetum; (b) tail of caudate nucleus; (c) stria terminalis; and (d) amygdaloid body.

Floor: (a) Collateral eminence raised by the collateral sulcus; and (b) hippocampus, medially (Fig. 29.6).

In the inferior horn, the line of ependymal invagination by the choroid plexus (i.e., the choroid fissure) lies between the stria terminalis and the fimbria.

LIMBIC SYSTEM

Introduction

The main objects of primitive life are food and sex. Food is necessary for survival of the individual, and sex, for survival of the species. The primitive brain is, therefore, adapted to control and regulate

A

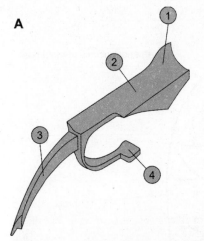

(A)
1. Anterior cornu of the lateral ventricle
2. Body of the lateral ventricle
3. Posterior cornu of the lateral ventricle
4. Inferior cornu of the lateral ventricle

B

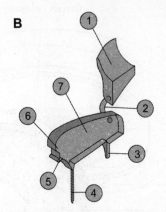

(B)
1. Anterior cornu of lateral ventricle
2. Interventricular foramen (of Monroe)
3. Pituitary recess
4. Aqueduct
5. Pineal recess
6. Suprapineal recess
7. Third ventricle

29.7: (A) Parts of the lateral ventricle (three dimensional) (B) Third ventricle connected to lateral ventricle via interventricular foramen. (Courtesy, Dr. S. Sircar, Medical Physiology, CBS Publishers and Distributers, New Delhi).

behaviour of the animal with regards to seeking and procuring of food, courtship, mating, housing, rearing of young, rage, aggression and emotions. The parts of the human brain controlling such behavioural patterns constitute the limbic system. These parts represent the phylogenetically older areas of the cortex (archipallium and paleopallium) which have been grouped in the past with the rhinencephalon and were earlier considered to be predominantly olfactory in function. However, their important role in controlling the behaviour patterns is now increasingly realized.

Constituent Parts

1. Olfactory nerves, bulb, tract, striae and trigone.
2. Anterior perforated substance.
3. Pyriform lobe, consisting of the uncus, the anterior part of the parahippocampal gyrus, and small areas in the region.
4. Posterior part of the parahippocampal and cingulate gyri.
5. Hippocampal formation, including the hippocampus, the dentate gyrus, the indusium griseum and longitudinal striae.
6. Amygdaloid nuclei.
7. Septal region
8. Fornix, stria terminalis, stria habenularis, anterior commissure.

Functions

1. It controls food habits necessary for survival of the individual.
2. It controls sex behaviour necessary for survival of the species.

3. It controls emotional behaviour expressed in form of joy and sorrow, fear, fight and friendship, and liking and disliking, associated with a variety of somatic and autonomic bodily alterations. This requires integration of olfactory, somatic and visceral impulses reaching the brain.

Following are the terms with their components related to limbic system.

1. Rhinencephalon: It comprises the following.

(i) Olfactory mucosa

(ii) Olfactory bulb

(iii) Olfactory tract—3 roots

(a) Medial root ends in subcallosal or parolfactory gyrus (Flow Chart 29.1A).

(b) Intermediate root ends in anterior perforated substance and diagonal band of Broca.

(c) Lateral, olfactory, root ends in pyriform lobe (uncus, anterior part of parahippocampal gyrus, cortex in region of limen insulae, dorsomedial part of amygdaloid nucleus) (Fig. 29.8).

2. Limbic lobe: Subcallosal gyrus + cingulate gyrus + parahippocampal gyrus.

3. Hippocampal formation: Hippocampus + dentate gyrus + part of parahippocampal gyrus (Flow Chart 29.1B).

4. Limbic System: Limbic lobe + hippocampal formation + amygdaloid nucleus + hypothalamus + anterior nucleus of thalamus.

5. Connecting pathways: Alveus, fimbria, fornix mamillary body, mamillothalamic tract, stria terminalis (Fig. 29.9).

6. Papez circuit : Hippocampal formation, fornix, mamillary body, thalamus, cingulate gyrus (Fig. 29.8, Flow Chart 29.1C).

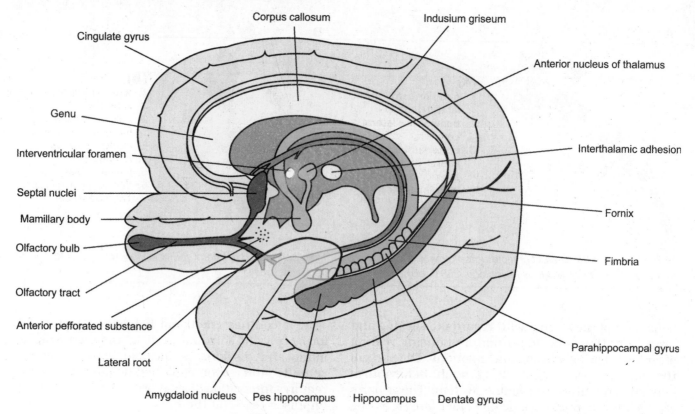

Fig. 29.8: *Rhinencephalon and Papez circuit.*

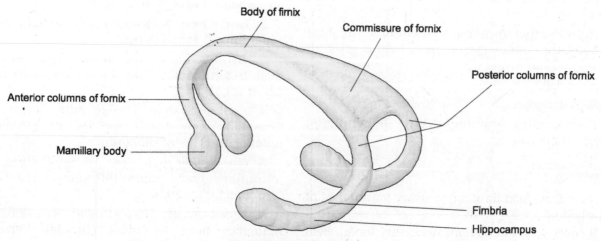

Fig. 29.9: *Parts of the fornix.*

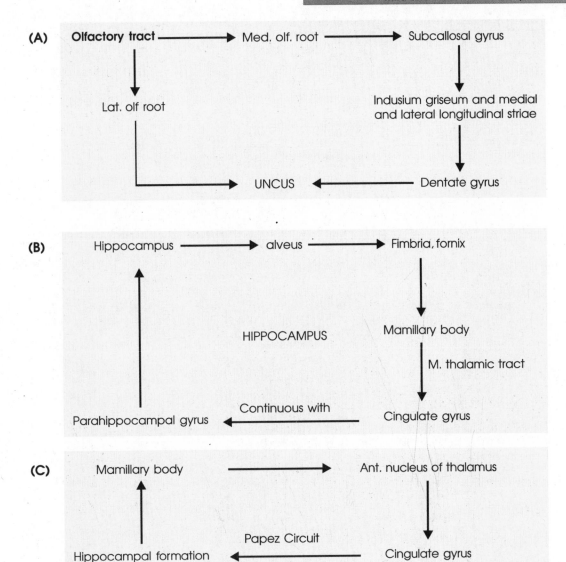

Flow Chart 29.1: *Connections of: (A) olfactory roots; (B) hippocampus; and (C) Papez circuit.*

1. Hippocampus can be regarded as the cortical centre for autonomic reflexes. Hippocampal-amygdala complex is related to the memory of recent events. Lesions of this complex are associated with a loss of memory for recent events only. Patient is unable to commit any new facts to memory and does not remember recent events. In spite of this his general intelligence remains unaltered.

2. Destruction of olfactory nerves results in loss of the sense of smell (anosmia).

3. A tumour, usually a meningioma, in the floor of anterior cranial fossa may interfere with the sense of smell because of pressure on olfactory bulb and the olfactory tract. It is necessary to test each nostril separately because the olfactory loss is likely to be unilateral.

4. A lesion that affects the uncus and amygdaloid body may cause, "uncinate fits" characterised by an imaginary disagreeable odour, by movements of lips and tongue, and often by a "dreamy state".

30

Some Neural Pathways

Course of pyramidal tracts responsible for voluntary movements is described here. The sensory pathways for exteroceptive, unconscious and conscious proprioceptive are outlined. In addition, the pathways of special sensations of sight, hearing, balance, smell and taste are briefly mentioned.

PYRAMIDAL TRACT
(Corticospinal and Corticonuclear Tracts)

This is a descending tract, extending from the cerebral cortex to various motor nuclei of the cranial and spinal nerves. It constitutes the upper motor neuron in the motor pathway from the cortex to voluntary muscles (Fig. 30.1).

Origin

Each pyramidal tract contains about one million fibres which originate from: (a) The motor area (Area 4) of the cortex; (b) premotor area (Area 6); and also (c) the somesthetic area (Areas 3, 2, 1). Certain notable features of the motor cortex are given.

1. The body is represented upside down. The areas for the legs and perineum lie in the paracentral lobule.

2. The angle of the mouth, tongue, larynx, the thumb and the great toe are represented by relatively large areas.

3. It is the movements which are represented in the cortex rather than the individual muscles.

Course of the Pyramidal Tract

The tract passes through the following parts of the CNS.

(1) Corona radiata; (2) internal capsule, occupying the genu and the anterior two-thirds of the posterior limb; (3) middle two-thirds of the crus cerebri of the midbrain; (4) basilar part of the pons; (5) pyramid of the medulla. In the lower part of the medulla, about 75 to 80% of the fibres cross to opposite side and descend as the lateral (crossed) corticospinal tract. About 20% fibres remain uncrossed and run down as the anterior (uncrossed) corticospinal tract. (6) Thus in the spinal cord, there are two corticospinal tracts: Lateral (crossed) and anterior (uncrossed). Ultimately most of the uncrossed fibres also cross to the opposite side before termination.

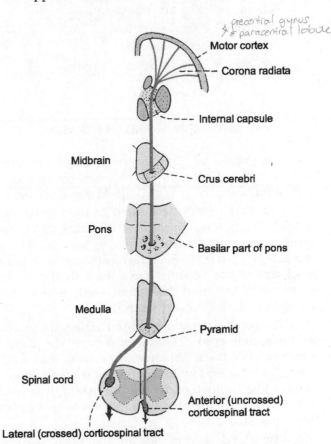

precentral gyrus & paracentral lobule

- Motor cortex
- Corona radiata
- Internal capsule
- Midbrain
- Crus cerebri
- Pons
- Basilar part of pons
- Medulla
- Pyramid
- Spinal cord
- Anterior (uncrossed) corticospinal tract
- Lateral (crossed) corticospinal tract

Fig. 30.1: *The corticospinal pathway.*

Termination

Before termination, all fibres of the pyramidal tract cross to opposite side. They terminate, mostly through an interneuron, in the motor nuclei of cranial nerves and in relation to the anterior horn cells of the spinal cord. The fibres which terminate in the motor nuclei of the cranial nerves collectively form the corticonuclear tract.

Functions

1. The pyramidal tract is concerned with voluntary movements of the body.

2. Possibly, it is also the pathway for superficial reflexes.

CLINICAL ANATOMY

Effects of Lesion of the Pyramidal Tract

Lesions above the level of decussation cause contralateral paralysis; while lesions below the decussation cause ipsilateral paralysis. It is an upper motor neuron type of paralysis which is characterized by the following.

1. Loss of power of voluntary movements.
2. Clasp-knife type of spasticity (hypertonia).
3. Tendon reflexes are exaggerated.
4. Superficial reflexes are lost.
5. Babinski's sign is positive.
6. Reaction of degeneration is absent.

PATHWAY OF PAIN AND TEMPERATURE

1. *Receptors:* (a) Free nerve endings for pain; (b) end bulbs of Krause for cold; and (c) organs of Ruffini for warmth, and of Golgi-Mazzoni for heat.

2. The *first neuron* is located in the dorsal root ganglia. Peripheral processes of neurons in the ganglia constitute the sensory nerves. These processes end in relation to the receptors. The central processes of the neurons pass through the dorsal nerve roots to enter the spinal cord, where they synapse with the second neuron.

3. The *second neuron* is located in the grey matter of the spinal cord. Their axons form the lateral spinothalamic tract. This tract is crossed. It ascends through the lateral white column of the spinal cord to enter the brainstem. In the brainstem, this tract is referred to as the spinal lemniscus to end in the thalamus (Fig. 23.7).

4. The *third neuron* lies in the posterolateral ventral nucleus of the thalamus. Fibres arising in

this nucleus pass through the internal capsule and the corona radiata to reach the somatosensory area (Areas 3, 1, 2) of the cerebral cortex.

PATHWAY OF TOUCH

1. *Receptors:* (a) Tactile (Messiner's) corpuscles; (b) Merkel's discs; and (c) free nerve endings around the hair follicles.

2. The *first neuron* is similar to that for pain and temperature pathway. The 2nd neuron are different for fine touch and for crude touch.

Pathway of Fine Touch

1. The central processes of the neurons in the dorsal nerve root ganglia enter the posterior white column of the spinal cord and form the fasciculus gracilis and the fasciculus cuneatus. These are uncrossed tracts (Fig. 23.7).

2. The second neuron lies in the nucleus gracilis or nucleus cuneatus. It gives off the internal arcuate fibres which cross to the opposite side through the sensory decussation. Reaching the other side they run upwards as the medial lemniscus. The medial lemniscus ends in the posterolateral ventral nucleus of the thalamus.

3. Fibres starting in the thalamus pass through the internal capsule and the corona radiata and end in the somatosensory area of the cerebral cortex (Areas 3, 1, 2).

Pathway for Crude Touch

1. The central processes of neurons in the dorsal nerve root ganglia terminate in the grey matter of the spinal cord (Fig. 23.7).

2. The second neuron lies in the spinal cord (mainly the posterior grey column). Axons of those neurons cross the midline and form the anterior spinothalamic tract. In the brainstem, this tract merges with the medial lemniscus.

3. The third neuron and termination of the pathway are the same as for fine touch (Fig. 23.7).

PATHWAY OF PROPRIOCEPTIVE (KINAESTHETIC) IMPULSES

1. *Receptors:* (a) Muscle spindles; (b) Golgi tendon organs; (c) Pacinian corpuscles; and (d) uncapsulated nerve endings.

2. The *first neuron* is similar to that for pain and temperature.

In their further course, the proprioceptive pathways are different for conscious and unconscious impulses.

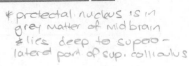

[handwritten note:] pretectal nucleus is in grey matter of midbrain & lies deep to superolateral part of sup. colliculus

Pathway for Conscious Proprioceptive Impulses

Their course is similar to that for fine touch described earlier (Fig. 23.7).

Pathway of Unconscious Proprioceptive Impulses

These impulses end in the cerebellum.

1. The first neuron has been described above.

2. The *second neuron* fibres are represented by three tracts, namely the posterior and anterior spinocerebellar tracts (from the lower limb and trunk) and the cuneocerebellar tract (posterior external arcuate fibres) from the upper limb.

The *posterior or direct spinocerebellar tract* contains ipsilateral fibres arising in the dorsal ((thoracic) nucleus of the spinal cord. It enters the ipsilateral cerebellar hemisphere through the inferior cerebellar peduncle (Fig. 23.8).

The *anterior or indirect spinocerebellar tract* is made up mainly of crossed fibres arising from the spinal grey matter (posterior grey column). The fibres ascend to the upper part of the pons and then turn down into the superior cerebellar peduncle to reach the cerebellum.

The *cuneocerebellar tract (posterior external arcuate fibres)* is functionally similar to the posterior spinocerebellar tract. It arises from the accessory (external) cuneate nucleus which receives afferents from the fasciculus cuneatus. The tract enters the ipsilateral cerebellar hemisphere through the inferior cerebellar peduncle.

VISUAL (OPTIC) PATHWAY

The visual pathways include structures which are concerned with the reception, transmission and perception of visual impulses. However, certain structures concerned with visual reflexes may also be conveniently mentioned here.

Structures in Visual Pathway

(1) Retina; (2) optic nerve; (3) optic chiasma; (4) optic tract, with its lateral and medial roots; (5) lateral geniculate body; (6) optic radiation; and (7) visual area in the cortex.

Structures Concerned with Visual Reflexes

(1) Pretectal nucleus; (2) oculomotor nucleus and nerve with ciliary ganglion; (3) frontal eye field; and (4) superior colliculus with tectobulbar and tectospinal tracts.

Retina

It is described in Chapter 19.

Optic Nerve

Optic nerve is made up of axons of ganglion cells of the retina. In a strict sense, the optic nerve is not a peripheral nerve because its fibres have no neurilemmal sheaths. It is a tract. Its fibres have no power of regeneration. The nerve is described in Chapter 7.

Optic Chiasma

In the chiasma, the nasal fibres (i.e. fibres of the optic nerve arising in the nasal, or medial half of the retina) including those from the nasal half of the macula, cross the midline and enter the opposite optic tract. The temporal (or lateral) fibres pass through the chiasma to enter the optic tract of the same side (Fig. 30.2).

Optic Tract

Each optic tract winds round the cerebral peduncle of the midbrain. Near the lateral geniculate body it divides into lateral and medial roots. The lateral root is thick and terminates in the lateral geniculate body. A few of its fibres pass to the superior colliculus, the pretectal nucleus and the hypothalamus. The medial root is believed to contain the supraoptic commissural fibres (Fig. 30.3).

Each optic tract contains temporal fibres of the same side and nasal fibres of the opposite side.

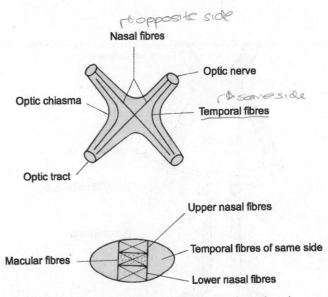

[handwritten annotations: "→ opposite side" near Nasal fibres; "→ same side" near Temporal fibres]

Fig. 30.2: *Fibres in the optic chiasma. (A) Superior view and (B) Sectional view.*

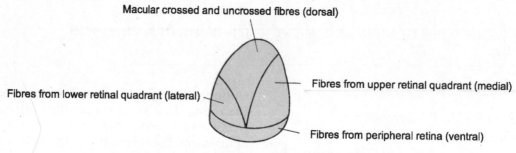

Macular crossed and uncrossed fibres (dorsal)

Fibres from lower retinal quadrant (lateral)

Fibres from upper retinal quadrant (medial)

Fibres from peripheral retina (ventral)

Fig. 30.3: *Section of the optic tract showing arrangement of its fibres.*

Lateral Geniculate Body

Lateral geniculate body receives the lateral root of the optic tract. Medially, it is connected to the superior colliculus, and laterally, it gives rise to the optic radiation.

The cells in this body are arranged in six layers. Layers 2, 3, 5 receive ipsilateral fibres, and layers 1, 4, 6 receive contralateral fibres (Fig. 28.15).

from opp. side

Optic Radiation (Geniculocalcarine Tract)

Optic radiation begins from the lateral geniculate body, passes through the retrolentiform part of the internal capsule, and ends in the visual cortex (Fig. 30.4).

Visual Cortex

The optic radiation in the striate area (Area 17) where the colour, size, shape, motion, illumination and transparency are appreciated separately. Objects are identified by integration of these perceptions with past experience stored in the parastriate and peristriate areas (Areas 18, 19).

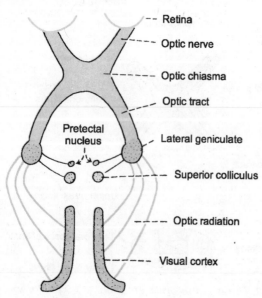

- - Retina

- Optic nerve

- Optic chiasma

- Optic tract

Pretectal nucleus

- Lateral geniculate

- Superior colliculus

- Optic radiation

- Visual cortex

Fig. 30.4: *The visual pathway.*

The area of the visual cortex that receives impulses from the macula is relatively much larger than the part related to the rest of the retina (Fig. 28.8).

Effects of lesion of different parts of visual pathways are depicted in Fig. 30.5.

Pathway of Light Reflex

→ pretectal; Edinger Westphal nucleus

Throwing light on the eye causes constriction of the pupil. This is mediated through the retina, the optic nerve, the optic chiasma, the optic tract, the lateral geniculate body, the pretectal nucleus, the Edinger-Westphal nucleus of the third nerve, the third cranial nerve itself, the ciliary ganglion, the short ciliary nerves, and the constrictor pupillae (Fig. 30.6).

Throwing light on one eye produces constriction of the pupil in both eyes (consensual reflex). This is due to bilateral connections of the pretectal nucleus with the Edinger-Westphal nuclei.

Pathway of Accommodation Reflex

Constriction of the pupil also takes place when looking at a near object. This is mediated through the retina, the optic nerve, the chiasma and tract, the lateral geniculate body, the optic radiation, the visual area of the cortex, the superior longitudinal association tract; the frontal eye field, the third nerve nucleus, the third cranial nerve, the ciliary ganglion, and the ciliaris and sphincter pupillae muscles.

Note that the pretectal nucleus is not involved in this reflex. In lesions of the pretectal nucleus, the light reflex is lost, but the pupil contracts on accommodation. This is called the Argyll-Robertson pupil.

PATHWAY OF HEARING
(Auditory Pathway)

1. The first neurons of the pathway are located in the spiral ganglion. They are bipolar. Their peripheral processes innervate the organ of Corti, while the central processes terminate in the dorsal and ventral cochlear nuclei.

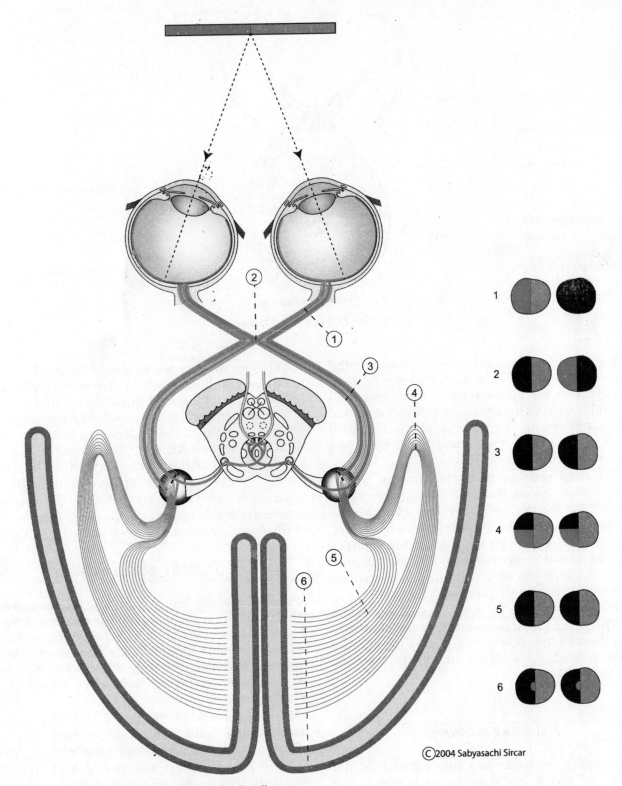

Fig. 30.5: Effects of lesions of different parts of visual pathways.

1. Lesion of the optic nerve causes **ipsilateral blindness**.
2. Mid-sagittal lesion of the optic chiasma causes **bitemporal hemianopia**.
3. Lesion of the optic tracts causes **contralateral homonymous hemianopia**.
4. Lesion of the temporal lobe affects the fibers of Meyer's loop coming from the lower half of the retina and causes **contralateral homonymous upper quadrantanopia**.
5. Lesion of the optic radiation causes **contralateral homonymous hemianopia**.
6. Lesion of the visual cortex causes **contralateral homonymous hemianopia** with **macular sparing**.

(Courtesy, Dr. S. Sircar, Medical Physiology, CBS Publishers and Distributers, New Delhi).

©2004 Sabyasachi Sircar

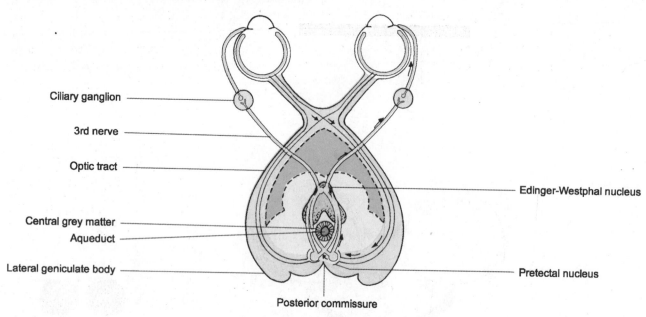

Ciliary ganglion

3rd nerve

Optic tract

Central grey matter

Aqueduct

Lateral geniculate body

Edinger-Westphal nucleus

Pretectal nucleus

Posterior commissure

Fig. 30.6: Pathway of light reflex.

2. The second neurons lie in the dorsal and ventral cochlear nuclei. Most of the axons arising in these nuclei cross to the opposite side (in the trapezoid body) and terminate in the superior olivary nucleus. (Many fibres end in the nucleus of the trapezoid body or of the lateral lemniscus.) Some fibres are uncrossed (Fig. 30.7).

3. The third neurons lie in the superior olivary nucleus. Their axons form the lateral lemniscus and reach the inferior colliculus (Figs 24.6, 24.9).

4. The fourth neurons lie in the inferior colliculus. Their axons pass through the inferior brachium to reach the medial geniculate body. (Some fibres of the lateral lemniscus reach the medial geniculate body without relay in the inferior colliculus.)

5. The fifth neurons lie in the medial geniculate body. Their axons form the auditory radiation, which passes through the sublentiform part of the internal capsule to reach the auditory area in the temporal lobe (Fig. 28.24).

VESTIBULAR PATHWAYS

The vestibular receptors are the maculae of the saccule and utricle (for static balance) and in the cristae of the ampullae of semicircular ducts (for kinetic balance). They are innervated by peripheral processes of bipolar neurons of the vestibular ganglion. This ganglion is situated in the internal acoustic meatus. The central processes arising from the neurons of the ganglion form the vestibular nerve which ends in the vestibular nuclei.

The second neurons in the pathway of balance lies in the vestibular nuclei. These nuclei send fibres: (a) To the archicerebellum through the inferior cerebellar peduncle (vestibulocerebellar tract); (b) to the motor nuclei of the brainstem (chiefly of the III, IV and VI nerves) through the medial longitudinal bundle; and (c) to the anterior horn cells of the spinal cord through the vestibulospinal tract (p. 326).

Through the vestibular pathway the impulses arising in the labyrinth can influence the movements of the eyes, the head, the neck and the trunk.

OLFACTORY (SMELL) PATHWAY

Receptors and the first neuron: (a) The *olfactory cells* (16–20 million in man) are bipolar neurons. They lie in the olfactory part of the nasal mucosa, and serve both as receptors as well as the first neurons in the olfactory pathway. (b) The *olfactory* nerves, about 20 in number, represent central processes of the olfactory cells.

Second neuron: (a) The mitral and tufted cells in the olfactory bulb give off fibres that form the *olfactory tract* and reach the primary olfactory areas.

Third neuron. These are located in the primary olfactory cortex which includes the anterior perforated substance, and several small masses of grey matter around it (Fig. 29.8).

Fourth neuron: Fibres arising in the primary olfactory cortex go to the secondary olfactory cortex (or entorhinal area) located in the anterior part of the parahippocampal gyrus. Smell is perceived in both the primary and secondary olfactory areas.

TASTE PATHWAY

(i) The taste from anterior two-thirds of tongue except from vallate papillae is carried by chorda tympani branch of facial till the geniculate ganglion. The central processes go to the tractus solitarius in the medulla.

(ii) Taste from posterior one-third of tongue including from the vallate papillae is carried by cranial nerve IX till the inferior ganglion. The central processes also reach the tractus solitarius.

(iii) Taste from posterior most part of tongue and epiglottis travel through vagus nerve till the inferior ganglion of vagus. These central processes also reach tractus solitarius.

(iv) After a relay in tractus solitarius, the solitario-thalamic tract is formed which becomes a part of trigeminal lemniscus and reaches postero-ventromedial nucleus of thalamus. Another relay here takes them to lowest part of postcentral gyrus, which is the area for taste (Figs 24.9, 24.10).

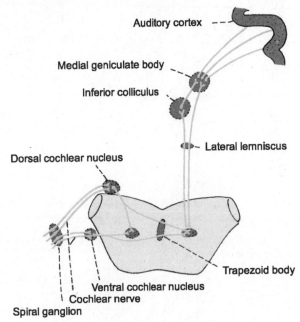

Fig. 30.7: *Auditory pathway.*

31

Blood Supply of the Spinal Cord and Brain

The nervous tissue is too delicate to bear anoxia beyond three minutes. The blood supply to nervous tissue per unit of tissue is maximum in the body. It shows the importance of the grey matter. The blood supply may be erratic due to haemorrhage, thrombosis or embolism of the arteries supplying the nervous tissue. Further the arteries are "end arteries" once these reach the deeper level. Neurons die, in bits and pieces; an individual also walks slowly and steadily towards death, and that is the end of this life—happy or sad.

BLOOD SUPPLY OF THE SPINAL CORD

The spinal cord receives its blood supply from three longitudinal arterial channels that extend along the length of the cord. The *anterior spinal artery* is present in relation to the anterior median sulcus. Two posterior spinal arteries (one on each side) run along the posterolateral sulcus (i.e. along the line of attachment of the dorsal nerve roots). In addition to these channels, the pia mater covering the spinal cord has an arterial plexus (called the *arteria vasocorona)* which also sends branches into the substance of the cord (Fig. 31.1).

The main source of blood to the spinal arteries is from the vertebral arteries (from which the anterior and posterior spinal arteries take origin). However, the blood from the vertebral arteries reaches only up to the cervical segments of the cord. The spinal arteries also receive blood through radicular arteries that reach the cord along the roots of spinal nerves. These radicular arteries arise from spinal branches of the vertebral, ascending cervical, deep cervical, intercostal, lumbar and sacral arteries.

Many of these radicular branches are small and end by supplying the nerve roots. A few of them, which are larger, contribute blood to the spinal

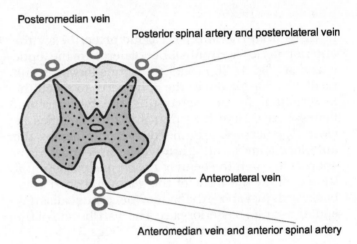

Fig. 31.1: *Blood supply of spinal cord.*

Posteromedian vein

Posterior spinal artery and posterolateral vein

Anterolateral vein

Anteromedian vein and anterior spinal artery

arteries. Frequently, one of the anterior radicular branches is very large and is called the *arteria radicularis magna*. Its position is variable. This artery may be responsible for supplying blood to as much as the lower two-thirds of the spinal cord.

The veins draining the spinal cord are arranged in the form of six longitudinal channels. These are anteromedian and posteromedian channels that lie in the midline; and anterolateral and posterolateral channels that are paired. These channels are interconnected by a plexus of veins that form a venous vasocorona. The blood from these veins is drained by radicular veins that open into a venous plexus lying between the dura and the vertebral canal (epidural or internal vertebral plexus) and through it into various segmental veins.

ARTERIAL SUPPLY OF THE CEREBRUM

The arteries supplying the brain are the internal carotid and vertebral arteries and their branches.

Cerebral Part of the Internal Carotid Artery and its Branches

After piercing the dura mater forming the roof of the cavernous sinus, the internal carotid artery gives off three large branches. These are the following.

(i) *Ophthalmic artery* (which supplies the orbit and is described in Chapter 7), and the

(ii) *Anterior and*

(iii) *Middle cerebral arteries* to the brain.

It also gives off two smaller branches that take part in supplying the brain: these are the

(iv) *Posterior communicating artery* and the

(v) *Anterior choroidal artery*.

Anterior Cerebral Artery

It arises from the internal carotid artery below the anterior perforated substance, lateral to the optic chiasma (Fig. 31.2). From here it runs forwards and medially crossing above the optic nerve to reach the longitudinal fissure separating the two cerebral hemispheres. Here the arteries of the two sides lie close together and are united to each other by the anterior communicating artery. The artery now turns sharply to reach the genu of the corpus callosum. It winds round the front of the genu and then runs backwards just above the body of the corpus callosum, ending near its posterior part. The distribution of the artery is considered in Table 31.1 (Figs 31.3–31.5).

Special mention must be made here of the recurrent branch of the anterior cerebral artery (artery of Heubner). This artery runs backwards and laterally to enter the anterior perforated substance.

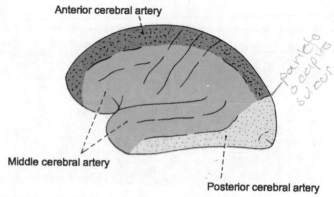

Fig. 31.3: *Arterial supply of the superolateral surface of the cerebral hemisphere.*

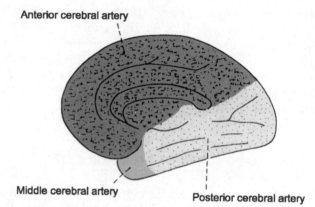

Fig. 31.4: *Arterial supply of the medial surface of the cerebral hemisphere.*

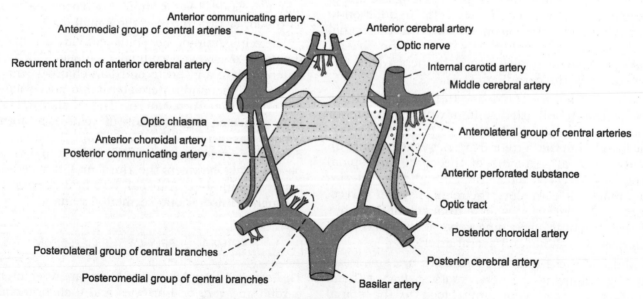

Fig. 31.2: *The circulus arteriosus or circle of Willis.*

Table 31.1: Important arteries of brain

Artery	Origin	Course	Branches Cortical	Branches Central
1. Middle cerebral	Largest and direct branch of ICA	In the lateral sulcus and on the insula	1. Orbital 2. Frontal 3. Parietal 4. Temporal	AL* central branches, arranged as medial and lateral striate artery
2. Anterior cerebral	Smaller terminal branch of ICA	Coextensive with corpus callosum. Two arteries are connected by the anterior communicating artery	1. Orbital 2. Frontal 3. Parietal, including paracentral artery	AM* central branches, including a Heubner's recurrent artery
3. Posterior cerebral	Terminal branch of basilar artery	Winds round cerebral peduncle to reach the tentorial surface of cerebrum	1. Temporal 2. Occipital 3. Parieto-occipital	1. PM* central branches 2. PL* central branches 3. Posterior choroidal
4. Posterior inferior cerebellar	Largest branch of vertebral artery	Tortuous course in relation of olive, lower border of pons and vallecula of cerebellum	It supplies : 1. Posterolateral part of medulla 2. Lower part of pons 3. Inferior surface of cerebellum	

* AL = anterolateral; AM = anteromedial; PM = posteromedial; PL = posterolateral.

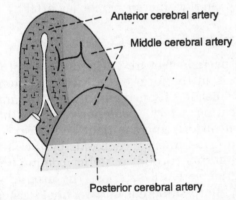

Fig. 31.5: *Arterial supply of the inferior surface of the cerebral hemisphere.*

Labels in figure: Anterior cerebral artery; Middle cerebral artery; Posterior cerebral artery.

Middle Cerebral Artery

After its origin from the internal carotid artery the middle cerebral artery runs laterally in the depth of the stem of the lateral sulcus. It curves on to the superolateral surface and runs backwards in the depth of the posterior ramus of the lateral sulcus. The main stem of the artery can be seen only by artificially separating the lips of the sulcus.

Posterior Communicating Artery

The artery runs backwards and anastomoses with the posterior cerebral artery, helping to complete circulus arterious.

Cranial Part of Vertebral Artery

The vertebral artery gives off the following branches.
  (i)   Meningeal
  (ii) Anterior spinal
  (iii) Posterior spinal
  (iv) Posterior inferior cerebellar
  (v)   Medullary

Basilar Artery and its Branches

The basilar artery is formed by the union of the right and left vertebral arteries, at the lower border of the pons. It ascends in the midline, ventral to the pons, and ends at its upper border by dividing into the right and left posterior cerebral arteries. It gives off the following branches.
  (i)   Pontine
  (ii) Labyrinthine (end artery)
  (iii) Anterior inferior cerebellar
  (iv) Superior cerebellar
  (v)   Posterior cerebral

Arterial Supply of the Cerebral Hemisphere

The anterior, middle and posterior cerebral arteries give rise to two sets of branches—cortical and central. The *cortical branches* ramify on the surface of the cerebral hemisphere and supply the cortex. Details of supply of individual areas of the cortex are given below. The *central* (or perforating) branches pass deep into the substance of the cerebral hemisphere to supply structures with it. They consist of four main groups—anteromedial, anterolateral, posteromedial and posterolateral.

Arterial Supply of the Cerebral Cortex

The cerebral cortex is supplied by cortical branches of the anterior, middle and posterior cerebral arteries.

The greater part of the *superolateral surface* is supplied by the middle cerebral artery. The areas not supplied by this artery are as follows: (i) A strip about 2 cm wide along the superomedial border extending from the frontal pole to the parieto-occipital sulcus is supplied by the anterior cerebral artery. (ii) The area belonging to the occipital lobe is supplied by the posterior cerebral artery. (iii) The inferior temporal gyrus is also supplied by the posterior cerebral artery.

The main artery supplying the *medial surface* is the anterior cerebral. The area of this surface belonging to the occipital lobe is supplied by the posterior cerebral artery.

The inferior surface is subdivided into orbital and tentorial surfaces.

The lateral part of the *orbital surface* is supplied by the middle cerebral artery, and the medial part by the anterior cerebral artery.

The *tentorial surface* is supplied by the posterior cerebral artery. The temporal pole is, however, supplied by the middle cerebral artery.

From the above description it will be clear that the main somatic motor and sensory areas are supplied by the middle cerebral artery except in their uppermost parts (leg areas) which are supplied by the anterior cerebral. The auditory area is supplied by the middle cerebral artery and the visual area by the posterior cerebral artery.

Arterial Supply of Other Parts of Cerebral Hemisphere

Internal capsule. It is supplied by the central branches of (i) the middle cerebral artery (lenticulostriate branches); (ii) the anterior cerebral artery (Heubner's recurrent branch); (iii) the posterior communicating artery; and (iv) the anterior choroidal artery (Fig. 31.6).

Corpus striatum: (i) Chiefly by the anterolateral central branches of the middle cerebral artery; and (ii) partly by the anteromedial central branches from the anterior cerebral and anterior communicating arteries.

Thalamus: (i) Chiefly by the posteromedial and posterolateral central branches of the posterior cerebral artery; and (ii) partly by the anteromedial central branches.

The Choroid Plexuses

The choroid plexuses of the lateral and third ventricles are supplied by the anterior choroidal artery (branch of internal carotid) and the posterior choroidal artery (branch of the posterior cerebral artery). The choroid plexus of the fourth ventricle is supplied by a branch from the posterior inferior cerebellar artery.

Anatomical Peculiarities of Cerebral Arteries

1. One peculiar feature is the presence of a free anastomosis in the form of the circulus arteriosus (circle of Willis). It is formed *anteriorly* by the anterior communicating artery, *posteriorly* by the basilar artery as it divides into the right and left posterior cerebral arteries, and *on each side* by the anterior cerebral, internal carotid, posterior communicating and posterior cerebral arteries. The arterial circle lies in the interpeduncular subarachnoid cistern. It equalizes pressure in the arteries of the two sides.

2. The second peculiarity is the existence of a 'blood–brain' barrier formed by structures between the blood and nerve cells of the brain. Thus the

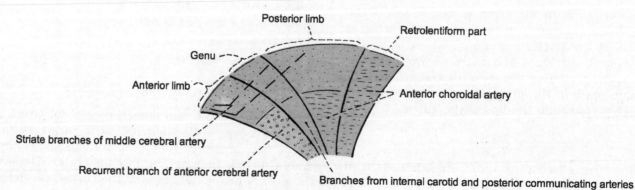

Fig. 31.6: *Arterial supply of the internal capsule.*

barrier is made up of: (i) the vessel wall; (ii) the arachnoid layer of the perivascular sheath; (iii) the perivascular space; (iv) the pial layer of the perivascular space; (v) the neuroglia and the ground substance of the brain. The barrier, at the capillary level, is reduced merely to the capillary endothelium with neuroglia and ground substance. It permits a selective passage of blood contents to nervous tissue. Toxic and harmful substances are ordinarily prevented from reaching the brain.

3. The third significant fact is that central branches of cerebral arteries are *end arteries.* Thrombosis of any one of them, invariably causes infarction. The cortical branches establish very poor anastomoses with each other: the anastomoses cannot compensate for any loss of blood supply to a particular area of the cortex.

VEINS OF THE CEREBRUM

Characteristics of the Veins

(1) The walls are devoid of muscle; (2) the veins have no valves; and (3) to maintain patency, some of them open into the cranial venous sinuses against the direction of blood flow in the sinus, e.g. the superior cerebral veins draining into the superior sagittal sinus (Fig. 31.7).

Groups of Veins

External Cerebral Veins

1. *Superior cerebral veins:* These are six to twelve in number. They drain the superolateral surface of the hemisphere. They terminate in the superior sagittal sinus (Fig. 31.7).

2. *Superficial middle cerebral vein:* This drains the area round the posterior ramus of the lateral sulcus. It terminates in the cavernous sinus, or at times into the sphenoparietal sinus. Through the superior and inferior anastomotic veins, it communicates with the superior sagittal and transverse sinuses. It also communicates with the deep middle cerebral vein.

3. *Deep middle cerebral vein:* This drains the surface of the insula and terminates in the basal vein.

4. *Inferior cerebral veins:* These are several in number. They are divided into orbital and tentorial veins. The orbital veins terminate in the superior cerebral veins or in the posterior sagittal sinus. The tentorial veins terminate in the cavernous or any other surrounding sinus.

5. *Anterior cerebral veins:* These are small veins which drain the corpus callosum and the anterior part of the medial surface of the hemisphere. They terminate in the basal vein.

Internal Cerebral Veins

There is one vein on each side. It is formed by the union of the thalamostriate and choroidal veins at the apex of the tela choroidea of the third ventricle (Fig. 31.8). The right and left veins run posteriorly parallel to each other in the tela choroidea, and unite together to form the great cerebral vein below the splenium of the corpus callosum.

Terminal Veins

1. *Great cerebral vein* This is a single median vein. It is formed by union of the two internal cerebral veins. It terminates in the straight sinus. Its tributaries include the basal veins, and veins from

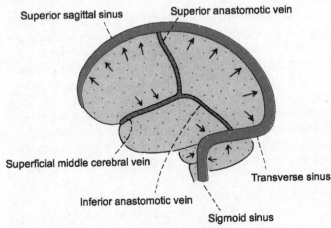

Fig. 31.7: *Veins on the superolateral surface of the cerebral hemisphere.*

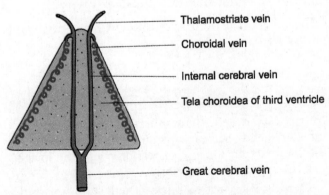

Fig. 31.8: *Superior view of the tela choroidea of third ventricle with its contents. The choroid plexus of the third ventricle is not shown.*

the pineal body, the colliculi, the cerebellum and the adjoining part of the occipital lobes of the cerebrum.

2. *Basal vein:* There is one vein on each side. It is formed at the anterior perforated substance by the union of the deep middle cerebral vein, the anterior cerebral veins, and the striate veins. It runs posteriorly, winds round the cerebral peduncle, and terminates by joining the great cerebral vein. Its tributaries include (apart from the veins forming it) small veins from the cerebral peduncle, interpeduncular structures, the tectum of the midbrain, and the parahippocampal gyrus.

Ultimately all veins drain into the various cranial venous sinuses which, in turn, drain into the internal jugular vein.

BLOOD SUPPLY OF THE CEREBELLUM

The superior surface of the cerebellum is supplied by the superior cerebellar branches of the basilar artery. The anterior part of the inferior surface is supplied by the anterior inferior cerebellar branches of the same artery. The posterior part of the inferior surface is supplied by the posterior inferior cerebellar artery.

The veins of the cerebellum drain into neighbouring venous sinuses.

BLOOD SUPPLY OF THE BRAINSTEM

The *midbrain* is supplied by branches from the posterior cerebral arteries, including their central branches, both posteromedial and posterolateral.

The *pons* is supplied by the pontine branches of basilar artery.

The *medulla* is supplied by (i) the medullary branches of the vertebral artery; and (ii) branches from the posterior inferior cerebellar artery.

The veins of the brainstem drain into neighbouring venous sinuses.

CLINICAL ANATOMY

1. *Hemiplegia* is a common condition It is an upper motor neuron type of paralysis of one half of the body, including the face. It is usually due to an internal capsule lesion caused by thrombosis of one of the lenticulostriate branches of the middle cerebral artery (cerebral thrombosis).

One of the lenticulostriate branches is most frequently ruptured (cerebral haemorrhage); it is known as Charcot's artery of cerebral haemorrhage. This lesion also produces hemiplegia with deep coma, and is ultimately fatal.

2. Thrombosis of Huebner's recurrent branch of the anterior cerebral artery causes contralateral *upper monoplegia.*

3. Thrombosis of the paracentral artery (terminal cortical branch of the anterior cerebral artery) causes contralateral *lower monoplegia.*

4. Thrombosis of the posterior inferior cerebellar artery causes *lateral medullary syndrome (Wallenberg's syndrome).* It is characterized by:

   a. Severe giddiness, due to involvement of the vestibular nuclei.

   b. Dysphagia, due to involvement of the nucleus ambiguus.

   c. Crossed hemianaesthesia, in which there is anaesthesia of one half of the body due to involvement of the lateral spinothalamic tract and of the opposite half of the face due to involvement of the nucleus of the spinal tract of the trigeminal nerve.

   d. Horner's syndrome, due to involvement of sympathetic pathways in the medulla.

   e. Cerebellar symptoms and signs.

5. *Pontine haemorrhage* is characterized by: (i) Paralysis (contralateral hemiplegia); (ii) deep coma; (iii) hyperpyrexia; and (iv) pinpoint pupil. It is invariably fatal.

6. Anastomotic and end arteries: In the circle of Willis, the blood in the three communicating arteries is normally static. Following occlusion of one of the three large arteries contributing to the circle, the other two compensate more or less completely, via communicating arteries. With occlusion of one internal carotid the other internal carotid may perfuse both anterior cerebral arteries. With occlusion of basilar each posterior cerebral artery may be perfused by the internal carotid of its own side.

Further anastomosis occurs between cortical branches of cerebral arteries, prior to perforation of the branches into brain substance. Once the cortical and central branches perforate, they become end arteries hardly communicating at capillary level.

7. Cerebral vascular disease is quite common in old age and manifests in different ways.

(a) Haemorrhage – cortical or subcortical

(b) Thrombosis

(c) Embolism.

8. Hypertensive encephalopathy, a manifestation of sustained elevation of diastolic blood pressure in the form of multiple diffuse small lesions distributed all over, results in a variegated picture of the circle of Willis (berry's aneurysm).

9. The arteries of the brain are supplied with sympathetic nerves which run onto them from carotid and vertebral plexuses. They are extremely sensitive to injury and readily react by passing into prolonged spasms. This by itself may be sufficient to cause damage to brain tissue since even the least sensitive neurons cannot withstand absolute loss of blood supply for a period more than 5–7 minutes.

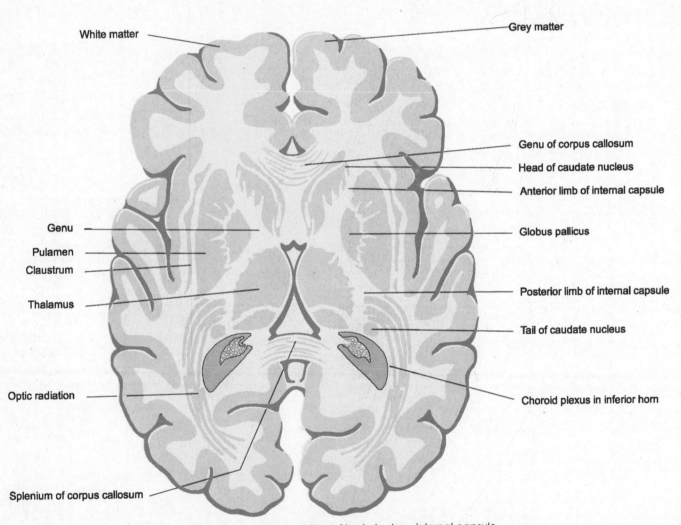

Fig. 31.9: Horizontal section of brain to show internal capsule.

32

Investigations in a Neurological Case, Surface Anatomy Radiological Anatomy and Evolution of Head

A neurological case needs to have a detailed clinical history, family history, and clinical examination besides the investigations.

INVESTIGATIONS REQUIRED IN A NEUROLOGICAL CASE

Study of brain is of importance in localising the lesion. Besides detailed history and clinical examination, the following investigations may have to be done according to the need of each case.

1. *X-ray skull:* Anteroposterior and lateral views (Fig. 20.1).

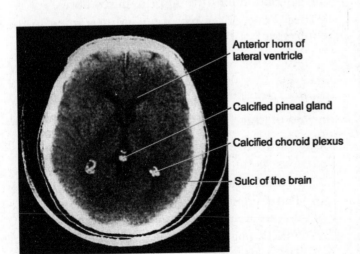

Fig. 32.1: *Normal CT scan.*

Anterior horn of lateral ventricle

Calcified pineal gland

Calcified choroid plexus

Sulci of the brain

2. *Lumbar puncture:* It is done between third and fourth lumbar vertebrae. This is clinically useful for diagnostic and prognostic purposes. It is also used for giving spinal anaesthesia.

3. *Computerised tomography or CT scan:* In this procedure, X-ray beam traces an arc at multiple angles around a section of the body. The resulting transverse section is reproduced by the computer on its monitor screen (Fig. 32.1).

4. *Magnetic resonance imaging:* The body is exposed to high energy magnetic field, which permits protons in tissues to arrange themselves in relation to the field. Then a pulse of radiowaves 'reads' these ion patterns and a colour-coded image is reproduced on the computer screen (Fig. 32.2).

5. *Sonography:* High frequency sound waves produced by wand (held in hand) get reflected off body tissues and are detected by the same instrument. The image, the *sonogram,* is reproduced on the computer screen. It is used to diagnose hydrocephaly or anencephaly during intrauterine life.

6. *Positron emission tomography (PET):* Substance emitting positrons is injected into the body which is taken up by tissues. Collision of positrons with electrons of body tissues produces gamma rays, detected by gamma cameras, put around the patient. Thus, PET scan is seen on computer screen. Activity of different areas of brain is visualised.

7. Angiography:

(a) *MR angiography:* This technique employs modification so that blood vessels can be visualised

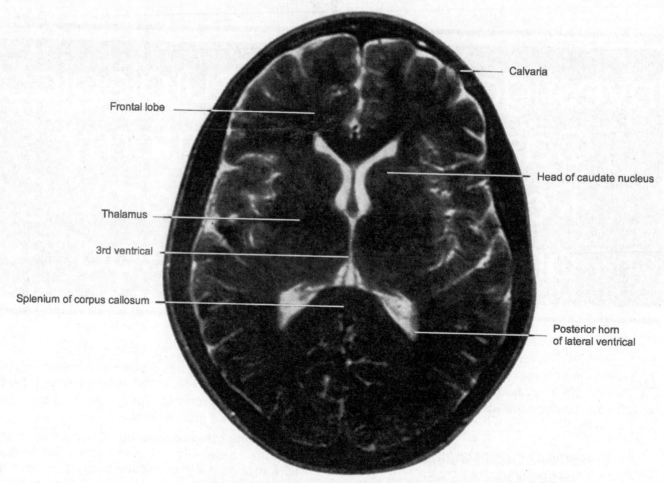

Calvaria

Frontal lobe

Head of caudate nucleus

Thalamus

3rd ventrical

Splenium of corpus callosum

Posterior horn
of lateral ventrical

Fig. 32.2: *MRI of the brain showing the ventricles.*

without injecting the dye. The conventional angiography is still preferred.

(b) *Angiography:* The contrast medium is injected into the common carotid or vertebral arteries. X-ray pictures taken immediately show the arterial pattern. The capillary and venous pattern is seen after a little time (Fig. 32.3).

(c) *Digital subtraction angiography (DSA):* In this procedure, low concentrations of contrast media are used. Bones and muscles are removed with the help of the computer. Ideal method is arterial DSA wherein diluted contrast medium is injected into the artery to see its course, branches and their diseases.

Because of these modern and safe procedures, the older techniques—pneumoencephalography, ventriculography and myelography have become obsolete.

8. *Electrophysiological methods:*

(a) *Electromyography (EMG):* This is the study of electrical activity accompanying the muscle contraction. It is also used to study the action of various muscles.

(b) *Electroencephalography (EEG):* The pattern of electrical activity of brain is analysed by putting electrodes in the scalp at different points and recording it in the machine.

(c) Nerve conduction studies done to estimate the rate of conduction through the nerve fibres.

These procedures may be used according to the requirement of the patient.

SURFACE ANATOMY

Borders of Cerebral Hemisphere

Mark the following points.

1. First point just superolateral to the inion.

2. Second point just superolateral to the nasion.

3. Third point at the zygomatic process of the frontal bone just above the eyebrow.

4. Fourth point at the pterion.

5. Fifth point at the middle of the upper border of the zygomatic arch (Fig. 1.8).

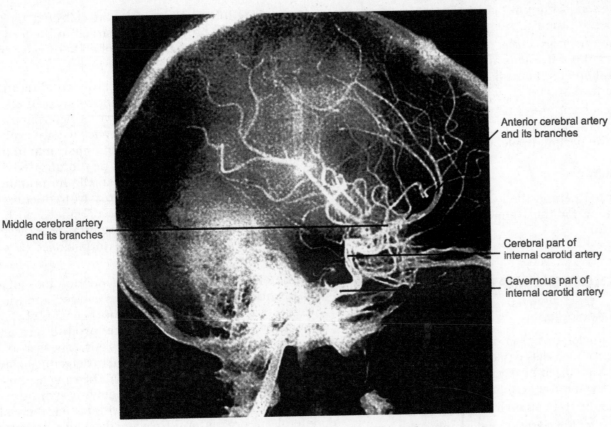

Middle cerebral artery
and its branches

Anterior cerebral artery
and its branches

Cerebral part of
internal carotid artery

Cavernous part of
internal carotid artery

Fig. 32.3: *Lateral view of carotid angiogram.*

The *superomedial border* is marked by joining points 1 and 2 by a paramedian line.

The *superciliary border* is marked by first joining points 2 and 3 by a line arching upwards just above the eyebrow, and then extending this line to point 4.

The *inferolateral border* is marked by first joining points 4 and 5 by a line convex forwards (temporal pole), and by then joining points 5 and 1 by a line convex upwards, passing just above the external acoustic meatus.

Central Sulcus

(1) First point 1.2 cm behind the midpoint of a line joining the nasion with the inion.

(2) Second point 5 cm above the preauricular point. The sulcus is marked by joining these points by a sinuously curved line running downwards and forwards making an angle of 70 degrees with the median plane.

Lateral Sulcus

The following points are used to mark the lateral sulcus and its rami.

(1) First point at the pterion.

(2) Second point 2 cm below the parietal eminence.

(3) Third point 2 cm above the pterion.

(4) Fourth point 2 cm in front of the pterion.

Point 1 (pterion) is also called the *Sylvian point*. Here the stem of the lateral sulcus divides into its three rami.

The posterior ramus of the lateral sulcus is about 7 cm long and can be marked by joining points 1 and 2.

The *anterior ascending ramus* is marked by joining points 1 and 3.

The *anterior horizontal ramus* is marked by joining points 1 and 4.

Superior Temporal Sulcus

This is marked by a line parallel and 1 cm below the posterior ramus of the lateral sulcus.

Functional Areas of Cerebral Cortex

1. The *motor area* is marked by a strip about 1 cm broad in front of the central sulcus.

2. The *sensory area* is marked by a strip about 1 cm broad, behind the central sulcus.

3. The *auditory area* is marked between the superior temporal sulcus and the posterior ramus of the lateral sulcus, immediately below the lower end of the central sulcus.

4. *The visual area* (the part extending on to the superolateral surface) is marked immediately in front of the occipital pole.

Cerebellum

It is marked behind the auricle, immediately below the marking for the transverse sinus described in Chapter 20.

RADIOLOGICAL ANATOMY OF THE BRAIN

Cerebral Angiography

Cerebral angiography is a radiological technique by which cerebral vessels can be visualized. The arterial system is visualized by carotid angiography, and the vertebral system by vertebral angiography.

Dye: About 10 to 12 ml of 30% pyelocil or diodone.

Technique: For carotid angiography, the common carotid artery is located at the carotid tubercle and the dye is injected percutaneously. A series of skiagrams are taken rapidly at intervals of 1 second. Within 2 seconds after the commencement of injection the dye reaches the cerebral arteries, and after 2 seconds it is in the veins. After another two seconds or so the dye passes into the intracranial venous sinuses. The skiagrams taken at different intervals provide arteriograms, venograms (or phlebograms) and sinograms.

Similarly for vertebral angiography, the dye is injected into the vertebral artery and skiagrams are taken as described above.

Indications : Cerebral angiography is helpful in diagnosis of intracranial tumours, haematomas, aneurysms and angiomas.

EVOLUTION OF THE HEAD

The head forms the *fore-end* of the body where all the special sense organs (eyes, ears, nose and tongue) are concentrated in and around the face. It is at this end of the body that the central nervous system shows its greatest development leading to the formation of the brain. The various sense organs keep the individual informed about the surroundings so that he can better adjust and sustain himself. The continuous inflow of information collected by the sense organs is processed and stored in the form of memory which forms the basis of all knowledge and experience.

Photosensitivity is one of the fundamental properties of protoplasm. This has resulted in evolution of the eyes which serve to determine the direction of movement with reference to light even in prevertebrate forms of life. In most mammals, however, vision appears to be dominated (in importance) by the sense of smell. In primates, including man, there is a progressive reduction in the importance of the sense of smell, with a concomitant increase in the importance of vision associated with the ability to perform skilled acts of a wide variety.

The evolution of the sense of *hearing* took place only when water dwelling species evolved into those with a terrestrial mode of life. This becomes obvious when we remember that the production and transmission of sound requires air. The sense of hearing greatly helped the animal in detecting hostile sounds made by enemies. In man, hearing assumed increasing importance in receiving sounds of articulate speech. Homologous with the ear there are lateral-line organs found in water dwelling vertebrates like fishes and amphibia. These organs are sensitive to vibration produced by water currents and help their owners in judging the depth and direction of movement of water, and also in detecting the presence of other animals in the neighbourhood.

The *sense of smell* (or *olfactory sense)* is one of the oldest sensibilities which made its appearance first in aquatic vertebrates, and was the first to receive cortical representation. Most of the primitive mammals are guided primarily and predominantly by their sense of smell; the other senses of touch, hearing and vision being merely accessory to the dominating influence of smell. Man has freely exploited this uncanny endowment of a sharp sense of smell in domesticated animals, especially in dogs. The sense of smell played a significant role in the animal's search for food; and for sex. With the adoption of an arboreal (= tree dwelling) mode of life by primates (monkeys and apes) the sense of smell became less important. This mode of life favoured a higher development of visual, tactile, acoustic, kinaesthetic, and motor functions in association with increasing intelligence. The reduced importance of the sense of smell has been associated with the loss of a projecting snout (the region of the mouth and nose) that is so typical of lower mammals. However, it is believed that the tactile function of the snout is more important than its olfactory function. The most important factor in the disappearance of the snout in primates and man appears to be the adoption of an erect posture in which the forelimbs are no longer required to support body weight, and are therefore free to perform various functions. (This is often referred to, by anthropologists, as *emancipation of the forelimbs*.)

Thus it would appear that the whole spectrum of human sensibilities is acquired by man from his animal ancestors. In fact man is inferior to many animals (dogs, cattle, etc.) in his acuity of the senses of smell, vision and hearing. However, the supremacy of man in the animal kingdom is due to the large relative size of his brain which has given him unlimited powers of thought, of reason and of judgement, highly developed speech, and hands that can achieve perfection at craftsmanship.

The anatomical features of the *human face* are a result of a series of changes that have occurred during evolution. The many changes observed are a result of two main factors. These are the progressive reduction in the size of the jaws; and a concomitant increase in the size of the cranial cavity in association with the increasing size of the brain. The alterations in the face and head are by-products of a change in posture from pronograde (four-footed), through orthograde to a plantigrade (two-footed) one. A pronograde animal (dog, cow) has large jaws and a small head. An orthograde animal (ape or monkey) has smaller jaws and a larger head than in pronograde animals. Plantigrade man has the smallest jaws and

the largest head. Thus the size of the jaws is inversely proportional to that of the head (Fig. 32.4).

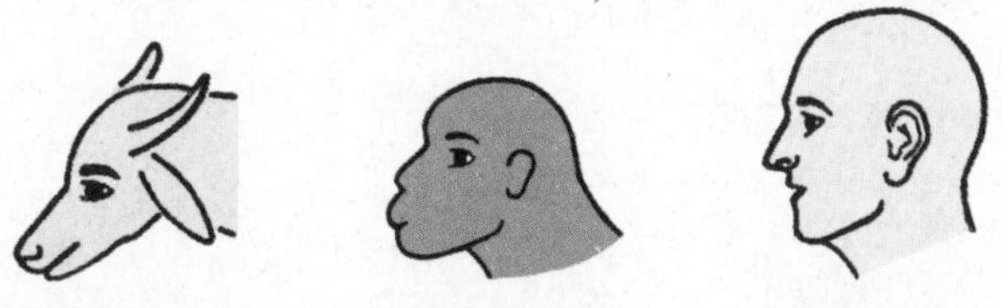

Reduction in jaw size is attributable to the liberty of movements of the upper limbs, and also to changed habit of eating cooked food, both of which have greatly relieved the jaws of their diverse functions (tactile feeling, holding, sorting, breaking, biting, tearing, chewing, piercing, fighting, etc.) seen in lower animals. The muscles acting on the jaws have obviously become smaller and weaker. The same is also true of muscles on the back of the neck. In pronograde animals these muscles support the weight of the head. In order to permit freedom of mobility to the tongue for articular speech in man, the alveolar arches are broadened and the chin is pushed forwards, making the mouth cavity more roomy. With recession of the jaws the oral aperture is reduced in size, and the lips are supported by a much better developed orbicularis oris. The distinctive external nose, with exuberant growth of cartilages forming the prominent dorsum, tip and alae is a characteristic human feature, although it appears to serve no special function. The eyes are directed forwards (and not laterally as in lower mammals). This change in direction of the eyes enables stereoscopic vision. The palpebral fissures are larger in man than in any other primate, and the bony orbits are decidedly smaller than in the great apes. Further, the interorbital distance is greater in man than in apes in whom the nasal root is greatly constricted. The supraorbital margins of man are markedly reduced remnants of the highly developed brow ridges of other primates. Then diminution in man is partly due to the receding jaws which relieve the ridges of their function as buttresses, and partly to the development of a prominent forehead (because of increase in the size of the cranial cavity). The forehead protects the eyes from above, a similar function being performed by the brow ridges in apes.

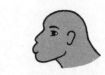

Pronograde cattle   Orthograde monkey   Plantigrade man

Fig. 32.4: *The size of the jaws relative to the size of the head.*

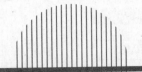

Appendix 2

Lateral Ventricle

The lateral ventricle comprises a central body and three horns—anterior, posterior and inferior. Their wall are enumerated.

Body or Central Part

Roof: Trunk of corpus callosum.

Floor: Superior surface of thalamus, thalamostriate vein, stria terminalis, body of caudate nucleus.

Medial: Septum pellucidum, body of fornix (Fig. 29.3).

Anterior Horn

Roof: Anterior part of trunk of corpus callosum.

Anterior: Genu and rostrum of corpus callosum.

Floor: Head of caudate nucleus (Fig. 29.4).

Medial wall: Septum pellucidum and column of fornix.

Posterior Horn

Roof and lateral wall: Tapetum of corpus callosum.

Medial wall: Bulb of posterior horn above and calcar avis below (Fig. 29.5).

Inferior Horn

Roof and lateral wall: Tapetum, tail of caudate nucleus, stria terminalis, amygdaloid nucleus.

Floor: Pes hippocampus, hippocampus, alveus, fimbria, dentate gyrus, collateral eminence (Fig. 29.6).

Third Ventricle

The third ventricle lies between the two thalami. The components of its boundaries and recesses are enumerated:

Anterior wall: Lamina terminalis, anterior commissure, anterior column of fornix (Fig. 29.2).

Posterior wall: Pineal body, cerebral aqueduct.

Floor: Optic chiasma, tubercinerium, infundibulum, mamillary body, posterior perforated substance, tegmentum of midbrain.

Roof: Ependyma, tela choroidea.

Lateral wall: Medial surface of thalamus, medial aspect of hypothalamus, epithalamus, interventricular foramen.

Recesses: Infundibular recess, optic recess, pineal recess, suprapineal recess (Fig. 29.7B).

Fourth Ventricle

The cavity of fourth ventricle is situated dorsal to pons and upper part of medulla oblongata and ventral to the cerebellum. Its boundaries, recesses, apertures and continuations are mentioned here:

Lateral Boundaries: Gracile tubercle, cuneate tubercle inferior cerebellar peduncles, superior cerebellar peduncles (Fig. 27.1).

Floor

Upper part: Facial colliculus on the dorsal surface of pons (Fig. 27.3).

Intermediate part: Vestibular nuclei, medullary striae.

Lower part: Upper part of medulla oblongata containing hypoglossal and vagal triangles.

Roof: Superior medullary velum, thin sheet of pia mater and ependyma with median aperture, inferior medullary velum (Fig. 27.2).

Recesses in roof: One median dorsal, two lateral dorsal and two lateral.

Apertures: One median — foramen of Magendie, two lateral — foramina of Lushka.

Continuity: Above with cerebral aqueduct
Below with central canal of spinal cord.

NUCLEAR COMPONENTS OF CRANIAL NERVES

CN I. Olfactory

Part of forebrain

CN II. Optic

Part of forebrain

CN III. Oculomotor

a. General somatic efferent column for 5 extraocular muscles.

b. General visceral efferent column for 2 sets of intraocular muscles (Chart A2.1).

c. General somatic afferent–spinal nucleus of CN V. It receives proprioceptive impulses from extraocular muscles.

CN IV. Trochlear

a. General somatic efferent column for supply of only superior oblique muscle.

b. General somatic afferent–spinal nucleus of CN V. It receives proprioceptive impulses from the superior oblique muscle.

CN V. Trigeminal

a. Special visceral efferent column for 4 muscles of mastication and 4 other muscles.

b. General somatic afferent:
  i) Spinal nucleus of CN V for pain and temperature from face.
  ii) Superior sensory nucleus of CN V for touch and pressure from face.
  iv) Mesencephalic nucleus of CN V for proprioceptive impulses from extraocular muscles and muscles of mastication.

CN VI. Abducent

a. General somatic efferent for lateral rectus.

b. General somatic afferent–spinal nucleus of CN V. It receives proprioceptive impulses from the lateral rectus muscle.

CN VII. Facial

a. Special visceral efferent for muscles of facial expression.

b. General visceral efferent for lacrimal, nasal, palatal and submandibular, sublingual glands (Chart A2.1).

c. Special visceral afferent and general visceral afferent (nucleus of tractus solitarius) for carrying taste from most of anterior two-thirds of tongue and afferents from glands supplied by it.

d. General somatic afferent from part of skin of auricle.

CN VIII. Vestibulocochlear

Special somatic afferent column:
  Two parts: Vestibular nuclei: Medial, superior, spinal, lateral.
  Cochlear nuclei: Dorsal and ventral.

CN IX. Glossopharyngeal

a. Special visceral efferent for one muscle of larynx — the stylopharyngeus.

b. General visceral efferent for parotid gland (Chart A2.1)

c. Special and general visceral afferent (nucleus of tractus solitarius) for sensations of taste from posterior one-third tongue and circumvallate papillae. Also carries general sensations from posterior one-third tongue, carotid body and carotid sinus.

d. General somatic afferent for proprioceptive fibres from the muscle.

CN X. + CN XI. Vagus and Cranial Part of CN XI

a. Special visceral efferent for muscles of larynx, pharynx and soft palate.

b. Special and general visceral afferents carry (nucleus of tractus solitarius) taste from posterior most part of tongue, epiglottis and afferents from foregut and midgut derivatives.

c. General visceral efferent for glands of respiratory system and gastrointestinal tract till right two-thirds of transverse colon.

d. General somatic afferent from skin of external auditory meatus.

CN XI. Spinal Part of Accessory Nerve

a. Special visceral efferent for sternocleidomastoid and trapezius.

b. General somatic afferent–spinal nucleus of CN V. It receives proprioceptive impulses from the above two muscles.

CN XII. Hypoglossal

a. General somatic efferent for all 4 intrinsic muscles of tongue and three extrinsic muscles — styloglossus, genioglossus and hyoglossus.

b. General somatic afferent–spinal nucleus of CN V. It receives proprioceptive impulses from the muscles of tongue.

EFFERENT PATHWAYS OF CRANIAL PART OF PARASYMPATHETIC NERVOUS SYSTEM

Preganglionic parasympathetic fibres are present in 4 cranial nerves e.g. cranial nerves III, VII, IX, X and along spinal nerves S2, S3, S4 . Four ganglia namely ciliary, pterygopalatine, submandibular and otic are concerned with efferent parasympathetic fibres. Their pathways are shown in Chart A2.1:

CLINICOANATOMICAL PROBLEMS

1. A 7-year-old boy has been having high grade fever for 5 days. One evening he complained of weakness in his right lower limb. Soon he could not support the weight.

   Clinicoanatomical problem:
   ❑ What is the probable diagnosis?
   ❑ Which part of the nervous system is affected?
   ❑ What type of paralysis is it and what are its features ?

   Ans. The likely diagnosis is the viral infection of poliomyelitis. The part of the nervous system affected is the anterior horn cells of the spinal cord from lumbar 2 to sacral 5 segments of spinal cord. This type of paralysis is the lower motor neuron paralysis. Muscles feel flaccid, tendon reflexes get absent, reaction of degeneration is seen. Later there is muscular atrophy. The limb becomes thinner and shorter than the opposite limb.

2. A 40-year-old obese man complains of nausea, vomiting, while eating, hoarseness of voice for 15 days, difficulty in walking on the right side, with inability to feel pain and hot and cold sensations from the limbs and trunk.

   Clinicoanatomical problem :
   ❑ Where is the lesion ?
   ❑ Which nuclei and fibres are involved?

   Ans. The symptoms in the present case are due to thrombosis of the largest branch of fourth part of vertebral artery, the posterior inferior cerebellar artery. The various nuclei involved are vestibular nuclei, inferior cerebellar peduncle, nucleus ambiguus and lateral spinothalamic tract of the opposite side.

3. A person suffering from syphilis complains of inability to close the eyes in response to light thrown in the eyes, whereas he can read and see nearby things.

   Clinicoanatomical problem:
   ❑ Where is the lesion?
   ❑ What is such a lesion called ?

   Ans. In such cases, the light reflex is lost, whereas accommodation reflex is retained. It is due to result of lesion in the vicinity of pretectal nucleus. Such a condition is called Argyll–Robertson pupil. The fibres of light reflex take following course:

   Retina-optic nerve—optic chaisma—optic tract—some fibres to pretectal nucleus—of both sides—Edinger-Westphal nucleus—3rd nerve nucleus—ciliary ganglion-short ciliary nerves—pupil constricts. The lesion in syphilis involves the pretectal nucleus, so light reflex is lost.

4. A 65-year-old person developed tremors in his hands. He cannot eat his food comfortably. His movements have slowed down, and walks by bending forwards. There is mostly a stare in his eyes with no emotional expression.

   Clinicoanatomical problem:
   ❑ What is the likely diagnosis ?
   ❑ What is the line of treatment ?

   Ans. The likely diagnosis is parkinsonism. In this condition, there is paucity of movements with lead-pipe rigidity. These are also associated with involuntary movements like tremors.

   The line of treatment is "L-dopa", given as a replacement therapy, because dopamine the normal neurotransmitter in globus pallidus is reduced in these conditions. Surgical treatment include pallidectomy to control tremors.

5. A hypertensive patient aged 60 years was taking the treatment very erratically. One night he felt severe headache and soon paralysis of both his right sided limbs.

   Clinicoanatomical problem :
   ❑ Where is the lesion ?
   ❑ Explain the genesis of his symptoms ?

   Ans. The hypertension should have been treated properly. Since the treatment was not done along the right lines, he suffered from haemorrhage of the left lateral striate arteries which supply the internal capsule. This lead to paralysis of his right half of the body. This is an

Chart A2.1

1. Edinger-Westphal nucleus → III nerve → Nerve to

   Inferior oblique
   ↓
   Branch to ciliary ganglion
   ↓
   Relay
   ↓
   Short ciliary nerves supply ciliaris
   and constrictor pupillae muscles

2. Superior salivatory nucleus of VII nerve　　→　　VIInerve
   ↓
   Chorda tympani branch
   ↓
   via lingual nerve
   ↓
   Submandibular ganglion
   ↓
   Relays to supply submandibular gland
   directly and sublingual salivary gland
   via lingual nerve

3. Lacrimatory nucleus of VII nerve　→　VII nerve → greater petrosal nerve
   + deep petrosal nerve (sympathetic)
   ↓
   nerve of pterygoid canal
   ↓
   Pterygopalatine ganglion
   ↓
   Relays to supply glands
   of nose, palate, pharynx
   and pass along maxillary nerve,
   ↓
   Zygomaticotemporal nerve, lacrimal
   nerve to supply lacrimal gland.

4. Inferior salivatory nucleus of → IX nerve → Tympanic branch
   ↓
   Tympanic plexus
   ↓
   Lesser petrosal nerve
   ↓
   Relays in otic ganglion
   ↓
   Fibres join auriculotemporal nerve → Parotid gland

5. Vagus carries preganglionic fibres for the glands in respiratory system and foregut and midgut derivatives of GIT.

6. S2, S3, S4 preganglionic fibres relay in the ganglia in the walls of the organs developing from hindgut and cloaca.

upper motor neuron type of paralysis with exaggerated reflexes, increased tone of the muscles, etc. It is quite a serious condition and is called "cerebral stroke".

MULTIPLE CHOICE QUESTIONS

Best response type

1. Lower end of filum terminale is attached to the dorsum of :
   a. Second lumbar vertebra
   b. Fifth lumbar vertebra
   c. Last sacral vertebra
   d. First coccygeal vertebra

2. Dura and arachnoid meninges extend upto the lower border of which of the following vertebra :
   a. Second lumbar
   b. Third lumbar
   c. Second sacral
   d. Fifth sacral

3. The grey appearance of spinal grey matter is due to the presence of :
   a. Neuronal body
   b. Neuroglia
   c. Neurites
   d. Blood vessels

4. Pyramidal fibres mostly arise from Brodmann's cortical area :
   a. 3, 1, 2
   b. 6
   c. 4
   d. 18

5. Which of the following tracts contains primary afferent neuron fibres
   a. Fasciculus gracilis and cuneatus
   b. Anterior spinothalamic
   c. Lateral spinothalamic
   d. Dorsal spinocerebellar

6. Substantia gelatinosa of spinal cord continues in medulla oblongata as :
   a. Nucleus of spinal tract of trigeminal
   b. Gracile nucleus
   c. Dorsal nucleus of vagus
   d. Cuneate nucleus

7. In the tegmentum of midbrain, the lemnisci are arranged from medial to lateral side as
   a. Medial, spinal, trigeminal, lateral
   b. Medial, lateral, spinal, trigeminal
   c. Lateral, trigeminal, spinal, medial
   d. Medial, trigeminal, spinal, lateral

8. In ratio of cerebellum to cerebrum in adults is:
   a. 1 : 4
   b. 1 : 8
   c. 1 : 16
   d. 1 : 20

9. Tela choroidea is defined as
   a. Double fold of pia mater
   b. Double fold of ependyma with vascular fringes
   c. Single layer of pia mater with ependyma
   d. Double fold of ependyma

10. The anterior limit of the median part of the forebrain is represented by
    a. Stria medullaris
    b. Stria terminalis
    c. Lamina terminalis
    d. Stria medullaris thalami

11. Which of the following sulcus of cerebral cortex is a limiting sulcus
    a. Central
    b. Calcarine
    c. Precentral
    d. Parieto-occipital

12. The subarachnoid space in the adult ends at the level of:
    a. Second sacral vertebra
    b. Second lumbar vertebra
    c. Second coccygeal vertebra
    d. First sacral vertebra

13. The internal vertebral venous plexus is seen in
    a. Subdural space
    b. Subarachnoid space
    c. Outside vertebral canal
    d. Epidural space

14. The cerebrospinal fluid enters into the blood stream at:
    a. Subarachnoid veins
    b. Arachnoid villi and granulations
    c. Cisterna magna
    d. Choroid plexus

15. The artery supplying the visual area of brain is
    a. Posterior cerebral
    b. Middle cerebral
    c. Anterior cerebral
    d. External carotid

16. Purkinje cells are situated in:
    a. Cerebral cortex
    b. Molecular layer of cerebellum
    c. Granular layer of cerebellum
    d. Nucleus emboliformis

17. Nucleus receiving impulses of taste is:
    a. Dorsal nucleus of vagus
    b. Spinal nucleus of trigeminal
    c. Nucleus ambiguus
    d. Nucleus of tractus solitarius

18. The number of tooth processes in the ligamentum denticulatum are:
    a. Ten
    b. Twenty-one
    c. Twenty
    d. Twenty-five

19. Match the structures on the left with their related structures on the right.
    a. Somatic afferent — i. Vestibulo-cochlear nerve
    b. Special somatic afferent — ii. Trigeminal
    c. Special visceral efferent — iii. Oculomotor
    d. Somatic efferent — iv. Accessory

20. Special features of the parts of brain:
    a. Olivary nucleus — i. Cerebellum
    b. Dentate nucleus — ii. Midbrain
    c. Facial colliculus — iii. Pons
    d. Substantia nigra — iv. Medulla oblongata

Answers to Multiple Choice Questions

1. d
2. c
3. a
4. c
5. a
6. a
7. d
8. b
9. a
10. c
11. a
12. a
13. d
14. b
15. a
16. b
17. d
18. b
19. a – ii   b – i   c – iv   d – iii
20. a – iv   b – i   c – iii   d – ii

Index

403

CBS Sure Success Books for Physiology

Highlights of the book

- 1400 questions that cover the syllabus systematically.
- Includes important questions with high yield in examinations.
- Format of questions includes the *Compare & Contrast* type.
- Questions organized chapterwise so that students can keep up with the class.
- Simple answers that are easy to understand, memorize and reproduce in examinations.
- Answers supported by flow charts and more than 300 two colour illustrations.
- Further details available in the textbook **Medical Physiology** by the same author.

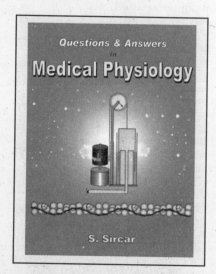

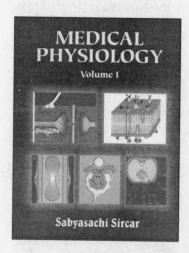

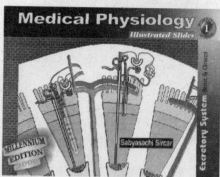

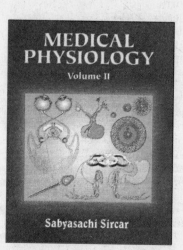

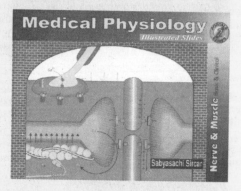

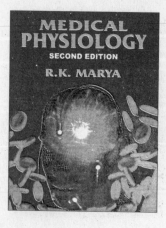

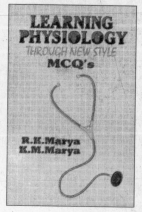

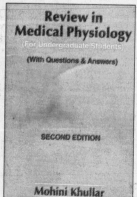

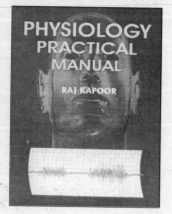